Reproductive and Developmental Toxicology on Macaca Fascicularis

Zhou Li · Sun Zuyue

Reproductive and Developmental Toxicology on Macaca Fascicularis

Springer

Editors
Zhou Li
Hubei Topgene Biotechnology Co., Ltd.
Wuhan, China

Sun Zuyue
The GBA National Institute
for Nanotechnology Innovation
Guangdong Canosafe Pharmtech Co., Ltd.
Guangdong, China

ISBN 978-981-92-3833-0 ISBN 978-981-92-3834-7 (eBook)
https://doi.org/10.1007/978-981-92-3834-7

Jointly published with Shanghai Scientific and Technical Publishers
ISBN of the Co-Publisher's edition: [XXXX

This Springer imprint is published by the registered company Springer Nature Singapore Pte Ltd.
The registered company address is: 152 Beach Road, #21-01/04 Gateway East, Singapore 189721, Singapore

If disposing of this product, please recycle the paper.

Summary

This book focuses on the basic theoretical knowledge of reproductive and developmental toxicology in cynomolgus monkeys, as well as on toxicity research and progress related to this field. It includes the cynomolgus monkey species introduction, reproductive system anatomy and histology, reproductive physiology, developmental characteristics, similarities with humans, animal welfare management, common techniques and methods for reproductive and developmental toxicology research of cynomolgus monkeys, fertility evaluation research in repeated drug toxicity test of cynomolgus monkey, and toxicity kinetics of cynomolgus monkey embryo and fetus developmental toxicity study combined with toxicokinetic study, enhanced perinatal developmental toxicity study combined with toxicokinetic study, developmental toxicology evaluation of juvenile cynomolgus monkey, and so forth. Classical cases are used to evaluate whether the test article is able to penetrate the blood–testis barrier, placental barrier, and blood–milk barrier of cynomolgus monkeys, and the methodological establishment, development, and validation of the above studies are carried out. The Appendices not only include relevant physiological background data on cynomolgus monkeys, but also display, for the first time, more than 130 normal and malformation maps of embryos, fetuses, bones, viscera, and bone density prepared by the chief editor's laboratory, as well as B-ultrasound pictures of pregnant uteruses and fetuses. The data are valuable and guidable.

Based on the research results of the "Major New Drug Creation of Major Scientific and Technological Projects" in the "13th Five-Year Plan," this book has high academic value and can provide important guidance and reference for drug developers and reproductive and developmental toxicity researchers.

Introduction

Reproductive and developmental toxicology of cynomolgus monkeys is the study of the reproductive and developmental toxicity of test article in cynomolgus monkeys and its mechanism of action, including the process of sperm and ovum formation, ovulation, mating, ejaculation, zygote formation, implantation, pregnancy, childbirth, and lactation, as well as reproductive and developmental toxicology studies from germ cell differentiation to whole cell growth, from embryonic cell development to individual organ formation, and from parental reproductive ability to progeny reproductive function (involving organ structure, physiological and biochemical functions, genetic and reproductive characteristics of parents and offspring reproductive systems).

Classic drug reproductive and developmental toxicology studies mainly include the fertility and early embryonic development (FEED) toxicity test, the embryo-fetal development (EFD) toxicity test, and the pre- and postnatal development (PPND) toxicity test. Reproductive and developmental toxicology research in cynomolgus monkey, one of the important branches of toxicology, aims to reflect the influence of the test article on the reproductive function and development process of cynomolgus monkey through toxicology tests and to predict its possible influence on the parental reproductive functions of human germ cells, conception, pregnancy, childbirth, lactation, and so forth and the adverse effects on embryo-fetal development and postnatal development of offspring.

With the support of the "Major New Drug Creation of Major Scientific and Technological Projects" in "13th Five-Year Plan," we have established the "Hubei Nonhuman Primate Reproductive and Developmental Toxicity Research Platform" at the Good Laboratory Practice (GLP) facility of Hubei Topgene Biotechnology Co., Ltd., Wuhan Branch, completed the system construction and verification of the reproductive and developmental toxicity platform of cynomolgus monkeys, and carried out a number of fertility evaluation studies combined with repeated dose toxicity tests (sexual maturity) in cynomolgus monkeys. A toxicity study of a monoclonal antibody administered to cynomolgus monkeys has also been performed, combined with the EFD tests and enhanced pre- and postnatal development (ePPND) toxicity tests of the blood–testis barrier, placental barrier, and blood–milk barrier. In addition, we inherit the theories and technologies of our predecessors, have learned many cutting-edge theories, technologies, and methods of drug reproductive and developmental toxicology at home and abroad, and have applied them to practical work. Therefore, we conceived the idea of writing a monograph to summarize our years of research results and experience in the field of drug reproductive and developmental toxicology.

Based on the guidelines for drug development such as NMPA (National Medical Products Administration)'s *Regulations on the Management of On-site Verification of Drug Registration*, *Measures for the Administration of Drug Registration*, *Quality Management Standards for Non-clinical Research of Drugs*, *Technical Guidelines for Reproductive Toxicity Research of Drugs*, and ICH S5(R3): *Detection of Reproductive and Developmental Toxicity for Human Pharmaceuticals*, this book is designed for the practical needs of person and researchers engaged in reproductive and developmental toxicology research of cynomolgus monkeys and safety evaluation of new drugs. Research on the reproductive and developmental toxicology of drugs is presented through experiments in reproductive and developmental toxicity studies in cynomolgus monkeys, combined with toxicokinetics study as complete and standardized as possible. It is hoped that this book can help staff in this field to understand the theory of drug reproduction and development toxicology in cynomolgus monkeys and master its technical specifications and operational methods. It will be a great encouragement to us if readers can get some help from this book.

In consideration of privacy and confidentiality, we have processed drug names and other sensitive information involved in the reproductive and developmental toxicity studies of cynomolgus monkeys conducted in our laboratory. For example, substitute "AAA, BBB, or CCC" for drug names and "×××" for company names, institution codes, and even study dates. Such treatment will not affect the authenticity, standardization, and science of the research content.

Please let us know if there are any mistakes in this book.

Jun 2024

Zhou Li
Sun Zuyue

Compliance with Ethical Standards

Funding: This study was funded by National Major Scientific and Technological Special Project for "Significant New Drugs Development" during the Thirteenth Five-year Plan Period (grant number 2018ZXO9201017-002).

Conflict of Interest: The author(s) declare no competing interests.

Ethical approval: All animal experiments conducted in this study complied with the Guide for the Care and Use of Laboratory Animals (2011) published by the US National Academy Press and the Regulations for the Administration of Laboratory Animals (revised in 2017) issued by the National Science and Technology Commission of China. The management, use, and related procedures involving animals were reviewed and approved by the Institutional Animal Care and Use Committee (IACUC).

Editors

Chief editors
Zhou Li
Sun ZuYue

Editorial board
Zhou Li Hubei Topgene Biotechnology Group Co., Ltd., Wuhan, China
Sun Zuyue The GBA National Institute for Nanotechnology Innovation; Guangdong Canosafe Pharmtech Co.
Yanjun Cui Hubei Topgene Biotechnology Group Co., Ltd.
Jia Yuling Shanghai Institute for Biomedical and Pharmaceutical Technologies
Tian Yichao Hubei Topgene Biotechnology Group Co., Ltd.
Pang Cong Hubei Topgene Biotechnology Group Co., Ltd.
Mao Shanshan Hubei Topgene Biotechnology Group Co., Ltd.
Lu Guocai Hubei Topgene Biotechnology Co., Ltd.
Zhou Wen Hubei Topgene Biotechnology Group Co., Ltd.
Wang Chun Hubei Topgene Biotechnology Group Co., Ltd.
Li Xingxia Hubei Topgene Biotechnology Group Co., Ltd.
Fang Pan Hubei Topgene Biotechnology Group Co., Ltd.
Xu Xu Hubei Topgene Biotechnology Group Co., Ltd.
Cao Min Hubei Topgene Biotechnology Group Co., Ltd.
Gong Xiashi Hubei Topgene Biotechnology Group Co., Ltd.

Picture
Xu Sichong Shanghai Institute for Biomedical and Pharmaceutical Technologies
Hou Yiwen Shanghai Institute for Biomedical and Pharmaceutical Technologies

Translator
Yue Jiaqi Hubei Topgene Biotechnology Group Co., Ltd.
Gu Yingying Hubei Topgene Biotechnology Group Co., Ltd.

Contents

About the Editors

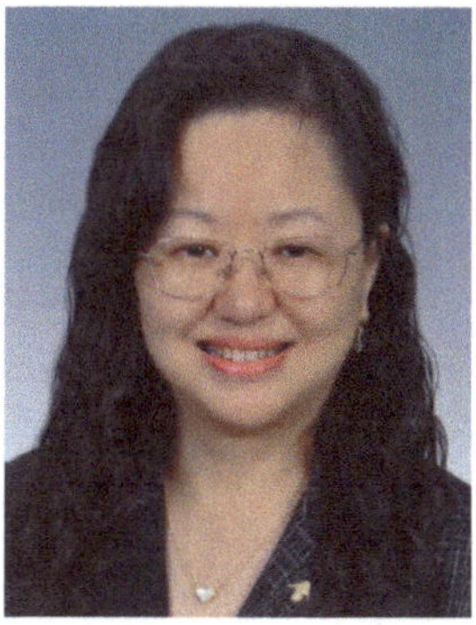

Li Zhou MD Research Fellow, Executive Vice President of Hubei Topgene Biotechnology Co., Ltd., General Manager of Wuhan Branch, Head of Hubei Engineering Research Center for Preclinical Research and Safety Evaluation of Drugs.

She works primarily in toxicological research and non-clinical safety evaluation of drugs. Her main social positions are as follows: About 20 academic positions, including Chairman of Committee of Reproductive & Developmental Toxicology, Chinese Society of Toxicology (CST), Chairman of Specialty Committee of Laboratory Animals and Toxicology of Chinese Association for Laboratory Animal Sciences, GLP Certified Expert of the Center for Food and Drug Inspection of NMPA and Expert of Center for Drug Evaluation, NMPA, GLP Inspection Expert for CNAS, Member of the Standing Committee of Specialty Committee of Toxicology Safety Evaluation of Biotechnological Drugs, CST, Executive Director of CST, Member of Chinese Association for Laboratory Animal Sciences.

She presided over or was responsible for the non-clinical safety evaluation projects and applications of over 300 new drugs. Nearly 100 new drugs have obtained clinical approval/clinical license or new drug certificate through NMPA review, and over 10 evaluated new drugs have obtained FDA and TGA clinical approval. She has hosted or participated in 10 national- and ministerial-level research projects; chaired the "Shanghai Professional and Technical Service Platform for Non-clinical Evaluation of Maternal and Child Drugs"; and, as the deputy team leader and sub-task leader, hosted the plan item "Establishment and Application of Key Technologies of Drug Non-clinical Reproduction and Developmental Toxicology" of "Major New Drug Creation of Major Scientific and Technological Projects" in the "13th Five-Year Plan" and the plan item "Establishment of Technical Platform for Preclinical Safety Evaluation in Line with International Norms For New Drug Research" of "Major New Drug Creation of Major Scientific and Technological Projects" in the "12th Five-Year Plan." She now hosts "Intermediate Stage Test Platform for Preclinical Research of Maternal and Child Drug Use in Wuhan" and "Intermediate Stage Test Platform for Clinical Research and Safety Evaluation of Pharmaceutical Department in Wuhan."

She edited and published six monographs and participated in editing five monographs.

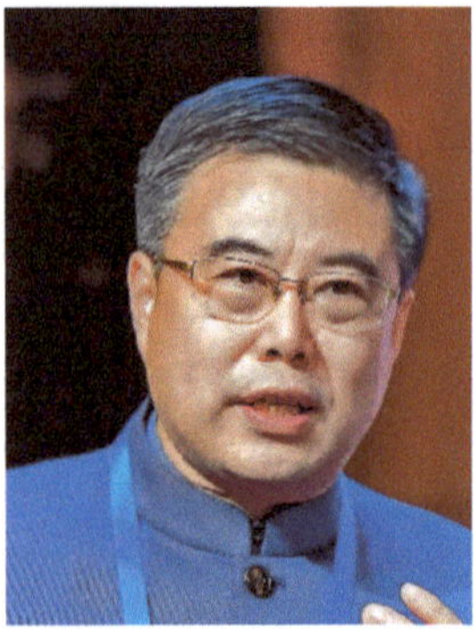

Sun Zuyue Doctor of Science, Chief Scientist of Shanghai Institute for Biomedical and Pharmaceutical Technologies, Research Fellow II, Doctoral Supervisor at Fudan University, Research Director of the National Centre for the Toxicology of Fertility Regulating Drug during 2006—2021, national excellent scientific and technological workers, enjoys the special government allowance issued by the State Council, and awarded the "Shanghai Leading Talents" by the Shanghai Municipal Organization Department of the Communist Party of China and the Shanghai Municipal Human Resources and Social Security Bureau.

In the past 20 years, Sun Zuyue has led the National Centre for the Toxicology of Fertility Regulating Drug and presided over the national research projects "Major New Drug Creation of Major Scientific and Technological Projects" in the "12th Five-Year Plan" and "13th Five-Year Plan." He led the center to win the title of "Drug Safety Evaluation Distinguished Platform" (only five in China), awarded by the National Major New Drug Creation of Major Scientific and Technological Projects Implementation Management Office. He was evaluated as the host of the three platforms, "Shanghai Professional Technical Service Platform for Non-clinical Evaluation of Drugs for Male Reproductive and Urinary Diseases" and "Shanghai Professional Technical Service Platform for Non-clinical Evaluation of Drugs for Women and Children" by the Shanghai Science and Technology Commission. The center is also a supporting unit of the Reproductive Toxicology Professional Committee of the CST and has become the most distinctive non-clinical safety evaluation center of drugs in China.

He was the sixth and seventh vice chairman of CST, first and second president of the Youth Committee of CST, honorary president of the Committee of Reproductive Toxicology of CST, vice president of the Committee of Toxicology on Traditional Chinese Medicine & Natural Medicine, CST, GLP inspector, and drug evaluation expert of NMPA.

He mainly engaged in drug reproductive pharmacology toxicology and drug non-clinical safety evaluation work, and presided over the completion of a total of 271 projects, including 19 national, provincial, and ministerial projects. He won the second prize and third prize of Shanghai Science and Technology Progress Award, the second prize of Science and Technology Award of Chinese Association for Laboratory Animal Science, the second prize of Huaxia Medical Science and Technology Award, the third prize of Science and Technology Progress Award of Chinese Pharmaceutical Association, and the silver prize of Science and Technology New Products Expo of China High-tech and New Products. He has applied for 39 science and technology patents, of which 27 have been authorized, 9 have been authorized as invention patents, and 6 have been transferred or authorized for use. He has published about 484 papers in various forms, edited 9 academic monographs, and contributed to the editing of 4 others.

Introduction to the Species of Cynomolgus Monkey

1

Tian Yichao

Abstract

This chapter introduces the species of cynomolgus monkey (*Macaca fascicularis*) in the context of nonhuman primates and the genus *Macaca*. It first outlines the general features, distribution, and classification of nonhuman primates and Old World monkeys, followed by an overview of macaques, including their phylogeny, evolutionary history, and species groups. The main focus is on cynomolgus monkeys, covering subspecies classification, morphological and anatomical characteristics, sensory perception, communication, social behavior, geographical and ecological distribution, habitat, feeding habits, reproduction, population status, conservation level, and relevant regulations in China. The chapter highlights the close biological similarity of cynomolgus monkeys to humans and their value as a nonhuman primate model in biomedical research and drug safety evaluation. It also emphasizes the high genetic diversity of the species, the importance of geographical origin, and the need for scientific breeding, population monitoring, habitat protection, and sustainable utilization. This chapter provides a useful reference for researchers, breeders, laboratory animal staff, and regulatory personnel.

Keywords

Cynomolgus monkey · *Macaca fascicularis* · Nonhuman primate · *Macaca* · Species characteristics · Biomedical research · Conservation and management

T. Yichao (✉)
Hubei Topgene Biotechnology Co., Ltd., Wuhan, China
e-mail: tianyichao@topgenebio.com

L. Zhou and Z. Sun (eds.), *Reproductive and Developmental Toxicology on Macaca Fascicularis*, https://doi.org/10.1007/978-981-92-3834-7_1

1.1 Introduction to Nonhuman Primates

Nonhuman primates (NHPs) may be one of the earliest recorded species used in scientific research. The very similar phylogenetic and physiological characteristics of nonhuman primates to human beings and the important role they play in the fields of biomedical, behavioral, and evolutionary research make them unique and valuable experimental animal models for scientific research.

Nonhuman primates are unique in that they are not domesticated species. Even those that are bred specifically for experimental research are not much different from their ancient ancestors. This allows researchers to better understand the biological characteristics of these animals when conducting experiments with them. In neuroscience, this understanding is integral to studying the structure and function of the nervous system and the mechanisms underlying related diseases.

For the breeder and researcher of nonhuman primates, it is essential to understand the natural environment in which these animals live. Even when raised in a laboratory, these animals still carry with them the effects of their natural environment on their biological evolution and development. Therefore, to better understand the results of the experiments, breeders need to consider the environments in which these animals live in the wild, as well as the behavioral changes they may exhibit in laboratory settings.

Nonhuman primates are native to Africa, Asia, Southern Europe (Spain), South and Central America, and their habitats range from tropical rainforests to semi-arid savannas and desert steppes. Although nonhuman primates are mainly found in the tropics, two species, the Rhesus macaque and the Japanese macaque, are also found in Beijing, China, and the northern part of Honshu, Japan, respectively.

New World monkeys are found in Central and South America and consist of four primate families: Cebidae, Aotidae, Atelidae, and Pitheciidae. Compared with the Old World monkeys, the New World monkeys are smaller in size and have less difference between the sexes; lack cheek pouches; have big toes that can be opposite; lack an ischial corpus callosum; and are arboreal.

The Old World monkeys in Africa and Asia in the Eastern Hemisphere belong to the family Cercopithecidae, which can be further subdivided into two subfamilies: the Cercopithecinae and the Colobinae. The Old World monkeys in the Eastern Hemisphere exhibit significant physiological and behavioral differences compared to those of the New World monkeys. They are usually larger, with significant size differences between males and females, and most species have buccal pouches for food storage. Their hands and feet are flexible, with opposable thumbs and big toes that provide a strong grip and enable adaptation to arboreal and other complex environments. The ischial corpus callosum supports them in sitting and lying in different environments. These monkeys can live in both arboreal and terrestrial environments, showing a diversity of ecological adaptations. The ability to meet physiological needs through dietary vitamin D2 highlights the body's ability to adapt to a variety of food sources. Together, this series of features depicts the unique and diverse biological characteristics of Old World monkeys in the Eastern Hemisphere and provides rich material for scientists to study the ecology, ethology, and evolution of primates [1].

A brief overview of several generic terms often used by nonhuman primatologists to describe or classify nonhuman primates [2].

- New world monkey: Describes or classifies the primates of South and Central America.
- Old world monkey: Describes the primates found in Africa and Asia.
- Prosimian: Describes or classifies primates in the Prosimii, such as lemurs and lorises. The word "prosimian" means "before monkeys" and reflects their original phylogenetic position in the primates.
- Monkey: Describes all primate species except prosimians and apes.
- Simian: Describes or classifies monkeys and apes.
- Great ape: Describes or classifies all nonhuman primates of the Hominidae, including chimpanzees, orangutans, and gorillas. Apes differ from monkeys in that they have no tail and can walk on two legs.
- Lesser ape: Describes or classifies all primates of the Cercopithecidae, including gibbons and Siamangs. Small apes are smaller than large ones, arboreal, tailless, and considered true brachiates.
- Macaque: Describes all primates belonging to the Macaca, including rhesus monkeys and cynomolgus monkeys.
- Baboon: Describes all primates belonging to the Baboon.
- Callitrichid: Describes or classifies primates of the callitrichid subfamily, including marmosets and tamarins.
- Marmoset: Describes or groups primates of the subgenus Marmoset and the Callimico goeldii genus of the Callitrichinae marmoset subfamily.
- Tamarin: Describes or classifies the primates of the Saguinus genus and the Lion Tamarin genus in the red-haired monkey subfamily.

1.2 Overview of Macaques

1.2.1 Basic Situation of Macaques

Macaques are one of the most adaptable and abundant species of Old World monkeys. They are the most widely distributed primate taxa outside of humans. There are 22 species of macaques, of which the Barbary macaques (also known as Mediterranean macaques) are found mainly in northwest Africa, including Morocco and Algeria, and Gibraltar (most likely introduced by humans). In addition, the remaining 21 macaque species are widely distributed across multiple regions of South, East and Southeast Asia, contributing to a diverse ecosystem. They even crossed Wallace's line and settled in Sulawesi and Timor. Fossil evidence further suggests that during the Pliocene-Pleistocene period, the historical range of macaques may have been wider, spanning most of Eurasia. Their range spans a variety of ecological settings, providing scientists with unique subjects for studying the evolution and adaptation strategies of primates across different geographic and ecological contexts [1].

The name macaque is derived from the Portuguese macaco (a), which in turn derives from the West African Bantu word (ma) kaku, meaning “monkey.” Macaques are medium-sized primates. The weight of female macaques is 3–11 kg, and that of male macaques is 5–18 kg. The weight differences between species are obvious. However, there is no significant sexual difference in macaques compared with their closely related baboons and mandrills. Basically, macaques are found mainly in the tropics, but their range is quite extensive, extending from Pulau Timor in the south to the northern island of Honshu in Japan. This characteristic makes the macaque a primate adapted to different climates and environments. The large latitudinal gradient it spans shows its adaptability to various ecosystems, with distributions ranging from tropical islands to temperate regions, providing scientists with a valuable opportunity to study temporal and spatial changes in animal ecology and physiology.

The central mountains of the Japanese island of Honshu are home to “snow monkeys” (Japanese macaques) that warm themselves in hot springs in winter; aside from them, most macaques live in various tropical forests and other broader tropical habitats in the Indian subcontinent, Southeast Asia, and Sundaland. Macaques are mainly arboreal, and several species have evolved into semi-terrestrial forms and undergone a series of physiological changes to adapt to life on land.

Macaca monkeys exhibit a variety of adaptive characteristics, and their body structure and living habits reflect differences in habitat and diet to some extent. In contrast, arboreal monkeys typically have relatively long hind limbs and long tails, which make it easier for them to balance on thin branches. The front and back legs of macaques are almost the same length, so they are easier to move on land. In addition, the tail of the macaque is relatively short, compared to the langurs of the same geographical distribution. This change in tail length may reflect their ecological adaptations across different environments and may also be related to their movement patterns and living habits [3].

In terms of diet, macaques mainly feed on fruits. Their diet is wide and includes other parts of the plant, such as leaves, flowers, seeds, bark, buds, and lichens, depending on their ecological environment. In addition, they ingest some invertebrates, such as insects and crustaceans, as well as small vertebrates, such as birds, reptiles and small mammals, and even eggs.

In the aspect of reproduction, some species of macaques show that females develop estrogen-dependent swelling of the pubic area or redness of the sexual skin during ovulation, which are often signs of ovulation.

Macaques are generally social animals, living in medium or large social groups that include several adult male and female macaques and their offspring. This social lifestyle helps them to work together, breed, and survive. Together, these characteristics constitute the ecological and behavioral characteristics of the macaques, providing useful evidence for scientists to further study the social structure and ecological adaptation of primates [4].

Females tend to be more domestic, while males will leave their natal groups when they reach adulthood. In groups, females live within a social network of relatives, and both males and females live under a strong hierarchy that often affects their access to resources and mating partners.

The ecological niche (the position and role of an organism in an ecosystem, including its adaptation to the environment, use of resources, and impact on other organisms) of macaques is highly diverse; some species exhibit clear ecological adaptability. Therefore, it is often observed that certain species are closely linked to human life and can make full use of resources provided to them, whether voluntarily or involuntarily.

While some macaque species may appear abundant in certain areas, the reality is that the prospects for most are not good. According to the IUCN Red List of Threatened species, of the 22 species of macaques, two are critically endangered, five are endangered, eight are vulnerable, two are near threatened, and five are of less concern. Among them, the less-concerned species include the two macaques most commonly used in biomedical research, the rhesus monkey and the cynomolgus monkey, which are also the two most widely distributed species.

However, genetic studies clearly indicate that the intraspecific variability of these two macaque species is extremely high and that there may be multiple (sub) species. Therefore, a new assessment of the conservation status of each (sub) species is necessary. In addition, the genetic genealogies of rhesus monkeys and cynomolgus monkeys also show significant differences, which may have implications for their use in biomedical research. It is important for biomedical research to understand patterns of genetic diversity among and within Macaca species. Nor should we overlook these significant taxonomic, ecological, physiological, and genetic differences in the macaques. In conclusion, Macaca includes not only macaques, but also the rhesus monkey and the cynomolgus monkey, which have their own unique characteristics and complexities [4].

1.2.2 Phylogenetic Characteristics of Macaques Among Primates

Macaca is one of the major lineages of the monkey family (Old World monkeys). The monkey family is the only surviving family of Halicmetus ruber and, together with the Hominoidea (man and ape), forms the Catarrhini. Thus, except for the large apes (chimpanzees, gorillas, orangutans) and small apes (gibbons), Old World monkeys are our closest living relatives [2].

According to fossil evidence and genetic analyses, about 32 million years ago, Cercopithecida and Hominoidea diverged into separate branches. By contrast, marmosets, squirrel monkeys, and night monkeys, the species widely used in biomedical research, belong to Platyrrhini (New World monkeys), which separated from the Catarrhini about 46 million years ago. Compared with New World monkeys, Old World monkeys are not only more closely related to humans but also more similar to humans in anatomy, physiology, genetics, physiological responses, and behavior. For this reason, Old World monkeys are regarded as the model of choice for biomedical research and drug safety evaluation. The Old World Monkey family consists of 23 genera and 159 extant species, making it by far the most diverse primate family. Based on differences in anatomy, morphology, and physiology (considering leaf-eating or frugivorous-eating features), the monkey family is divided into two subfamilies: leaf-eating monkeys (Colobinae) and frugivorous cheek pouch monkeys (Cercopithecinae).

Cheek pouch monkeys are found mainly in Africa, while in Asia, only macaques have cheek pouches. Cheek pouch monkeys can be further divided into baboons and vervet monkeys based on differences in anatomy, morphology, behavior, and genetics. The baboon family, which includes macaques, baboons, mangabeys, and other related species, is more adapted to land life and more robust. In contrast, the vervet monkeys are generally smaller and more elongated, and are mainly arboreal, with fewer terrestrial species. Among them, the African green monkey (Chlorocebus) is widely used in biomedical research. Both macaques and baboons in the baboon family are important models for biomedical research, used in studies of simian immunodeficiency virus, drug safety studies, risk assessment, and xenotransplantation.

1.2.3 Evolutionary History of Macaca

Macaca contains 22 species and 37 taxonomic units, making it one of the most diverse Old World monkey genera. Scholars have divided macaques into several groups of species. However, over the past 50 years, there have been conflicting accounts of the number and composition of species groups. According to recent reports, dividing macaques into seven genera may provide a more complete picture of their evolutionary history. Of the seven species groups, three are monotypic species groups, meaning that each population contains only one species (Mediterranean macaques, stump-tail macaques, and cynomolgus macaques), and four polytypic species groups, meaning that a group contains multiple species (*Macaca silenus*, Macaca nigra, *Sri Macaca sinica*, and *Macaca mulatta*). This new classification system is expected to more accurately reveal the diversity and divergence of macaques over the long course of their evolution [5].

The Mediterranean macaque population includes only the Barbary macaques that are distributed in northwest Africa and Gibraltar. Other populations originated in Africa, separated from Mediterranean macaques about 5.5 million years ago, and subsequently migrated to Asia. This process of separation and migration highlights the geographic diversity and evolution of macaques, providing scientists with valuable clues about their evolution and adaptability.

Around 4.5 million years ago, the ancestors of living Asian macaques first split into two main branches. The first branch includes the populations of *Macaca silenus* and *Macaca nigra*; alternatively, the two populations can be merged into one, or even placed in the same population as the Mediterranean macaque. The second branch covers the remaining species groups (the stump-tail Macaque population, the cynomolgus monkey population, the *Macaca sinica* population, and the Rhesus population). In the early recognition, the Rhesus macaque species was included in the cynomolgus macaque population, and the stump-tailed macaque in the Toque Macaque or cynomolgus macaque population.

The lion-tailed monkey population separated from the *Macaca nigra* population about three million years ago. There are five genera in the lion tail monkey population: The *Macaca silenus* from southern India, the *Macaca nemestrina* from Sundaland, also known as the Southern Pigtail Macaque, the *Macaca leonina* from the vast mainland of Southeast Asia, the *Macaca siberu* from Siberu Island, and the *Macaca pagensis* from Sipura Island and the Northern and Southern Pagai Islands.

Until recently, three genera, the northern pig-tailed macaque, *Macaca siberu*, and *Macaca pagensis*, have been recognized as subspecies of the Southern Pigtail Macaques. However, the Pagai macaques of the Mentawai Islands appear to exhibit syn-genealogy, in which macaques form sister lineages with other members of the genus, rather than including all descendants from a common ancestor. As a result, it has been suggested that the Mentawai Islands may have served as a refuge for rainforests during the Pleistocene, from which all living members of the genus may have originated. Within this genus, the lion-tailed monkeys, northern pigtailed monkeys, Siberut monkeys, and southern pigtailed monkeys share a common ancestor. The analysis of this evolutionary relationship provides a deeper understanding of the differentiation and adaptive evolution of macaques across different geographical and ecological environments.

Interestingly, southern Pigtail macaques from Borneo form a clear cluster with the Celebes crested macaque, and genetic data suggest a link between the same species in Sumatra and Peninsular Malaysia, suggesting a cross between remote southern Pigtail macaques and ancient Celebes crested macaques.

Two to three million years ago, the ancestors of Celebes crested macaques invaded Sulawesi and quickly divided into six neighboring species (Celebes crested macaque, Gorontalo macaque, Heck's macaque, Tonkean macaque, Moor macaque, and booted macaque). Due to the rapid differentiation, many mysteries remain in the phylogenetic relationships among these six species. In almost all areas of contact between the two species, the frequency of natural interbreeding appears to be relatively high. This suggests that the chiasma between species may involve complex genetic and ecological factors, raising further questions for scientists to investigate and help solve these puzzles.

In the second major clade, Toque macaques, first diverging about 3.5 million years ago, consists of five species, namely the Toque macaque in Sri Lanka, the Bonnet macaque in southern India, the *Macaca munzala* in Andhra Pradesh, India, and the Tibetan macaque in China, as well as the Assamese macaque, which is widely distributed from Nepal in the west to northern Vietnam in the east.

There is only one species in the stump-tail macaque species group, which is widely distributed in Southeast Asia. The stump-tailed macaque is probably a hybrid species that arose between the ancestors of the Toque macaque and rhesus monkey populations. Genetic data suggest that the species groups of stump-tail monkeys and rhesus monkeys are related. Y chromosome data provide strong evidence for classifying the stump-tail macaques into the population of Toque macaques.

Studies of autosomal sequence data and reverse-sequence integration suggest an intermediate position between the two parental lineages. In addition, several morphological features found in stump-tail macaques are simultaneously observed in populations of Toque macaques or rhesus monkeys. This observation suggests that stump-tailed macaques may share morphological characteristics with both the Toque macaque population and the rhesus monkey population. These results also provide further clues to the complex relationships among these macaque genera and highlight the importance of integrating morphological, genetic, and molecular biology data to reveal the evolutionary history of the species. Therefore, the current persuasive evidence indicates that stump-tail macaques with chimeric genomes are indeed the product of two-way hybridization.

The rhesus monkey species group consists of three genera: Japanese macaque, Chinese macaque, and Rhesus macaque. Rhesus macaques are the most widespread, found from Afghanistan in the west to eastern China. Although many subspecies have been described, rhesus macaques have been recognized as monotypic in recent taxonomies, primarily due to intraspecific confounding and a lack of data. This means that Rhesus monkeys are considered to belong to the same genus in the current systematic classification, with no internal subspecies or other further classification. However, such classifications may change with new data and research findings, especially in addressing issues of missing and confounding data. Molecular biological data indicate that the Formosan rock macaque in Taiwan, China, and the Japanese macaque originated from the western population of rhesus monkeys. The sea level rose one million years ago, disrupting the gene flow between these rhesus monkeys and those on the mainland, ultimately leading to allopatric speciation in Japan and Taiwan, China. In contrast, gene flow between western and eastern rhesus monkey populations continued until about 160,000 years ago.

1.3 Species Characteristics of Cynomolgus Monkey

Macaca fascicularis, also known as the *Wacaca fascicularis*, cynomolgus macaque, and long-tailed macaque, is a species of animal in the genus Macaca spp. Cynomolgus monkeys are highly similar to human beings in biological and behavioral characteristics and genetic material homology, and have developed a central nervous system and other organizational structures like human beings. In addition, it has digestive, circulatory, and respiratory systems similar to humans, making it an ideal animal model for studying human health and disease. Cynomolgus monkeys have become the standard macaque model in pharmacological and toxicological research and are used in studies of diabetes, cardiovascular diseases and infectious diseases [6].

1.3.1 Subspecies Differentiation

The cynomolgus monkey population is a monotypic species group, containing only one species, the cynomolgus monkey. It belongs to Macaca, Cercopithecinae, Catarhini, Anthropoidea, Primates, Mammalia. The cynomolgus monkey exhibits a high degree of diversity and has a relatively wide distribution area. Based on differences in fur color, the cynomolgus monkey has been divided into ten subspecies (Table 1.1).

Table. 1.1 Subspecies classification of cynomolgus monkeys

SI no.	Common name	Scientific name
1	Myanmar long-tailed macaque	*Macaca fascicularis aurea*
2	Dark-crowned long-tailed macaque	*Macaca fascicularis atriceps*
3	Cynomolgus macaque	*Macaca fascicularis fascicularis*
4	Con Son long-tailed macaque	*Macaca fascicularis condorensis*
5	Karimunjawa long-tailed macaque	*Macaca fascicularis karimondjawae*
6	Simeulue monkey	*Macaca fascicularis fusca*
7	Philippine long-tailed macaque	*Macaca fascicularis philippinensis*
8	Laisa long-tailed macaque	*Macaca fascicularis lasiae*
9	Nicobar long-tailed macaque	*Macaca fascicularis umbrosa*
10	Maratua long-tailed macaque	*Macaca fascicularis tua*

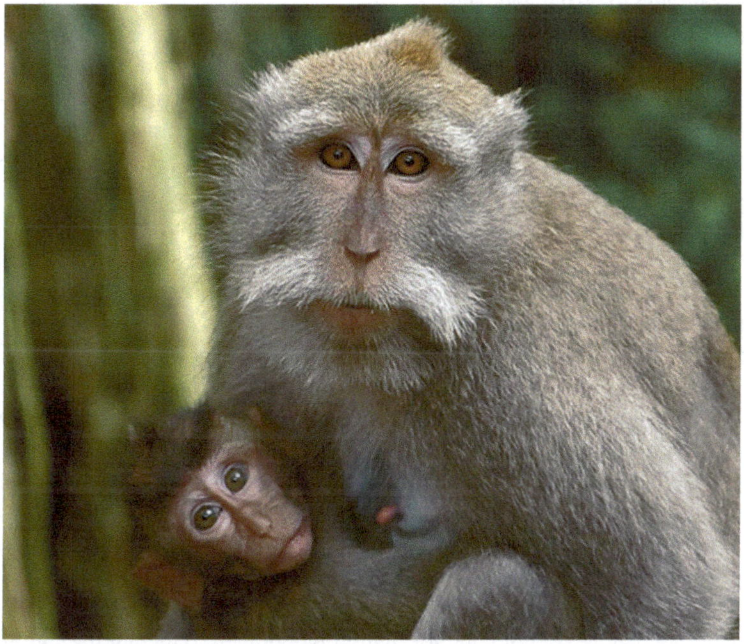

Fig. 1.1 Cynomolgus monkey, with small, pointed hair on the head or gray whiskers

1.3.2 Morphological Characteristics

The cynomolgus monkey and the rhesus monkey both belong to the genus Macaca and are the most common nonhuman primate experimental animals. However, they are slightly smaller than the rhesus monkeys. Its body length generally does not exceed 50 cm (usually 40–47 cm), and the tail length is 1–1.5 times the length of the head and body, with small, pointed hair on the head or gray whiskers (Fig. 1.1). Among all macaque species, they have the longest tails, and they often search for food in and under water, including crustaceans (such as crabs and shellfish).

The cynomolgus monkey mainly communicates vocally and visually. Visual means are crucial for communication between animals at close distances, including facial expressions, body postures, and gestures. These characteristics help them convey information, maintain social structures, and communicate in social interactions [7].

The cynomolgus monkey is medium-sized and exhibits pronounced sexual dimorphism. The most obvious differences can be found in the larger body, snout (maxilla and mandible), and canine tooth sizes of male animals. The skull of the cynomolgus monkey enlarges, and the foramen magnum orients downward to adapt to an upright trunk; the length of the nose shortens, the eye sockets are closer together, and the face is more forward, resulting in an overlapping field of vision (binocular vision) to provide better depth perception. The bones of its eye sockets are intact. In the brain of the cynomolgus monkey, the cerebral cortex and cerebellum continue to develop, a process related to visual and tactile acuity.

In the cynomolgus monkey, most rotational movements of the back occur in the thoracic region, while most bending movements occur in the lumbar region. It has a tail that can be curled, which plays an important role in movement. The versatility of the limbs enables the cynomolgus monkey to perform a wider range of activities and serve functional purposes. The forelimbs are anatomically and functionally closer to the human arms, with a complete shoulder girdle, including well-developed clavicles and scapulae, and the radius and ulna are well-developed and separate. These characteristics and the joint structure of the forelimbs provide the shoulders and forearms with a considerable range of motion, which is crucial for movement, grasping, eating, grooming, and activities in the habitat.

Meanwhile, the pelvic girdle of the hind limbs of the cynomolgus monkey is more similar to that of other quadrupedal animals, rather than the short and wide bipedal pelvic girdle of humans. The tibia and fibula develop independently and are similar in shape to those of humans. These characteristics and the shape of the patella make the hind limbs of the cynomolgus monkey structurally closer to those of humans. These anatomical characteristics enable the cynomolgus monkey to perform various movements and behaviors in its ecological environment. Usually, the lengths of the forelimbs and hind limbs of the cynomolgus monkey are approximately equal. The hands and feet of the cynomolgus monkey have obvious grasping abilities; that is, their hands and feet can grasp, hold, and/or manipulate objects. The thumbs and big toes of the cynomolgus monkey are functionally opposed; that is, the thumb or big toe can touch other fingers or toes on the same hand or foot, and there are nails on their fingers.

Male cynomolgus monkeys have well-developed scrotums, and their testicles are located within the scrotum. The skin on the ischial tuberosity of the pelvis is covered by a callus-like structure called the ischial callus (Fig. 1.2). The ischial callus is a physiological structure unique to the cynomolgus monkey and is usually considered to be related to its sitting posture. The ischial callus is a bony growth on the ischial bone, forming a cushion-like structure in the cynomolgus monkey.

The cynomolgus monkey usually sits in trees or on the ground to eat, rest, or socialize. The presence of the ischial callus may provide additional support, enabling the

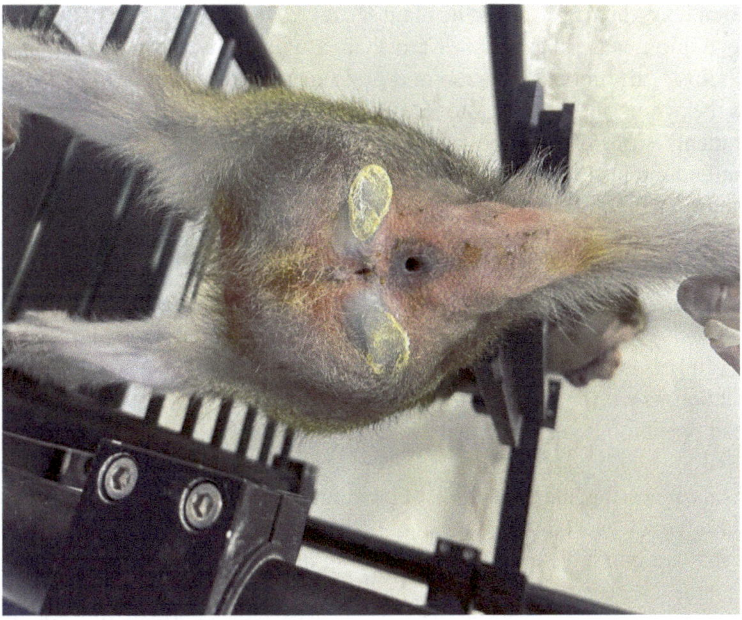

Fig. 1.2 The skin on the ischial tuberosity of the pelvis of the cynomolgus monkey is covered by the ischial callus (callus-like structure)

cynomolgus monkey to sit more comfortably. Such an adaptive structure helps them carry out various behaviors more effectively in their natural environment.

Although the wild environment influences seasonal breeding, the cynomolgus monkey tends to breed year-round. Female cynomolgus monkeys have a single uterus and usually give birth to only one offspring. The reproductive characteristics of the cynomolgus monkey exhibit unique life-cycle features. They have a relatively long gestation period. In addition, the postnatal period (from birth to puberty) of the cynomolgus monkey often involves an extended developmental process that may facilitate the development of its social skills, because the cynomolgus monkey needs to engage in complex social learning. During puberty, the cynomolgus monkey typically undergoes a period of rapid growth and development. This is a critical developmental period, marking the individual's entry into adulthood and accompanied by significant changes in body shape, physiology, and behavior. This stage may be of great significance for the social and reproductive behaviors of the cynomolgus monkey, as it requires the development of mature behavioral abilities that adapt to social and survival requirements [8].

The sensory world of the cynomolgus monkey is very similar to that of humans. The perceptual abilities used and the associated communication signals play important roles in interactions between the cynomolgus monkey and its environment, as well as between other cynomolgus monkeys and humans. A basic understanding of these sensory systems and the related communication signals is crucial for managing these complex animals. Vision is the main sense of the cynomolgus monkey. The eyes of the cynomolgus monkey are forward-facing, with an overlapping field of vision, which helps with binocular vision and good depth perception. This visual mode enables the cynomolgus monkey to locate predators, move quickly in complex forest environments, skillfully manipulate plant materials, and capture fast-moving insects and small mammals [9].

Cynomolgus monkeys have excellent color vision, can recognize ripe fruits and young leaves, and have the sexual receptivity to discriminate between skin color changes. Like humans, cynomolgus monkeys have a trichromatic visual system, enabling them to see green, blue, and red, which gives them greater accuracy in finding food and recognizing social signals. In addition, cynomolgus monkeys have a well-developed sense of smell, which plays an important role in food discrimination and selection, as well as in social behavior. Their good taste makes them more inclined to choose sweet foods, ensuring that the selected foods taste delicious, especially ripe fruits [10].

In terms of hearing, the upper limit of hearing frequency of cynomolgus monkeys is 40–42 kHz, which exceeds the range of human hearing. This allows them to hear some sounds that are inaudible to humans, including ultrasound generated in a laboratory environment. These superior perceptual abilities help the cynomolgus monkey better adapt to its natural environment, find food and interact more efficiently with different survival challenges.

Cynomolgus monkeys have a variety of sensory receptors in their skin and subcutaneous tissue that respond to touch, heat, cold, pressure, and pain. As a result, they behave based on these feelings, including how to interact with their environment. In addition, touch or haptic interaction is an important means of communication in cynomolgus monkeys.

Communication is crucial in the functioning of cynomolgus monkey societies, including intra- and inter-group interactions. It maintains group cohesion during migration and identifies predators and food resources. Cynomolgus monkeys use a variety of ways to communicate, including scent, vocalization, touch, and visual signals. It is of great significance to study the communication and behavior of cynomolgus monkeys in the natural environment. The communication signals of cynomolgus monkeys are usually specific rather than a simple, predictable response to a class of events or signals. Therefore, it is important to consider not only the signal itself but also the environment in which it occurs [11].

A typical example is "mutual grooming behavior" or "social grooming behavior," which has both hygienic and social functions and can reflect and/or be associated with different types of events. From a hygienic perspective, mutual grooming behavior plays an important role in removing dirt, debris, and ectoparasites from animal fur. Mutual grooming is regarded as an important social behavior in macaque monkeys' social interactions, which may be related to a variety of situations and social relationships. "Mutual grooming" may reflect social structure and organization within the group and may also help establish and maintain social bonds between animals of different ranks, as well as serve as a method of reconciliation after aggression. Mutual grooming behavior is associated with the release of endorphins that can reduce heart rate and anxiety, and has a calming effect on both the grooming and the groomed, playing an important role in social and behavioral interactions in cynomolgus monkeys. This behavior can occur in a variety of contexts, including expressing intimacy, reducing tension, strengthening social bonds, and establishing social hierarchy. Therefore, a thorough understanding of the background and environment of mutual grooming behavior is crucial to understanding the dynamics and complexity of macaque social behavior. This behavior may be part of social communication in macaques, providing a way to exchange information in a variety of social situations [12].

In one case, mutual grooming behavior may indicate that two animals are relaxed and interact in a positive way; In other cases, however, mutual grooming may indicate an act of aggression and be associated with the release of tension. In addition, communication between cynomolgus monkeys may involve multiple modes; for example, they may use squeals accompanied by fearful expressions to signal fear.

The use of vocalizations is an important method of communication among cynomolgus monkeys. The vocal signals of cynomolgus monkeys are innate and unique. The sounds produced by the cynomolgus monkey include purring, barking, cooing, and screeching. Figure 1.3 shows a screaming cynomolgus monkey. They make connected sounds to keep the group together. These calls are known as "long calls" and consist of multiple distinct sound pulses or syllables. Many cynomolgus monkeys use sound to communicate when they spot food. They may produce a purring sound when they find a low-quality food source, and a harmonious, high-pitched trill when they find a high-quality food source.

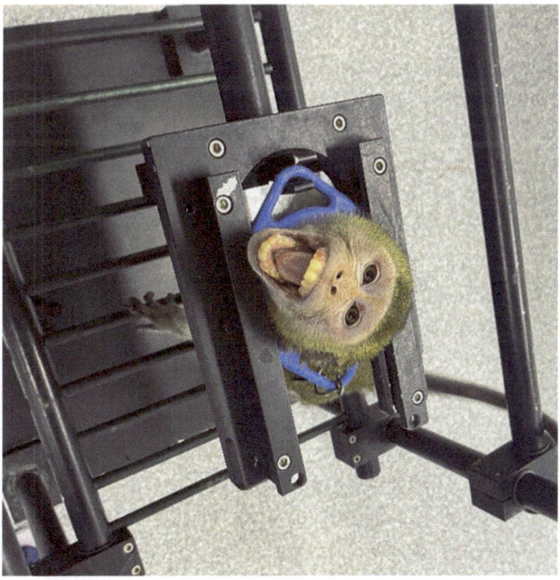

Fig. 1.3 Scream of a cynomolgus monkey

This vocal communication may serve a variety of functions in macaque social groups. First, by making specific sounds, the cynomolgus monkeys can convey information about the quality of their food to other members of the group. This facilitates information sharing within social groups, allowing other members to quickly understand the availability and value of food. Second, through different vocal expressions, cynomolgus monkeys may be able to adjust their behavior within social groups, such as attracting other members to share food or maintaining social order. This vocal communication may be an important means of communication in the social system of cynomolgus monkeys, contributing to group collaboration and efficient resource use. Cynomolgus monkeys also emit audible signals in front of predators to raise alarms, and each alarm call makes a different response from the animals in the group.

While the facial expressions of a cynomolgus monkey may be similar to those of a human, the meanings can be quite different. Examples include fearful grins/faces, yawns, and stares. The fearful face is a very common expression in cynomolgus monkeys, with teeth clenched together or slightly opened, and lips contracted. This facial expression resembles a human smile and can be misinterpreted as a sign of happiness; in fact, the animal is communicating fear and/or anxiety.

Yawning, a common facial expression in cynomolgus monkeys, may have nonsocial implications, such as fatigue observed in humans; it can also have social significance, such as signaling a threat. To interpret a yawn, it is necessary to consider the context in which the facial expression occurs and the extent to which the lips are drawn back to expose the canine teeth. Studies have shown that in captive cynomolgus monkeys, nonsocial yawns account for 90% of the total. This yawn has been observed in animals of all ages and genders, suggesting that it may be related to a general physiological or behavioral state. Social yawns are much less frequent, accounting for about 10% of yawns, and are mostly expressed by adult males. This social yawning may be related to social interactions, threatening behavior, or other group relationships.

Humans often stare at an object out of interest; However, cynomolgus monkeys may stare with or without their mouths open as a sign of threat or aggression. People who keep or work with primates for extended periods should avoid making direct eye contact with cynomolgus monkeys, as this may be perceived as a threat by the animals. Posture can also play an important role in communication between animals. The physical submission posture commonly found in cynomolgus monkeys is called "display," in which the animal in a submissive position raises its tail and exposes ("shows") its rear end/buttocks and genitals to the dominant animal. Using this body position relieves the tension between the two animals. Another aggressive body posture of the cynomolgus monkey includes hair standing up, a stiff body, and moving toward the aggressive animal or object. This aggressive posture makes the animal appear larger than it really is and is often accompanied by aggressive facial expressions. Animal caregivers who regularly work with cynomolgus monkeys should have a basic understanding of common signals indicating aggressive and submissive behavior. This understanding is an important tool for staff and cynomolgus monkey interactions, allowing animal caregivers to play an important role in providing feedback on social interactions of cynomolgus monkeys living in groups and pairs [13].

1.3.3 Distribution Range (Including Geographical Distribution and Ecological Distribution)

Seven of the ten subspecies of the cynomolgus monkey live on small islands, with only three species having relatively large ranges: the cynomolgus macaque, Philippine long-tailed macaque, and Myanmar long-tailed macaque. In fact, the most widely distributed species is the cynomolgus macaque, and most of the distribution range of the cynomolgus monkey genus is contributed by the cynomolgus macaque (southern Vietnam, Cambodia, southern Thailand; South to the Malay Peninsula, Sumatra, Borneo, Java and Bali; As far east as Timor and the southern islands of the Philippine archipelago). It is therefore not surprising that the internal (genetic) variability of the cynomolgus macaque is high, which explains why geographical origin can be so important for animals used in biomedical and experimental research. In the cynomolgus macaque, there is a large genetic difference between the Asian continental and Sunda species, whereas the association with both lineages is observed in the Sumatran species. In addition to exhibiting genetic variation in local populations, genetic evidence also reveals that cynomolgus monkeys on the Asian mainland have been genetically infiltrated by Rhesus macaques. About 30% of the genomes of cynomolgus monkeys in mainland Asia are derived from rhesus monkeys.

This ancient gene flow tends to be unidirectional, from rhesus monkeys to cynomolgus monkeys, and not the other way around. Even today, gene flow in rhesus and cynomolgus monkeys is widespread, spanning Vietnam, Laos, Thailand, and possibly even Myanmar [14].

The first generation of cynomolgus monkeys in most breeding centers in China and Vietnam probably came from mainland Asian populations that had been genetically admixed with rhesus macaques, while those from Indonesia (except those from Sumatra) were likely to be "pure" indigenous cynomolgus monkeys. However, due to the wide distribution of cynomolgus monkeys in Indonesia, and especially the isolation of certain island populations, genetic variation among them is also evident. Although there are two subspecies of cynomolgus monkey in the Philippines (Philippine long-tailed macaque and cynomolgus macaque), they are generally referred to collectively as "Philippine long-tailed macaques" or Philippine cynomolgus monkeys. It is likely that breeders of Philippine cynomolgus monkeys have interbred the two subspecies, resulting in a mixture of taxonomic and genetic traits between them. In contrast, the population characteristics of Mauritius cynomolgus monkeys are well preserved and have homogeneity. The Mauritius cynomolgus monkey population originated from several early individuals (probably from the island of Sumatra) who arrived in the sixteenth or seventeenth century.

1.3.4 Habitat

Cynomolgus monkeys primarily live in trees and are found across Southeast Asian islands and other regions, including southern Bangladesh, Myanmar, Thailand, Malaysia, Indonesia, Singapore, Laos, Cambodia, Vietnam, Brunei, and the Philippines.

Beyond Southeast Asia, they can also be found on the island of Mauritius. Cynomolgus macaques inhabit primary forests, secondary forests, coastal forests, mangrove swamps, marshes, and riverside forests at altitudes of up to 6000 feet. Although they prefer forest areas near water sources, they are also found in secondary forests near human settlements.

1.3.5 Living Habits

Cynomolgus monkeys are considered frugivorous monkeys, and most of their food comes from ripe, fleshy fruits in the wild. They also eat insects, stems, leaves, flowers, seeds, grass, mushrooms, bird eggs, tree bark, frogs, and invertebrates such as shrimps, clams, crabs, and octopuses. Cynomolgus monkeys living near human settlements will eat crops and beg for food from humans.

1.3.6 Reproduction Methods

Cynomolgus monkeys generally live in multi-male/multi-female groups consisting of 8–30 animals. Females remain in the group where they were born and form a dominance hierarchy based on matrilineal kinship. The status of females in the group remains relatively stable throughout their lives and is passed on to their female offspring.

In cynomolgus monkey society, males usually leave their natal group at ages 4.5–6 years and join another group. This migratory behavior may occur multiple times, and males may move between different groups throughout their lives in search of suitable mating opportunities. In the new group, males will exhibit certain social behaviors and a hierarchical structure.

Male cynomolgus monkeys exhibit a clear social hierarchy in the new group, and the highest-ranking male typically has greater access to reproductively capable females. This social hierarchy may be established through competition, threats, and friendly interactions, ultimately forming a social hierarchy within the group. This social structure is of great significance for males in obtaining reproductive rights and increasing their chances of successful reproduction.

The hierarchical status of males is dynamic and will change over time as a dominant male is replaced by another. The mating season of cynomolgus monkeys mostly occurs in autumn. The gestation period of female cynomolgus monkeys is generally 6–7 months, and they give birth to one offspring per litter. The infant macaques are mainly cared for by their mother macaques [15].

1.3.7 Population Status

Cynomolgus monkeys are an important resource for biomedical research and are widely used in fields such as pharmacology and toxicology. Especially at present, they are used extremely frequently in nonclinical research on biological products, such as safety assessments of antibody drugs and vaccines, and pharmacodynamic and pharmacokinetic studies.

Currently, the captive breeding of cynomolgus monkeys in China has witnessed rapid development. The population of captive-bred cynomolgus monkeys has been steadily increasing, ensuring the nonclinical testing of a large number of new drugs and delivering significant social and economic benefits. Previously, due to various factors, several new challenges have emerged in areas such as the protection, captive breeding, management, and import and export of cynomolgus monkeys, mainly including weak technical strength at each link, a relatively single business model, and insufficient development momentum. The breeding conditions at some individual breeding bases are relatively backward, and the quality of cynomolgus monkeys cannot be effectively guaranteed [16, 17].

With the alignment of China's new drug access system with international standards, a large number of drugs, especially biological products, must undergo nonclinical evaluation studies in nonhuman primate species before going on the market. The expansion of the market demand for cynomolgus monkeys has also spurred the vigorous development of the domestic cynomolgus monkey breeding industry. To improve the quality of cynomolgus monkeys, it is essential to intensify reproductive research on captive cynomolgus monkeys [18].

Global biomedical research requires a large number of cynomolgus monkeys every year, and the United States is the main importer. Since 2020, due to the intensive research and development of vaccines, biopharmaceuticals, and antibody drugs, domestic demand for cynomolgus monkeys has surged. Generally speaking, only cynomolgus monkeys over 3 years old can be used for the research and development of new drugs. The closure of the import and export channels for foreign cynomolgus monkeys has led to a situation where it is "hard to get a single macaque." Due to the skyrocketing price of cynomolgus monkeys, some cynomolgus monkey breeding institutions are currently selling any available macaques, even breeding macaques, resulting in a sharp reduction in the population of cynomolgus monkeys in China, an aging population bias, and a preponderance of male macaques. This has also led to a continuous decline in the slaughter rate of cynomolgus monkeys, a further decline in the supply of cynomolgus monkeys, and a continuously high price [19].

To evaluate the population status of cynomolgus monkeys and protect the resources, the number of the wild population has always been an important issue of concern. However, due to the great difficulty of obtaining wild population data, particularly the lack of reliable statistical data in some countries, it is very difficult to conduct a comprehensive assessment of the current status of the global cynomolgus monkey population. The protection and management of cynomolgus monkey resources should not only involve legislation and law enforcement but also require effective, dynamic monitoring of its population, social, and age structures, habitat, and protection measures, ultimately achieving the purpose of scientific protection and sustainable utilization of cynomolgus monkey resources [20].

1.3.8 Protection Level

China has listed cynomolgus monkeys as the national second-class protected animal and the vulnerable species in the *List of National Key Wild Animals* (Table 1.2) and the *China Red Data Book of Endangered Animals*. Cynomolgus monkeys are also protected by the Wildlife (Protection) Act of Bangladesh, the Wildlife (Protection) Act of India, and the National Parks and Wildlife Protection Act of Nepal, and are currently protected by China's *Wildlife Protection Regulations* and *Regulations on*

Table. 1.2 Protection level of cynomolgus monkeys in the List of National Key Wild Animals

Common name	Scientific name	Protection level	Note
Chordate phylum	Chordata		
Mammalia	Mammalia		
Primates	Primates		
Lorisidae	Lorisidac		
Ashy slow loris	*Nycticebus bengalensis*	Class 1	
Pygmy loris	*Nycticebus pygmaeus*	Class 1	
Old world monkey	Cercopithecidae		
Stump-tail macaque	*Macaca arctoides*	Class 2	
Assamese macaque	*Macaca assamensis*	Class 2	
Taiwan macaque	*Macaca cyclopis*	Class 1	
Northern pig-tailed macaque	*Macaca leonina*	Class 1	Its original Chinese name is "Tun Wei Hou"
White-cheeked macaque	*Macaca leucogenys*	Class 2	
Rhesus monkey	*Macaca mulatta*	Class 2	
Southern Tibet macaque	*Macaca munzala*	Class 2	
Tibetan stump-tailed macaque	*Macaca thibetana*	Class 2	
Nepal gray langur	*Semnopithecus schistaceus*	Class 1	
Indochinese gray langur	*Trachypithecus crepusculus*	Class 1	
Black leaf monkey	*Trachypithecus francoisi*	Class 1	
Phayre's leaf monkey	*Trachypithecus phayrei*	Class 1	
Capped monkey	*Trachypithecus pileatus*	Class 1	
White-headed black langur	*Trachypithecus leucocephalus*	Class 1	
Shortridge's capped langur	*Trachypithecus shortridgei*	Class 1	
Yunnan snub-nosed monkey	*Rhinopithecus bieti*	Class 1	
Guizhou snub-nosed monkey	*Rhinopithecus brelichi*	Class 1	
Sichuan golden snub-nosed Monkey	*Rhinopithecus roxellana*	Class 1	
Myanmar snub-nosed monkey	*Rhinopithecus strykeri*	Class 1	

the Protection of Endangered Species of Animals and Plants. Meanwhile, cynomolgus monkeys have been listed in the 2008 Red List of Threatened Species of the International Union for Conservation of Nature (IUCN) as a least concern (LC) species and are also included in the *Convention on International Trade in Endangered Species of Wild Fauna and Flora* [21].

As a nationally protected second-class animal, the production, purchase, transportation, and use of cynomolgus monkeys require strict supervision and approval from the national administrative department. Take the handling of transportation approval documents for cynomolgus monkeys by provincial scientific research units as an example. First, the scientific research unit must possess an "Experimental Animal Use License" issued by the provincial department of science and technology, and this use license must cover nonhuman primates. Second, before using cynomolgus monkeys, the unit must sign a purchase contract with the animal production factory and submit the "Application Form for Administrative License Matters of Wildlife Protection and Management" and the specific contents involved to the relevant competent departments of the government and hand over to the provincial forestry administrative departments in the form of written documents. Among them, the forestry administrative department at the district or city level where the scientific research unit is located will complete the corresponding paperwork after review and submit it to the provincial forestry administrative department. After the administrative departments review the application level by level, the provincial forestry bureau will issue the "Administrative License Decision Document" authorizing the scientific research institution to purchase and transport animals from the provincial cynomolgus monkey production factory. If the cynomolgus monkey production factory is located in an area outside the province, the same process is required to obtain the "Administrative License Decision Document" issued by the provincial forestry bureau before the cynomolgus monkeys can be transported. A validity period is specified for the "Administrative License Decision Document," and it varies by province, ranging from 1 to 6 months. During transportation, ensure the transportation time falls within the validity period.

Cynomolgus monkeys have attracted attention for their unique characteristics and wide distribution. This medium-sized primate is known for its long and powerful tail, well-developed ischial callosities on the buttocks, and relatively small body size. It is highly adaptable, able to move nimbly on land and forage in the water, demonstrating diverse ecological roles.

Cynomolgus monkeys provide extremely valuable experimental models for medical research. In the biomedical field, especially in drug research and development and disease research, cynomolgus monkeys, as experimental subjects, play an important role, which makes the protection and management of their natural habitats particularly urgent.

Looking ahead, the global community needs to strengthen cooperation and promote the health and stability of the cynomolgus monkey population through scientific research and protection plans. Meanwhile, we should strengthen our understanding of their value in medical applications and commit to promoting the comprehensive protection of this species to support the sustainable development of biodiversity.

Ethical Approval

This chapter is a review of previously published accounts; as such, no animal or human studies were performed.

References

1. Groves CP (2005) Order primates. In mammal species of the world: a taxonomic and geographic reference. Hopkins University Press, Baltimore, MD
2. Wolfensohn S (2010) Old world monkeys. Wiley-Blackwell, Oxford, UK
3. Turnquist JE, Minugh-Purvis N (2012) Functional morphology. Academic Press, Waltham, MA
4. Fortman JD, Hewett TA, Bennett BT (2002) Important biological features. In: The laboratory nonhuman primate. CRC Press, Boca Raton, FL
5. Harding JD (2013) Progress in genetics and genomics in nonhuman primates. ILAR J 54:7781
6. Johnson DO, Johnson DK, Whitney RA (2012) History of the use of nonhuman primates in biomedical research. Academic Press, Waltham, MA
7. Ghazanfar AA, Cohen YE (2009) Primate communication: evolution. In: Encyclopedia of neuroscience. Elsevier Press, Oxford, UK
8. Tardif S, Carville A, Elmore D et al (2012) Reproduction and breeding of nonhuman primates. Academic Press, Waltham, MA
9. Zuberbuhler K (2012) Primate communication. Nat Educ Knowledge 3(10):83
10. Surridge AK, Osorio D, Mundy NI (2003) Evolution and selection of trichromatic vision in primates. Trends Ecol Evol 18:198205
11. Williams LE, Berstein IS (2012) Study of nonhuman primate social behavior. Academic Press, Waltham, MA
12. Gruete CC, Bissonette A, Isler K et al. (2013) Grooming and group cohesion in primates: implications for the evolution of language. Evol Hum Behav 34(1):618
13. Honess P (2013) Behavior and enrichment of long-tailed (cynomolgus) macaques (*Macaca fascicularis*). Charles River Laboratories, Wilmington, MA
14. Guangmei Y, Guojie Z, Fang X et al. (2011) Genome sequencing and comparison of two nonhuman primate animal models, the cynomolgus and Chinese rhesus macaques. Nat Biotechol 29(11):10191025
15. Wang Hong, Xuewei Fu, Zhigang Chen et al. (2017) Study on the reproductive patterns and performance of rhesus monkeys and cynomolgus monkeys in Kunming area. Chin J Comparat Med 27(7):3439
16. Sibbal LR (2001) Nonhuman primates: a critical role in current disease research. ILAR 42(2):7484
17. Kalin NH (2003) Nonhuman primate models to study anxiety, emotion regulation, and psychopathology. Ann NY Acad Sci 1008:189200
18. Liang Bin (2011) Progress on nonhuman primate models of diabetes mellitus. Zool Res 32(1):911996
19. Bolton ID (2015) Basic physiology of *Macaca fascicularis*. In: The nonhuman primate in nonclinical drug safety development and safety assessment. Academic Press, Waltham, MA
20. Buck WR (2015) Comparative physiology, growth, and development. In: The nonhuman primate in nonclinical drug development and safety assessment. Academic Press, Waltham, MA
21. Jennings M, Prescott MJ (2009) Refinements in husbandry, care and common procedures for non-human primates: ninth report of the BVAAWF/FRAME/RSPCA/UFAW Joint Working Group on Refinement. Lab Anim 43(Suppl1):147

Anatomy and Histology of the Reproductive System in Cynomolgus Monkeys

2

Yanjun Cui

Abstract

This chapter describes the anatomy and histology of the reproductive system in cynomolgus monkeys. It covers the male reproductive system, including the testes, epididymis, vas deferens, seminal vesicles, prostate, bulbourethral gland, and penis, with emphasis on testicular descent, tunica albuginea, testicular septa and lobules, seminiferous tubules, rete testis, spermatogenic cells, Sertoli cells, Leydig cells, and the 12 stages and 14 steps of the spermatogenic cycle. It also describes the female reproductive system, including the ovaries, oviduct, uterus, cervix, vagina, and mammary glands, focusing on the ovarian cortex and medulla, follicular development, atresia, corpus luteum, oviductal mucosa, endometrial cycle, myometrium, cervical glands, vaginal epithelium, and mammary gland structure. The chapter provides detailed anatomical and histological references for reproductive and developmental toxicity studies, breeding, and biomedical research in cynomolgus monkeys.

Keywords

Cynomolgus monkey · Reproductive system · Anatomy · Histology · Testis · Epididymis · Spermatogenesis · Ovary · Uterus · Mammary gland

The reproductive system is a general term for the organs closely related to reproductive functions in an organism. It is divided into male and female types. The male and female reproductive systems not only differ in their anatomical and histological

Y. Cui (✉)
Hubei Topgene Biotechnology Co., Ltd., Wuhan, China
e-mail: cuiyanjun@topgenebio.com

L. Zhou and Z. Sun (eds.), *Reproductive and Developmental Toxicology on Macaca Fascicularis*, https://doi.org/10.1007/978-981-92-3834-7_2

structures but also in their functions. There are slight differences in the composition of reproductive systems among laboratory animal species. The following is a description of the anatomical and histological structure of the male and female reproductive systems in cynomolgus monkeys.

2.1 Male Reproductive System

The male reproductive system in nonhuman primates is highly similar to that of humans. It consists of the internal and external genitalia, with primary functions including sperm production and androgen secretion. The internal genitalia include the testes, the duct system (epididymis, vas deferens, and ejaculatory ducts), and accessory glands (such as the seminal vesicles and prostate). The external genitalia consist of the scrotum and penis [1, 2].

2.1.1 Testes

In adult animals, the testes are located in the scrotum, just below the pubic symphysis, with one on each side. Their main functions are sperm production and androgen secretion. In most mammalian species, the testes descend from the abdomen into the scrotum during fetal or neonatal development. In cynomolgus monkeys, the position of the testes changes with the animal's age. In nonhuman primates, testicular descent occurs at birth, but shortly thereafter, the testes ascend into the inguinal canal, followed by a postnatal regression phase. Around the age of 3 years, the testes descend again, and their size increases (Fig. 2.1).

The testes of the cynomolgus monkey (Fig. 2.2) have an oval appearance, with a covering membrane. From the outside to the inside, this membrane consists of the visceral layer of the tunica vaginalis, the tunica albuginea, and the vascular layer.

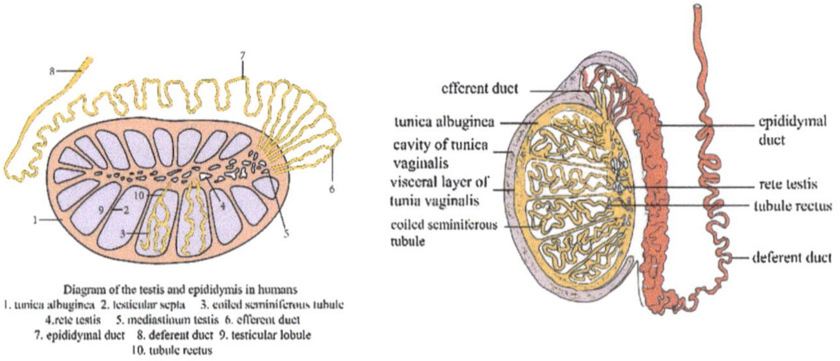

Fig. 2.1 Diagram of the testis and epididymis in cynomolgus monkeys and humans (left: cynomolgus monkey, right: human)

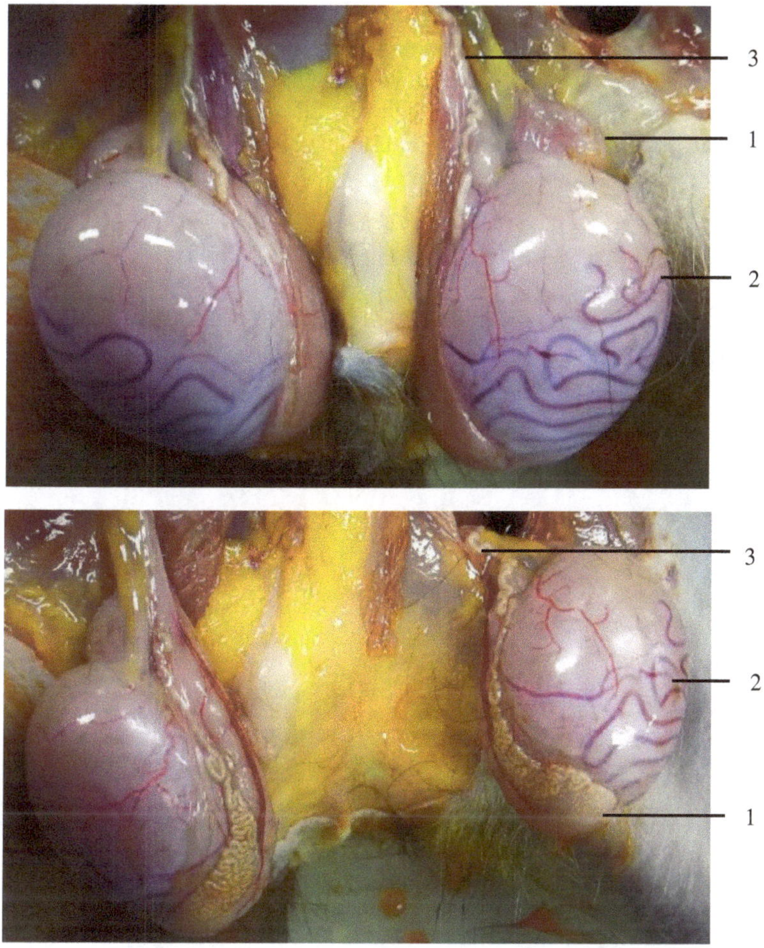

Fig. 2.2 Views of the ventral (left) and dorsal (right) sides of the testis and epididymis in a 5-year-old cynomolgus monkey. 1. Epididymis; 2. Testis; 3. Vas deferens

The visceral layer of the tunica vaginalis and the parietal layer of the tunica vaginalis within the scrotum form a narrow space known as the tunica vaginalis cavity, which contains a small amount of fluid that serves a lubricating function.

The deeper layer is the tunica albuginea, composed of dense connective tissue, containing a large number of collagen fibers and fibroblasts. The tunica albuginea extends radially into the substance of the testis, forming the testicular septa that divide the testicular parenchyma into several conical lobules. Each lobule contains coiled and elongated seminiferous tubules. Near the deep portion of the testicular septa, the seminiferous tubules become short and straight, forming the straight tubules, which converge within the testicular septa to connect and form the rete testis.

In humans, the rete testis is primarily located along the posterior border of the testes, whereas in rats and mice it is more superficial, directly beneath the tunica albuginea.

In cynomolgus monkeys and dogs, the rete testis is located within the testicular septa (Figs. 2.1, 2.3, and 2.4). Its vascular layer is thin and loose, richly vascularized, and tightly connected to the testicular parenchyma, extending into the spaces between the seminiferous tubules. The tissue between the seminiferous tubules is loose connective tissue, known as the interstitial tissue of the testes. The structure of the testicular lobules varies among species. Dogs and monkeys have distinct septa and lobular structures,

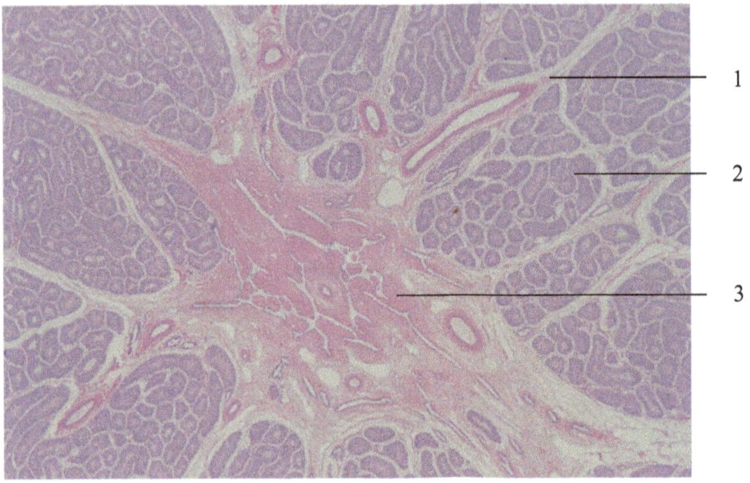

Fig. 2.3 Testicular septa, lobules, and rete testis in a 4-year-old cynomolgus monkey (HE staining, ×200). 1. Testicular septa; 2. Testicular lobules; 3. Rete testis

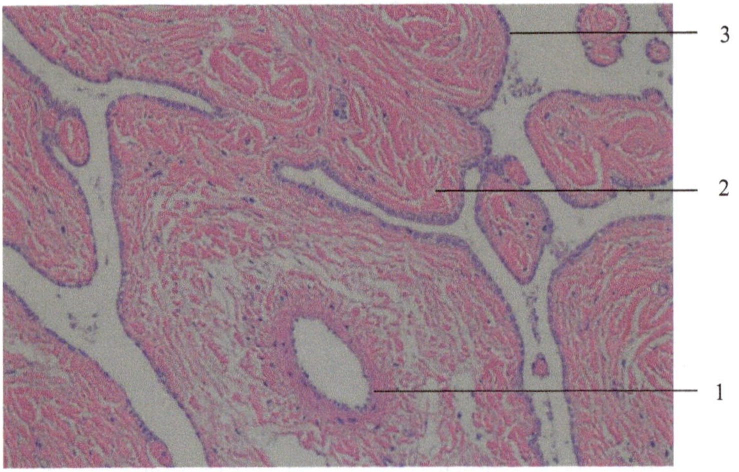

Fig. 2.4 Rete testis in a 4-year-old cynomolgus monkey (HE staining, ×200). 1. Blood vessels within the testicular septa; 2. Connective tissue within the testicular septa; 3. Rete testis (single-layer cuboidal epithelium)

with straight seminiferous tubules and the rete testis within the septa. In contrast, rats and mice lack septa or lobular structures, with the straight seminiferous tubules and rete testis located on the dorsal inner side of the testes.

The substance of the testis consists of seminiferous tubules (Figs. 2.5 and 2.6), with the lumen covered by germinal epithelium. The germinal epithelium is composed of spermatogenic cells and Sertoli cells. The spermatogenic cells continuously proliferate

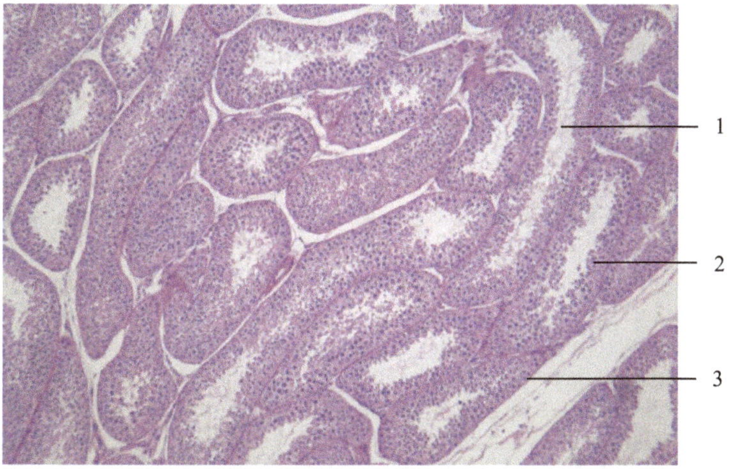

Fig. 2.5 Testis of a 5-year-old cynomolgus monkey (HE staining, ×100). 1. Lumen of seminiferous tubules; 2. Germinal epithelium of seminiferous tubules; 3. Basement membrane of seminiferous tubules

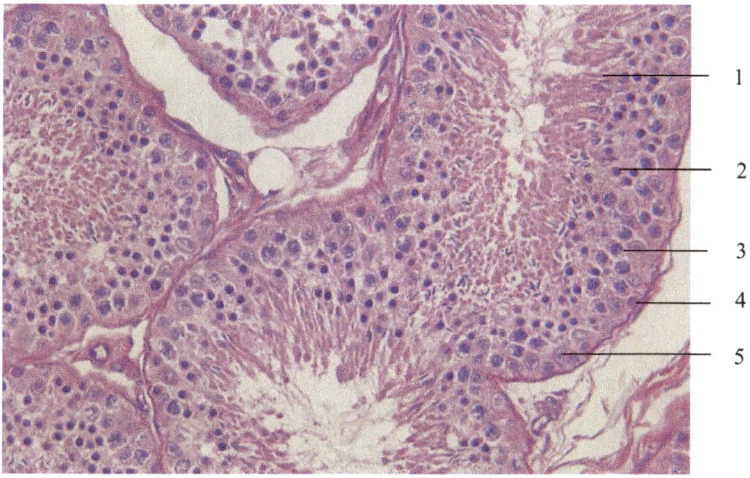

Fig. 2.6 Testis of a 5-year-old cynomolgus monkey (HE staining, ×400). 1. Elongated spermatocytes; 2. Round spermatocytes; 3. Spermatogonia; 4. Spermatogenic cells; 5. Sertoli cells

and differentiate into mature sperm, while the Sertoli cells are distributed between them. Sertoli cells do not proliferate but serve supportive, secretory, nutritional, and phagocytic functions, and are regulated by gonadal hormones.

The spermatogenic cells at different developmental stages are arranged in layers from the basal layer of the seminiferous tubule to the lumen, in the following order: spermatogonia, primary spermatocytes, secondary spermatocytes, spermatids, and spermatozoa (Fig. 2.7). In the cynomolgus monkey, spermatids can be classified into 14 types, and the spermatogenic epithelium cycle is divided into 12 stages [3]. The emergence of a new generation of sperm from primary spermatocytes (Step 1) is used to define the first morphological stage (Stage I), while the production and division of secondary spermatocytes is defined as the final stage of the spermatogenic cycle (Stage XII). The spermatogenesis time in cynomolgus monkeys, from spermatogonia to fully developed elongated spermatids, takes 42 days, with each cycle of spermatogenic epithelium (comprising 12 morphological stages) lasting approximately 10.5 days. The 12 different morphological stages of sperm and the 14 developmental steps are shown in Fig. 2.8.

The sperm production process in all mammals is fundamentally the same, involving the continuous division and maturation of precursor stem cells (spermatogonia), followed by meiosis (spermatocytes). During meiosis, these cells undergo DNA replication and meiosis to form haploid germ cells (spermatids). These cells then undergo a complex morphological transformation, changing from round spermatids (cells with a normal appearance) to elongated, flagellum-like cells with a head, body, and tail (mature sperm cells). Mature sperm are released from the seminiferous epithelium

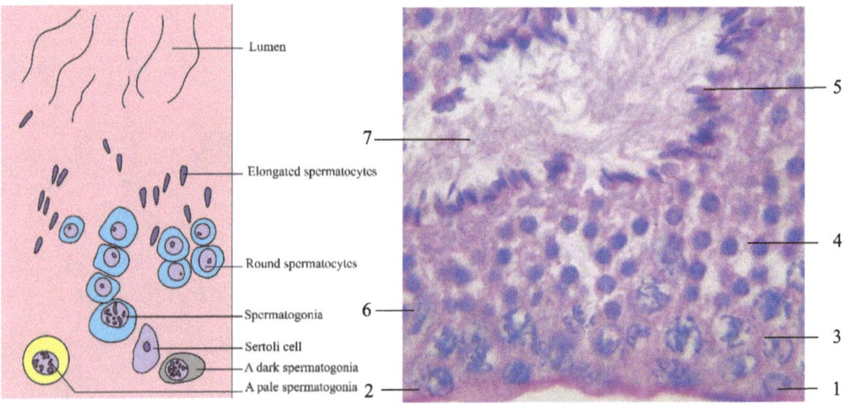

Fig. 2.7 Cross-section of the normal testis of a mature cynomolgus monkey, showing different cell types present during spermatogenesis (the top image is a schematic; the bottom image is PAS-stained, ×1000). From the basement membrane to the lumen of the seminiferous tubule, the following cell types are visible: spermatogonia (two subtypes of type A spermatogonia, namely dark A spermatogonia (1) and light A spermatogonia (2)), spermatocytes (3), round spermatids (4), elongated spermatids (5), and Sertoli cells (6), the nuclei of Sertoli cells are large and elongated, located near the basement membrane, while their cytoplasm extends toward the lumen of the seminiferous tubule (7), making close contact with other cell types

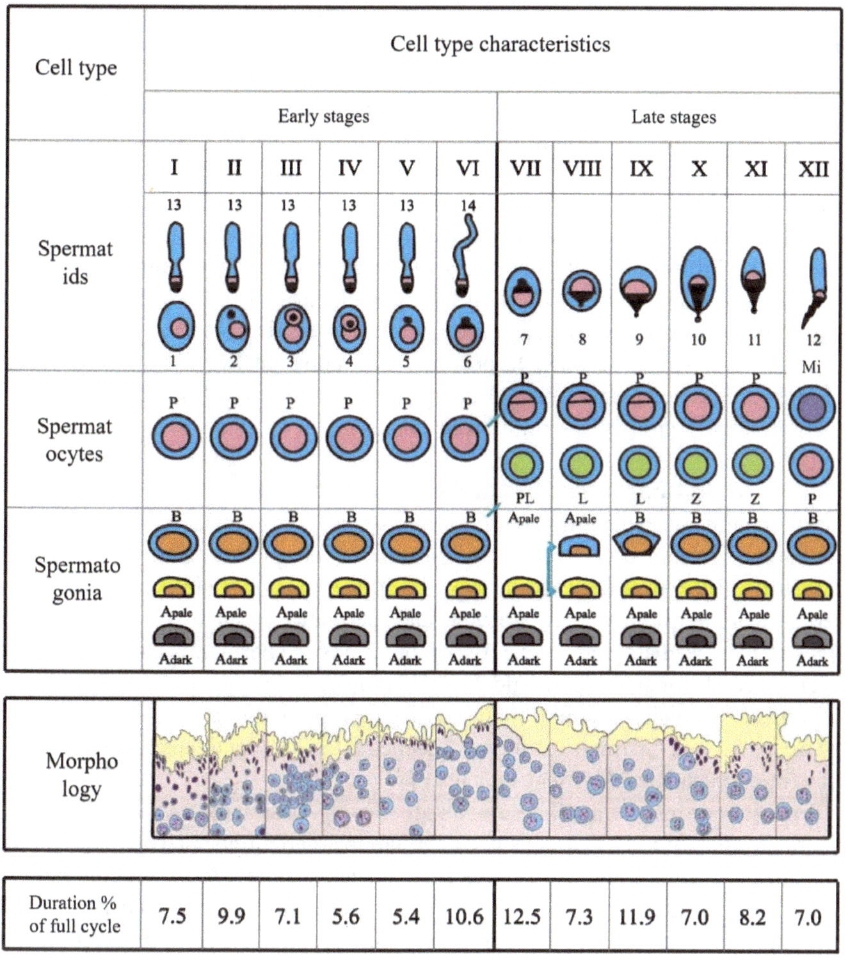

Fig. 2.8 The stages of the spermatogenic cycle in cynomolgus monkeys. In the cycle diagram, the cells proceed from the left side to the right side, completing the process of sperm release. This includes spermatogonia, primary spermatocytes (PL, L, Z, P), and spermatids at stages 1–14. The numbers I–XII represent the 12 morphological stages, while numbers 1–14 indicate the different steps of spermatid development. The spermatogenic cycle is divided into early stages I–VI, with two generations of spermatids, and late stages VII–XII, with only one generation of spermatids. The bottom row of the diagram shows the duration of each stage in the complete spermatogenic cycle, expressed as a percentage of the total cycle length. Adark, Type A dark spermatogonia; Apale, Type A pale spermatogonia; B, Type B spermatogonia; PL, Primary spermatocytes at the preleptotene stage; L, Primary spermatocytes at the leptotene stage; Z, Primary spermatocytes at the zygotene stage; P, Primary spermatocytes at the pachytene stage

(spermiation) and are transported through the seminiferous tubules to the rete testis for collection, then pass through the efferent ducts to the epididymis. The process is the same across species, with only slight differences in the characteristics of various cell types, the process dynamics and regulatory pathways.

Different types of germ cells (spermatogonia, spermatocytes, and spermatids) are arranged in a highly organized, layered manner within the seminiferous tubules. These cells are structurally and metabolically supported by somatic cells, namely Sertoli cells, which surround each germ cell with cytoplasmic projections that are not readily discernible under the light microscope. Sertoli cells are located on the basement membrane of the seminiferous tubules and extend throughout the entire seminiferous epithelium. Tight junctions between Sertoli cells divide the seminiferous tubule into luminal and basal compartments, forming the main structure of the blood-testis barrier. Sertoli cells play a crucial role in forming and maintaining the microenvironment necessary for spermatogenesis, providing support and nutrients to the germ cells. When germ cells are absent from the seminiferous tubules, leaving only Sertoli cells lining them, the true extent of Sertoli cells becomes more apparent. Spermatogenesis occurs in a highly regulated manner, with four generations of germ cells always developing synchronously in any given seminiferous tubule.

2.1.1.1 Main Characteristics of Cell Types and Stages

The spermatogenic cycle is divided into early stages I–VI and late stages VII–XII. In the cynomolgus monkey, the cells at each stage of the spermatogenic cycle include spermatogonia (Type A dark spermatogonia, Type A pale spermatogonia, and B-type spermatogonia), primary spermatocytes, and spermatids at stages 1–14. In the early stages of the spermatogenic cycle, two generations of spermatids can be observed (i.e., round and elongated spermatids), whereas in the late stages, only one generation of spermatids is visible (either round or elongated spermatids).

Spermatogonia: Spermatogonia are classified into type A and type B based on their differentiation and developmental stages.

Type A Spermatogonia: These cells are closely associated with the basement membrane and are present at all stages, though in small numbers. The nucleus contains fine granular chromatin and one or two nucleoli. Type A spermatogonia can be further divided into two subtypes: Type A dark spermatogonia (Ad) and Type A pale spermatogonia (Ap). Ad spermatogonia are in mitotic arrest and are considered reserve stem cells, whereas Ap spermatogonia are mitotically active, self-renewing, and give rise to the first generation of differentiating type B spermatogonia. The distinction between the two subtypes is based on staining characteristics, nuclear density, nuclear size (approximately 6.4 μm for Ad and 8.4 μm for Ap), and the content of PAS-positive substances in the cytoplasm. Ad spermatogonia have a higher content of PAS-positive material. The mitotic divisions of Ap spermatogonia occur during stages VII, VIII, and IX of the spermatogenic cycle.

Type B Spermatogonia: Type B spermatogonia are the primary progenitor cells. The characteristic feature of these cells is the presence of a nucleolus located at the center of the nucleus, along with deeply stained chromatin clumps or granules distributed along the nuclear membrane. These features allow them to be distinguished from type A spermatogonia. Type B spermatogonia undergo four rounds of mitotic division within a single spermatogenic cycle, producing four generations of differentiated cells, namely B1, B2, B3, and B4. After each mitotic division, the cell number doubles. The mitotic division of B1 occurs mainly during stage IX, B2 during stage

XII, B3 during stage II, and B4 during stage IV. These cells are difficult to distinguish from each other using conventional staining methods.

Primary spermatocytes: Primary spermatocytes are divided into the preleptotene (PL), leptotene (L), zygotene (Z), and pachytene (P) stages. Newly formed diploid preleptotene primary spermatocytes have nuclei that are indistinguishable from those of type B spermatogonia. However, as the chromosomes replicate during the preleptotene stage to form tetraploid cells, the nuclei of these spermatocytes are characterized by linear chromatin clumps. As they progress through prophase of meiosis, the chromatin clumps gradually thicken and become more condensed.

Pachytene primary spermatocytes: These cells develop from zygotene primary spermatocytes during stage XII. They are located closer to the tubular lumen than other primary spermatocytes and contain a large, round nucleus with chromatin arranged in thick, rope-like strands. The nucleolus is large and dark. As tetraploid cells progress through pachytene, the size of the primary spermatocytes gradually increases. After a very brief diploid and terminal differentiation phase, they undergo the first meiotic division to form diploid secondary spermatocytes, which then quickly enter the second meiotic division to become haploid spermatids.

Spermatids: Spermatids develop after the second division of secondary spermatocytes during stage XII. Meiosis is characteristic of stage XII and is easily identifiable. Steps 1–14 of spermatid development are distinguished by details of the acrosome. The acrosome can only be observed after PAS staining, and even then, structures such as the acrosomal granule and early acrosomal cap remain very small and difficult to discern in routine sections. The latter seven steps can be distinguished by the shape of the spermatids, as shown in Fig. 2.9.

2.1.1.2 The Stages of Spermatogenesis are as Follows

Stage I: At this stage, Step 1 round spermatids are present (Fig. 2.10), but they lack distinct features due to the invisibility of the pre-acrosomal granules. At this stage, there are also elongated spermatids, which are Step 13 spermatids. These are flattened with a paddle-shaped nucleus, partially covered by the acrosomal system (fused head cap and acrosome). These cells are fully condensed and dark in appearance. The apical region is rounded, and the spermatids are arranged in clusters. Step 13 spermatids are the nearly final stage of spermatid development and are typically found from stage I to stage V.

Stage II: Step 2 round spermatids (Fig. 2.11) are present at this stage, with the initial formation of the pro-acrosomal vesicles. The vesicles contain pre-acrosomal granules. These small pro-acrosomal vesicles fuse to form a single large vesicle containing a fusion granule, which is in contact with the nucleus. The prominent Golgi apparatus is a relatively large eosinophilic structure within the cytoplasm. Step 13 elongated spermatids, still present at this stage, have a more loosely arranged cluster.

Stage III: Step 3 round spermatids show acrosomal vesicles attached to the nuclear membrane (Fig. 2.12). Step 13: elongated spermatids are still present.

Stage IV: Step 4 round spermatids show acrosomal vesicles that flatten against the nuclear surface (Fig. 2.13), forming a cranial structure. Step 13: elongated spermatids are also present.

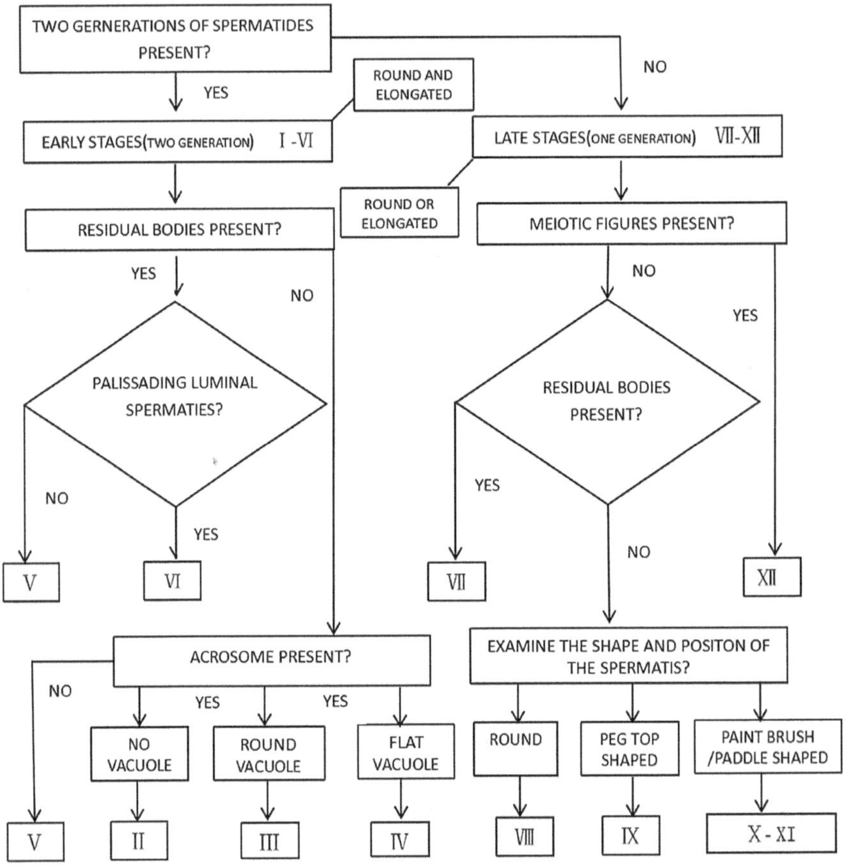

Fig. 2.9 Decision tree for rapidly identifying the spermatogenic stages of cynomolgus monkey in PAS-stained cross-sections

Stage V: In Step 5, round spermatids, the acrosomal granules begin to spread across the nuclear membrane, forming a small acrosomal cap (Fig. 2.14). At this stage, Step 13 spermatids have begun to condense a portion of the cytoplasm, which becomes visible as small cellular remnants known as the residual body of the spermatogenic cell (also observed in stages VI and VII).

Stage VI: In Step 6, round spermatids, the acrosomal cap covers about one-quarter of the nuclear surface. At this stage, Step 14 elongated spermatids are visible, representing fully developed sperm being released from the testis. Residual bodies are a prominent feature of this stage (Fig. 2.15).

Stage VII: In Step 7, round spermatids, the acrosomal cap extends to its maximum size, covering about one-third of the nuclear surface. Step 14: elongated spermatids are released into the lumen (spermiation). From this stage onward, only one generation of spermatids is present. Residual bodies remain clearly visible at the boundary of

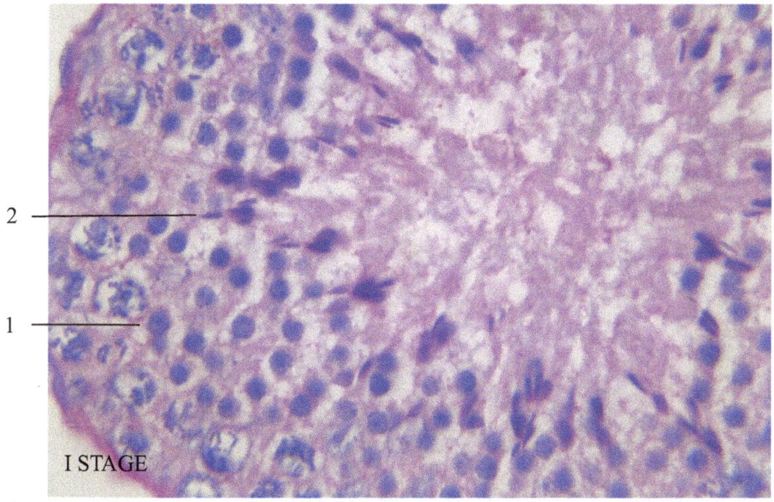

Fig. 2.10 Cross-section of the seminiferous tubules in the spermatogenic cycle of the cynomolgus monkey at stage I. Step 1: round spermatids are present, with no visible pre-acrosomal granules; Step 13: elongated spermatids are also present (PAS staining, ×1000). 1. Step 1 spermatids; 2. Step 13 spermatids

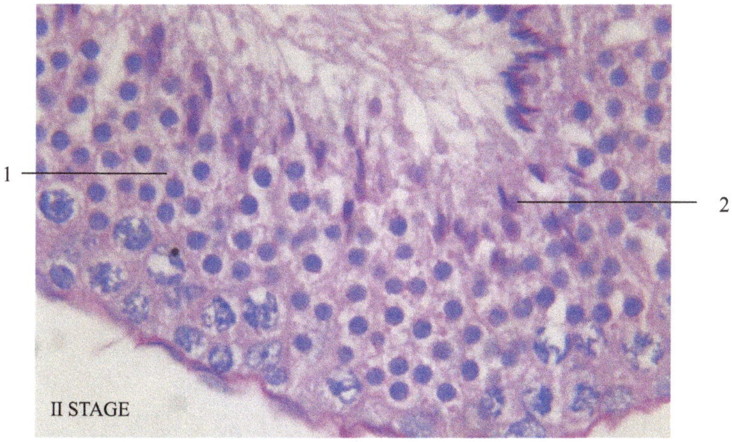

Fig. 2.11 Cross-section of the seminiferous tubules in the spermatogenic cycle of the cynomolgus monkey at stage II. Step 2 round spermatids are present, with visible pre-acrosomal vesicles, and Step 13 elongated spermatids are also present (PAS staining, ×1000). 1. Step 2 spermatids; Step 13 spermatids

the lumen space (Fig. 2.16). Ultimately, they are either expelled through the lumen or engulfed by Sertoli cells.

Stage VIII: In Step 8 spermatids, the acrosomal cap faces the basal membrane (Fig. 2.17). At this stage, the spermatids are still round.

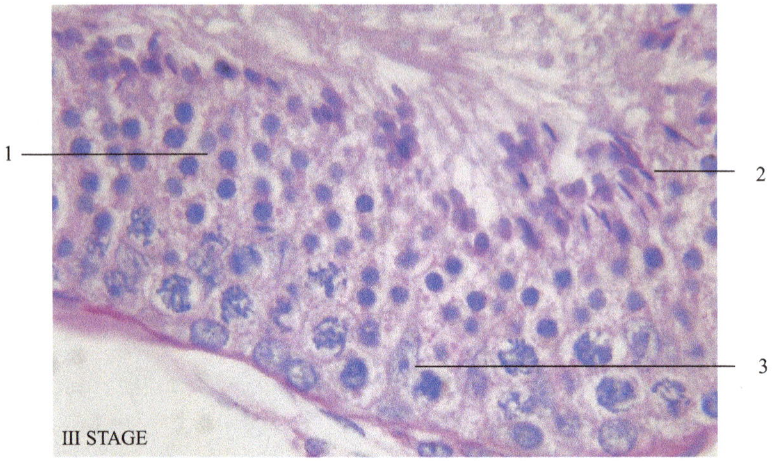

Fig. 2.12 Cross-section of the seminiferous tubules in the spermatogenic cycle of the cynomolgus monkey at stage III. Step 3 round spermatids are present, with acrosomal vesicles containing small granules adhering to the nuclear membrane; Step 13 elongated spermatids are still present (PAS staining, ×1000). 1. Step 3 spermatids; 2. Step 13 spermatids; 3. Sertoli cells

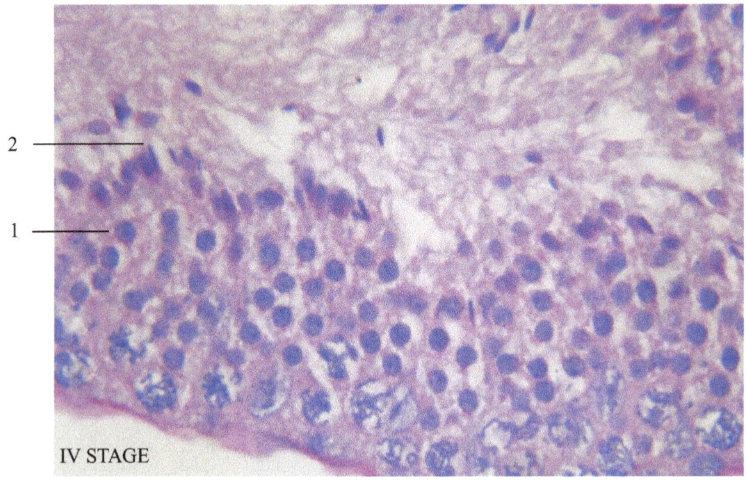

Fig. 2.13 Cross-section of the seminiferous tubules in the spermatogenic cycle of the cynomolgus monkey at stage IV. Step 4 round spermatids are present, with acrosomal vesicles flattening, and step 13 spermatids are also present (PAS staining, ×1000). 1. Step 4 spermatids; 2. Step 13 spermatids

Stage IX: In Step 9 spermatids, the nucleus elongates, and the portion covered by the acrosomal cap takes on a conical shape, resembling a spiral (Fig. 2.18).

Stage X: In Step 10 spermatids, the nucleus continues to elongate, and the tip becomes noticeably sharp (Fig. 2.19).

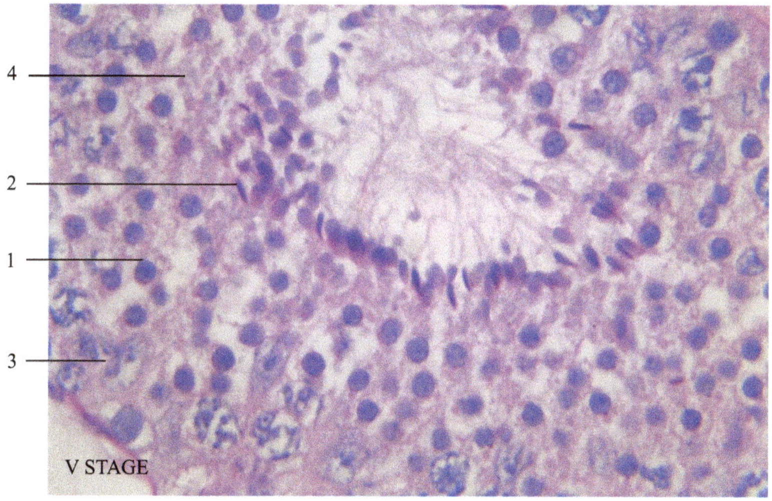

Fig. 2.14 Cross-section of the seminiferous tubules in the spermatogenic cycle of the cynomolgus monkey at stage V. Step 5 round spermatids are present, with a small acrosomal cap, along with Step 13 elongated spermatids and a few residual bodies (PAS staining, ×1000). 1. Step 5 spermatids; 2. Step 13 spermatids; 3. Sertoli cells; 4. Residual bodies

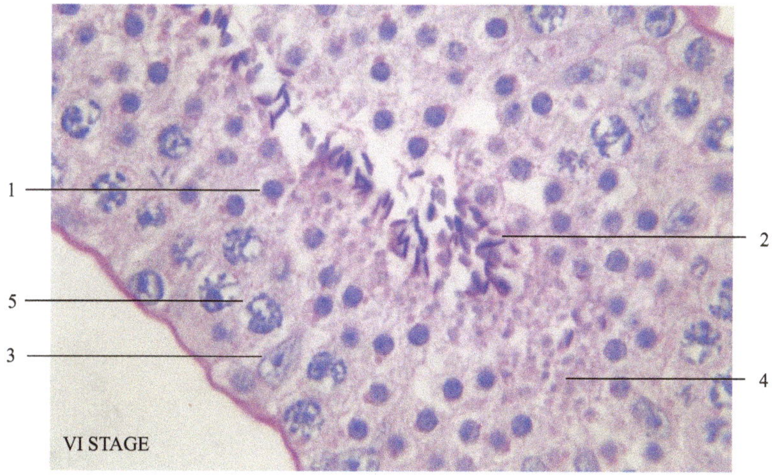

Fig. 2.15 Cross-section of the seminiferous tubules in the spermatogenic cycle of the cynomolgus monkey at stage VI. Step 6 round spermatids are present, with the acrosomal cap covering about one-quarter of the nuclear surface, along with step 14 elongated spermatids and abundant residual bodies (PAS staining, ×1000). 1. Step 6 spermatids; 2. Step 14 spermatids; 3. Sertoli cells; 4. Residual bodies; 5. Pachytene primary spermatocytes

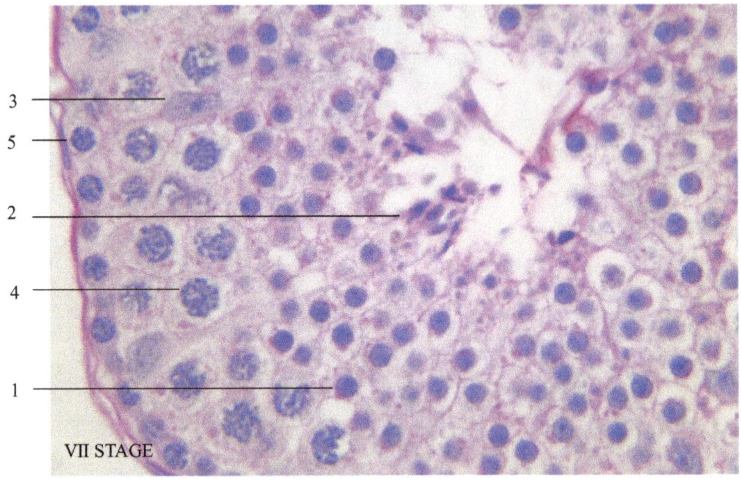

Fig. 2.16 Cross-section of the seminiferous tubules in the spermatogenic cycle of the cynomolgus monkey at stage VII. Step 7 round spermatids are present, with the acrosomal cap covering one-third of the nuclear surface, along with some residual bodies (PAS staining, ×1000). 1. Step 7 spermatids; 2. Step 14 spermatids and residual bodies; 3. Sertoli cells; 4. Pachytene primary spermatocytes; 5. B-type spermatogonia

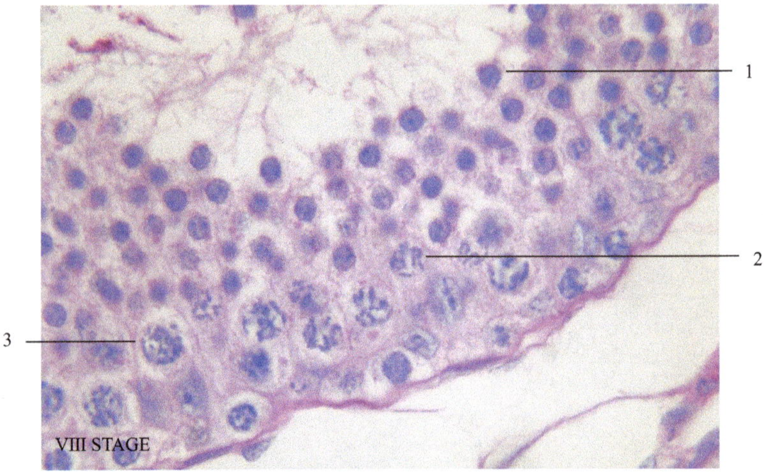

Fig. 2.17 Cross-section of the seminiferous tubules in the spermatogenic cycle of the cynomolgus monkey at stage VIII. Step 8 round spermatids are present, with a transparent acrosomal cap facing the basal membrane (PAS staining, ×1000). 1. Step 8 spermatids; 2. Leptotene primary spermatocytes; 3. Pachytene primary spermatocytes

Stage XI: In Step 11 spermatids, the nucleus continues to elongate and becomes significantly flattened, forming a brush/propeller-like shape (Fig. 2.20).

Stage XII: In Step 12 spermatids, the nuclear flattening is completed. The apex becomes rounded, and meiosis of the primary spermatocytes is a characteristic feature

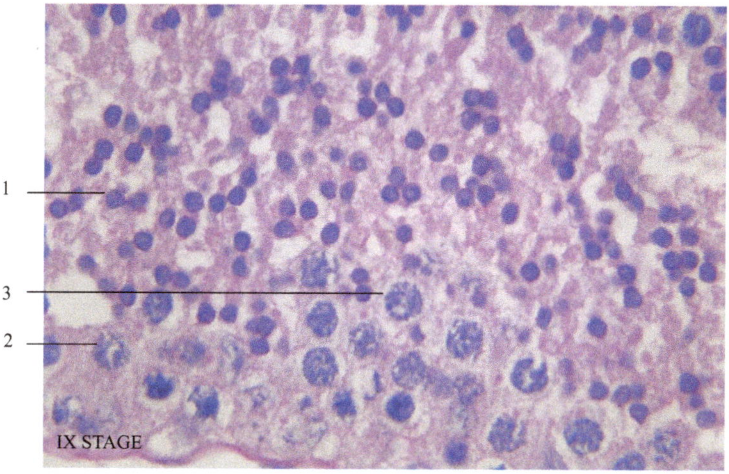

Fig. 2.18 Cross-section of the seminiferous tubules in the spermatogenic cycle of the cynomolgus monkey at stage IX. Step 9 spermatids with a spiral shape are present (PAS staining, ×1000). 1. Step 9 spermatids; 2. Leptotene primary spermatocytes; 3. Pachytene primary spermatocytes

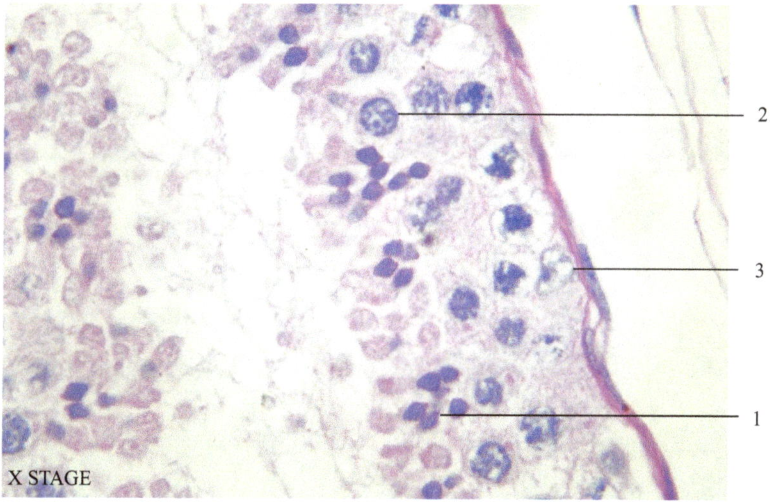

Fig. 2.19 Cross-section of the seminiferous tubules in the spermatogenic cycle of the cynomolgus monkey at stage X. Step 10 spermatids are present, with elongated spermatids displaying a clearly pointed tip (PAS staining, ×1000). 1. Step 10 spermatids; 2. Pachytene primary spermatocytes; 3. Sertoli cells

of this stage (Fig. 2.21, as shown in the meiotic diagram). This marks the initiation of the process leading to the formation of the first step spermatids in the subsequent cycle.

The testicular stroma is the loose connective tissue between the seminiferous tubules, which contains not only interstitial cells but also phagocytic cells, myoid cells, blood

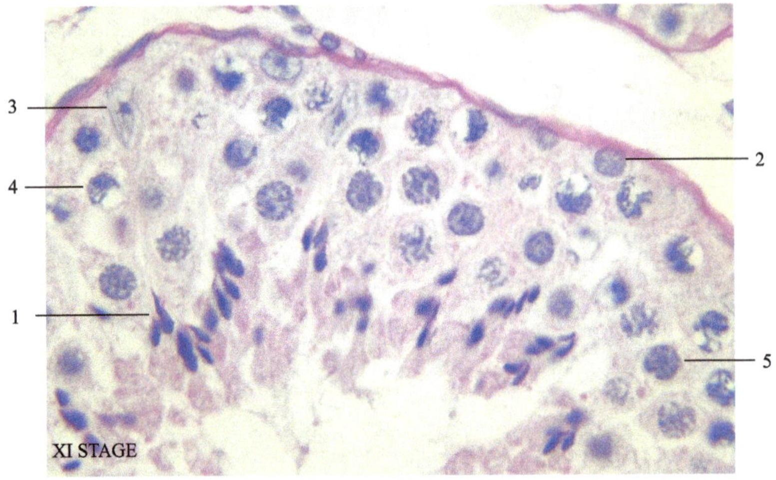

Fig. 2.20 Cross-section of the seminiferous tubules in the spermatogenic cycle of the cynomolgus monkey at stage XI. Step 11 elongated spermatids are present, with the nucleus exhibiting a brush/propeller-like shape (PAS staining, ×1000). 1. Step 11 spermatids; 2. Ap spermatogonia; 3. Sertoli cells; 4. Zygotene primary spermatocytes; 5. Pachytene primary spermatocytes

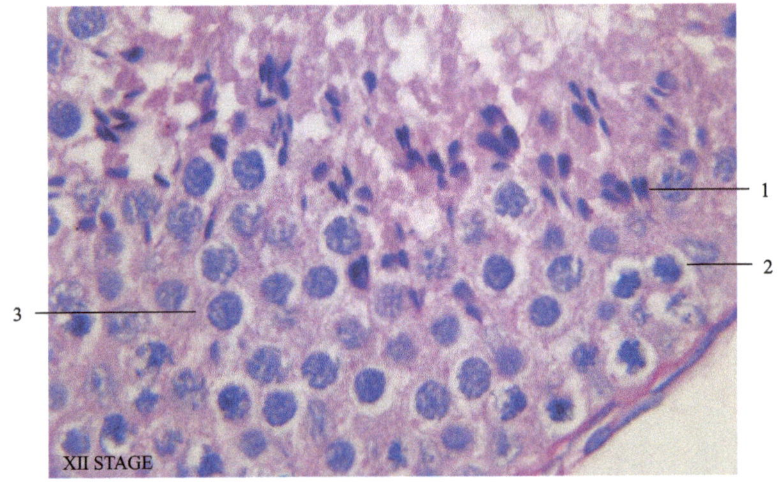

Fig. 2.21 Cross-section of the seminiferous tubules in the spermatogenic cycle of the cynomolgus monkey at stage XII. Step 12 spermatids are visible, with a brush/propeller-shaped nucleus and meiosis occurring (PAS staining, ×1000). 1. Step 12 spermatids; 2. Mitosis; 3. Pachytene primary spermatocytes

vessels, and lymphatic vessels [4, 5] (Fig. 2.22). The endothelial cells of the capillaries in the stroma have pores, and the interstitial fluid is rich in proteins and other nutrients. The spermatogenic epithelium absorbs nutrients from the stroma via osmosis.

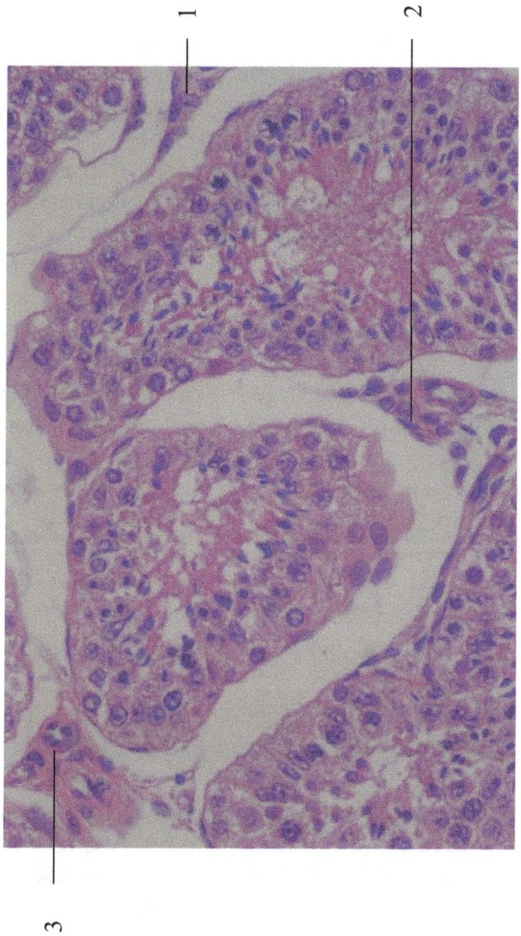

Fig. 2.22 Testicular stroma of a cynomolgus monkey (4 years old) (HE staining, ×400). 1. Interstitial cells; 2. Myoid cells; Blood vessels

Cynomolgus monkey Leydig cells (LC) are scattered and evenly distributed in the testicular interstitium between the seminiferous tubules. The Leydig cells are large in size, with a round or polygonal shape. The nucleus is round and centrally located, and the cytoplasm is strongly eosinophilic. The cytoplasm is rich in smooth endoplasmic reticulum and mitochondria. The interstitial cells secrete androgens, which promote spermatogenesis and the development and differentiation of male reproductive organs. Macrophages/phagocytes are typically thought to account for about 25% of the interstitial cell population in adult mice and rats, and they are widely believed to originate from monocytes in the circulating blood. Another possibility is that they are derived from a small number of progenitor or primitive cells that migrated to the testes early in development. In mature testes, macrophages influence the steroidogenesis of testicular interstitial cells by secreting 25-hydroxycholesterol, which is taken up by adult Leydig cells and used for testosterone synthesis [6].

The structure of Leydig cells in mammalian testes shows interspecies differences [7]. The literature divides the interstitial tissue of mammalian testes into three main categories: Category 1: Leydig cells are small in size (constituting 1%–5% of the total testicular volume), with minimal interstitial connective tissue but relatively abundant peritubular lymphoid tissue. This type is represented by rats, mice, and guinea pigs. Category 2: Leydig cells are widely distributed within loose connective tissue. The representative species for this category include nonhuman primates and humans. Category 3: Leydig cells are densely arranged, almost filling the interstitial space, accompanied by loose lymphatic vessels and a small amount of interstitial tissue. This type is represented by pigs and miniature pigs. In humans, characteristic protein crystals (Reinke crystals) can be found in the cytoplasm of Leydig cells, a feature not commonly observed in laboratory animals.

2.1.1.3 The Characteristics of Immature and Prepubertal Testes are as Follows

In immature testes, only Sertoli cells and undifferentiated spermatogonia are present. The seminiferous tubules have a small cross-sectional diameter, with narrow lumens. The testicular weight is low, and spermatogonia (Ad and Ap) are typically located on the basement membrane, though some may be found in the center of the tubule. Until the prepubertal stage, the testicular weight and seminiferous tubule diameter increase gradually. In prepubertal testes, growth occurs rapidly, and the lumen diameter of the seminiferous tubules enlarges. The first generation of B-type spermatogonia appears, and successive mitotic divisions of B1 to B4 spermatogonia can produce 16 spermatocytes. The mitotic activity of spermatogonia marks the beginning of spermatogenesis. Under the microscope, immature testes show seminiferous tubules filled with Sertoli cells and some spermatogonia. In prepubertal testes, additional cell types are present, including Sertoli cells, spermatogonia (A-type and B-type), primary spermatocytes in prophase, and some round spermatocytes (fewer than in mature testes). However, elongated sperm are not yet present.

During this period, the testicular morphology shows significant individual variation between animals of the same age. In some animals, the testes exhibit complete spermatogenesis, producing mature sperm, while in others, spermatogenesis may be incomplete. Even within a single testis, there can be considerable variation, with areas where spermatogenesis is fully developed, areas where germ cells are partially absent, and areas with fewer germ cells. In prepubertal and postpubertal testes, spermatogenesis may still be suboptimal (lacking certain germ cell populations), and shedding of degenerating germ cells into the lumen may be a normal occurrence.

2.1.2 Epididymis

The anatomy and position of the epididymis in the cynomolgus monkey are similar to those in other common laboratory animals. It consists of two bean-shaped structures attached to the surface of the testes, connecting the testes to the vas deferens. Anatomically, the epididymis is divided into three parts: the caput (head), corpus (body), and cauda (tail) of the epididymis (Figs. 2.23 and 2.24). The caput epididymis is crescent-shaped and consists of efferent ducts from the testis and the epididymal duct. The corpus epididymis is narrow and serves as the site for sperm storage and the acquisition of motility, composed mainly of the epididymal duct. The cauda epididymis is club-shaped, anatomically connected to the vas deferens, and histologically composed of the epididymal duct.

The epididymis is the site for sperm storage and maturation. The epithelial cells of the epididymal duct have both absorptive and secretory functions. They secrete various glycoproteins, steroids, and phospholipids, which contribute to sperm maturation. Additionally, the epididymal epithelium can phagocytose residual bodies and degenerated sperm.

The efferent ductules are lined by a single layer of cuboidal to pseudo-stratified columnar epithelium, surrounded by a multilayered smooth muscle layer and elastic fibers. The unabsorbed fluid within the efferent ductules is largely absorbed by the

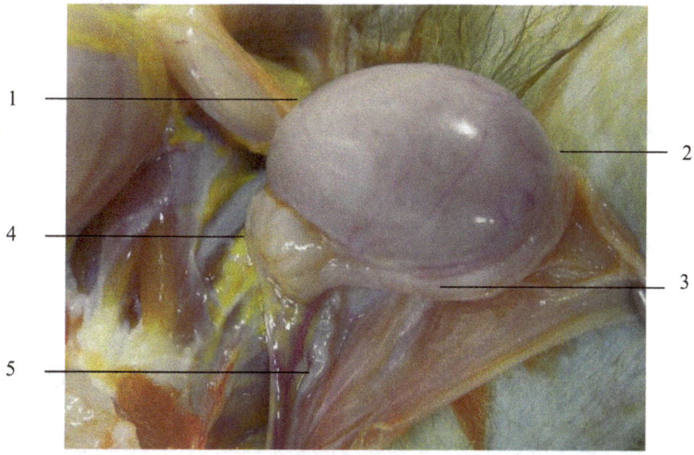

Fig. 2.23 Gross photograph of the testes, epididymis, and vas deferens of a 5-year-old cynomolgus monkey. 1. Testis; 2. Caput (head) of the epididymis; 3. Corpus (body) of the epididymis; 4. Cauda (tail) of the epididymis; 5. Vas deferens

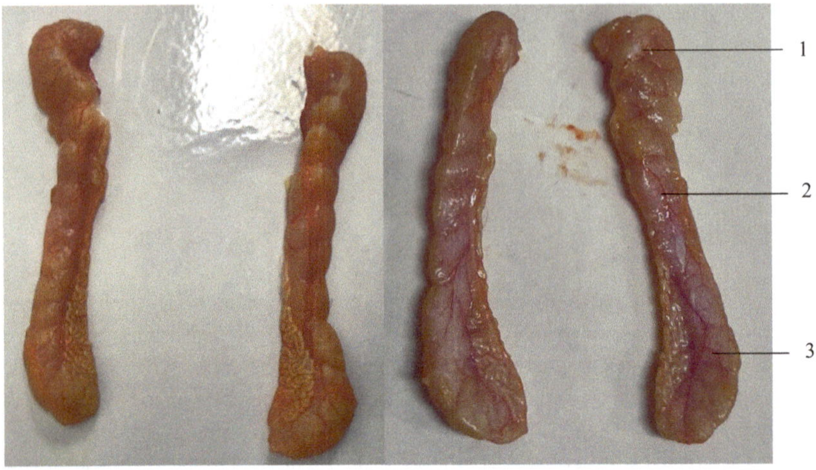

Fig. 2.24 Gross photograph of the epididymis of a 5-year-old cynomolgus monkey, viewed from the dorsal side (left) and ventral side (right). 1. Caput (head); 2. Corpus (body); 3. Cauda (tail)

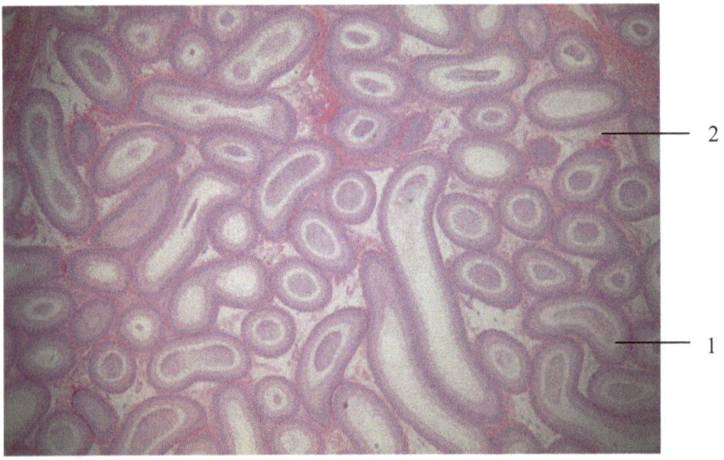

Fig. 2.25 Epididymis, epididymal ducts, and interstitial composition of a 5-year-old cynomolgus monkey (HE stain, ×40). 1. Epididymal duct; 2. Epididymal interstitium

epididymal ducts in the head of the epididymis. The epididymal duct is covered by pseudo-stratified columnar epithelium, composed of principal cells and basal cells. The basal cells are small, round or oval, located close to the basement membrane, and are generally considered reserve cells. The principal cells are columnar in shape, with long, coarse microvilli and stereocilia on their apical surface, and are involved in secretion and absorption. From the head to the tail of the epididymis, the wall of the epididymal duct and smooth muscle gradually thicken, the principal cells and stereocilia decrease in height, and the lumen gradually enlarges (Figs. 2.25–2.28).

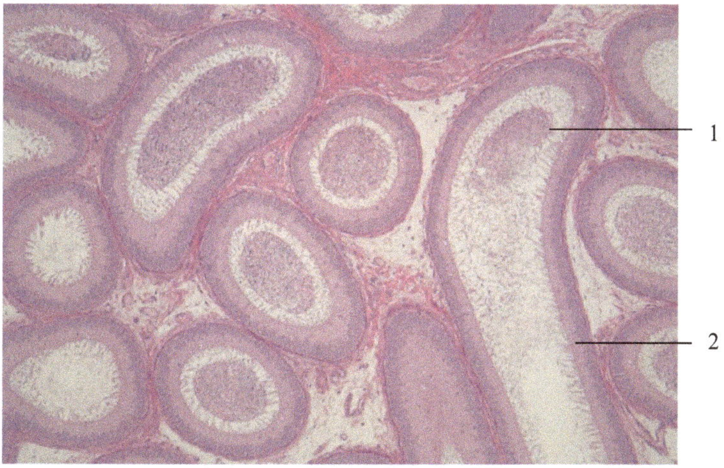

Fig. 2.26 Epididymis of a 5-year-old cynomolgus monkey, showing the epididymal duct epithelium covered by pseudo-stratified columnar epithelium, composed of principal cells and basal cells. A large number of sperm are visible within the epididymal duct lumen (HE stain, ×100). 1. Sperm in the lumen; 2. Pseudo-stratified columnar epithelium

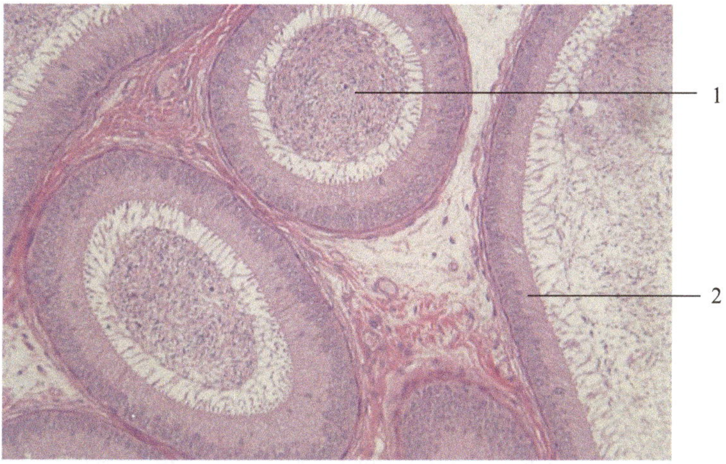

Fig. 2.27 Epididymis of a 5-year-old cynomolgus monkey, showing the epididymal duct epithelium covered by pseudo-stratified columnar epithelium, composed of principal cells and basal cells. A large number of sperm are visible within the epididymal duct lumen (HE stain, ×200). 1. Sperm; 2. Epididymal epithelium, pseudo-stratified epithelium

2.1.3 Vas Deferens

The vas deferens is a muscular tube that extends from the epididymal duct and opens into the urethra. In large animals, the distal end of the vas deferens is dilated,

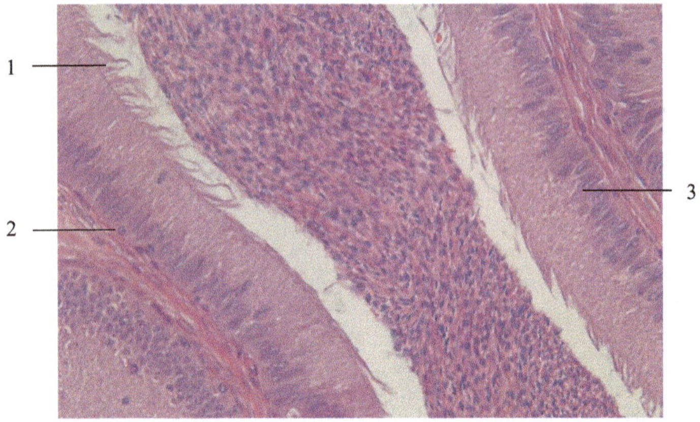

Fig. 2.28 Epididymis of a 5-year-old cynomolgus monkey, showing principal cells as tall columnar cells, and basal cells as small, round or oval cells near the basement membrane. These cells together form the epididymal epithelium. The epithelial surface shows long, coarse microvilli as well as stereocilia (HE stain, ×400). 1. Microvilli; 2. Basal cells; 3. Principal cells

forming the ampulla of the vas deferens. Secretions from the seminal vesicles and prostate are emptied into the ampulla, from where they enter the urethra. The urethra runs the entire length of the penis and serves to expel both urine and semen from the body.

The wall of the vas deferens consists of the mucosa, muscular layer, and adventitia, with a well-developed muscular layer that aids in ejaculation. The mucosa forms irregular longitudinal folds, and the epithelial lining is composed of either a single layer or pseudo-stratified columnar epithelial cells. The muscular layer includes three layers: an inner longitudinal layer, a middle circular layer, and an outer longitudinal layer. The inner longitudinal layer is relatively thin, while the middle circular layer is the thickest. The adventitia is made up of loose connective tissue, rich in blood vessels and nerves.

2.1.4 Seminal Vesicle

The seminal vesicle is located behind the bladder and above the prostate, and is a paired, lobular, sac-like organ. Its primary function is to secrete substances such as fructose, prostaglandins, and proteins, which make up semen. Among these, fructose provides energy to enhance sperm motility.

The seminal vesicle consists mainly of the mucosal layer and the muscular layer. The epithelial lining of the mucosa is either a single layer of columnar epithelium or pseudo-stratified columnar epithelium, composed of principal cells and basal cells. The lamina propria is made up of connective tissue, containing a small number of fibroblasts, moderate amounts of collagen fibers, reticular fibers, a large quantity of elastic fibers, and a rich vascular network. The muscular layer mainly consists of an inner layer of irregularly arranged circular and oblique smooth muscle fibers, and an outer layer of longitudinal smooth muscle tissue. The outer membrane is a thin layer of loose connective tissue containing small nerve ganglia (Figs. 2.29 and 2.30).

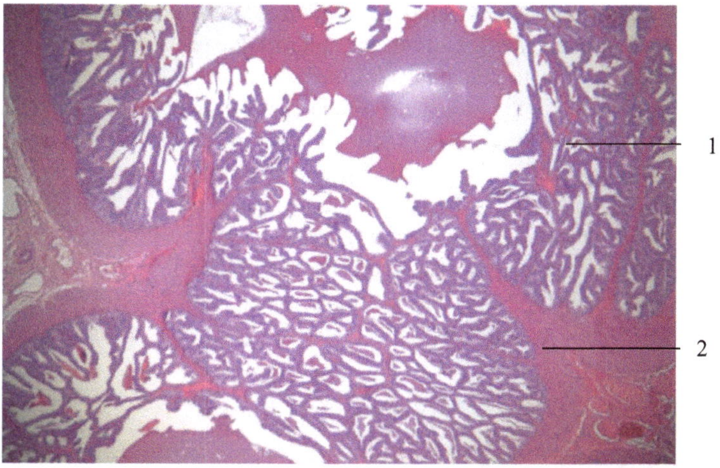

Fig. 2.29 Seminal vesicle of a 5-year-old cynomolgus monkey. The seminal vesicle is composed of the mucosal layer, muscular layer, and outer membrane (HE staining, ×40). 1. Mucosal layer; 2. Muscular layer

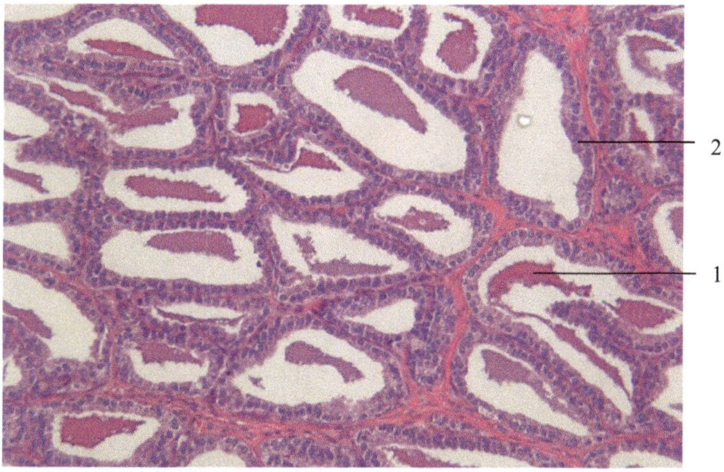

Fig. 2.30 Seminal vesicle of a 5-year-old cynomolgus monkey. The epithelial lining of the glandular lumen of the seminal vesicle is a single layer of columnar epithelium (HE staining, ×200). 1. Secretions in the glandular lumen of the seminal vesicle; 2. Epithelium of the glandular lumen of the seminal vesicle

2.1.5 Prostate Gland

The prostate is shaped like a chestnut, with its upper end closely connected to the base of the bladder and its lower end located on top of the urogenital diaphragm. The region between the upper and lower ends is referred to as the prostatic body. Depending on the species, the prostate may form a discrete gland or be diffusely distributed around the urethra, with glandular ducts passing through the urethral wall and into the urethra. In species such as dogs, monkeys, and rats, the prostate forms a discrete gland. In monkeys and rats, the prostate surrounds the urethra, whereas in dogs, the urethra lies slightly dorsal to the prostate. The capsule and stroma of the prostate can be divided into three layers, from outer to inner: the vascular layer, fibrous layer, and muscular layer. The connective tissue and smooth muscle of the capsule extend into the glandular parenchyma, subdividing it into lobes and contributing to the formation of the stromal matrix surrounding the gland (Figs. 2.31–2.33).

The glandular tissue is primarily composed of acinar glands of varying sizes, which are serous tubular-alveolar glands. The secretions are rich in proteolytic enzymes and acid phosphatase. Protein-like coagula with a pinkish staining can be observed in the glandular lumen.

2.1.6 Bulbourethral Gland

The bulbourethral gland is located on the lateral sides of the membranous part of the urethra, above the posterior portion of the bulbourethral bulb, and on both sides of the rectum. Its secretions contribute to the composition of semen and represent the initial portion of the ejaculate, lubricating the urethra. Bulbourethral glands are absent in monkeys.

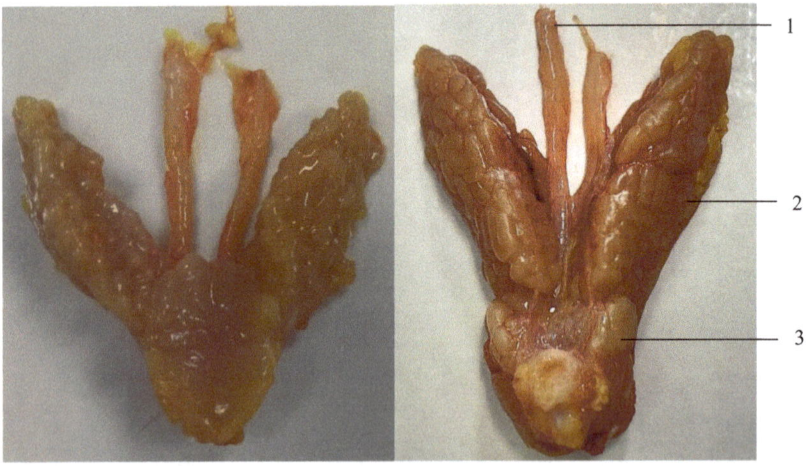

Fig. 2.31 Gross photograph of the prostate, seminal vesicle, and vas deferens in a 5-year-old cynomolgus monkey; The left side shows the dorsal view, and the right side shows the ventral view. 1. Vas deferens; 2. Seminal vesicle; 3. Prostate gland

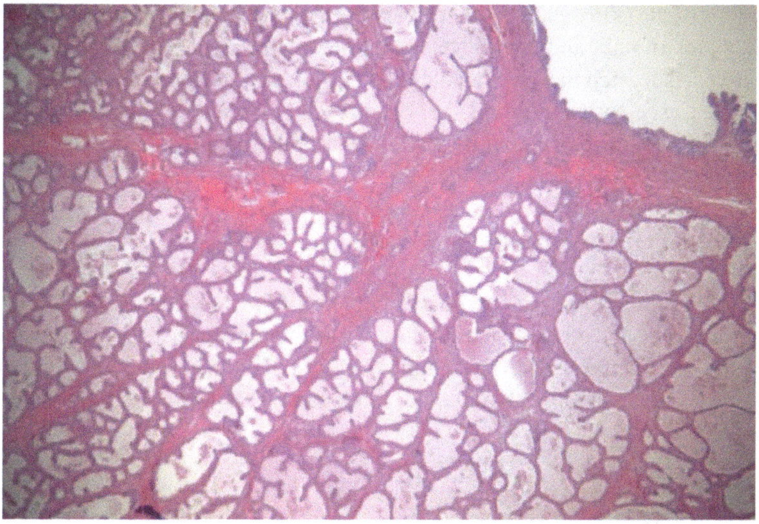

Fig. 2.32 Prostate of a 5-year-old cynomolgus monkey; the prostate consists of acinar glands of varying sizes, arranged in a tubular and alveolar structure (HE staining, ×40)

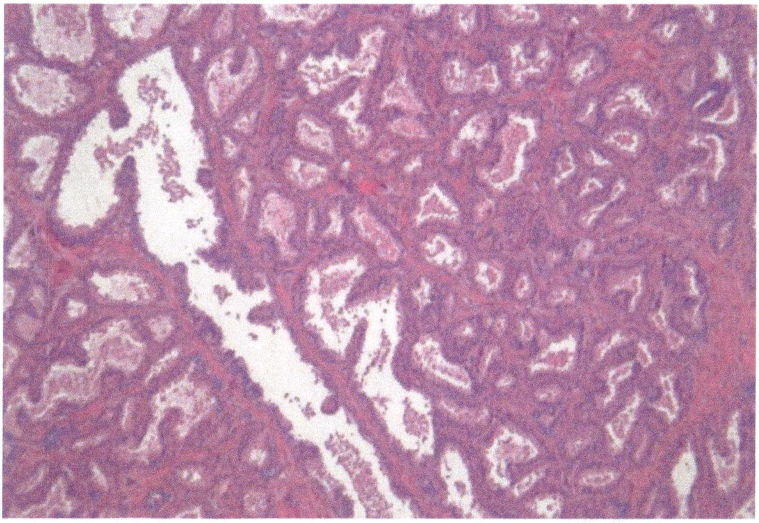

Fig. 2.33 Prostate of a 5-year-old cynomolgus monkey; the prostate consists of acinar glands of varying sizes, arranged in a tubular and alveolar structure (HE staining, ×100)

2.1.7 Penis

The penis is located in front of the scrotum, originating from the ischiatic arch and is enclosed within the prepuce. Its structure consists of two corpora cavernosa and one corpus spongiosum, all surrounded by skin and subcutaneous loose connective tissue.

The dermis of the skin contains scattered smooth muscle bundles, with no subcutaneous fat, a lack of hair, and well-developed sweat glands. Beneath the skin lies loose connective tissue, rich in nerve bundles and blood vessels. Below the capsule, dense connective tissue forms the tunica albuginea. The tunica albuginea of the corpora cavernosa is well-developed, while that of the corpus spongiosum is relatively thin.

2.2 Female Reproductive System

The female reproductive system primarily consists of the internal reproductive organs, external genitalia, and other related structures. The internal reproductive organs include the vagina, uterus, fallopian tubes, and ovaries [1, 2, 4, 5]. The external genitalia consist of the mons pubis, labia majora, labia minora, clitoris, and the vestibule of the vagina (Fig. 2.34).

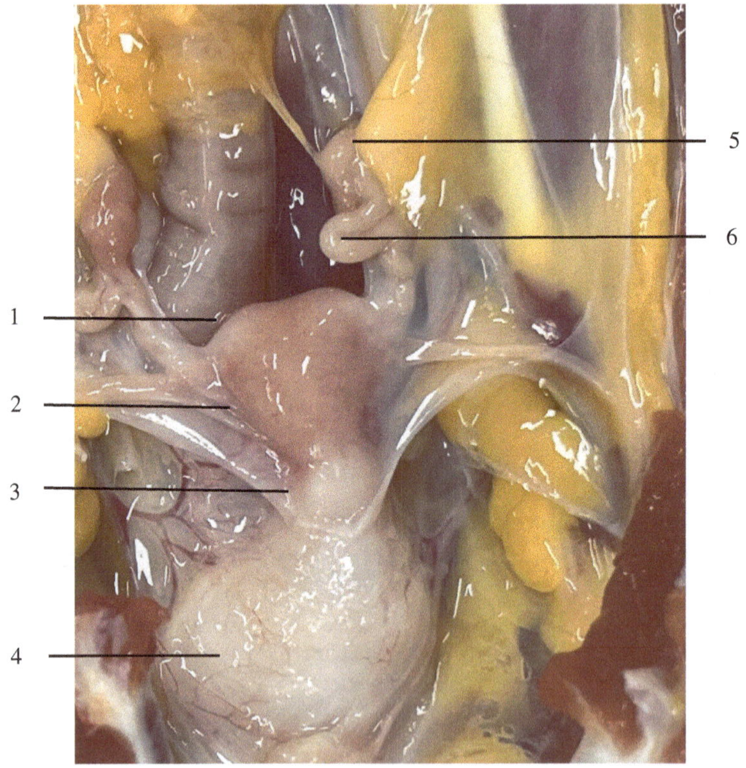

Fig. 2.34 Gross photograph of the ovary, fallopian tube, and uterus in a 3-year-old cynomolgus monkey. 1. Fundus of the uterus; 2. Body of the uterus; 3. Cervix of the uterus; 4. Vaginal fornix; 5. Ovary; 6. Fallopian tube

2.2.1 Ovary

The ovaries of the cynomolgus monkey are paired organs located below the kidneys, on either side of the pelvic inlet. Since the cynomolgus monkey exhibits unilateral ovulation, one ovary often shows a significant change in size relative to the other. Occasionally, small protrusions on the surface may be seen, corresponding to sites of ovulation.

The primary function of the ovary is to produce oocytes (eggs) and secrete estrogen and progesterone. The ovary is typically divided into the cortex, medulla, and capsule. In the cynomolgus monkey, the boundary between the cortical and medullary regions is clearly defined. The capsule, also known as the tunica albuginea, is a fibrous connective tissue layer covered by a single layer of flat, cuboidal, or columnar mesothelial cells. In the cynomolgus monkey, the tunica albuginea is not very distinct. The cortex contains germ cells at various stages of development, follicles, and interfollicular connective tissue. The medulla is located centrally within the ovary and is composed of connective tissue, containing stromal cells, blood vessels, lymphatic vessels, and nerve fibers.

The follicle is the main component of the ovary, and its development and maturation are continuous processes, typically divided into the primordial follicle, primary follicle, secondary follicle, and mature follicle stages. Usually, each follicle contains a single oocyte, but occasionally, multiple oocytes can be observed within a single follicle in the cynomolgus monkey (Figs. 2.35–2.37).

Primordial follicle: The primordial follicle is in a dormant state, numerous in number, small in size, and located in the superficial layer of the ovarian cortex. Its morphology is characterized by a centrally positioned oocyte surrounded by a single layer of flat follicular cells. The oocyte has a large, round nucleus with a prominent nucleolus, sparse chromatin, and weakly eosinophilic cytoplasm. The follicular cells are small and flat, with a flattened, deeply staining nucleus, and a basal membrane is present between the cells and the surrounding connective tissue, though it is not clearly defined.

Primary follicle: The primary follicle is composed of a single layer to several layers of cuboidal or columnar follicular cells surrounding the oocyte, with the follicular cells near the basal membrane being cuboidal or columnar in shape. The primary oocyte increases in size, and its nucleolus becomes deeply stained. A homogeneous, eosinophilic zona pellucida begins to form between the oocyte and the follicular cells. The inner layer of the theca folliculi starts to form. Follicles that grow without the appearance of a lumen between the follicular cells are classified as primary follicles.

Secondary follicle: As the follicle continues to develop, the oocyte reaches its maximum size. The follicular cells proliferate and increase to several layers. One or more irregular follicular cavities appear between the follicular cells, and these cavities contain follicular fluid. As the follicular cavity enlarges, the oocyte is positioned on one side of the cavity. The zona pellucida becomes more distinct, and a corona radiata forms. A layer of follicular cells adjacent to the zona pellucida becomes columnar and arranges radially around the primary oocyte, forming the corona radiata. The follicular cells surrounding the follicular cavity are densely arranged in a granular layer, known as the granulosa layer. The granulosa cells near the basal membrane are columnar and

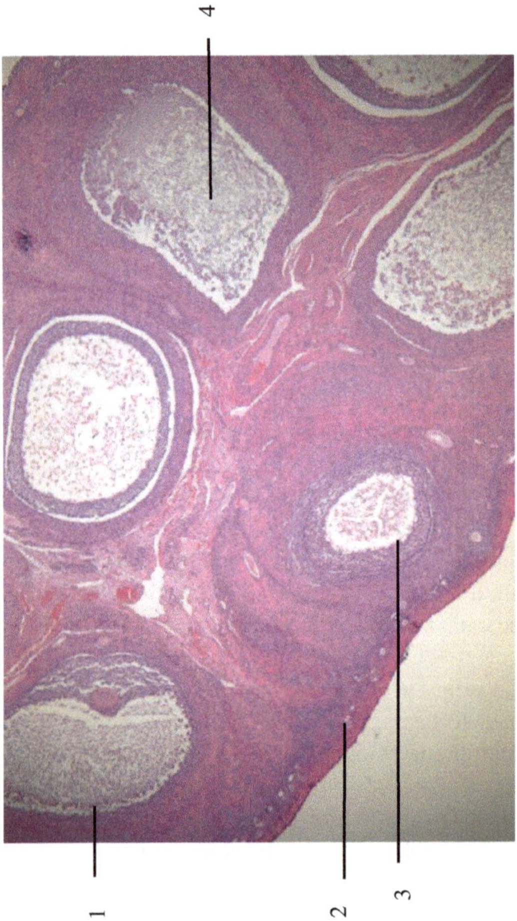

Fig. 2.35 Ovary of a 3-year-old cynomolgus monkey. Various types of follicles at different stages of development, along with a corpus luteum formed after ovulation, are visible (HE staining, ×40). 1. Mature follicle; 2. Primordial follicle; 3. Corpus luteum; 4. Atretic follicle

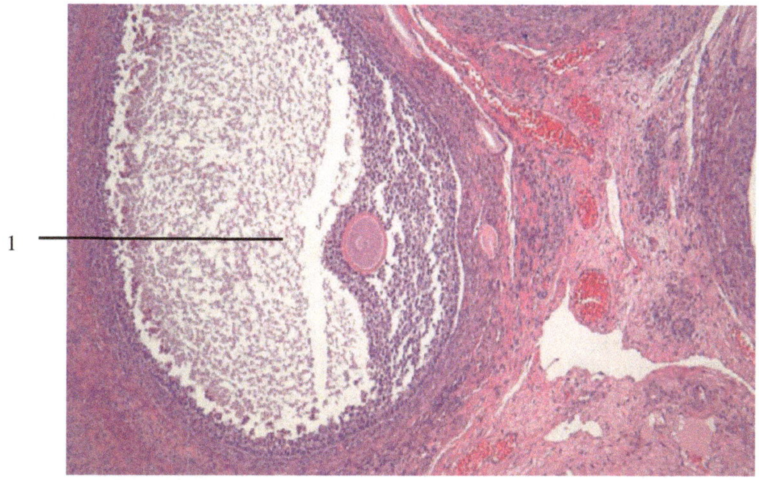

Fig. 2.36 Ovary of a 3-year-old cynomolgus monkey. A mature follicle in the process of development is visible (HE staining, ×100). 1. Mature follicle in development

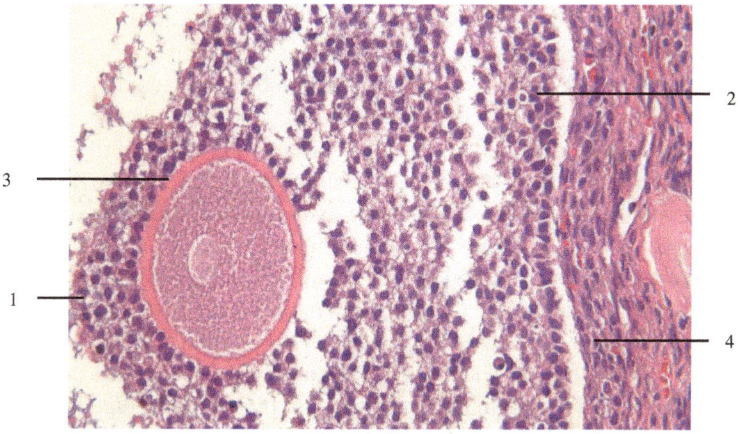

Fig. 2.37 Ovary of a 3-year-old cynomolgus monkey; a mature follicle in the process of development is visible (HE staining, ×400). 1. Cumulus oophorus; 2. Granulosa layer; 3. Zona pellucida; 4. Theca folliculi

are oriented perpendicular to the membrane. The granulosa layer is avascular, and nutrients are supplied to the oocyte through the spaces between the granulosa cells. The spindle-shaped cells in the connective tissue surrounding the basal membrane of the follicle proliferate and differentiate to form theca folliculi. The theca folliculi is divided into an inner and outer layer, with the inner layer becoming more distinct, while the outer layer begins to form.

Mature follicle: The follicle reaches its maximum size, and a central antrum and cumulus oophorus are formed. The follicle wall protrudes and bulges towards the ovarian surface. The follicular fluid increases dramatically, and multiple follicular cavities merge to form a single antrum, known as the central antrum, while the granulosa layer becomes thinner. The cumulus oophorus contains the primary oocyte, zona pellucida, and corona radiata. The inner and outer layers of the theca folliculi further differentiate, and there is no distinct boundary between them. The inner layer consists of numerous oval or polygonal cells, capillaries, fibroblasts, and collagen fibers. A prominent basal membrane is present between the inner layer and the granulosa cells. The outer layer has fewer cellular components, with more fibrous tissue and a small amount of smooth muscle, and it merges with the surrounding ovarian stroma.

Atretic follicle: During each reproductive cycle, multiple primordial follicles begin to grow and develop, but usually, only a few follicles mature and undergo ovulation. Therefore, the vast majority of follicles degenerate during development, forming atretic follicles. Degeneration can occur at any stage of follicular development. When primordial and primary follicles undergo atresia, both the oocyte and follicular cells undergo degeneration, atrophy, and apoptosis. The follicle becomes morphologically irregular and eventually either disappears or calcifies. In the case of secondary and mature follicles undergoing atresia, the follicular wall collapses, the zona pellucida shrinks and disappears, and the oocyte also degenerates and vanishes. Atretic follicles may contain degenerated oocytes, follicular cells, fibroblasts, connective tissue, and calcification foci.

Corpus luteum: After ovulation, the follicular wall, along with the blood vessels, collapses into the follicular cavity. Under the influence of luteinizing hormone, it gradually develops into a large, highly vascularized endocrine cell mass, which appears yellow to the naked eye and is known as the corpus luteum. The majority of the corpus luteum cells are derived from the granulosa cells of the follicle. These luteal cells are large, polygonal, with lightly stained cytoplasm and lipid droplets, and are called granulosa luteal cells. These cells are located in the center of the corpus luteum and primarily secrete progesterone and relaxin. The luteal cells derived from theca cells of the follicle are smaller, round or polygonal, more deeply stained, and less numerous. These are called theca luteal cells, located at the periphery of the corpus luteum, primarily secreting estrogen. The blood vessels and lymphatic vessels from the theca folliculi also proliferate, forming a rich network of blood vessels and lymphatic vessels within the corpus luteum. If the oocyte is fertilized, the corpus luteum continues to develop and enlarge under the influence of human chorionic gonadotropin (hCG) from the placenta until pregnancy is completed. If the oocyte is not fertilized, the luteal cells undergo degeneration and necrosis, and are phagocytized and digested by macrophages, leading to the regression of the corpus luteum. Connective tissue gradually proliferates, replacing the corpus luteum and forming white scar tissue visible to the naked eye. Some luteal cells may differentiate into stromal cells (Figs. 2.38 and 2.39).

2.2.2 Oviduct

The oviduct is a muscular conduit primarily responsible for transporting the oocyte and providing a microenvironment for fertilization. Its anatomical structure is typically

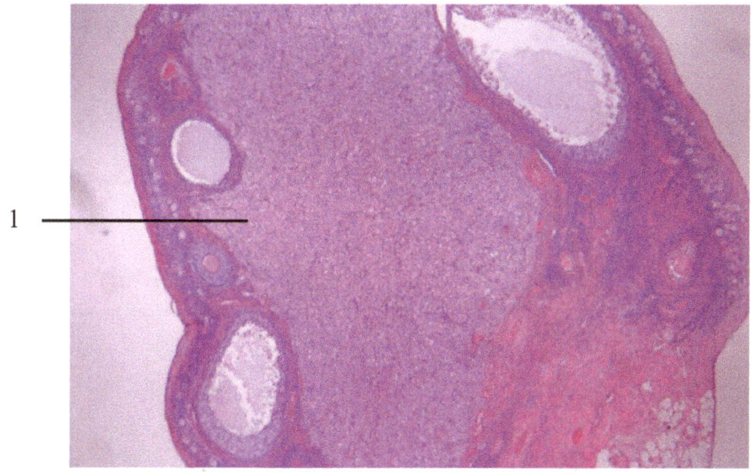

Fig. 2.38 Corpus luteum in the ovary of a 3-year-old cynomolgus monkey (HE staining, ×40). 1. Corpus luteum

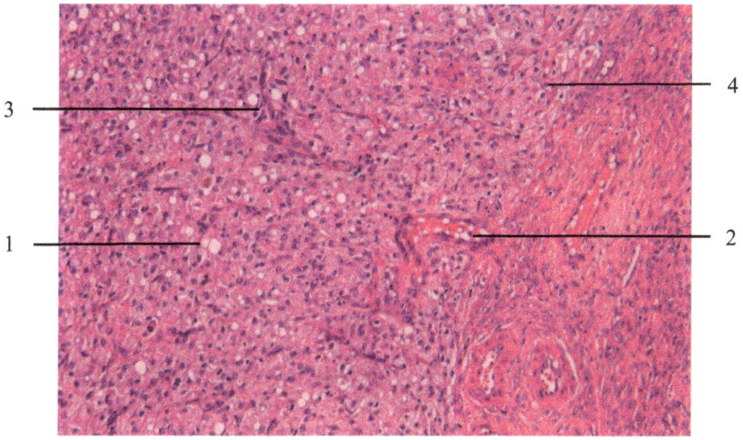

Fig. 2.39 Corpus luteum in the ovary of a 3-year-old cynomolgus monkey (HE staining, ×200). 1. Granulosa luteal cells; 2. Blood vessels; 3. Fibrous connective tissue; 4. Theca luteal cells

divided into the infundibulum, ampulla, isthmus, and uterine portion. The infundibulum begins at the ovary and opens into the abdominal cavity.

The wall of the oviduct consists of three layers: the mucosa, muscularis, and serosa (Figs. 2.40 and 2.41). The mucosa forms numerous longitudinal and branching folds, and the cross-sectional lumen is irregular. The mucosa is composed of a loose connective tissue lamina propria and a single layer of columnar epithelium. The epithelium consists of secretory cells and ciliated cells. The infundibulum and ampulla are rich

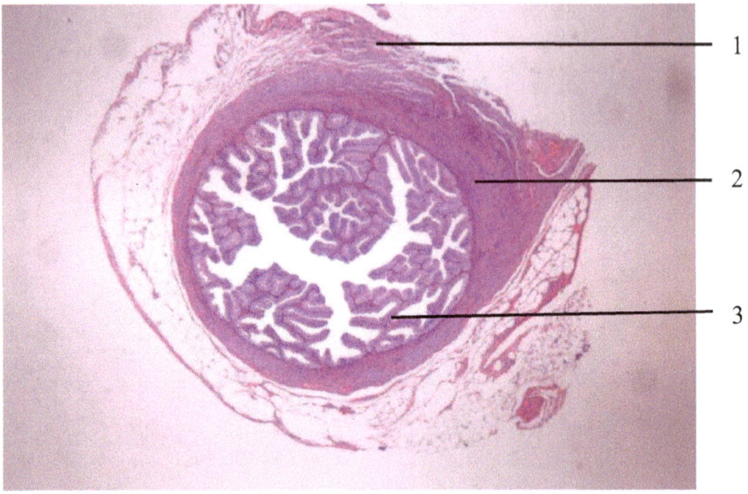

Fig. 2.40 Oviduct of cynomolgus monkey (3 years old) (HE staining, ×40). 1. Serosa layer; 2. Muscularis layer; 3. Mucosa layer

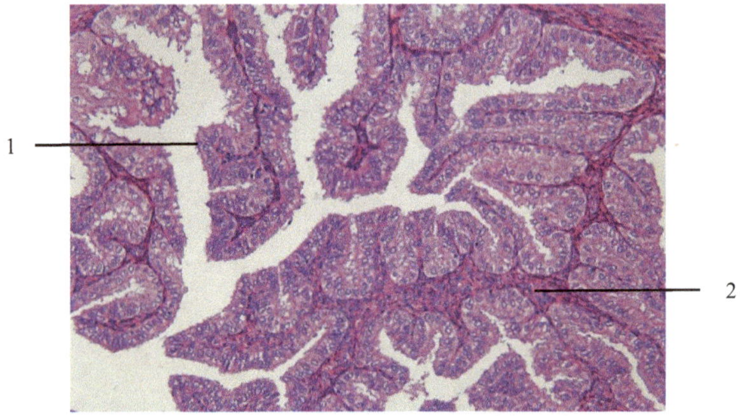

Fig. 2.41 Mucosa layer of the oviduct in a cynomolgus monkey (3 years old) (HE staining, × 200). The mucosa is composed of a lamina propria (loose connective tissue) and a single layer of columnar epithelium. The epithelium consists of secretory cells and ciliated cells. 1. Single layer of columnar epithelium; 2. Lamina propria (loose connective tissue)

in ciliated cells. The cilia beat towards the uterus, aiding the transport of the oocyte. Secretory cells are scattered between the ciliated cells, with microvilli on their free edges. The secretory cells release their secretions onto the mucosal surface through apocrine secretion, forming oviductal fluid that nourishes the oocyte. The muscularis consists of inner circular and outer longitudinal smooth muscle fibers. The serosa is made up of mesothelium and loose connective tissue and is rich in blood vessels.

2.2.3 Uterus

The uterus is a muscular, hollow organ where fetal development occurs. In the cynomolgus monkey, the uterus is pear-shaped and divided into the cervix and the uterine body. The uterine wall consists of the endometrium, myometrium, and serosa (Figs. 2.42–2.45). The endometrium is composed of a single layer of columnar epithelium

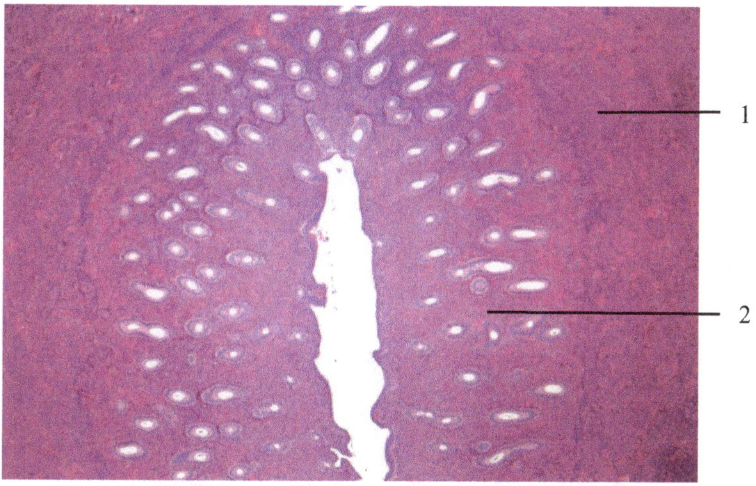

Fig. 2.42 Cynomolgus monkey (3.5 years old) uterus, divided into the endometrium, myometrium, and serosa (HE stain, ×40). 1. Myometrium; 2. Endometrium

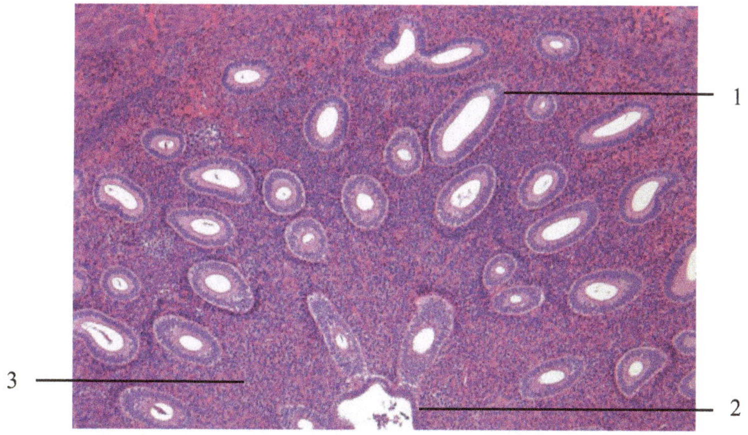

Fig. 2.43 Cynomolgus monkey (3.5 years old) endometrium, the stroma of the endometrium contains abundant uterine glands. The uterine glands are tubular and have their origin from the epithelial layer of the endometrium, with branching at the terminal ends. The stromal cells in the endometrial stroma are spindle-shaped or stellate, with small cytoplasm and large, round nuclei (HE stain, ×100). 1. Uterine glands; 2. Endometrial epithelium; 3. Stromal cells of the endometrium

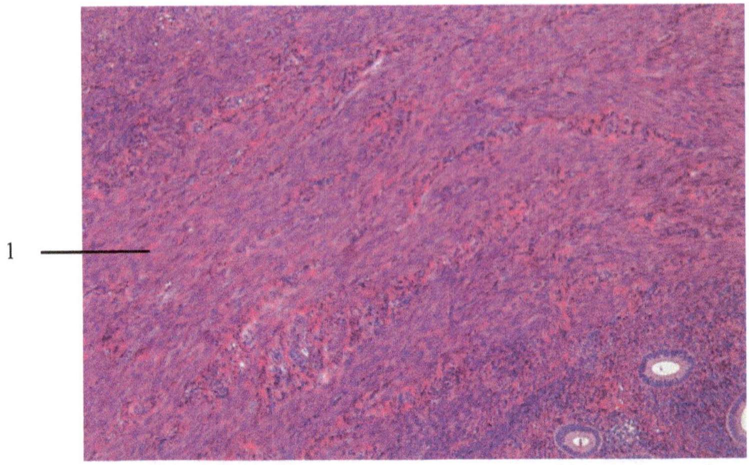

Fig. 2.44 Cynomolgus monkey (3.5 years old) myometrium (HE stain, ×100). 1. Myometrium, divided into the inner circular layer, outer longitudinal layer, and middle oblique layer

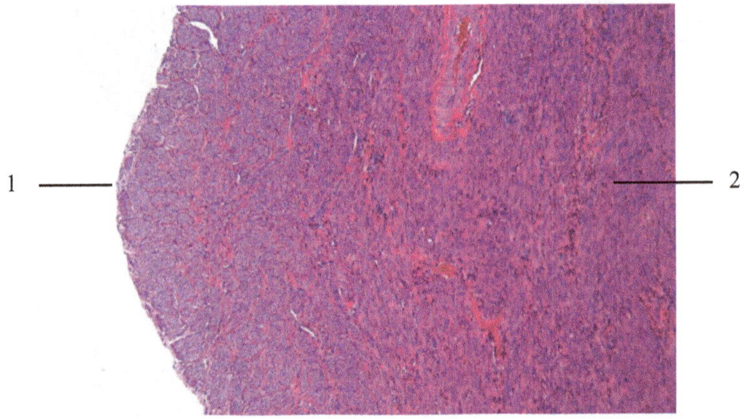

Fig. 2.45 Cynomolgus monkey (3.5 years old) myometrium and serosa (HE stain, ×100). 1. Serosa, a thin layer; 2. Myometrium

and the lamina propria. The glandular epithelium mainly consists of secretory cells that secrete via apocrine secretion. The lamina propria contains abundant uterine glands, blood vessels, lymphatic vessels, nerves, and stromal cells. The uterine glands are tubular and continue with the epithelial layer at the basal end, where they branch. The stromal cells in the lamina propria are spindle- or star-shaped, with scant cytoplasm, large round nuclei, and collagen secretion, resembling fibroblasts. Basal cells have a lower degree of differentiation and proliferate and differentiate in response to changes during pregnancy and the estrous cycle [8].

The myometrium is thick and continuous with the muscular layers of the fallopian tubes and vagina. It can be divided into layers such as the outer longitudinal, inner circular, and middle oblique layers, although the boundaries between them are indistinct. The connective tissue in the myometrium contains undifferentiated mesenchymal cells, which can differentiate into smooth muscle cells during pregnancy, undergoing proliferation and hypertrophy. Progesterone promotes the enlargement of smooth muscle cells and inhibits smooth muscle contraction. Estrogen stimulates the proliferation of smooth muscle cells, increasing their number. After delivery, the smooth muscle cells of the uterus gradually atrophy, shrink, or undergo apoptosis, and the connective tissue is degraded and absorbed, allowing the uterus to return to its original state.

The cynomolgus monkey uterus mucosa is divided into the superficial functional layer and the deeper basal layer. After entering the myometrium of the uterine wall, the uterine artery branches into the endometrium to form the spiral arteries. The spiral arteries form a network of capillaries and capillary sinusoids in the superficial part of the functional layer of the endometrium, which then drain into the corresponding veins. The spiral arteries are sensitive to hormonal stimulation and are involved in the cyclical changes of the endometrium.

The cyclical changes of the cynomolgus monkey endometrium can be divided into three stages: the proliferative phase, the secretory phase, and the menstrual phase.

The proliferative phase, also known as the follicular phase, is primarily influenced by estrogen. During this phase, the ovarian follicles develop and mature, with the granulosa cells secreting estrogen. Under the influence of estrogen, the uterine mucosal epithelium proliferates, and the endometrium undergoes growth and rebuilding. The uterine glands proliferate and increase in number, with the glandular lumens initially large and straight, gradually becoming more curved or spiral-shaped. The endometrial and glandular epithelia are pseudostratified columnar, with prominent mitotic figures in both epithelial and stromal cells.

The secretory phase, also known as the luteal phase, is primarily influenced by progesterone. After ovulation, the corpus luteum forms, and the luteal cells secrete progesterone. Under the influence of both progesterone and estrogen, the uterine mucosa continues to proliferate and thicken. The uterine glands expand and become more curved, with the glandular lumens exhibiting a serrated appearance in cross-section, filled with mucous secretions. The epithelial cells of the mucosa become hypertrophic and columnar, with no significant mitotic activity. The apical cytoplasm appears irregular. Occasionally, glycogen and lipid droplets may accumulate in the cytoplasm, both above and below the nucleus, giving it a vacuolated appearance. Stromal cells also become hypertrophic, and mitotic activity in the stroma disappears.

The menstrual phase, also known as luteal regression, occurs if the egg is not fertilized. The corpus luteum undergoes degeneration and atrophy, leading to decreased levels of estrogen and progesterone secreted by the ovaries. The uterine mucosal arteries constrict, causing ischemia, necrosis, and shedding of the mucosal surface. As a result, the mucosa becomes thinner.

The cervix is composed of the outer membrane, muscular layer, and mucosa. The outer membrane consists of fibrous connective tissue. The muscular layer is made up of smooth muscle interspersed with abundant connective tissue. In the cynomolgus monkey, the cervical mucosa contains numerous cervical glands and branched tubular glands that secrete mucus. The mucosal epithelium consists of a single layer of columnar cells, consisting mainly of secretory cells and a small number of basal cells. Basal cells are scattered between the columnar cells and the basement membrane; they are small, poorly differentiated, and have proliferative and reparative functions. At the external cervical os, the single-layer columnar epithelium transforms into stratified squamous epithelium, with a mixed structure of mucus-secreting cells and stratified squamous epithelium. The cyclic morphological changes in the cervical mucosa are less pronounced (Figs. 2.46 and 2.47).

Vagina is a fibrous and muscular tubular structure. The vagina consists of three layers: the external membrane, the muscular layer, and the mucosal layer. The mucosal layer is covered by stratified squamous epithelium, and the lamina propria is composed of fibrous elastic connective tissue, without any glandular structures. The muscular layer is made up of interwoven smooth muscle fiber bundles. The external membrane is composed of dense connective tissue and extends into surrounding structures (Figs. 2.48 and 2.49).

In cynomolgus monkeys, the vaginal epithelium undergoes changes throughout the estrous cycle. These changes can be used to distinguish different stages of the estrous cycle in cynomolgus monkeys from vaginal epithelial tissue sections and vaginal secretion smears.

2.2.4 Mammary Gland

The position and number of mammary glands vary by species. Monkeys have one pair of mammary glands, rats have six pairs, mice have five pairs, and dogs have five or six pairs. The mammary gland is a compound tubuloalveolar gland derived from the

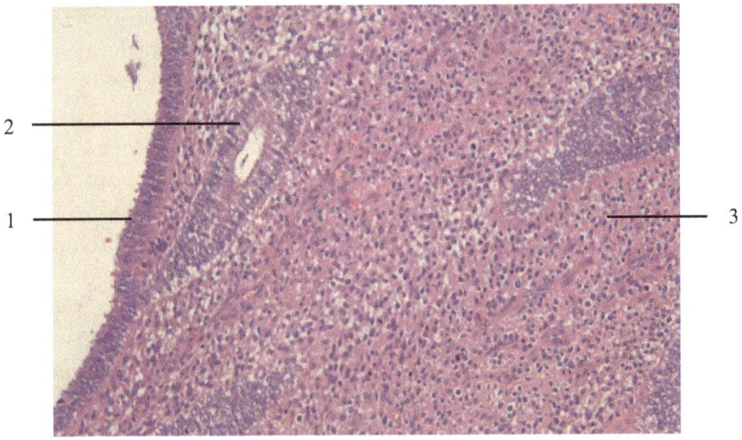

Fig. 2.46 Cynomolgus monkey (3.5 years) cervical mucosal layer (HE staining, ×200). 1. Single-layer columnar epithelial lining; 2. Cervical glands; 3. Fibrous connective tissue

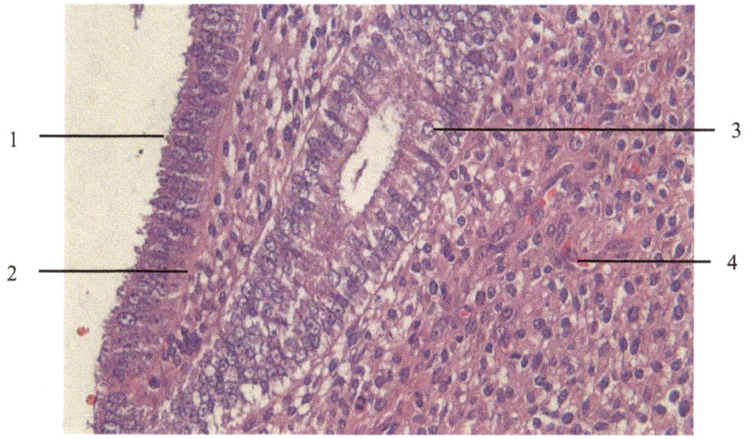

Fig. 2.47 Cynomolgus monkey (3.5 years) cervical mucosa, epithelial lining and lamina propria (HE staining, ×400). 1. Single-layer columnar epithelial lining; 2. Basement membrane of columnar epithelium; 3. Cervical glands; 4. Capillaries in connective tissue

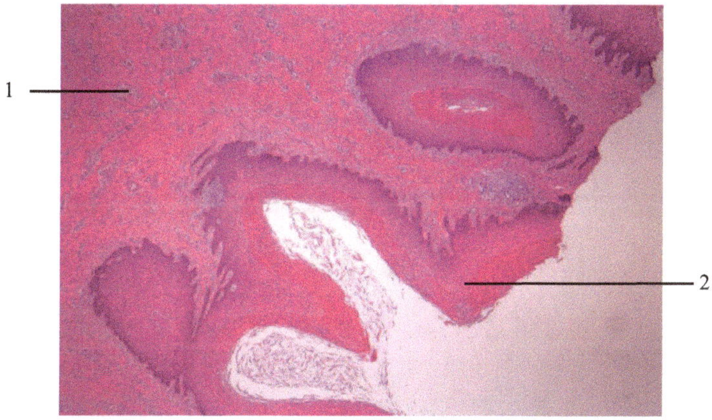

Fig. 2.48 Cynomolgus monkey (3.5 years) vagina composed of the outer membrane layer, muscle layer, and mucosa layer (HE staining, ×40). 1. Muscle layer; 2. Mucosa layer

ectoderm, a type of sweat gland and a characteristic tissue of mammals. In sexually mature female animals, the mammary glands are well-developed and produce milk. Male animals have underdeveloped mammary gland tissue, with only a small amount of glandular tissue present.

The mammary gland is composed of lobules, ducts, and the nipple, with less adipose tissue in the stroma compared with rodents (Figs. 2.50–2.53). The lobules secrete milk and are composed of a single layer of cuboidal epithelium, which becomes flattened after secretion. The various levels of mammary ducts are lined with a single layer or

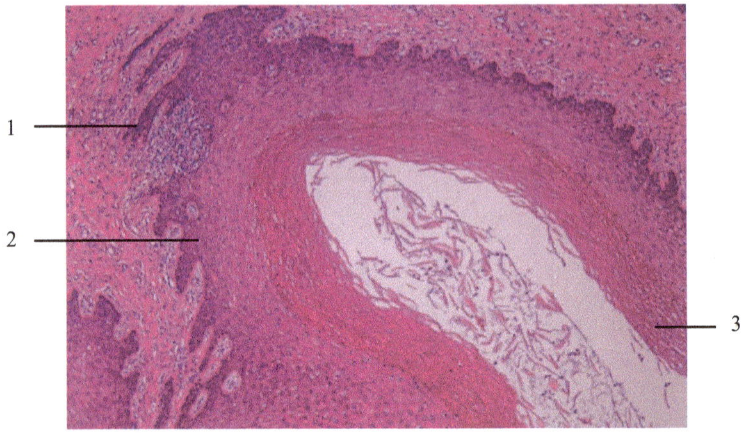

Fig. 2.49 Cynomolgus monkey (3.5 years) vaginal mucosa, covered by stratified squamous epithelium (HE staining, ×100). 1. Basal cell layer; 2. Spinous cell layer; 3. Keratinized layer

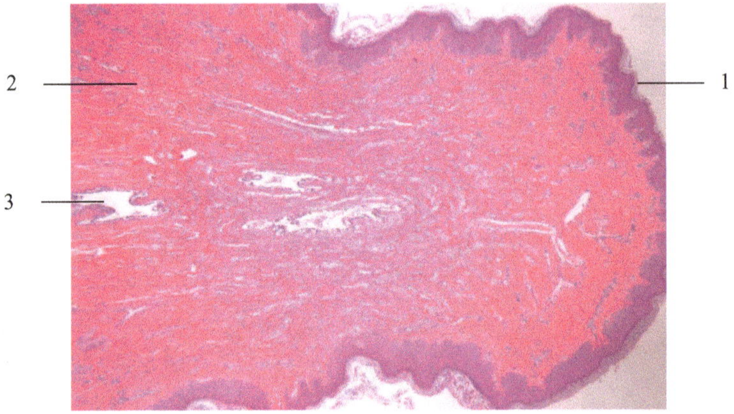

Fig. 2.50 Cynomolgus monkey (3 years old) nipple (HE staining, ×40). 1. Nipple epithelium; 2. Connective tissue; 3. Mammary duct under the nipple

pseudo-stratified cuboidal or columnar epithelial cells. Between the epithelial cells of the lobules and ducts and the basement membrane, there are myoepithelial-like cells. These myoepithelial-like cells contract to facilitate milk secretion and also secrete components that form the basement membrane. The main ducts and nipple ducts are lined with stratified squamous epithelium [9].

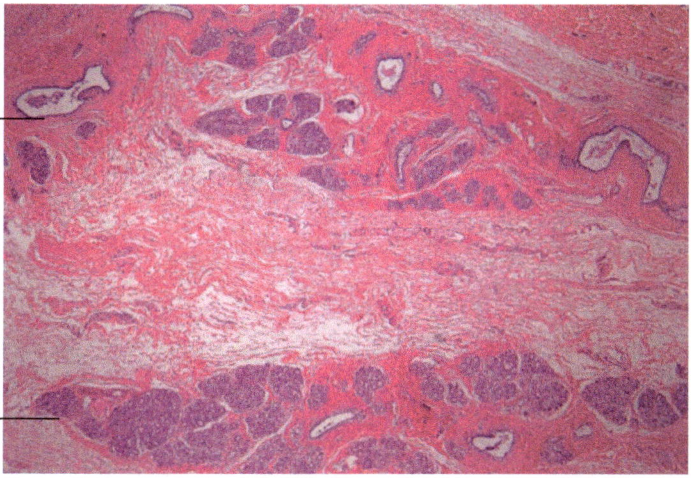

Fig. 2.51 Female cynomolgus monkey (3.5 years old) mammary gland tissue beneath the nipple. The mammary tissue is well-developed, with scattered tubular-alveolar glands and duct structures (HE staining, ×100). 1. Tubulo-alveolar gland; 2. Duct structure

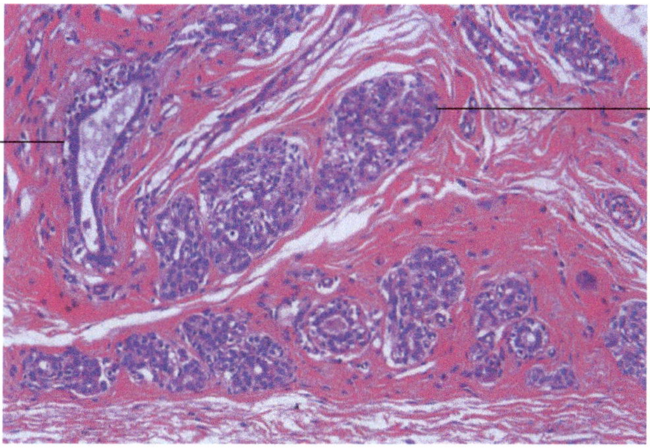

Fig. 2.52 Female cynomolgus monkey (3.5 years old) mammary gland tissue beneath the nipple. The mammary tissue is well-developed, with scattered tubular-alveolar glands and duct structures (HE staining, ×200). 1. Mammary tubulo-alveolar gland; 2. Duct structure

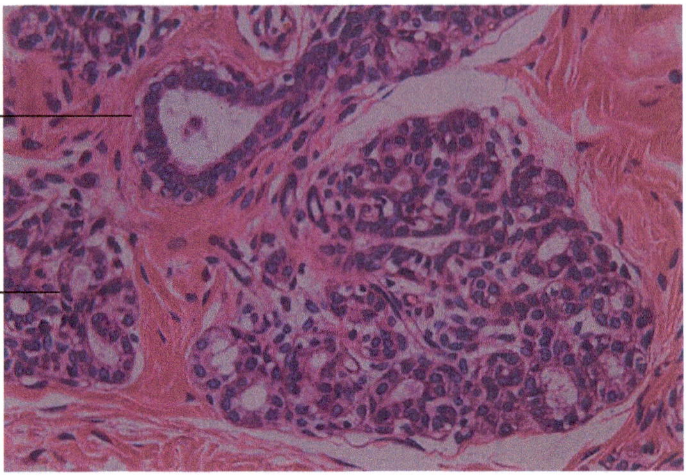

Fig. 2.53 Female cynomolgus monkey (3.5 years old) mammary gland tissue beneath the nipple. The mammary tissue is well-developed, with scattered tubular-alveolar glands and duct structures (HE staining, ×400). 1. Mammary tubulo-alveolar gland; 2. Duct structure

Ethical Approval

This chapter is a review of previously published accounts; as such, no animal or human studies were performed.

References

1. Xiantang L, Nasir Khan K, Burkhardt JE (2018) Functional histology of laboratory animals. Science Press, Beijing
2. Chuan Q, Wei D, Yanfeng X (2017) Color atlas of comparative histology of laboratory animals. Science Press, Beijing
3. Yingmao G, He L, Jicheng L et al (2015) Histology and embryology. People's Medical Publishing House, Beijing
4. Cen Xiaobo, Hu Chunyan, Du Yanchun et al (2011) Color atlas of histopathology in non-human primates. People's Medical Publishing House, Beijing
5. Sahota PS,Popp JA, Hardisty JF (2018) Toxicologic pathology: nonclinical safety assessment. Translated by Jianjun L, Hemei W, Kejian L et al Beijing Science and Technology Press, Beijing
6. Graves P (2018) Histopathology of preclinical toxicity studies interpretation and relevance in drug safety evaluation. Translated by Hemei W, Jianjun L, Junwen Q, et al Beijing Science and Technology Press, Beijing
7. Dreef HC, Van Esch E, Rijk EPCTDE (2007) Spermatogenesis in the cynomolgus monkey (*Macaca fascicularis*): a practical guide for routine morphological staging. Toxicol Pathol 35:395–404

8. Svingen T, Koopman P (2013) Building the mammalian testis: origins, differentiation, and assembly of the component cell populations. Genes Dev 27:24092426. https://doi.org/10.1101/gad.228080.113
9. Fawcett Don W, Neaves William B, Flores Martha N (1973) Comparative observations on intertubular lymphatics and the organization of the interstitial tissue of the mammalian testis. Biol Reprod 9:500–532

Reproductive Physiology of Cynomolgus Monkeys

3

Zhou Wen

Abstract

The cynomolgus monkey (*Macaca fascicularis*), a nonhuman primate closely related to humans that reproduces year-round, is an important laboratory animal whose reproductive physiology underpins breeding management, reproductive toxicology assessment, and research on human reproductive medicine. This chapter systematically describes the reproductive physiology of the cynomolgus monkey, including (1) external morphological characteristics such as fur color and cheek pouches, together with basic biological parameters; (2) sex determination, and species differences and seasonal variations in reproductive cycles; (3) endocrine regulation of reproduction by the hypothalamic–pituitary–ovarian–uterine axis, and the detection and application of major reproductive hormones; (4) cyclic changes in sexual skin in response to hormonal fluctuations; (5) oogenesis, follicular development, and ovulation, including morphological changes and hormonal markers; (6) semen collection and characteristics, sperm morphology, and motility analysis; and (7) the reproductive system, pregnancy diagnosis, and parturition management. By comparing reproductive parameters such as age at sexual maturity, ovarian cycle length, gestation period, and semen characteristics of cynomolgus monkeys with those of other nonhuman primates, including rhesus macaques, baboons, squirrel monkeys, and tamarins, this chapter summarizes key techniques for hormonal monitoring of the ovarian cycle, ovulation induction, semen collection and analysis, and pregnancy diagnosis by palpation and ultrasonography, and discusses the advantages and limitations of nonhuman primates as models for human reproductive research. This provides a

Z. Wen (✉)
Hubei Topgene Biotechnology Co., Ltd., Wuhan, China
e-mail: zhouwen@topgenebio.com

L. Zhou and Z. Sun (eds.), *Reproductive and Developmental Toxicology on Macaca Fascicularis*, https://doi.org/10.1007/978-981-92-3834-7_3

reference for laboratory management, breeding practice, and reproductive biology research on cynomolgus monkeys.

Keywords

Cynomolgus monkey · Reproductive physiology · Reproductive cycle · Endocrine regulation · Follicular development and ovulation · Semen analysis · Pregnancy diagnosis

This chapter primarily introduces the external characteristics of the cynomolgus monkey, normal reproductive physiology, sex determination, reproductive cycles, endocrine system, sexual skin, oogenesis, ovarian and follicular development, ovulation, semen, sperm morphology, capacitation, fertilization and implantation, placenta and embryo development, pregnancy diagnosis, and parturition.

3.1 External Characteristics of the Cynomolgus Monkey

The external characteristics of the cynomolgus monkey include fur coloration that varies from yellow, gray, to brown, ranging from gray-brown to reddish-brown. The fur on the abdomen and the inner sides of the limbs is light white, with a crown of hair that falls backward. The ears are upright, and the eyes are black. The nose is flat with very narrow nostrils. On both sides of the face, there are well-developed cheek pouches (Fig. 3.1–3.4).

3.2 Sex Determination and Reproductive Cycle

3.2.1 Sex Determination

In addition to certain inherent sexual characteristics specific to nonhuman primates, the sex of adult nonhuman primates can typically be determined by observing the external genitalia. Males have a prominent penis and a pendulous scrotum, which, in most species, is located behind the penis (Fig. 3.5). Females have a vulva, and the distance between the anus and the genitalia is shorter than in males (Fig. 3.6). However, in some species, age-related changes in the external genitalia may make it difficult for an inexperienced observer to accurately determine the sex of certain nonhuman primates [1].

To accurately distinguish the sex of nonhuman primates, the following points should be noted:

There is significant variation in the size of the labial folds and clitoris among female individuals across species, especially among New World monkeys. A typical example is the spider monkey, where the clitoris of adult females is more prominent and

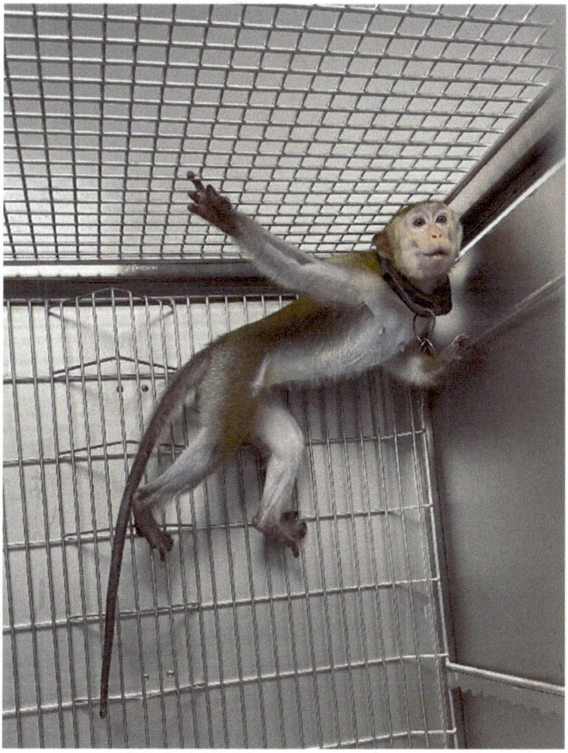

Fig. 3.1 Female cynomolgus monkey, 3.5 years old, appearance

pendulous than the penis of adult males. By examining the perineum for the presence of a scrotum, adult females with slender genitalia can be differentiated from males [2].

It is difficult to distinguish the sex of newborn or juvenile tamarins, macaques, and squirrel monkeys because the external genitalia of both sexes are similar in size, and females may have a pseudo-scrotum or genital pad. To correctly identify the sex of these juvenile animals, the external genitalia can be separated to reveal a rounded preputial opening (male) or a slit-like vaginal opening (female) [1].

In all nonhuman primates, the testes descend into the scrotum either before birth or shortly after birth. After the initial descent, there is considerable variation across species regarding whether the testes remain in the scrotum or retract back into the inguinal canal or abdomen before puberty. In many species, the testes return to the inguinal canal or abdominal cavity and do not descend into the scrotum again until puberty. This can make it more difficult to accurately determine the sex of juvenile nonhuman primates. The typical age at which the testes fully descend in common species is as follows: Tamarins: 8–11 months; Rhesus macaques: around 3 years of age; cynomolgus monkeys and baboons: around 4 years of age [2].

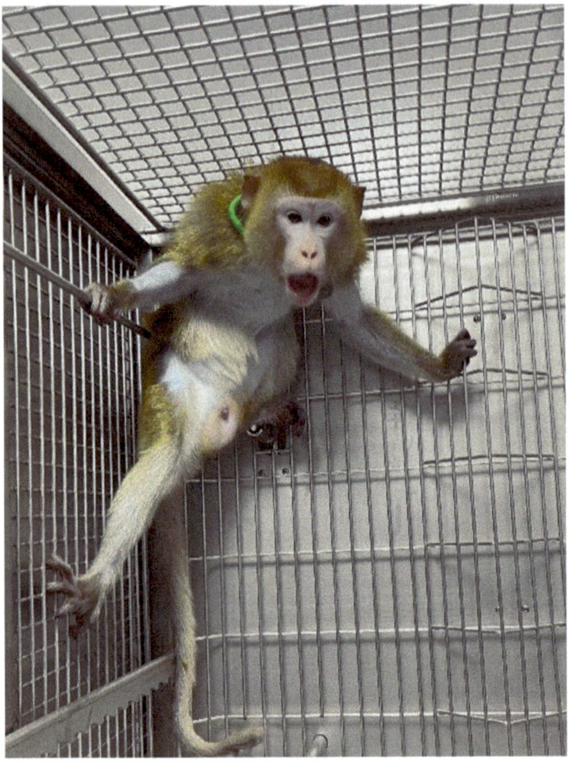

Fig. 3.2 Male cynomolgus monkey, 3.5 years old, appearance

3.2.2 Reproductive Cycle

The reproductive cycle and its seasonal variations in nonhuman primates vary by species. New World monkeys do not experience menstruation; thus, their reproductive cycle is referred to as the estrous cycle, the period from the beginning of one estrus phase to the beginning of the next [1]. The female reproductive cycle is typically measured from the time of sexual receptivity to the time just before ovulation. When predicting ovulation, female tamarins often do not exhibit noticeable changes in appearance, behavior, or vaginal cytology.

Tamarins are not considered seasonal breeders, as they mate and reproduce year-round under captive conditions. Additionally, tamarins experience postpartum estrus and have relatively short gestation periods, typically giving birth twice per year [2].

Female squirrel monkeys typically do not exhibit the typical behavioral changes associated with estrus, but ovulation can be determined through changes in vaginal cytology. Newly born offspring generally appear about 5 months after mating, with the mating season lasting approximately 3 months. In the Northern Hemisphere, the mating season typically occurs between December and March, with most offspring

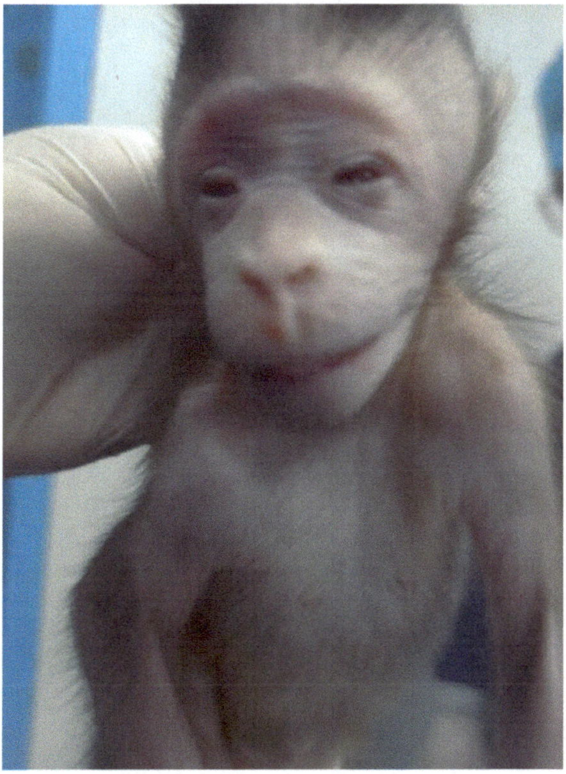

Fig. 3.3 Male cynomolgus monkey, 2 months old, appearance

being born between May and August. At the start of the breeding season, both male and female squirrel monkeys experience an increase in body weight (with males gaining up to 15%). Other physical changes in males at the onset of the breeding season include an increase in trunk width, enlargement of the testes, and increased spermatogenesis. These changes are referred to as the "fat male" condition and are associated with higher androgen levels. During the breeding season, some behavioral changes are observed, including reduced aggressive responses, increased sexual interactions, genital exposure or examination, and mating [2]. In contrast, during the nonbreeding season, sexual interactions between male and female squirrel monkeys are generally uncommon.

The external genitalia of female owl monkeys and specific changes in vaginal cytology are not observable, making it difficult to determine whether ovulation occurs. Owl monkeys mate throughout their estrous cycle and, under captive conditions, reproduce year-round. However, in the wild, these behaviors are typically seasonal [2].

Species in the Eastern Hemisphere (such as baboons and macaques) exhibit a true menstrual cycle, where the endometrial lining of the uterus undergoes periodic shedding. The menstrual cycle is measured from the first day of one menstruation to the first day of the next; the first day of the cycle is typically the first day of menstrual bleeding.

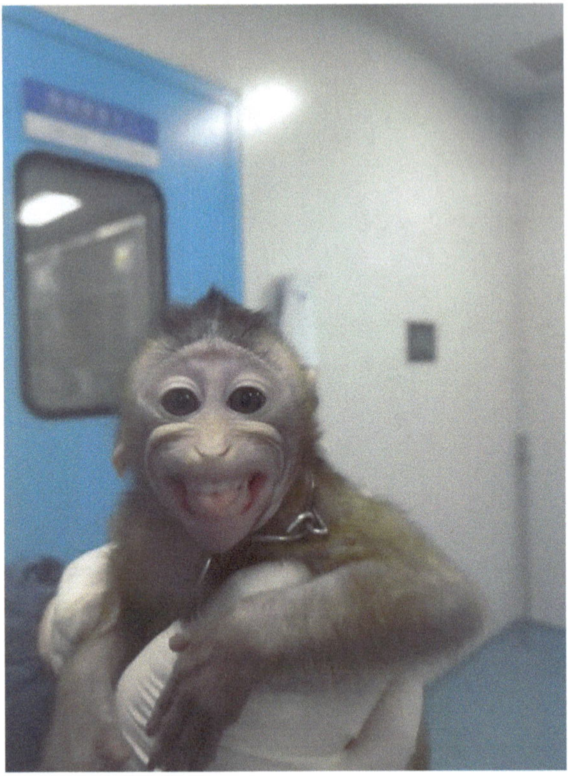

Fig. 3.4 Male cynomolgus monkey, 4 months old, appearance

The onset of menstruation can be determined by visually inspecting the external genitalia or through vaginal smears. The duration and frequency of menstruation can vary due to species differences and individual variation. For example, baboons have a distinct menstrual period, while Green monkeys have very little menstruation, which is usually only detectable through vaginal smears. The menstrual cycle typically lasts 4–5 weeks, with increased mating activity during ovulation and the mid-cycle phase [1].

The breeding seasons of macaques vary. Rhesus macaques are seasonal breeders with a distinct birthing season. Cynomolgus monkeys and baboons mate and reproduce year-round. Green monkeys exhibit seasonal breeding in the wild, but in captivity, they breed year-round. The breeding season for North American rhesus macaques typically occurs between October and February, with a peak in births from March to July. Although rhesus macaques do not ovulate during the nonbreeding season, they do continue to menstruate. Menstrual cycles outside of the breeding season tend to be more irregular compared to those during the breeding season [2].

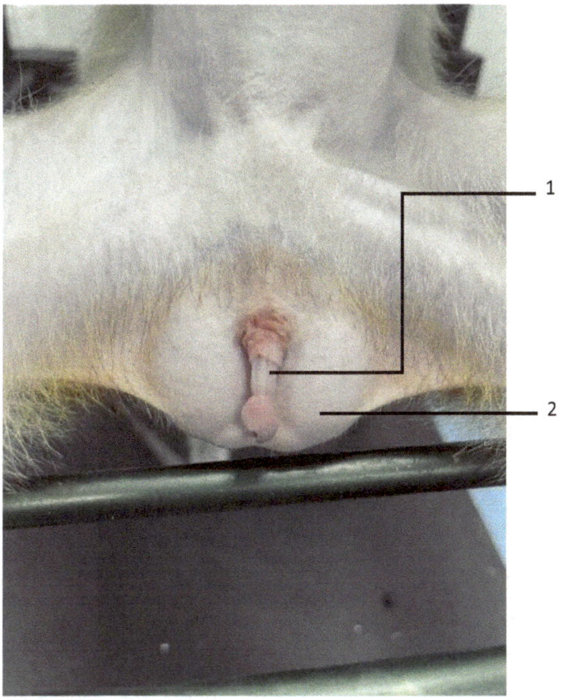

Fig. 3.5 Male cynomolgus monkey external genitalia. 1. Penis; 2. Scrotal gland

3.3 The Endocrine System and its Functional Regulation

Sociosexual behavior is related to the female's ovarian cycle. Hormones influence sexual desire, and male sexual demands on females are associated with ovulation. Dixson suggests that sexual function is a direct stimulus that enhances female sexual attractiveness. This attractiveness is based on hormonal changes, such as how sexual skin reflects fluctuations in estrogen and progesterone levels [3].

The term "hypothalamic-pituitary-ovarian-uterine axis" provides a good description of the regulatory mechanisms in female reproduction. External factors such as mating partners, stress, and light exposure can influence the secretion pattern of gonadotropin-releasing hormone (GnRH), which in turn stimulates the pituitary to secrete gonadotropins (Gn), such as follicle-stimulating hormone (FSH) and luteinizing hormone (LH). GnRH stimulates steroid production and other hormones in the ovaries, inducing follicular growth, ovulation, and LH formation. Typical hormones can be detected in bodily fluids and secretions to estimate the follicular phase and the ovulatory and luteal phases [3].

1. Major hormones: The main hormones related to the ovaries include estrogen (E), progesterone (P), relaxin (RLN), growth hormone (GH), prostaglandins (PG), and

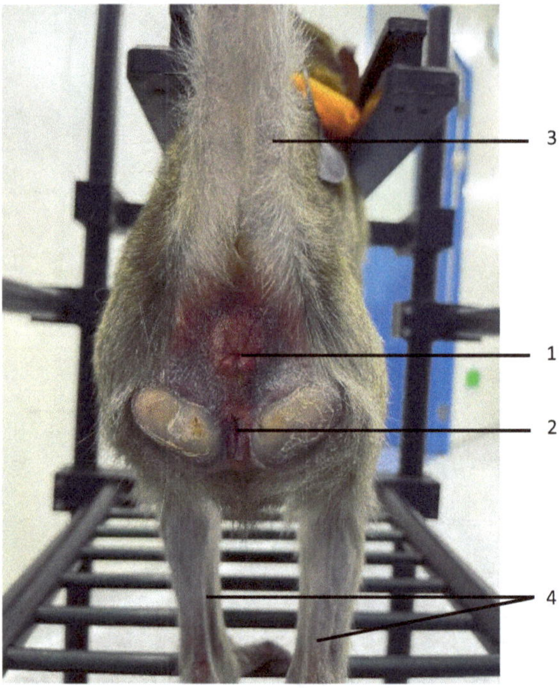

Fig. 3.6 Female cynomolgus monkey external genitalia. 1. Anal area; 2. Vulva; 3. Tail; 4. Hindlimbs

inhibin (INH). Estrogen is primarily secreted by the pre-ovulatory follicles during the follicular phase and reaches its highest plasma levels just before and after ovulation. These changes induce behavioral changes, as well as alterations in vaginal epithelial cells, perianal skin color, and skin swelling. Overall, all the changes induced by estrogen make the female more attractive to the male. However, when progesterone levels increase during the luteal phase, the female's receptivity decreases, indicating that progesterone has a negative impact on mating behavior. In New World species, sexual activity can be directly suppressed by administering progesterone. Estrogen stimulates LH secretion, and both hormones peak just before and after ovulation, then decline. Ovulation can be identified by measuring the increase in estradiol (E2) and LH in blood or urine prior to ovulation. This helps with the routine management, assisted reproduction, and pregnancy of nonhuman primates [3].

In humans and most catarrhines (named after their narrow nasal septum and downward-facing nostrils, previously classified as the suborder Anthropoidea or Apes), estrogen levels in urine or serum increase significantly prior to ovulation. However, due to the time lag in metabolic pathways, it is difficult to determine the exact timing of ovulation using urine samples alone. In contrast, there is no clear estrogen pattern in the blood tests or skin swelling in tamarins, nor are there noticeable changes in vaginal cytology. A sensitive parameter for predicting ovulation is the estrogen metabolites in urine (such as estrone-3-sulfate, which can be used to determine the cycle stage) [3]. Estrogen can also be measured directly, but it is necessary to analyze changes in creatinine alongside it to account for the effects of urine concentration and volume.

2. Hormone testing: Hormonal analysis of urine or feces can provide noninvasive monitoring of the ovarian cycles in captive and wild nonhuman primates during both pregnancy and nonpregnancy. To better interpret the results, information on urinary metabolites, metabolic pathways, and the temporal relationships among changes is needed [6].

Noninvasive monitoring of the ovarian cycle during both pregnancy and nonpregnancy can be achieved by detecting immunologically active E1C, 17β-estradiol, and pregnanediol in blood. Hormonal testing in blood requires the use of a blood collection device to puncture the animal's body and collect blood samples, which are then analyzed to detect hormone levels [3]. In general, hormonal analysis is primarily used for cycle monitoring; except for pregnancy markers such as chorionic gonadotropin (CG) or relaxin, individual hormone results alone are not sufficient to provide adequate data for cycle monitoring.

After ovulation, a new corpus luteum forms, and this corpus luteum produces the main hormone of the luteal phase, progesterone. Therefore, progesterone is a good indicator for monitoring ovulation and luteinization. The presence of human chorionic gonadotropin (CG) or relaxin can confirm the luteal phase and early pregnancy. Relaxin is produced by the uterus and placenta, and during implantation and early pregnancy, both relaxin and CG levels increase significantly, making them important early pregnancy markers. Both hormones can be detected in serum samples from tamarins and proboscis monkeys, and the result of either hormone can provide information about the pregnancy status of individual primates. Relaxin levels differ between normal pregnancy and pregnancy loss; in pregnancy loss, the decline in relaxin levels occurs later than in normal pregnancy. Therefore, relaxin is one of the indicators used to monitor placental status and fetal health. Typically, serum relaxin concentration provides both pathological and physiological information about the pregnancy [3].

3. Hormones and social status: The social status of nonhuman primates is closely related to changes in hormone levels. In nonhuman primates, a reduction in LH secretion is typically due to a lack of pulsatile LH release, which is suppressed by the endogenous secretion of GnRH from the hypothalamus, thereby inhibiting the pituitary's response to GnRH. For example, removing individuals from a nonhuman primate group can lead to a rapid increase in plasma LH levels in females, resulting in ovulation. Typically, proboscis monkey (New World monkeys, named because they were discovered in the Americas) can exhibit both physiological and behavioral disturbances, leading to the maximal social control over female reproductive capability. In a study of tamarins, females in the group ovulated, but because one female held a dominant social position, no other females became pregnant. This form of social suppression is also commonly observed in baboons [3].

In female primates with subordinate social status, elevated plasma prolactin or cortisol levels are also associated with suppressed reproductive function. However, certain reproductive conditions in females are related to cortisol responses. For example, exogenous estrogen administration increases cortisol levels in humans, and elevated cortisol during the ovulatory phase can predict ovulation in both humans and tamarins.

4. Fetal endocrinology: Research has shown that by day 100 of gestation, the hypothalamic-pituitary-gonadal (HPG) axis begins to function in male rhesus monkey fetuses. Studies on fetal gonadectomy have shown that in developing male rhesus monkey fetuses, testosterone (T) or its metabolite, dihydrotestosterone (DHT), can feed back to regulate luteinizing hormone (LH) secretion. The duration of this feedback regulation has also been documented. For instance, on day 60 of gestation, the plasma testosterone levels in the fetal umbilical artery of male rhesus monkeys averaged 2100 pg/mL; by day 100, this decreased to 1000 pg/mL, and then increased to approximately 1500 pg/mL by day 160 of gestation. Testicular tissue collected from male rhesus monkeys at gestational days 45 and 60 was capable of converting 14C pregnenolone into testosterone and androstenedione. Plasma levels of testosterone and androstenedione in male rhesus monkey fetuses decreased from 66 ng/100 mL to 43 ng/100 mL between days 100 and 120 of gestation, and reached 140 ng/100 mL by day 150. Androgen secretion by the fetal testis before birth plays a crucial role in the development of the epididymal duct. At day 130 of gestation, the epididymal epithelium was almost undifferentiated. However, the secretion of androgens at this stage induced cell differentiation, leading to the formation of structures similar to those found in the adult cells, including static ciliated cells in the body and tail of the epididymis. Following birth, as androgen levels decline, the epithelial cells regress to an undifferentiated state, which persists until puberty, when androgen levels increase again [3].

5. Endocrinology of neonatal and juvenile monkeys: The androgen levels in newborn rhesus monkeys decline sharply after birth and continue to decrease until puberty. Reports have shown that the FSH levels in juvenile rhesus monkeys are 2.4 ng/mL $\pm$ 0.8 ng/mL, in pubertal males are 6.4 ng/mL $\pm$ 1.8 ng/mL, and in adult males are 16.1 ng/mL $\pm$ 1.8 ng/mL. LH in male rhesus monkeys was undetectable before puberty but increased to 16.2 ng/mL $\pm$ 3.1 ng/mL during puberty. In juvenile Green monkeys (*Cercopithecus aethiops*), GnRH secretion is correlated with LH secretion, but this response is age-dependent, with sustained testosterone secretion until the onset of sperm maturation. Plasma inhibin and androgen-binding protein (a protein secreted by Sertoli cells) in male cynomolgus monkey aged 1.5–2.5 years are significantly lower than those in adult males. Inhibin B is detectable in rhesus monkeys at 1 week of age, and its levels increase with rising plasma FSH in neonates, then gradually decline, though it remains detectable until 1 year of age. In adult males, the levels are higher than any values observed before 1 year of age [3].

3.4 Sexual Skin

Many nonhuman primates from Asia, Africa, and Europe show sexual skin, which is typically associated with the perineal region. The skin in this area undergoes changes in response to hormonal fluctuations. Variations in sex hormone levels across the menstrual cycle among species may lead to noticeable differences in the color and responsiveness of the sexual skin. The following describes some of these interspecies differences.

The sexual skin of female cynomolgus monkeys is located at the base of the tail. This tissue exhibits slight swelling during the mid-phase of the menstrual cycle, which is near the time of ovulation [1].

The sexual skin of female rhesus monkeys undergoes a series of changes during puberty. Sexual skin typically involves the perineal region and the distal tail end of the hind limbs, but it may also appear at the tail end of the abdomen and on the forehead of the animal. The outer sides of the tail end on the hind limbs may show folds in the sexual skin. As the animal enters puberty, the skin in the perineal area and hind limbs becomes swollen. When the swelling subsides, the skin in these areas turns red. In adult animals, the color of this skin changes with the hormonal fluctuations of the menstrual cycle, being most pale during menstruation. In some animals, the sexual skin becomes slightly swollen near the time of ovulation [1].

Baboon and chimpanzee sexual skin undergoes very distinct changes. In these species, the size of the sexual skin shows significant cyclic variation associated with different phases of the menstrual cycle. Near the onset of menstruation, the perineal area is flat, whereas near ovulation, the skin becomes highly swollen. At the peak of swelling, just before ovulation, the skin in the perineal area appears smooth, shiny, and deep red (Fig. 3.7). The cyclical changes in sexual skin can be used to estimate the timing of ovulation in these species [1].

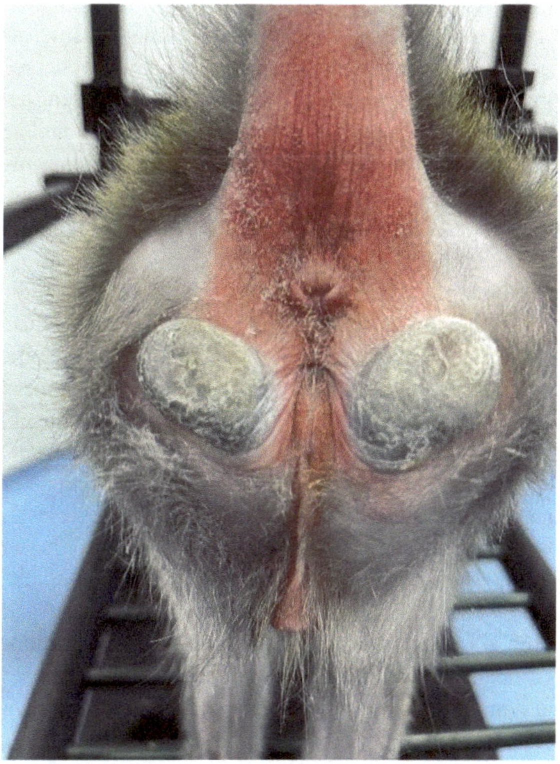

Fig. 3.7 Perineal skin of a cynomolgus monkey near menstruation

The sexual skin of female cynomolgus monkeys is red and located at the base of the tail. This area exhibits mild to pronounced swelling.

Green monkeys (*Cercopithecus aethiops*) lack sexual skin and do not show cyclic swelling of sexual skin associated with the menstrual cycle [1].

3.5 Oogenesis, Follicular Development, and Ovulation

Walter Heape (1855–1929), of the University of Cambridge, is regarded as the father of modern reproductive biology. His major work involved demonstrating the production of oocytes and embryos in rabbit models, and he even employed embryo transplantation to produce viable offspring. During his travels to India, Heape became interested in studying rhesus monkeys and brought five of them back to his home in the United Kingdom. He then studied their menstrual cycles and compared rhesus monkeys' reproductive information with that of humans, publishing the first scientific report in this field.

Subsequently, in 1933, Hartman's research demonstrated that ovulation in rhesus monkeys occurs on the 13th day of a 28-day menstrual cycle. Later, in his 1945 study, he found that the optimal time for mating was on the 11th or 12th day. The concept of capacitation time, proposed by Hartman based on these studies, was not widely recognized until 1951 [3].

Until around 1960, many researchers conducted numerous studies on rhesus monkeys. Although issues such as pronounced seasonal ovulation were present, a wealth of background information had accumulated on the species, providing a solid foundation for using rhesus monkeys as models for human fertilization and early embryonic development. In the late 1970s, India banned the export of rhesus monkeys, leading researchers to turn to other nonhuman primates as models for human studies. Today, Cynomolgus monkeys and long-tailed macaques have gradually replaced rhesus monkeys in most research.

Although the number of nonhuman primates used in various studies has declined, a large number of nonhuman primates are still used in experiments, including species from Asia, Africa, and Europe (such as rhesus monkeys, cynomolgus monkeys, long-tailed macaques, baboons, and green monkeys), as well as apes (chimpanzees), prosimians (lemurs and tarsiers), and New World species (squirrel monkeys, marmosets, and capuchins). Currently, many endangered species are no longer used as animal models in human research. Over the years, the breeding and reproduction of nonhuman primates, particularly those with regular mating cycles, have provided a wealth of information on their estrous and menstrual cycles for human studies.

In 1981, diZerega and Hodgson, and in 1982, Hodgson et al., defined the endocrine processes involved in the selection of the dominant follicle and its subsequent ovulation. Research in macaques confirmed that follicular development occurs prior to ovulation. Significant advancements in laparoscopy techniques in the 1960s made nonhuman primate models highly valuable for studying human developmental processes [3].

3.5.1 Oocyte and Follicular Morphology

As ovulation approaches, the dominant follicle protrudes from the ovarian surface, and blood vessels increase. The follicular structure consists primarily of a fluid-filled cavity, with granular cells arranged within the cavity. These cells eventually transform into luteal cells after ovulation. At the base of the follicle is a small cluster of granulosa cells known as the cumulus oophorus, which extends from the follicular wall, surrounding the oocyte. The basic composition of the oocyte is: ① a loosely packed layer of large granulosa cells; ② a layer of small granulosa cells tightly adjacent to the oocyte; ③ a glycoprotein layer directly surrounding the oocyte, known as the zona pellucida. The structure is illustrated in Fig. 3.8. During ovulation, the oocyte is expelled from the follicle, and the cumulus oophorus cells facilitate capacitation of the oocyte through the wave-like movements of cilia at the fimbrial end of the fallopian tube. The endocrine system controls these processes, including follicular development, oocyte capacitation, ciliary growth affecting oocyte transport, and the muscle activity of the female reproductive tract [3].

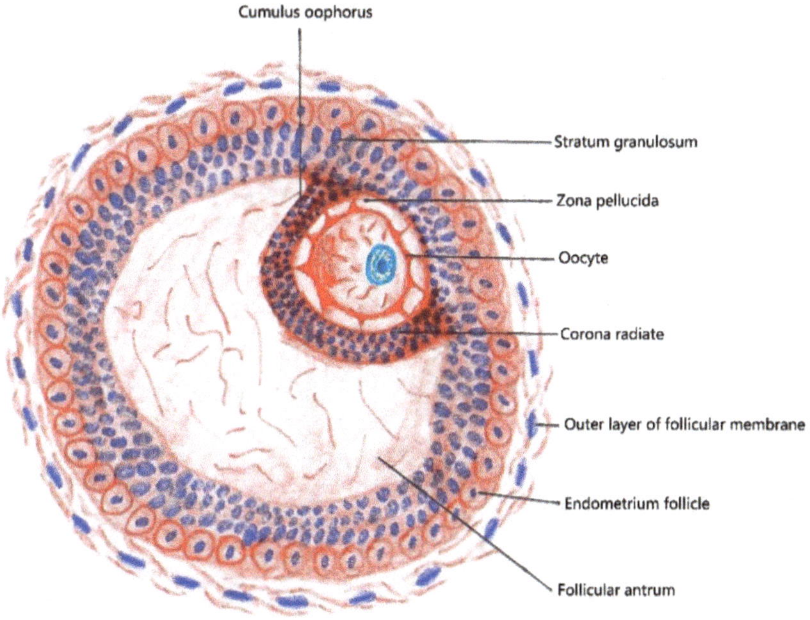

Fig. 3.8 Structure of the primate follicle

3.5.2 Activity of the Ovarian Epithelium Before Ovulation

The use of laparoscopy allows for precise observation of changes on the surface of the follicle. Studies in cynomolgus monkeys and squirrel monkeys have shown that morphological changes in the follicle occur within 24–36 h prior to ovulation. These changes occur within a fixed time window, making it more reasonable and accurate to predict natural ovulation timing. Weick et al. studied the endocrine changes associated with ovulation in macaques, finding that LH secretion forms a continuous, symmetrical peak, with maximum plasma concentrations ranging from 42 to 81 ng/mL. FSH exhibits a similar secretion pattern, with peak levels ranging from 67 to 230 ng/mL, occurring either simultaneously with the LH peak or 3 h after. The average duration of these fluctuating secretions is about 50 h [3]. Estradiol levels peak 9–15 h before the LH peak. As estradiol concentrations rise, plasma LH levels also increase significantly. Plasma progesterone and testosterone concentrations are very low (below 0.1 ng/mL) until at least 15 h after the LH surge, or 6–9 h after the peak in estradiol. A small progesterone peak occurs within 6 h after the LH peak, followed by a continuous decline over the next 18 h, before increasing sharply (in relation to luteal secretion). The hormonal cycle changes are shown in Fig. 3.9. The earliest time for ovulation generally occurs about 28 h after the LH peak [3].

When selecting an appropriate animal model for research, it is essential to consider the differences in reproductive information across species. Given the menstrual

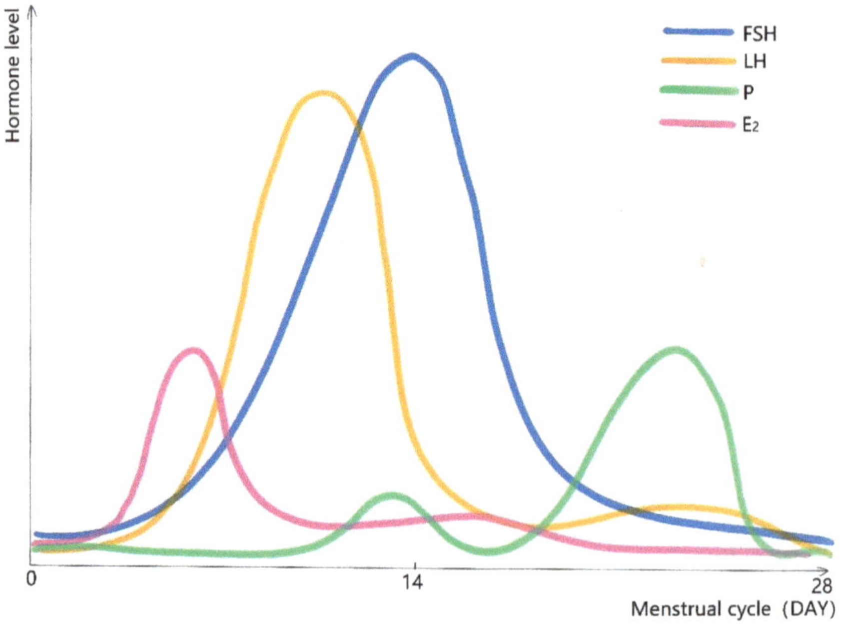

Fig. 3.9 Hormonal fluctuations during the menstrual cycle in macaques

cycle and evolutionary relationship to humans, an increasing number of nonhuman primates are being used as models for human studies. These theoretical foundations are valuable in many research fields, though there are some exceptions [3]. For example, compared to humans, nonhuman primates typically have a more superficial implantation site. To identify a more suitable model, researchers may also use guinea pigs to study implantation. Not all nonhuman primates have menstrual cycles (many New World primates do not), and some species exhibit abnormally active luteal phases. Although many nonhuman primates have menstrual cycles similar in duration and characteristics to those of humans, the vast majority have shorter gestation periods, and many exhibit seasonal reproductive responses that do not occur in humans. When conducting such studies, it is important to fully understand these differences, not only between nonhuman primates and humans but also among different nonhuman primate species. Typically, the rhesus macaque is the most commonly used nonhuman primate model in human reproductive research. However, this species experiences a period of anovulation during the summer, sometimes referred to as "summer infertility," which makes it less suitable for ovulation studies [3]. In contrast, macaques such as cynomolgus monkeys, rhesus monkeys, and long-tailed macaques ovulate and become pregnant year-round, making them more suitable for research on ovulation.

Two days before ovulation, the ovarian surface reveals the sites of follicular development, and the entire area becomes swollen and darkened, with ovarian volume increasing by approximately 35%. Within 30 h before ovulation, star-shaped blood vessels appear on the surface of the follicle. By 8–10 h before ovulation, these vessels become more prominent, and the follicle forms a cone-shaped or stigma appearance. At this point, the fimbrial membrane of the fallopian tube moves to enclose the developing follicle, preparing for ovulation from the ovarian surface. Two to 3 h before ovulation, the base of the follicle lightens in color, which may indicate the secretion of LH and progesterone before ovulation [3]. Observations of 78 actual ovulations in cynomolgus monkeys showed that the ovulation time could be determined within 24 h for 19 of these events.

A similar vascular pattern has also been observed in squirrel monkeys, but with a notable difference: prior to ovulation, there is more widespread hemorrhaging at the base of the follicle. As a result, the scattered vascular pattern is harder to observe. In owl monkeys (infant monkeys), the follicle forms a very prominent protrusion on the ovarian surface, with follicular blood vessels visible at the base of the follicle, occasionally extending near the apex of the follicle. Unlike cynomolgus monkeys, squirrel monkeys, and owl monkeys do not exhibit a clear transparent area (stigma). In Japanese macaques, baboons, and chimpanzees, a generally similar follicular development pattern is observed. In capuchins, star-shaped blood vessels are distinctly visible around 24 h before ovulation, while the concentrations of estradiol peak and progesterone also slightly increase at the same time.

According to research reports, 10 h before ovulation, as estradiol decreases and progesterone increases, the follicle takes on a conical shape, and the follicular wall hemorrhages. A characteristic of ovulation is that the fimbriae of the fallopian tube closely adhere to the surface of the follicle, maintaining this attachment for at least 2 h.

The follicular diameter before ovulation in nonhuman primates varies with body size. In humans, the follicle diameter is approximately 10 mm. Other nonhuman primates have the following follicle diameters: gorillas, 7 mm; rhesus macaques, 6.3–6.6 mm; baboons, 6 mm; gibbons, 5–6 mm; and New World monkeys, 5–6 mm. Across these species, the number of granulosa cells is similar, and the difference in follicle size is primarily due to fluid secretion into the antrum. The inner layer of the follicular membrane typically consists of two to four cell layers. The overall size of the ovaries is generally proportional to body size. An exception is the proboscis monkey, which exhibits unusual follicular development characterized by the invagination or folding of the follicular wall into the follicular antrum [3].

Exogenous steroid administration is commonly used to stimulate and mimic the normal reproductive cycle. In most macaque species, exogenous estradiol leads to an increase in LH levels, and serum progesterone levels rise a few hours after the LH surge begins, as well as just before LH peaks. In most macaques, FSH shows a secondary peak 2–3 days after the LH peak. The significance of the second FSH surge remains unclear, but it may enhance the synthesis of progesterone and estrogen after ovulation [3].

3.5.3 Ovulation

Over the years, various methods have been used to induce ovulation. Steroid drugs are often used to alter the menstrual cycle, typically involving gonadotropins (LH and FSH) or related compounds such as Pregnant Mare Serum (PMS), human menopausal gonadotropin (hMG), human chorionic gonadotropin (hCG), and various release factors or synthetic compounds to induce oocyte/follicle maturation and ovulation. In studies with cynomolgus monkeys, administration of 0.5 mg/day of progesterone can block ovulation and prevent the LH peak [3]. This principle is the foundation of synchronizing the reproductive cycles of certain laboratory or captive species, which has been crucial in the development of "human contraceptive pills." When progesterone administration is stopped, and estradiol is injected, the animals' LH levels and ovulation rates increase significantly.

Several nonhuman primate species exhibit seasonal variations in their response to ovulation induction therapy. For example, the rhesus macaque shows a clear seasonal influence on ovulation, which needs to be taken into account in breeding programs or studies of basic reproductive phenomena. The seasonal response is even more pronounced in squirrel monkeys. When animals receive an ovulation regimen of 5 mg progesterone for 5 consecutive days, followed by 1 mg FSH and one injection of hCG for 4 consecutive days, seasonal reactions naturally occur. However, in the Northern Hemisphere, this method is ineffective in July, August, and September. Overcoming this seasonal response requires a variety of techniques and a more gradual approach to better mimic the natural cycle. Prior treatment with estradiol and progesterone before FSH/hCG therapy can increase ovulation rates. Alternatively, simply increasing the

FSH dose from 1 to 2 mg/day or extending the duration from 4 to 5 days can result in higher ovulation rates [3].

Researchers have extracted gonadotropins from various captive animals and used them in nonhuman primates to induce ovulation, achieving varying degrees of success. Ovulation induced by LH has species-specific requirements, while FSH from different sources can be used to stimulate follicular growth in nonhuman primates. Therefore, many hormones used in nonhuman primates are either derived from primates or synthesized using modern techniques. For primates, the most commonly used hormone is FSH, which is sourced from hMG or pituitary compounds from either humans or nonhuman primates. hCG is most commonly used to induce ovulation. Additionally, clomiphene citrate, a nonsteroidal estrogen compound that increases endogenous FSH release, is used in both humans and nonhuman primates, though its application makes it difficult to control the exact timing of ovulation. In cynomolgus monkeys, a "staircase" method can be used to increase hMG levels, with close monitoring of urinary estrogen levels. Once estrogen secretion reaches normal pre-ovulatory levels (around 7 mg) and has been sustained for 24 h, hMG treatment can be stopped to allow estrogen levels to decline. A single injection of 500 IU of hCG is then administered to induce ovulation. The required dose of hMG to induce follicular development varies among animals. In baboons, the hMG-hCG regimen typically induces a single ovulation, although some studies have reported that increasing hCG levels can lead to multiple ovulations [3].

Overuse of gonadotropins and related drugs can lead to antibody responses, reducing the effectiveness of the drug or, in some cases, making it ineffective in subsequent treatments. This is most evident with the use of pregnant mare serum (PMS). This compound can induce "superovulation" (the production of more than the normal number of eggs/embryos) in many animal species, but it is only effective after a limited number of treatments. It should not be used unless the animal is expected to be euthanized after a single trial. For other compounds, preliminary experiments are recommended to determine the minimal effective dose (MED) required to promote follicular growth and ovulation. For example, in squirrel monkeys, the FSH dose used is approximately 1 mg per day, administered continuously for 4 days. For hCG in squirrel monkeys, the minimal effective dose (MED) ranges from 100 to 250 IU. In sheep, the clinical dose typically used is 1500–2000 IU, with the MED around 100 IU. Interestingly, in human in vitro fertilization (IVF) procedures, hCG doses of 5000–10,000 IU are commonly administered, which is approximately seven times the amount required to induce ovulation in cattle. When rabbits are given excessive hCG to induce ovulation, there is a 9.7% chance that blastocysts on day 6 will show chromosomal defects. Studies have shown that the overuse of gonadotropins can be harmful [3]. Luteinizing hormone-releasing hormone (LHRH) or GnRH, used in many nonhuman primates and humans, triggers an LH response. In female fetuses, infants, and prepubertal animals, exposure to LHRH can stimulate LH release. In chimpanzees, LHRH antagonists can block the release of gonadotropins, just as they do in humans [3].

3.6 Semen Characteristics, Sperm Morphology, and Motility

In general, the male reproductive system of nonhuman primates (NHP) is similar to that of humans both macroscopically and histologically. For example, the gonadal somatic index (the ratio of gonad weight to body weight) in green monkeys is 0.36, which is similar to other nonhuman primates [3]. The average weight of human testes is approximately 16 or 32 g. The gonadal index in a 70 kg male human is only 0.04, which is about ten times lower than that in NHPs. The external morphology and histology of the seminiferous tubules have been studied in several NHP species and are considered to be highly similar to those in humans. Spermatogenesis in the human spermatogenic epithelium is spiral. In New World and Eurasian Old World primates, spermatogenesis exhibits a similar spiral wave pattern, but there are slight variations among NHP species. Weinbauer suggests that the common marmoset, because its testicular tissue is similar to that of humans, may serve as a new animal model for experimental studies of human spermatogenesis. This suggests that New World primates could be relevant models for human studies [3].

The process of sperm maturation in the epididymis is essentially the same in both NHPs and humans. Histological data on the development of sperm movement along the epididymis show that sperm motility and maturation are similar in both NHPs and humans. Additionally, the motility of the sperm head is negligible, with no forward movement. In contrast, the sperm tail exhibits high motility, and this motility continues to improve as the sperm passes through the epididymal tail.

In summary, from both a gross anatomical and histological perspective, the male reproductive system of NHPs is very similar to that of humans. The primary difference is that, compared to humans, NHPs (such as rhesus monkeys) produce sperm in larger quantities and more efficiently on a daily basis.

1. Semen collection and semen characteristics: The definition of semen quality and fertility, as well as a thorough understanding of the status of semen samples, plays a crucial role in related research. Semen analysis in NHPs should be conducted using standards similar to those for human semen analysis, preferably employing internationally recognized methods. The resulting data can then be analyzed alongside fertility status. In this regard, the best approach to determining the fertility status of a specific NHP is to observe its mating with several different females within a population (which has been shown to successfully produce offspring). The semen parameters can then be compared with those of humans to establish a relevant model [3].

In most cases, humans obtain semen manually, but in certain special circumstances, such as spinal cord injuries, semen can be obtained through rectal probe electrostimulation or penile vibratory stimulation. Rectal probe electrostimulation and penile vibratory stimulation are the two main methods for obtaining ejaculation. While penile vibratory stimulation is a more humane method for collecting semen from NHPs and may produce higher-quality semen, the success of these methods typically depends on the operator. Generally, under ketamine anesthesia, rectal probe electrostimulation is used to obtain high-quality semen samples from macaques [3].

The semen of NHPs generally consists of two main components: the liquid portion and the coagulum. The liquefaction process of the coagulum is very slow, and it will not completely liquefy in vitro. Trypsin can be used to fully liquefy the coagulum components for accurate sperm concentration measurements. Additionally, adding 1% streptomycin to Eagle's medium can successfully liquefy the coagulum in the semen of cynomolgus monkeys. This method does not generally affect the sperm within the body, in contrast to sperm found in the vaginal canal after natural mating [3].

Although the viscosity of semen in humans and NHPs differs, there are many similarities. Harrison studied the semen parameters in cynomolgus monkeys and rhesus monkeys, while Kraemer, Vera Cruz, Bornman, and others conducted similar studies in baboons. In studies of chacma baboons, only minor modifications to the procedure are needed to apply human sperm imaging techniques to evaluate semen quality. Valerio and Dalgard were the first to report on the semen characteristics of green monkeys. Seier et al. conducted an in-depth study of the semen characteristics from 91 ejaculations of 47 green monkeys using electrostimulation, and established a sperm profile for ten sexually mature males (proven "fathers") and for green monkeys with unknown fertility status. Hiyaoka and Cho developed a method for inducing ejaculation in green monkeys through manual manipulation of the penis, with semen volume, sperm density, and motile sperm percentage all falling within the range of various parameters measured by Seier et al. using rectal probe electrostimulation [3].

2. Sperm motility analysis: The most common sperm abnormality in humans is teratospermia, specifically irregular head morphology. In contrast, sperm head abnormalities are rarely observed in most NHP species, whereas midpiece abnormalities are more common. Additionally, the average sperm motility percentage in various NHP species and humans falls within a very narrow range.

Significant progress has been made in sperm motility quantification in most mammals, especially in humans. Studies have reported that computer-assisted sperm analysis (CASA) has been applied to the semen analysis of nonhuman primates (NHPs). Some studies still rely on subjective evaluation of sperm motility, which may lead to significant inter-laboratory variability. Establishing standards for normal sperm directional motility in NHPs is particularly important, as it not only provides accurate baseline data for sperm motility in specific species but also, when combined with the physical and biochemical parameters of semen, helps to establish cutoff points for fertility assessments. This is especially important in the contexts of sperm capacitation, male fertility assessment, contraception, and reproductive toxicology research.

Sperm motility parameters of ejaculated sperm as measured in seminal plasma and the culture medium, Ham's F10,after about 10 minutes immersion at 36°C. When sperm are incubated in the medium for a short period, their swimming velocity increases. In humans, linear movement decreases, while the amplitude of the sperm head oscillation increases. In normal, fertile semen samples, more than 20% of human sperm become highly active (with very fast swimming speed) within 1–3 h of incubation. Hyperactivation is an important parameter, indicating that sperm capacitation is occurring. If sperm are not capacitated, they cannot undergo the acrosome reaction, which is a prerequisite for fertilization. Hyperactivation has already been observed in macaque sperm. It has been demonstrated that sperm from green monkeys undergo hyperactivation in capacitation media, such as human tubal fluid. This finding has been applied in both in vitro studies and human clinical research, including in vitro fertilization (IVF), gamete intrafallopian transfer (GIFT), and intrauterine insemination (IUI).

Tests for sperm motility, function, and fertilizing ability, such as the hypo-osmotic swelling test (HOS), cervical mucus penetration test, acrosome reaction, and sperm zona binding test, are important adjuncts in human semen analysis. However, these methods are rarely applied in nonhuman primates (NHPs). Nevertheless, Lohiya et al. [4] successfully performed the HOS test in a study on fertility in langur monkey sperm. Mdhluli et al. [8] further demonstrated the four classifications of peanut agglutinin (PNA) labeling, which depict various stages of the human acrosome reaction, with similar classifications found in owl monkeys. Hewitson and Schatten, using rhesus macaque pairs, showed that the cellular structures involved in fertilization during in vitro fertilization (IVF) and intracytoplasmic sperm injection (ICSI) in rhesus macaques closely resemble those in humans. Indeed, NHP models may be useful for determining experimental safety, improving current reproductive strategies, and developing new techniques. Additionally, Sutovsky et al. suggested that the similarities between rhesus macaque and human fertilization provide a systematic model for studying the cellular and molecular biology of human reproduction.

The results from NHP models indicate that great caution is needed when conducting clinical research, such as ICSI. Studies have shown that rhesus macaque sperm can bind to exogenous DNA and retain their full reproductive capacity during ICSI. However, there are concerns that ICSI could theoretically transmit infectious agents [5]. Additionally, embryos fertilized via ICSI in rhesus macaques may exhibit abnormalities in nuclear reprogramming, leading to asynchronous chromatin decondensation in sperm and delays in DNA synthesis. This has raised concerns that the ICSI procedure might cause chromatin damage during DNA decondensation. It is suggested that, before the global adoption of ICSI and other assisted reproductive techniques, there is a need for well-designed, optimized nonclinical evaluations [6].

3.7 Reproductive System, Pregnancy, and Parturition

1. Reproductive system: Multiple reproductive systems are used for breeding nonhuman primates (NHPs) for biomedical research. The reproductive system employed depends on factors such as species, facilities, space limitations, labor constraints, production requirements, and the specific needs of the research project.

The mating system of captive tamarins is typically either a single female and a single male, or a small group with one reproductive female, her mate, and their offspring. In other words, family members, including the male and older offspring, participate in caring for the young. This system is also known as cooperative breeding or cooperative care [2].

The owl monkey follows a monogamous mating system, with one female and one male forming a pair. This pair forms a small group consisting of an adult reproductive monkey and up to three infants or juveniles. In breeding, the adult male owl monkey primarily takes care of the infants, while the female's role is mainly limited to nursing.

Due to their territorial nature, it is necessary to physically separate paired tamarins or owl monkeys from other breeding pairs to prevent conflicts [2].

Squirrel monkeys are highly adaptable to various living environments. For reproductive purposes, squirrel monkeys can form small or large groups, typically consisting of 12–16 females and one to two males [1].

Species such as the American cynomolgus monkey, rhesus macaque, and baboons breed successfully in free-range environments (such as enclosures and islands) as well as in large outdoor cages or captive enclosures with multi-male/multi-female groups. The best breeding results for a single male and multiple females are typically achieved in smaller indoor or outdoor enclosures. Initially, pairing is done with a male-to-female ratio of 1: (10–12), and this ratio can be adjusted based on species needs, as well as the size and configuration of the enclosure. For African green monkeys, breeding is more successful when one male is paired with two to six females [2].

To support specific research projects, some species of American primates are kept separately after mating and co-housed only for a few days during the female's ovulation period. With the development of ultrasound-based methods for predicting fetal development, mating in nonhuman primates has gradually become less reliant on timing to specific periods.

The method for determining the optimal mating time (ovulation period) for rhesus macaques and cynomolgus monkeys is to calculate the average length of the last three menstrual cycles, then divide by 2 and subtract 3. Mating is then initiated on the calculated date, with the male and female co-housed for 2–3 days. It is important to note that during the nonbreeding season, the menstrual cycle of rhesus macaques can be irregular.

For baboons, the optimal mating time is calculated based on the last three menstrual cycles, with the average number of days for the sexual swelling to subside subtracted by 3. Since baboons typically ovulate 1–2 days before the sexual swelling subsides, mating is initiated on the calculated date, with the male and female co-housed for 3–4 days.

2. Pregnancy diagnosis: In a laboratory setting, the most commonly used methods for pregnancy diagnosis are palpation and ultrasound examination. Palpation techniques have been widely applied to determine pregnancy in various species. Experienced researchers can detect pregnancy in tamarins, owl monkeys, and squirrel monkeys by palpating the 4–5 mm area of the uterus on the ventral side of the tail and abdomen during the 4th or 5th week of gestation. Additionally, artificial palpation techniques are commonly used to estimate fetal age and expected delivery date in these species [7].

In American species, abdominal palpation can be used during the mid- to late stages of pregnancy to determine pregnancy. However, during the early stages of pregnancy, it is recommended to use bimanual rectal palpation to confirm pregnancy. Experienced researchers can determine pregnancy as early as day 16 of gestation in rhesus macaques and baboons [2].

In recent years, ultrasound diagnostics have become an important tool for promoting the reproduction of nonhuman primates. Ultrasound examinations can be used as early as day 14 and day 18 of gestation to determine pregnancy in rhesus macaques, cynomolgus monkeys, and baboons. Embryonic heartbeat can be first detected in rhesus macaques and cynomolgus monkeys between days 21 and 25 of gestation, and in olive baboons on day 27 [2]. Ultrasound can confirm pregnancy as early as day 25 of gestation in squirrel monkeys and day 30 in tamarins. Moreover, by day 39 of pregnancy, fetal heartbeats are easy to detect in both squirrel monkeys and tamarins [2]. Therefore, the use of ultrasound diagnostics extends far beyond pregnancy detection. Diagnostic ultrasound can also be used to assess fetal viability, estimate fetal age, evaluate fetal development, determine placental location, diagnose reproductive diseases such as endometriosis, and support various research projects [2].

3. Parturition: Nonhuman primates exhibit very similar parturition behaviors. Reports indicate that species from Asia, Africa, and Europe show behavioral changes prior to giving birth, including restlessness, changes in eating and sleeping habits, frequent urination, and genital touching. Typically, nonhuman primates give birth in a squatting or upright position, often during the night or early morning, delivering a single infant.

If signs of parturition appear during the day, it may indicate complications with the delivery, and veterinary consultation should be sought. A normal delivery usually lasts 1–4 h, and the majority of infants are born head-first. Licking or cleaning the newborn is a common behavior in many species, and chewing on the placenta is also typical. Female American monkeys will assist their infants in finding the nipple, whereas female tamarins and squirrel monkeys rarely help their newborns find the nipple [1].

Ethical Approval

This chapter is a review of previously published accounts; as such, no animal or human studies were performed.

References

1. Fortman JD (2017) The laboratory nonhuman primate. CRC Press
2. Tardif S, Carville A, Elmore D et al (2012) Reproduction and breeding of nonhuman primates. Elsevier
3. Wolfecoote S (2005) The laboratory primate. J Phys D Appl Phys 33(23):3083
4. Lohiya NK, Manivannan B, Mishra PK et al (2002) Chloroform extract of Carica papaya seeds induces long term reversible azoospermia in langur monkey. Asian J Androl 4(1):10
5. Chan AW, Luetjens CM, Dominko T et al (2000) Foreign DNA transmission by ICSI: injection of spermatozoa bound with exogenous DNA results in embryonic GFP expression and live rhesus monkey births. Mol Hum Reprod 6(1):2633
6. Hewitson L, Simerly C, Dominko T et al (2000) Cellular and molecular events after in vitro fertilization and intracytoplasmic sperm injection. 53(1):95104
7. Hubrecht R, Kirkwood J, Hubrecht R et al (2010) The UFAW handbook on the care and management of laboratory and other research animals. Wiley Blackwell
8. Mdhluli MC (2003) Toxicological and antifertility investigations of oleanolic acid in male vervet monkeys (Chlorocebus aethiops). Unpublished PhD, University ofthe Western Cape

4 Development of Cynomolgus Monkey

Jia Yuling

Abstract

This chapter systematically illustrates the developmental characteristics of cynomolgus monkeys, including intrauterine development, extrauterine development, and pubertal development. As an important nonhuman primate model, cynomolgus monkeys exhibit high similarity to humans in reproductive physiology, embryonic development, metabolism and nervous system. The section on intrauterine development describes key biological events of early embryogenesis such as gametogenesis, fertilization, cleavage, blastocyst formation and implantation, summarizes critical gestational-day milestones for organogenesis, and compares the differentiation profiles of immune organs including the spleen and thymus during embryonic and fetal stages. For extrauterine development, the postnatal developmental timelines of the nervous system (motor function, fine motor performance, cognition, reflexes, social behaviors, sleep–wake cycle, etc.), skeletal system, and tooth eruption are elaborated, with cross-species comparisons among rats, dogs, and humans. Regarding pubertal development, the concepts of puberty and sexual maturity are defined. The pubertal processes of female and male cynomolgus monkeys are interpreted from the perspectives of neuroendocrine regulation, histomorphology, and function. Core mechanisms are presented, such as activation of the hypothalamic–pituitary–gonadal axis, graded testicular development, and the male masculinization programming window. Individual and population-related variations in the timing of sexual maturation across cynomolgus macaque strains are also highlighted. This chapter provides

J. Yuling (✉)
Shanghai Institute for Biomedical and Pharmaceutical Technologies, Shanghai, China
e-mail: jiayuling@kexing.com

L. Zhou and Z. Sun (eds.), *Reproductive and Developmental Toxicology on Macaca Fascicularis*, https://doi.org/10.1007/978-981-92-3834-7_4

fundamental background information for non-clinical reproductive and developmental toxicity assessment using nonhuman primates.

Keywords

Cynomolgus monkey · Nonhuman primate · Embryonic development · Organogenesis · Extrauterine development · Puberty · Reproductive development · Model animal

Old World monkeys, found in Africa and Asia, tend to be larger than New World monkeys, and many Old World monkeys live primarily on land rather than in trees. The Old World monkeys most commonly used in biomedical research belong to Cercopithecoidea, which includes macaques, baboons, gibbons, and mangabeys. The nonhuman primate (NHP) is the most widely distributed of the nonhuman primates. In nonclinical trial facilities in North America, Old World monkeys (primarily cynomolgus or rhesus monkeys) are often the preferred NHP model.

Nonhuman primates have been used for research for decades, with macaques and cynomolgus monkeys being the most commonly used NHPs. Cynomolgus monkey and rhesus monkey belong to the genus Rhesus, and the reproductive physiology and embryonic development characteristics of this species are very similar to those of humans. Embryonic and fetal development in cynomolgus monkeys and rhesus monkeys is very similar, so background data for both can often be used in common. At the same time, their reproductive organs and reproductive ways are highly similar to humans, with structures similar to the human pear-shaped uterus, ovaries, and fallopian tubes, as well as similar menstrual cycles, which is an important model to study human reproductive development.

On the other hand, the high similarity between NHP and humans in the metabolic system, nervous system, and brain structure makes NHP an ideal model animal for the study of human diseases, especially nervous system diseases, and NHP is being widely used in biomedical research, becoming a bridge connecting basic research and clinical translational applications.

Like other mammals, the early development of NHP begins with the oosperm. After the sperm and egg combine, they first form a totipotent zygote. The zygotic genome begins a reprogramming process, and the embryo continues to proliferate and differentiate into cells, eventually developing into an animal with more than 200 cell types. The development process before the embryo is implanted into the endometrium, from the oosperm to the blastocyst, is called preimplantation development. This process in primates (human or monkey) usually takes 6–7 days, during which the embryo will undergo a series of important biological events, such as maternal zygotic transformation (MZT), zygotic genome activation (ZGA), cell lineage differentiation, germ layer differentiation, etc. Development after fertilization is also a reprogrammed process of the zygotic genome, which depends on the sequential expression of the maternal material and zygotic genome carried by the oocyte, and is guided by a series of complex molecular mechanisms. Epigenetic modification mechanisms such as DNA, histone methylation/demethylation, and gene imprinting are used to ensure normal gene expression [1].

In the history of life sciences, the study of the early development of mammalian embryos has attracted much attention, but it was not until reliable methods of in vitro culture and embryo manipulation were developed that mammalian developmental biology blossomed as a discipline. In the early stage, in vitro research of embryos mainly relies on embryo morphology and the establishment of in vitro culture conditions, such as in vitro fertilization, germ cells, and embryo cryopreservation. With the development of advanced imaging technology and genome sequencing technology, humans have gradually gained a clearer understanding of the development of mammalian preimplantation embryos at the molecular level.

4.1 Intrauterine Development of Cynomolgus Monkeys and Their Characteristics

4.1.1 Early Embryonic Development of Cynomolgus Monkeys

1. *Gametogenesis.* The development and differentiation of gamesters forming primordial germ cells (PGC) marks the origin of gametes and is required for sexual reproduction. During the development of mammalian embryos, PGC development begins in the ectoderm, then migrates to the developing genital ridge, and when it reaches the embryonic gonad, it undergoes sex-specific differentiation and becomes a gamete (female oocyte or male sperm) precursor. The sex determination of the PGC is independent of its own sex chromosomes, and the type of gamete (egg or sperm) it eventually develops into is determined by its gonadal environment. Expression of gonadal cells containing XY sex chromosomes, SRY (Y chromosome sex-determining gene), and SOX9 (transcription factor SOX9 protein antibody) induces germ cells to develop into male gametes (sperm). If there is no expression of the SRY gene, the germ cell will develop into a female gamete (eggs).

After several mitoses in the developing ovary, the female PGCs enter meiosis I phase and develop into primary oocytes, and then into primordial follicles after birth. For male animals, primordial germ cells continue to proliferate and gradually differentiate into spermatogonium in the developing testis, while somatic cells continue to divide and proliferate, spermatogonium are surrounded by somatic cells to form spermatogenic tubule cords. It is not until puberty that the primordial germ cells begin to develop further.

(1)Female gametogenesis (egg development): Primate gametes develop from PGC, which form early in fetal development, originate in the yolk sac wall of the embryo, and gradually migrate to the gonadal region. In female animals at the sixth week of embryonic development, the yolk sac wall enters the ovary, differentiates into oocytes, and is covered by a layer of flat epithelial cells. These cells are called follicular cells and are derived from stromal or epithelial cells of the ovary. The oocytes are encapsulated by follicular cells to form a primordial follicle. At this time, the oocytes in the follicle are mononuclear, and the nucleolus has obvious eccentricity. Monolayer follicular cells are connected to form clusters and form single-leaf primary follicles. Follicular cells are also called granulosa cells. The primary oocyte and its granulosa cell secrete a glycoprotein substance that forms a thick membrane between the two, i.e., the zona pellucida, to separate the oocyte from the granulosa cell (Fig. 4.1).

The early development of follicles is not significantly influenced by hormones, but as puberty approaches, the continued maturation of follicles depends on the action of gonadotropin FSH. At this time, the surface of the follicular cells already has FSH receptors, and when blood-borne FSH is "bound" to the FSH receptor, the stimulated follicular cells will produce a small amount of estrogen. The most obvious sign of further follicle development is the formation of follicular cavities: small fluid-filled cavities begin to appear between the multiple layers of granulosa cells in the follicle, which gradually fuse together to become a large cavity, and the follicle in this process is called a secondary follicle. The oocyte is then gradually enlarged, pushing the oocyte to the side of the follicle. The granulosa cells surrounding the oocyte are now called cumulus cells. When the follicle expands, the ovarian stromal cells surrounding the granulosa cells form a layer of the inner lining of the follicle, and outside the membrane, some of the fibrous tissue is compressed into another membrane, called the outer membrane. At this point, the follicle is fully mature and is called a mature follicle (also called a Graafian follicle or vesicular follicle).

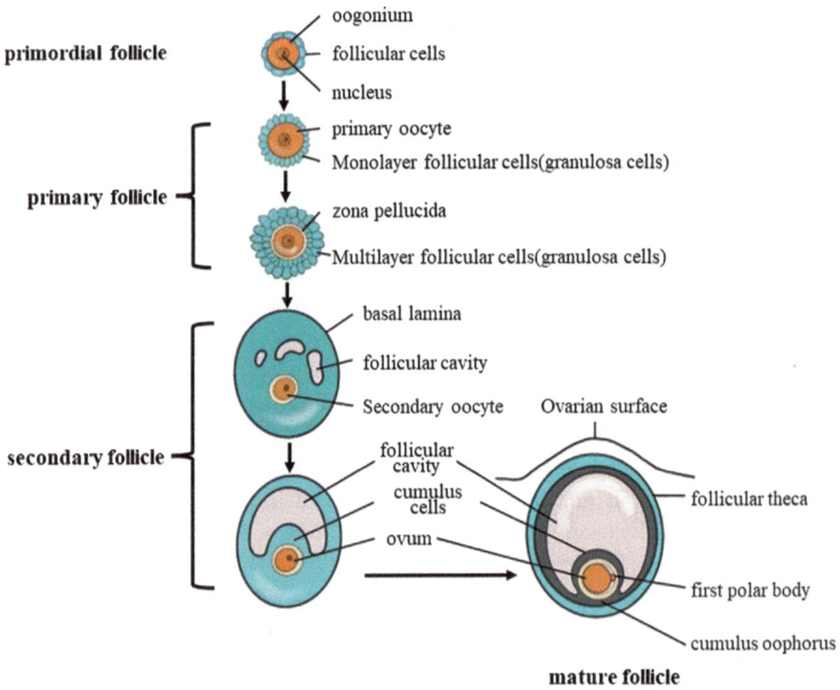

Fig. 4.1 Schematic diagram of follicle development

The maturation process of oocytes is shown in Fig. 4.2. The female germ cells of mammals develop in the fetal stage and stop before the first meiosis. In the ovarian cycle of sexually mature female animals, the primary oocyte completes the first meiosis, forming the secondary oocyte and releasing the first polar body. The secondary oocyte enters the second meiotic phase, and ovulation occurs when the chromosomes are arranged in the middle phase, at this time the cell cycle remains in the second meiotic phase until fertilization occurs. At fertilization, the oocyte completes the second meiosis, forming a mature oocyte and releasing the second polar body.

(2) Male gametogenesis (spermatogenesis): Gametogenesis in male NHP is usually divided into three stages: spermiogenesis, meiosis, and spermatogenesis. In the fetal period, the yolk sac wall reaches the testicular tissue at the sixth week of embryonic development, after which it lies dormant until puberty. During puberty, PGCs differentiate into type A spermatogonium cells. Type A spermatogonia undergo asymmetric mitosis, one of which retains the properties of type A spermatogonia and thus maintains the number of germ stem cells, and the other forms type B spermatogonia and enters the sperm differentiation pathway (Fig. 4.3). Stimulated by retinoic acid (A derivative of vitamin A), type B spermatogonia enter meiotic phase I, and DNA replicates to form primary spermatocytes. Meiotic phase I lasts for a long time, during which the early phase of division lasts for about 24 days (such as humans), and is divided into leptotene phase, zygotene stage, pachytene stage, diplotene phase, and diakinesis according to different developmental stages. During this period, paternal and maternal genetic material is exchanged and recombined. After the primary spermatocyte

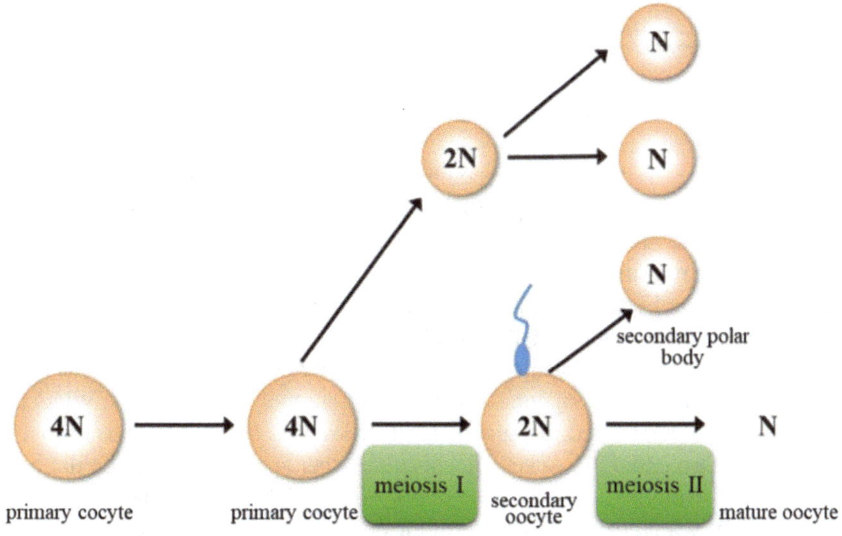

Fig. 4.2 Meiosis during oocyte development. In the process of oocyte formation, most of the mRNA in the cytoplasm has a translation function, while some mRNA does not. In the late stage of oocyte formation and the early stage of embryo, oocytes activate translation by precisely adding poly A

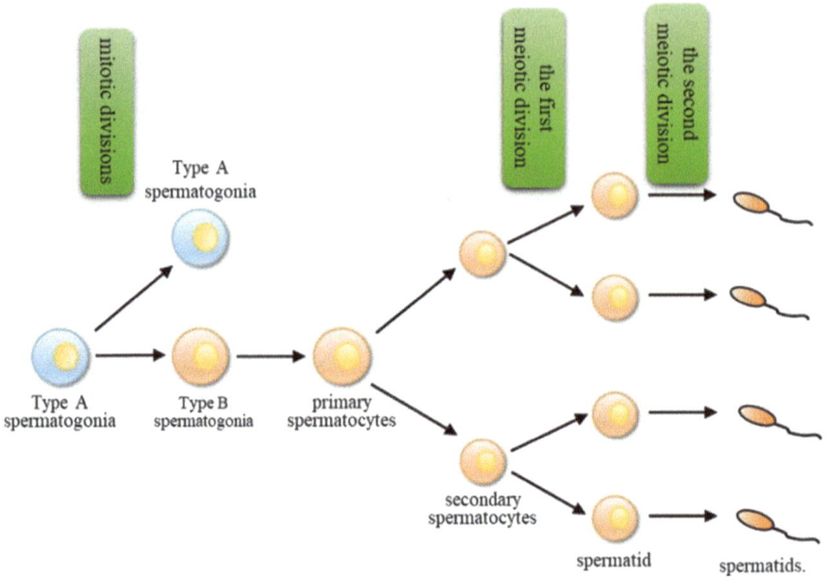

Fig. 4.3 Spermatogenesis. Process: Type A spermatogonium becomes one type B spermatogonium and one type A spermatogonium by mitosis, among which the type B spermatogonium is further developed into the primary spermatocyte, and the primary spermatocyte eventually develop into four mature sperm after two meiosis

completes the meiosis phase I, two secondary spermatocytes are formed and are connected by a cytoplasmic bridge, and the secondary spermatocytes immediately enter and complete the meiosis phase II, forming sperm cells, and the duration is short (For example, it takes about 5 h in humans) because the second meiosis does not require DNA replication and chromosome recombination. After the formation of sperm cells, they will undergo a series of morphological changes to form sperm, which first enter the spermatogenic tubule lumen, and then enter the accessory gonad and gradually develop into mature sperm.

2. *Fertilization.* Fertilization in mammals occurs in the ampulla of the fallopian tube of the female individual, and sperm bind to the zona pellucida of oocytes during meiosis II, triggering the acrosomal reaction and releasing acrosomal enzymes. With the aid of acrosomal enzymes, sperm penetrate the zona pellucida. When the zona pellucida is penetrated, it causes a cortical reaction of oocytes, thus changing the membrane potential of oocytes, inactivating other sperm receptors on the zona pellucida, and avoiding the occurrence of polyspermy. The sperm entering the zona pellucida fuses with the cell membrane of the oocyte, and the nuclear contents of the sperm enter the cytoplasm of the oocyte. The sperm nuclear structure further forms the precursors of the male prokaryote, while the tail and mitochondria degenerate. The mitochondria in the zygote come from the mother, the oocyte, but because the oocyte loses the centriole during meiosis, the formation of the zygote depends on the

centriole of the sperm. In this process, the secondary oocyte completes the second meiosis to form a mature egg, and the first and second polar bodies are released at the same time, and the cell nucleus in the cell develops into the female pronucleus. When the male and female pronuclei fuse, the fertilization process is completed, the zygote is formed, and the fertilized egg enters the cleavage stage (Fig. 4.4).

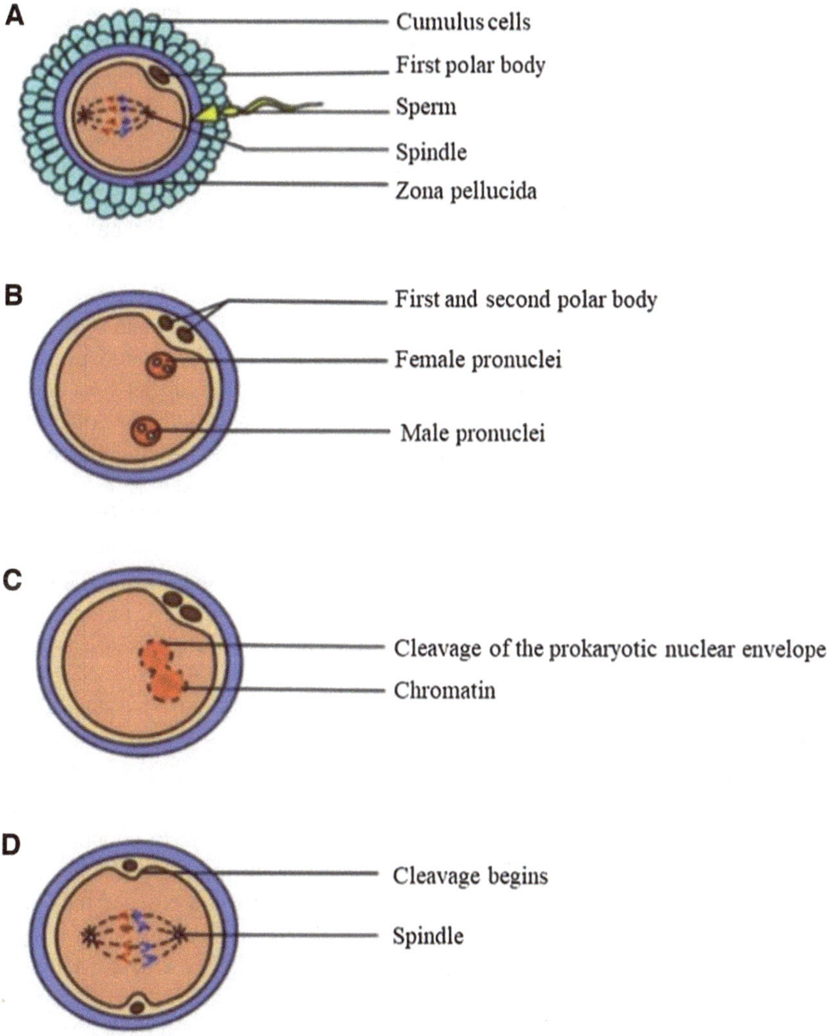

Fig. 4.4 Fertilization process of the oocyte. (**A**) After sperm entered the oocyte cytoplasm through the cumulus cells and the zona pellucida, the oocyte began the second meiosis. (**B**) After fertilization, the oocyte expels the second polar body, and the female and male pronuclei form. (**C**) The female and male prokaryotes were close to each other and fused to form diploid prokaryotes. (**D**) The fertilized egg begins its first mitosis

3. *Cleavage*. Cleavage refers to the series of mitoses that a fertilized egg undergoes during development, through which the egg cell distributes a large amount of ooplasm into several small cells. There are many types of cleavage in the animal kingdom, primates are secondary with little yolk, and cleavage type is total cleavage, that is, each meiosis changes from one cell to two cells. A characteristic of the cleavage process is asynchronous division, i.e., the time it takes for one cell to divide compared to other cells is different, so the total number of cleavage cells in an embryo may be odd at some time. During cleavage, the cell volume does not increase, but the ooplasm of the fertilized egg is continuously distributed to the daughter cells. Compared with other stages of development, the number of cells in the cleavage stage increases much faster. The result of this division is a rapid increase in the ratio of nucleus to cytoplasm. However, the distribution of ooplasm to each cleavage cell during the division process is not uniform, and the nuclei of each blastomere may be in different cytoplasmic environments, resulting in differences in the fate of subsequent cells.

After three rounds of cleavage, the embryo enters the eight-cell stage, and it has been confirmed that the activation of zygotic genes in primate embryos occurs around the eight-cell stage. At this time, another important change is that the cleavage cells begin to densify, that is, the cleavage cells move closer to each other and form tighter cell connections. Morphologically, the cleavage cells are compressed into each other, the boundaries become blurred to form a sphere of cells, and the gap between the cells and the zona pellucida becomes larger. This is due to the plasma membrane of the basal and parietal surfaces of cleavage cells beginning to differ when densification occurs, and the outer basement membrane is distinguished from the apical plasma membrane by the tight junctions, gap junctions, and localization of epithelial Ca^{2+}-dependent adhesion molecules (Ecadherin), which cause cleavage cells to shrink toward the center. This process is accompanied by changes in the hardness of the plasma membrane and the composition and distribution direction of the cytoskeleton. At the same time, the cells become polarized, and the cleavage cells have begun to differentiate in both directions of the trophectoderm and the inner cell mass (Fig. 4.5).

4. *Blastocyst formation*. When the blastocyst forms the morula, the fluid gradually enters the interior of the cell mass to form the hollow blastocyst cavity of the embryo. At this point, cells differentiate into two broad categories: a small, tightly packed inner mass called an inner cell mass, which will eventually develop into a fetus; The outer cell mass forms a spherical structure of a single layer of cells, called the trophoblast, which will develop into the placenta. The main reason for the formation of the blastocyst cavity is that Na+ is actively transported to the center of the embryo, and the change of osmotic pressure leads to water entering the center of the embryo and forming the cavity. The formation and expansion of the blastocyst cavity are crucial for embryo hatching and subsequent development. The fluid in the blastocyst cavity contains various factors that affect the proliferation and differentiation of the inner cell mass, and these factors will affect the formation of various germ layers after implantation.

The embryo remains enclosed in the zona pellucida until a day or two after the formation of the blastocyst, when the blastocyst cavity expands rapidly. The embryo enters the uterus during this process, and the expansion of the blastocyst cavity thins the zona pellucida. At the same time, proteolytic enzymes produced by the trophectodermal

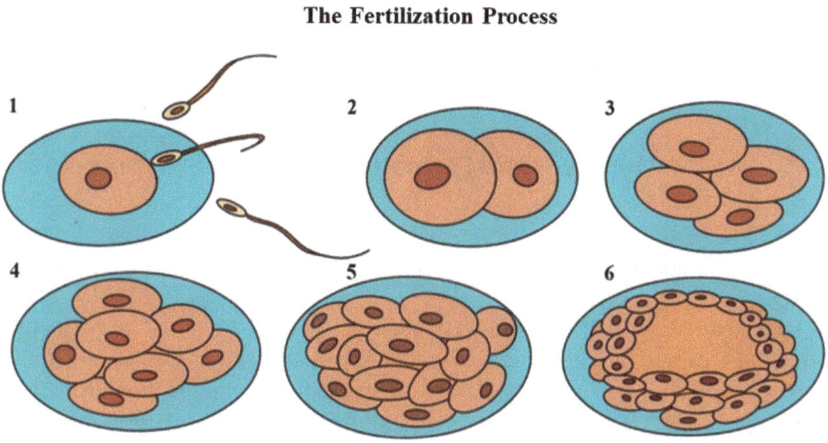

Fig. 4.5 Embryonic development of macaque monkeys before implantation. 1. Sperm–egg union, 2. two-cell stage, 3. four-cell stage, 4. eight-cell stage, 5. morula, 6. expanded blastocyst

cells digest part of the zona pellucida, opening a gap in the zona pellucida, and the blastocyst begins to detach from it. This process is called blastocyst hatching.

5. *Implantation*. After implantation, the hatched blastocyst contacts with the endometrium of the corresponding part of the uterus and implants (also called implantation), which is the process of further development, movement, and contact with the uterine wall of the embryo in the later stage of the blastocyst. During the secretory phase of the female animal's menstrual cycle, progesterone is secreted by the luteal cells of the ovaries, prompting the endometrium to react and be highly sensitive to foreign body stimulation and pressure, in preparation for receiving the embryo. After implantation, the mother's uterus provides nutrients to the fetus, so that the embryo can successfully carry out tissue differentiation, organ formation, and eventually develop into a fetus. Therefore, implantation is an important stage to establish the connection between the embryo and the mother.

Embryo implantation in higher mammals can be divided into three types based on how closely the embryo is connected to the uterus: surface implantation, eccentric implantation, and intramural implantation. Surface implantation refers to trophoblast cells that only make contact with the maternal uterine epithelium and do not embed deep in the endometrium, a type found in eutherian animals such as cattle, sheep, cats, dogs, and pigs. Eccentric implantation refers to the local projection of the trophectoderm and internal parietal mesoderm that are embedded in the endometrial folds, and rodents such as mice and rats belong to this type. Embryo implantation in primates is intramural implantation, also known as complete interstitial implantation, which means that after the blastocyst hatches, part of the inner cell mass contacts the uterine epithelium, trophoblast cells dissolve the uterine epithelium, and the blastocyst is completely implanted in the superficial layer of the mucous lamina propria. The shallow layer, also called the functional layer, is composed of a sponge layer and a dense layer. After the blastocyst invasion, the trophoblast ectodermal cells divide and become large multinuclear giant cells. After the formation of nucleosomes, the remaining trophoblast ectodermal cells become cytotrophoblast.

4.1.2 The Development and Formation of Organs in Cynomolgus Monkeys

Table 4.1 summarizes the key time points of intrauterine development of cynomolgus monkeys.

The menstrual cycle of cynomolgus monkeys is similar to that of humans, about 28 days. The duration of spermatogenesis is 40–46 days, compared to 64–74 days in humans. Organogenesis is similar in humans and cynomolgus monkeys (20–50 days of gestation). After organogenesis, cynomolgus monkeys undergo a more rapid development relative to humans, and at birth, cynomolgus monkeys may be more fully developed than humans [2].

The lymphoid organ system and lymphocyte anatomical region division in cynomolgus monkeys show that development begins in the second trimester (GD_{65}) and takes on an adult morphology in the first trimester. By GD_{100}, the fetus has developed well enough morphology and bones.

Through the pregnancy study data of 5167 control groups, it was confirmed that the gestation period of cynomolgus monkeys was about 160 days (134–184 days).

1. *Embryonic period.* The embryonic period is the time when major organs are formed. The embryonic period of cynomolgus monkeys is 20–50 days of gestation, and it is estimated that the embryonic period of humans is 20–56 days of gestation.

The embryonic period is a period of rapid cell division, including cell differentiation, organ development, and formation. The sequence and timing of organogenesis in humans and cynomolgus monkeys are very similar. Because rapid development occurs during organogenesis, this period is extremely susceptible to teratogens and can lead to severe congenital malformations.

The cardiovascular system is the first major system in which the embryo develops and functions. Fetal heartbeats in humans and cynomolgus monkeys can be detected by ultrasound as early as day 22 of gestation. At the end of the major organogenetic period, the crown–rump length of human and cynomolgus embryos is approximately 30 mm long and weighs about 8 g, with distinct human (or NHP) characteristics. At this point, all major organs are in place [3].

2. *Fetal stage.* The fetal stage begins at the end of organogenesis (week 8 in humans and week 7 in cynomolgus monkeys) and is marked by closure of the hard palate. In the early fetal period, primary ossification centers appear in the bones, early genitals appear, red blood cells migrate from the liver to the spleen, and urine begins to form. This initial stage is followed by a period of rapid bone ossification and sexual differentiation. In cynomolgus monkeys, the development of some organ systems is accelerated during the fetal period relative to humans (Table 4.2).

Table 4.1 Key developmental events in intrauterine development of cynomolgus monkeys

No.	Developmental events		Cynomolgus monkeys
1	Embryonic development	Implantation	GD_{9}
2		Primitive streak	GD_{17}
3		Ten-somite stage	GD_{23}
4		Lower limb buds	GD_{28}
5		Hand (forepaw) rays	GD_{35}
6		Palatal folds uniting	GD_{46}
7	Nervous system	Neural plate	GD_{20}
8		Neuropores closed	$GD_{25–27}$
9		Three brain vesicles	GD_{25}
10		Cerebral hemispheres	GD_{29}
11		Cerebellum	GD_{36}
12		Olfactory bulbs	GD_{38}
13	Eye and ear	Optic vesicle forming	GD_{23}
14		Lens separated	GD_{32}
15		Optic nerve fibers present	GD_{39}
16		Cochlea appearing	GD_{37}
17		Optic capsule cartilaginous	GD_{42}
18	Heart and great arteries	Fusing heart tubes	GD_{22}
19		S-shaped heart	GD_{25}
20		Septation occurring	GD_{28}
21		Foramen oval present	GD_{34}
22		Truncal septation comple te	GD_{36}
23		Aortic arch arteries forming	$GD_{22–30}$
24	Gastrointestinal system	Intestinal pocket	Foregut: $GD_{20.5}$; Hindgut: ——
25		Membranes perforate	Oral: $GD_{27–28}$; Anal: ——
26		Liver	Anlage: $GD_{24–26}$; Epithelial Cords: –
27		Gall bladder	$GD_{28–29}$
28		Stomach appears	$GD_{28–29}$
29		Umbilical hernia	Begins: $GD_{33–34}$; Reduced: $GD_{47–48}$
30	Kidney	Metanephros	$GD_{38–39}$
31	Spleen	Spleen demarcation	GD_{80}
32		Thymic primordia	GD_{35}
33	Parturition	Gestation period	GD_{167}
34		Eating	At birth (GD_{167})
35		Taste	At birth (GD_{167})

Note: The embryonic and fetal development of cynomolgus monkeys and rhesus macaques are very similar, so the background data can usually be used in common. *GD* gestational days

Table 4.2 Timing of some major postnatal developmental events in cynomolgus monkeys and humans

Organ system	Cynomolgus monkeys	Human
Kidney	By birth	By birth
Lung	By birth	2–8
Heart	By birth	By birth
Bone		
Appearance of secondary ossification centers	Birth–6 months	6 months–12 years
Epiphyseal fusion	5–9 years	11–20 years
Reproductive system		
Puberty	3–6 years	8–14 years
Immune system		
Spleen and lymph node development	By birth	By birth
Immunocompetence	Birth–3 months	Birth–3 months
Central nervous system		
Locomotor development	7 weeks	9–13 months
Fine motor development/ dexterity	6 months	1.5–13 years
Sensory and reflex development	Birth–1 year	Birth–1 year
Cognitive development	3 weeks–3 years	1 months–9 years
Communication	Birth–1 year	Birth–2 years

Lungs: The lungs of cynomolgus monkeys mature during fetal life to accommodate gas exchange. The bronchioles and alveoli are separated, and the degree of vascularization increases.

Kidneys: The kidneys of cynomolgus monkeys develop in the fetal stage. The immune systems of humans and cynomolgus monkeys appear to develop similarly. This can also be confirmed when comparing the immune system development of humans and cynomolgus monkeys as a percentage of the total gestation period. During the fetal period, the number of various immune cells in the immune organs increases, and the cells gradually gather to reach their final anatomical position. It has been shown that cynomolgus fetal cells at GD_{70} produce IgG, IgM, and IgA. Cells in the gastrointestinal tract secrete IgG and IgA, while cells in the thymus and spleen secrete IgM.

During the embryonic, fetal, and neonatal stages, the fetus continues to grow rapidly. The embryogenetic period (organogenesis) is generally considered to be the time interval between implantation (formation of the ectodermal nerve plate) and closure of the hard palate (Table 4.3).

3. *Spleen development.* When the spleen develops at GD_{65}, a large number of lymphocytes begin to differentiate, accompanied by more and more lymphatic tissue partitions, respectively, specific T-cell areas and B-cell areas, and at GD_{80}, peripheral lymphatic organs appear. At GD_{75}, the largest proportion of lymphocytes in the

Table 4.3 Derivation of various organs from primary germ layers of the embryonic inner cell mass

Endoderm	Mesoderm	Ectoderm (trophoblast)
Liver	Vertebrae	Brain
Pancreas	Muscle	Spinal cord
Serous, mucous, and gastric glands	Dermis of skin, bone, and cartilage	Pituitary
Epithelium of the digestive tube, respiratory system, and bladder	Connective tissue, blood, and blood vessels	Neural crest cells, retina, and lens adrenal medulla
Thyroid	Urinary and reproductive apparatus	Enamel of teeth
Parathyroid	Epithelia of the adrenal cortex, spleen, and lymph nodes	Enamel of teeth
Pancreatic islets	/	Epithelium of oral, nasal, olfactory, genital and anal cavities
Thymic corpuscles	/	Epithelium of skin and its derivatives—hair, nails, sweat, sebaceous, and mammary glands

embryonic spleen is $CD20^{+}$B cells, and the number of T cells is very low. At GD_{145}, the ratio of white pulp to red pulp is 1:1, similar to that of a mature primate spleen. At GD_{80}, a large number of B and T cells are scattered in the lymph nodes. During the development of GD_{145}, the B-cell follicular area and the T-cell paracortex area expand. There are a large number of $CD20^{+}$B cells and $CD3^{+}$T cells in the membrane propria of the small intestine at GD_{80}. In the later stages of fetal development (from GD_{100} to GD_{145}), the direction of lymphoid aggregation is B cells toward the lumen side and muscle layer, where T cells are in the contralateral.

4. *Thymus development.* Thymus development is influenced by thymus epithelial cells, thymus lymphocytes express T-cell receptors (TcR), undergo a series of selections, eliminate autoreactive cells, and eventually migrate out of the expressed TcR tissue and a set of specific membrane glycoproteins to determine the phenotype and predict the function of these cells. Disturbances in T-cell development during these important stages can alter the evolution of "self" versus "nonself" identification, leading to autoimmune diseases or increased susceptibility to infection. Thymocyte cells are produced rapidly after sexual maturity in all vertebrates.

In 1975, Tanimura and Tanioka reported that fetal thymus tissue had been demonstrated to develop in rhesus monkeys. The thymus primordium is separated from the pharyngeal pouch and proliferates at $GD_{37–48}$. These studies show that differentiation of lymphokines occurs within the thymus at $GD_{50–73}$ and maturation of the fetal lymphatic system occurs at $GD_{100–133}$. In 2002, Hendrickx in the same laboratory reported that studies in cynomolgus monkeys showed that the cortex and medulla of the thymus are distinguishable at GD_{65}, all regions of the fetal thymus, with most of the thymocytes being $CD3^+$, while $CD20^+B$ cells are scattered at the corticomedullary junction. The number of $CD20^+B$ cells at the corticomedullary junction increased in the $GD_{100-145}$ fetus, while the number of $CD3^+$ thymocytes remained consistent throughout the gestation period. In the same study, flow cytometry analysis of lymphocyte subsets showed a slight increase in single positive thymocytes ($CD4^+/CD8^-$ and $CD4^-/CD8^+$) and a slight decrease in double positive thymocytes ($CD4^+/CD8^+$) between GD_{80} and GD_{145} (86%–76%).

4.2 Extrauterine Developmental Process and Characteristics of Cynomolgus Monkeys

Cynomolgus monkeys are born with mature lungs compared to humans. In humans, more than 85% of the alveoli develop after birth, and the lungs do not fully mature until about 2–8 years of age (Table 4.2). Several of the most commonly used endpoints for the functional development of the central nervous system (CNS) at birth in cynomolgus monkeys are also more developed [4].

The development of kidneys and hearts after birth appears to be very similar in humans and cynomolgus monkeys. Nephrogenesis is completed at birth, renal function matures after birth, and glomerular filtration rate and concentration capacity increase. From the 4th week to the 39th week after birth, the clinicopathological parameters of cynomolgus monkeys remained almost unchanged except for changes in gamma-glutamyltransferase and an increase in blood urea nitrogen, indicating that kidney function in newborn rhesus monkeys is well developed early. In humans, the kidneys remain in functional development until 1 year of age.

After birth, the major organ systems in which cynomolgus monkeys and humans continue to experience growth and maturity are the growth of bones, the development of central nervous system function, the acquisition of immune capacity, and sexual maturity.

Bone development begins with the appearance of the primary ossification center before birth and continues after birth until the appearance of the secondary ossification center and the longitudinal bone growth on the epiphyseal growth plate, which finally fuses when the bone develops to adulthood. At birth, monkeys have more ossification centers than humans. It is estimated that the bone age of cynomolgus monkeys at birth is similar to that of humans aged 5–6 years, and within 6 months of birth is similar to that of humans aged 7 years. The growth plate fusion of different bones varies with age and sex, but cynomolgus monkeys are about 5–9 years old.

After birth, the development of the reproductive system of cynomolgus monkeys is similar to that of humans, characterized by the initiation of the secretion of reproductive-related hormones during the perinatal period, followed by the suspension of the reproductive endocrine system until the onset of puberty. The sexual maturity time of female cynomolgus monkeys is 3–4 years old, and that of male cynomolgus monkeys is 4–6 years old.

The development of the immune system after birth is similar in cynomolgus monkeys and humans. Nonhuman primates are born with more mature immune systems than rodents and acquire immunity after birth. Human and cynomolgus monkey newborns have higher serum concentrations of IgG and lower concentrations of IgM and IgA at birth. The IgG in the serum of newborns is mainly derived from the mother, and the levels of IgM and IgA gradually increase after birth. The concentration of IgG will decrease during the first 6 months of life due to the removal of antibodies produced by the mother, and then increases as the infant begins to produce IgG on its own. The key time points of extrauterine development of cynomolgus monkeys are shown in Table 4.4.

Table 4.4 Key developmental events in extrauterine development of cynomolgus monkeys

No.	Developmental events		Cynomolgus monkeys
1	Adult body size		Rhesus monkey: 8 years, chimpanzee: ~11 years
2	P450 enzyme development		Develops in utero; detected in the liver and adrenal at early fetal stages
3	Brain	Adult brain weight	7 years
4		Presence of external granular layer	Disappears at 2–3 months
5	Functional neurological landmarks	Sexual differentiation of the brain	Testosterone surge in males within 2 weeks postnatal
6		Fully mature prefrontal cortex (synaptogenesis and myelination complete)	Adolescence/early adulthood 4–7 years
7	Postnatal neurogenesis and synaptogenesis	Postnatal neurogenesis	20% of neurogenesis in the dentate gyrus occurs after birth; neurogenesis slows with age, but a small amount continues throughout life. Neurogenesis in the cerebellum is complete at 2–3 months of age
8		Peak of the overall brain synaptogenesis	GD_{40}–PND_{61}
9		Duration of synaptogenesis	Synaptogenesis continues for the first two postnatal months, and slowly tapers off
10		Pruning of synapses	The number of synapses increases during early childhood, plateaus until puberty, then decreases to adult levels due to pruning. The peak number of synapses is reached prior to puberty. At this point, there are approximately 40% more synapses than in the adult

PND postnatal day

This section describes the development of the nervous system, skeletal system, and tooth eruption in cynomolgus monkeys in detail.

4.2.1 Nervous System

In terms of brain development, the growth peak in rhesus monkeys occurs before birth, while the growth peak in rats and humans occurs after birth. However, one important area where cynomolgus monkeys are more similar to humans is the pattern of synaptogenesis. This pattern is specific to the cerebral cortex of nonhuman primates. There are three main phases of synaptogenesis: the rapid synaptic growth phase, the plateau phase of synapse formation, and the regressive phase, when the number of synapses decreases and is recombined. In the human cerebral cortex, a 2-year-old child has about twice as many synapses as an adult. Synaptic proliferation and branching peak at the age 3, but half of synapses will disappear by age 15–16. Nonhuman primates exhibit a similar pattern of synaptogenesis [5].

This section focuses on the behavioral detection of central nervous system development in cynomolgus monkeys, but does not include neuroanatomical or neurochemical aspects. It is generally accepted that the developing nervous system is qualitatively different from the adult system. The human central nervous system is relatively late maturing; that is, it does not have all the functions of the mature central nervous system at birth, but has a fairly long development after birth, and the human central nervous system must go through a considerable developmental stage after birth to reach the mature state of adulthood.

The CNS maturation process of cynomolgus monkeys is divided into eight aspects: ① motor development; ② fine motor development; ③ sensory and reflex development; ④ cognitive development; ⑤ communication; ⑥ social games; ⑦development of fear response; and ⑧ development of the sleep cycle. The following will be introduced in detail from these aspects [4].

1. *Motor development.* It is normal for infant monkeys to be dependent on their mothers during the first 3 days of life. Soon after, the infant monkey can lift its chest off the ground by extending its arms and head. Amazingly, infant monkeys can get down on all fours 4 days after birth. At about 3 weeks of age (and in some cases as early as the end of the first week), the position of the torso becomes more parallel to the ground (i.e., more like an adult). Young monkeys can be observed standing on 2 ft at 7 weeks of age. Young monkeys develop motor abilities in both horizontal (i.e., the ground) and vertical (i.e., climbing and jumping) planes. During the first 2 weeks of life, the infant monkey advances horizontally by extending or grasping the limbs in an outward extended position (i.e., limbs extending away from the midline of the body). From 5 to 11 weeks of age, the extension of the limbs becomes more exaggerated, and the knees are relatively extended compared to the adult state. Knee flexion, extension, and adduction of the limbs (i.e., limbs extending toward the midline of the body) begin at week 7, but consistency of movement is not observed until about 12 weeks of age [6].

Infant cynomolgus monkeys begin to have the ability to climb at the age of 2 days. However, by the end of weeks 1 and 5, the ability to regress or turn around and return

Table 4.5 Summary of locomotor development

Ability	Human	Rat	Dog	NonhumanPrimate(Rhesus monkey)
Crawling	PND_{270} (about 9 months)	PND_3–PND_{12}	PND_4–PND_{20}	PND_4–PND_{49}
Walking	PND_{396} (about 13 months)	PND_{12}–PND_{16}	PND_{20}–PND_{28}	PND_{49}

began to manifest itself, respectively. Even the most adventurous cynomolgus monkeys do not attempt to jump until they are 5 weeks old.

At 4 weeks of age, infant cynomolgus monkeys can squat down on 2 ft with the help of their tails.

In humans, rats, dogs, and nonhuman primates, motor capacity is not developed until after birth (Table 4.5). In rats, dogs, and humans, there appears to be a more progressive process of rostro-caudal maturation that results in the shoulder being higher than the pelvis. In contrast, nonhuman primates develop faster than humans after birth. Therefore, the motor development of rats, dogs, and NHP can be evaluated in toxicity studies in young animals. However, studies on NHP species need to be carefully designed to accommodate the rapid development of motor function.

2. *Fine motor development*. Nonhuman primates show fairly rapid fine motor and dexterity development after birth. The ontogenetic development of newborn cynomolgus monkeys, such as relatively independent finger movements, requires further development and connectivity of functional cortical motor neurons. Although corticospinal fibers reach all levels of the spinal cord before birth, and there may be substantial innervation of the gray matter in the intermediate regions, important cortical motor neuronal connections associated with the motor nucleus are not present at birth [7].

The relatively independent finger movements of cynomolgus monkeys occurred at around 3 months of age. Thereafter, both anatomical and physiological development of the corticospinal system continue for a considerable period of time, which usually coincides with the maturation of motor skills. Fine finger movements are not observed until functional cortical motor neuron connections are well constructed, and rapid changes in the physiological properties of the corticospinal system coincided with the period of precision grip maturity (3–6 months). However, corticospinal development continues long after relevant functional indicators of flexibility detection mature, and these changes may help improve speed and coordination in hand tasks.

At 6 months of age, all the basic operations in adult monkeys are already present in young monkeys. During the first 8 weeks, the movements that often occur are gentle, including sustained visual orientation and target contact. Later movements are more powerful, such as grasping. The activity rate increased significantly from birth to 6 months of age. The increased activity during the first 8 weeks to the second 8 weeks may be due to increased alert and active time, reduced time spent in the arms of the female monkey, improved postural control and endurance, and the onset of independent movement. The change in form is largely attributed to postural factors and neuromuscular development, resulting in more precise targeting and control of movement at the 5th and 6th months of age.

Infant monkeys develop fine motor skills rapidly. At 14 weeks of age, infant monkeys showed good fine motor skills, including hand-to-mouth coordination, two-handed coordination (using one hand to lift the transparent beaker and turn it upside down while retrieving the task reward with the other hand), and finger-to-thumb opposition. Due to differences in the maturity of motor systems at birth, these results may not easily generalize to humans. Newborn monkeys are more developed in motor function than human newborns. For example, monkeys can crawl a few days after birth.

Fine motor and dexterity development is usually long-term (Table 4.6). Human newborns do not have the ability to make fine finger movements, and these abilities may not appear for several months after birth. For example, precise coordination, such as grasping and lifting objects, may not fully mature until the second decade of life. Although NHPs develop much faster than humans, postnatal development of fine motor activity in humans and NHPs follows a similar pattern.

3. *Sensory and reflex development.* The sensory systems develop sequentially. In many species, the function of the auditory system precedes the visual system. In addition, the functions of touch and smell usually precede those of the auditory system. Conditioned responses to various sensory modes develop in the same order, i.e., conditioned responses usually appear in the sense of smell, then in hearing, and finally in vision. While electrophysiological and histological research tools are very useful in determining the initiation of the functional sensory system, the importance of sensory function is ultimately related to behaviors that are detected as sensorimotor reflexes [8]. Unfortunately, the limitation of this approach is that the development of the sensorimotor system depends on the maturation of the motor and sensory systems. Therefore, it is not always possible to completely separate the development of a particular sensory system from that of the motor system.

In nonhuman primates, there is a tendency for those species that achieve higher levels of functioning to have longer juvenile periods. It takes about 18 months for a tree shrew to reach adulthood, and the juvenile growth period lasts even longer, such

Table 4.6 Summary of fine motor development and dexterity

Fine motor development	Approximate postnatal age ability emerges
Human	
Palmar grasping reflex	PND < 2 months
Prehension	5–9 months
Precision grip	1.5–13 years
Rat	
Fine motor development	PND_2–PND_{32}
NHP	
Fine motor development	11 weeks
Precision grip	3–6 months
Manipulations	6 months

as 2–3 years for cynomolgus monkeys and 8 years for gorillas. Infant cynomolgus monkeys exhibit a rooting reflex at birth, with a peak at PND_4 and PND_{10}, disappearing. At birth, infant cynomolgus monkeys have other responses, including hand and foot grasping and gripping. From birth, if the infant is placed on its back, it will quickly turn to the right to achieve ventral contact.

The somatosensory system is functional at birth; young monkeys have a response to needling at birth. While these systems are functional at birth, they can still be refined during development. For example, infant monkeys reach adult threshold levels at 10 weeks of life and are able to distinguish differences in texture and size, suggesting that the tactile sensory system, while functioning at birth, continues to develop after birth. In nonhuman primates, auditory responses can be observed at birth, indicating that the functional auditory sensory system develops before birth, while at PND_{10}, infant monkeys show a startle response to sudden sounds.

Humans can track their mothers with their eyes at birth, track a moving object within a few days of birth, and locate a small object at PND_{13}. The retinal images of cynomolgus monkeys are well focused at birth and can rapidly reach adult level by 9 weeks after birth.

The sensory and reflex systems of rats, dogs, and nonhuman primates develop in a sequence similar to that of human infants. For example, the taste system of newborn animals is important for selective uptake, and smell and taste are the first two sensory systems to be developed. Behavioral responses in humans and rats suggest the presence of functional taste and smell systems at birth, and that smell may function in the uterus. Although the sequence of development of the sensory and reflex systems may be similar, some systems differ relative to the time of development at birth. In general, rats, dogs, and humans tend to develop slowly after birth and have a well-defined neonatal period during which they rely on their mothers for shelter and food. In contrast, nonhuman primates tend to be better developed at birth. For example, at birth, monkeys have more developed tactile, auditory, and visual systems than humans or rats. This may reflect the need for rapid development after birth in nonhuman primates. Within 3 months of birth, infant cynomolgus monkeys develop from a state of complete dependence on their mother to a state of relative independence.

Although nonhuman primates are precocious in reflex and sensory behavior, with the exception of vision and taste, all common laboratory animal species (such as rats and dogs) are relatively developed at birth. Thus, the assessment of somatosensory development in juvenile toxicity studies provides limited reference value because these systems are fully developed during human gestation (Table 4.7).

4. *Cognitive development.* In many species, some learning abilities appear early in life, such as classical conditioned reflex. However, the acquisition of more complex learning abilities, such as delayed response or spatial learning, is gradual and improves progressively as the animal develops. Learned responses also play an important role in social interaction and ontogeny in many species, including playful behavior development and fear of strangers. In addition, normal sleep–wake rhythms also mature in the early postnatal period [9].

In 1959, Harlow et al. assessed the development of learning in rhesus monkeys. The conditioned avoidance task began on the third day of life. The infant monkeys

Table 4.7 Postnatal sensory and reflexive development in different species

Activity	Human	Rat	Dog	NHP
Eating/rooting	Birth	Birth	Birth	Birth
Surface righting		PND_1–PND_{11}	–	Birth
Grasping/clasping	Birth–2 months	–	–	Birth
Orientation	–	PND_9–PND_{11}	–	3 weeks
Air righting	–	PND_{15}–PND_{18}	–	5 weeks
Olfaction	–	Birth	Birth	
Taste	Birth	Birth	Birth	Birth
Tactile	Birth	Vibrissa placement: $PND_{12.5}$; nociceptive PND_{21}; tail flick PND_{10}–PND_{25}	Proprioceptive: PND_1; air puff: PND_{10}; Nociceptive: PND_1–PND_{18}; adultlike nociceptive response: PND_{21}	Pinprick: GD_{167}; mature: 10 weeks
Auditory	Birth	ASR: PND_{12}; inhibition of ASR : PND_{21}–PND_{42}	ASR: PND_{19}–PND_{25}	Auditory: Birth ; ASR: PND_{14}–PND_{25}
Visual	Visual tracking: birth; perception: mature in 2 months ; acuity: mature in 4–6 months	Phototaxis response: PND_5; eyes open: PND_{14}–PND_{16}; visual placing: PND_{17}	Visual orientation: PND $_{21}$–PND_{25}	Visual tracking: Birth; visual orientation: PND_{13}; acuity: improves during first 2 months of life; mature: 1 year

showed improvement (i.e., improved learning ability) over 5 consecutive days of testing. However, when memory tests were performed at 23 days of age, a considerable degree of learning loss was observed.

Two groups of newborn rhesus monkeys (the first group started training at birth and the second group started training at day 11) were trained on a black and white discrimination task, i.e., object discrimination. Newborn monkeys learn this task quickly. In the group that began training at birth, 90% accuracy was achieved from 9 days of age. The second group was rewarded for climbing either of the two grey slopes in the first 10 days of life. On day 11, the black and white slopes were replaced. By the second test day (day 12), the infants were able to distinguish. Interestingly, in the reverse discrimination task, when the first reverse discrimination task was performed, the infant monkeys made a lot of errors and showed severe emotional disorder (such as hesitation, vocalization, urination, and defecation). Although 11-day-old infants can solve the black and white discrimination task, the ability to solve the triangle circle discrimination requires that the CNS be more mature. Infant monkeys of 20–30 days of age may need 150–200 tests to complete the triangle circle discrimination task. The development of more complex object discrimination abilities (i.e., 3D objects with different color, form, size, and material) was assessed in rhesus monkeys at 30, 60, 90, 120, 150, and 366 days of age. Animals were tested 25 times/day, 5 days a week, for 4 weeks. The number of tests required for 10 consecutive correct responses decreased with age and approached the performance of adult monkeys at 120–150 days of age.

In the delayed response task, the animals were first shown a food reward, and then the food was hidden under one of two identical containers during the delay. Rhesus monkeys were tested at 60, 90, 120, or 150 days of age. Over time, all four groups showed an increasing ability to solve delayed response tasks. However, Harlow noted that the ability to solve the problem of delayed response was better in animals aged 125–135 days than in animals aged 60–90 days. In addition, half of the monkeys aged 200–250 days performed perfectly at the task. Obviously, the ability to solve the problem of delayed response matures later than the ability to solve object recognition tasks.

So far, two conclusions can be drawn from the monkey data. First, certain learning abilities appear early in a monkey's life, such as conditioned avoidance or black and white discrimination. The ability to solve problems may be present as early as 1 day of age, and within a few days of age, performance changes from accidental levels to near 100% accuracy. Second, the development of certain more complex learning abilities is gradual and progressively improved, such as delayed response learning and some discrimination learning tasks (such as color, pattern, or shape discrimination). It is worth noting that extensive early training for complex tasks, such as delayed response tasks, does not promote task completion rates, and the ability to successfully complete tasks is related to age. That is, even though young animals were trained more extensively than older animals, they did not perform as well as older monkeys.

The learning ability of rats, dogs, monkeys, and human infants changes during development. In all species assessed, the ability to regulate reflex behavior exceeds learning behavioral responses. The study suggests that the sequence of behavioral development reflects the sequence of maturation from the caudal side of the body to the rostral side. It is well known that the subcortical structure is sufficient to support many instances of Pavlovian conditioned reflex, and that the lower center of the sensory system is sufficient to support primitive reflex behavior. Higher learning centers (such as the hippocampus and prefrontal cortex) are necessary to acquire more complex behaviors. Thus, in all common laboratory animal species, assessment of cognitive function in juvenile toxicity studies can provide insight into the development of mature individuals in these systems (Table 4.8). Newborn and young animals generally take longer to learn specific tasks than adults. In addition, the accuracy of learning the task is usually not equal to adulthood. This means that even if the task can be completed in infancy, it is by no means mature in learning function, that is, not enough to reach the level of adult performance. Finally, attention, learning, and memory are closely related to the maturation of many of the sensory systems mentioned above.

5. *Communication*. There are three different emotional vocalizations in cynomolgus monkeys: play calls, fear and pain cries, and food satisfaction. Emotional vocalizations are dominant in the first 6 months of life and come in the form of single syllables or phrases. After 6 months of age, the number of monosyllabic and two-syllable pronunciations increases significantly, and there are differences in pitch, timbre, and tone. Sounds of similar pitch are combined in different ways to change phrases in the lab

Table 4.8 Summary of cognitive development

Learning task	Approximate postnatal age ability emerges
Human	
Classical conditioning	20–30 days old
Operant conditioning	2–18 months
Long-term recall	13–20 months
Implicit learning	<5 years
Explicit learning	5–9 years
Rat	
Appetitive learning	PND_1
Associative learning (olfactory)	PND_2–PND_8
Active avoidance	PND_9–PND_{12}
Passive avoidance	PND_{10}–PND_{21}
Sequential learning (Biel maze)	PND_{17}–PND_{23}
Proximal cued learning (Morris water maze)	PND_{17}
Spatial learning (Morris water maze)	PND_{35}–PND_{40}
Dog	
Associative learning (olfactory)	PND_1–PND_6
Visual discrimination	5–16 weeks
Delayed response task	12–16 weeks
NHP	
Conditioned avoidance	PND_3–PND_8
Black–white discrimination task	PND_9–PND_{12}
Color, pattern, or shape discrimination	PND_{20}–PND_{150}
Delayed response task	PND_{60} (rudimentary performance)
	PND_{125}–PND_{135} (improved performance) and PND_{200}–PND_{250} (flawless performance)

according to specific situations. During the first year of life, the number of phrases increases to four or five, but never to seven or eight, as is heard in adulthood [10].

Assessment of communication development in juvenile toxicity studies in rats and dogs (and to some extent nonhuman primates) is unlikely to provide important insights because communication in these species appears to be primarily about expressing distress (Table 4.9). The development of language in humans is an important part of the maturation of the central nervous system.

6. *Social games*. Social games are a means by which individuals gain information about their social environment. By playing with peers, individuals learn norms of social communication, social dominance, and social integration, where performance of errors usually has neither aversive nor fatal consequences.

There are two forms of play in cynomolgus monkeys: action play and social play. As long as young monkeys are able to move easily (i.e., repeat actions such as jumping, running, and climbing), they can finish play behavior. At about 4 weeks of age, young monkeys can bounce on wire mesh. Young monkeys begin social play at about 5 weeks

Table 4.9 Summary of communication

Communication	Approximate postnatal age ability emerges
Human	
"Coos" in response to voices	2 months
Babble with inflection	8 months
Imitates sound	9–10 months
Can understand or say 2 or 3 words with meaning	12 months
Begins to join words together	21–24 months
Rat	
Ultrasonic vocalizations	PND_7–PND_9
USV (maximum)	PND_{13}
Dog	
Distress vocalizations	3–3.5 weeks
Whining vocalizations	4–5 weeks
NHP	
Emotional vocalizations (1 or 2 syllables)	0–6 months
Emotional vocalizations (3, 4, or 5 syllables)	6 months–1 year

Table 4.10 Summary of social play

Social play	Approximate postnatal age ability begins to emerge
Human	40 weeks to 1 year
Rat	PND_{14}–PND_{28}
Dog	3–5 weeks
NHP	5–9 weeks

of age. They avoid and chase older monkeys that are allowed to run freely around the room. Despite having plenty of food in their cages, infant monkeys at about 6 weeks of age begin stealing food from another cage, which is a well-established behavior for adult monkeys. Between 7 and 9 weeks of age, infant monkeys approach each other with open arms and gently pat each other, signaling the beginning of rough rolling and biting. Among juvenile cynomolgus monkeys, males generally prefer intense wrestling and fake biting more than females.

Assessment of social play development in juvenile toxicity studies may provide some insight. Postnatal development of social play in all common laboratory species such as rats, dogs, and NHP (Table 4.10). In conventional screening studies, methods for assessing social game development are complicated because cross-species methods are not easily compared.

7. *Development of fear response*. At about 2.5 months of age, infant monkeys separated from their mothers become agitated, make frequent distress calls, and show a marked increase in corticotropic hormone response. At the same time, infant monkeys also begin to show fear reactions to threatening images, strange objects, and new

things encountered at this age. If a person enters a caged monkey's room, the animal will become silent and stiff, both signs of fear of the unfamiliar.

There has been a great deal of work studying the central nervous system responses related to fear development. The stiffness response appears to be influenced by the gamma-aminobutyric acid system, while distress calls are influenced by the opioid system. Both the anterior cingulate cortex and the amygdala have a high density of opioid receptors, and both are involved in distress calls. At 2.5 months of age, ablation of the bilateral amygdala significantly reduces the fear response to new situations. Animals show fear of unfamiliar places, and it takes control animals three times as long to leave a familiar cage and enter an unfamiliar one as animals with a damaged amygdala. The monkeys with the amygdalotomy also show significantly less fear response to photos of monkey faces expressing fear.

The amygdala is involved in animal emotions and species-specific social behavior. In adult animals, the amygdala is involved in determining whether an object or organism is potentially dangerous. If the amygdala detects danger, it will coordinate various other brain regions to produce a typical avoidance response to avoid the danger. Thus, the amygdala contributes to understanding dangers in the environment. The amygdala of 2-week-old cynomolgus monkeys was selectively damaged, the cynomolgus monkeys were tested at 6–8 months of age, and the monkeys were observed to have a reduced fear of new objects, such as rubber snakes. During social interactions, the neurologically damaged animals showed more fearful behaviors than the uninjured control group. These studies suggest that amygdala damage in newborns separates the system mediating social fear from the system mediating fear of inanimate objects. Thus, damage to the amygdala in early development affects social behavior differently than damage produced in adulthood, by reducing fear of inanimate objects and increasing fear during social behavior.

Assessment of fear response development may provide some reference for juvenile toxicity studies, as fear response development occurs after birth in all common laboratory animal species (Table 4.11). Methods for assessing fear response development are not widely used in screening toxicity studies.

8. *Development of sleep cycles*. The sleep–wake cycle is acquired in many species and is generally considered to be a key behavior for cognitive development. In contrast to the sleep/wake patterns of adult monkeys, young monkeys are less defined. At 28 days of age, newborn monkeys already sleep more frequently at night than during the day. Although adult-like sleep–wake cycles can occur after birth, the use of sleep–wake cycles as a method in juvenile toxicity studies

Table 4.11 Summary of fear response

Fear response	Approximate postnatal age ability begins to emerge
Human	7–9 months
Rat	PND_{20}–PND_{30}
Dog	3–7 weeks
NHP	2.5–4 months

provides very limited insight because their development is unknown (Table 4.12).

4.2.2 The Skeletal System

Bone is a dynamic connective tissue, and postnatal skeletal development in all species reflects its multiple tasks in vivo. The bones of all mammals serve two major functions: to provide mechanical support as part of the locomotor apparatus, and to ensure a safe environment for the vital organs in the body. In addition, bone, as a store of calcium and phosphorus, is also involved in metabolic pathways related to mineral homeostasis. Bone matrix is also a reservoir of growth factors and cytokines released locally and systemically during bone resorption (autocrine, paracrine, and endocrine). Bone provides a safe and stable environment for bone marrow.

After birth, important features of bone growth are reflected in different types of bone. This section focuses on the postnatal growth and development of the upper limb bones (humerus, non-weight-bearing bone), lower limb bones (femur, weight-bearing bone), and craniofacial bones (mandible, non-weight-bearing bone with intermittent mechanical loading) [11].

When studying the time of the emergence and fusion of secondary ossification centers in rhesus monkeys, it will be noted that there are more ossification centers in monkeys than in humans at birth. In general, skeletal ossification in newborn rhesus monkeys is similar to that of a 5- to 6-year-old human. It takes 5.25 years for male and 6.5 years for female rhesus monkeys to complete limb ossification [12].

The postnatal ossification of the long and short bone centers occurs 12–20 months earlier in chimpanzees than in humans.

4.2.2.1 Humerus

Male rhesus monkeys are born with two separate ossification centers present in the epiphysis of the proximal humerus. In the epiphyseal region of the distal humerus, a secondary ossification center is present at birth. Two additional centers develop in the distal humerus during the first postnatal month. By 9 months after birth, the different centers of the proximal and distal epiphysis of the humerus form a single secondary ossification center within their respective regions. Fusion of the proximal epiphysis and diaphysis occurs at the age of 6 years in males and 4.75–5.5 years in females. The postnatal union of the distal epiphysis of the diaphysis occurs between 3.4 and

Table 4.12 Summary of sleep–wake cycle

"Semi-adultlike" sleep cycle	Approximate postnatal age ability begins to emerge
Human	3–15 months
Rat	PND_{15}–PND_{23}
Dog	2–4 weeks
NHP	2–8 days

4.5 years of age in male monkeys. Fusion of the distal epiphysis occurs in female monkeys within about 2 years after birth [13].

Table 4.13 shows the time of appearance and fusion of humeral epiphyses in rhesus and cynomolgus monkeys.

4.2.2.2 Femur

At birth, the rhesus monkey has epiphyseal ossification centers in the femoral head. The epiphyseal ossification center of the distal femur is also present at birth [14]. In addition, secondary ossification centers develop in the lesser trochanter of the femur at 6 months after birth.

In male rhesus monkeys, fusion of the proximal and distal femoral epiphysis occurs around 6 and 5.25 years of age, respectively. Fusion of the proximal and distal femoral epiphysis occurs at 4.75 years of age in female rhesus monkeys.

The time of the appearance of fusion in the femoral epiphysis of rhesus and cynomolgus monkeys is shown in Table 4.13.

Table 4.13 Timing of secondary ossification center appearance and epiphyseal fusion in rhesus and cynomolgus monkey

Bone	Male		Female	
	Secondary ossification center appearance	Epiphyseal fusion	Secondary ossification center appearance	Epiphyseal fusion
Rhesus monkey				
Humerus				
Proximal epiphysis	Birth	4–6 years	Birth	4–5.25 years
Distal epiphysis	Birth–1 month	2 years	Birth	1.75–2 years
Femur				
Proximal epiphysis				
Lesser trochanter	6 months	2.75–3.75 years	6 months	–
Head	Birth	3–3.75 years	Birth	2.25–3.25 years
Medial epicondyle	–	3–3.75 years	–	2.25–2.5 years
Distal epiphysis	Birth	4–5.75 years	Birth	3.25–4.25 years
Cynomolgus monkeys				
Humerus				
Proximal epiphysis	<5 months	6 years	<4 months	4.75–5.5 years
Distal epiphysis	<5 months	3.4–4.5 years	<4 months	2.25 years
Femur				
Proximal epiphysis	<5 months	6 years	<4 months	4.75 years
Distal epiphysis	<5 months	5.25 years	<4 months	4.75 years

4.2.2.3 Mandible

During the postnatal growth of the monkey mandible, a substantial increase in the overall dimensions of the mandible occurs due to a process of growth and remodeling from infancy to adulthood. Skeletal growth occurs on essentially all surfaces of the primate mandible during postnatal development.

The following discussion is mainly from a 1975 study by McNamara and Graber et al. [15], which mainly studied the development of the mandible in rhesus monkeys after birth. In this study, four groups of monkeys, of different ages, were evaluated for 6 consecutive months. Infant monkeys aged 5.5–7 months, juvenile monkeys aged 18–24 months, adolescent monkeys aged 45–54 months, and adult monkeys aged 72 months were included in the study.

The mandible of the rhesus monkey grows most rapidly during infancy. The growth rate of the mandibular condyle process is the fastest in the juvenile period, and the growth rate slows down with the aging of the animal. Specifically, condyle processes were 5.92, 4.47, 3.00, and 1.07 mm in infant, juvenile, adolescent, and adult monkeys, respectively, during the 6-month experimental observation period [16].

During postnatal development, bone deposition occurs along the posterior margin of the ramus, and bone resorption occurs along the anterior margin of the ramus. In infant monkeys (5.5–13 months of age), the width of the branches increased the most. Compared with animals older than 18 months of age, the posterior margin bone deposits of the mandibular branch in infant monkeys were four times higher than those of the anterior margin bones. As animals age, the posterior margin of ramus bone deposition decreases. The width of the mandibular ramus showed little variation in adult monkeys. In addition, bone deposits occur along the posterior margin of the condyle process.

Remodeling of the mandibular angle was observed in infant, juvenile, and adolescent monkeys. However, remodeling of the mandibular angle was not observed in adult monkeys. Juvenile monkeys showed the greatest change in mandibular angle during the 6-month observation period of the trial. The mandibular angles of infant, juvenile, and adolescent monkeys decreased by an average of 6.2°, 2.4°, and 1.7° during the 6-month observation period.

4.2.3 Tooth Eruption

Like other mammals, cynomolgus monkeys have two sets of teeth, namely 20 deciduous teeth and 32 permanent teeth: the first set is called the primary teeth or dentition, which precedes the second set of teeth; the second set of teeth is known as the permanent teeth or second dentition. These teeth are heteromorphic, and their shape varies according to their different functions, such as cutting, piercing, and grinding. Different tooth types are named, from the anterior midline to the posterior line, and the four types of teeth are incisors, canines, premolars, and molars, denoted as I (incisors), C (canines), P (premolars), and M (molars), respectively. It should be noted that molars are present only in the permanent dentitions of nonhuman primates. Permanent teeth are indicated in capital letters, and the number indicating the tooth position of the tooth type is usually followed by the letter name. For example, permanent incisors are abbreviated I, numbered backward from the midline, I1 for the central incisor, and I2 for the lateral incisor. Primary teeth are usually expressed by lowercase letters, preceded by "d" and followed by the sequence of numbers representing teeth, for example, d1 and d2 refer to primary central and lateral incisors, respectively [17].

Each animal species has a unique developmental pattern, with a specific sequence and a specific schedule for tooth formation and eruption. The crown is always formed before root extension. In nonhuman primates, there is considerable variation in the time of crown formation, as well as the sequence and schedule of eruptions. Before the permanent tooth replaces the deciduous tooth, the root of the deciduous tooth will be absorbed, and the crown of the deciduous tooth will be extruded by the replacement deciduous tooth. In general, the occlusal pair of teeth (upper and lower) erupts more or less simultaneously. Tooth eruption occurs when the root grows.

In many, but not all, nonhuman primate species, premolars are the first permanent teeth to develop. Premolars erupt before the deciduous teeth are replaced and are usually associated with weaning. In humans and many great apes, the third molar is the last to develop. However, this is not common in nonhuman primates. In species with strong dental dimorphism, there may be a pronounced "dimorphism," with males maturing later than females. This will affect the age of teething, especially permanent canine teeth.

Teeth keep an indelible record of their own development, which can be read from the microstructure of tooth enamel. Disruption of enamel matrix formation can lead to enamel defects or hypoplasia. Once the crowns are fully formed, the shape of the crown cannot be changed unless it is damaged and worn. Teeth of different animal species differ in enamel relative thickness and enamel prismatic structure, which may affect the functional life of teeth. In some species, even in the wild, the buccal crown normally wears down to the root of the tooth during an individual's lifetime. As enamel wears down and dentin is exposed, the first layer of dentin is replaced by a second, extending the functional life of the tooth [18].

At about 5 months of age, all the deciduous teeth of cynomolgus monkeys emerge, and at 4.5 years of age, all the deciduous teeth are replaced by permanent teeth. Usually, male monkeys have permanent teeth at about 6.5 years old, while females do not until about 7 years old. Since then, as the animal ages, the tooth surfaces of various types of teeth will be subjected to varying degrees of wear.

1. *Deciduous tooth order and age*. In cynomolgus monkeys, the first deciduous teeth are the lower and upper median incisors (I1), followed by the lateral incisors (I2). Males erupt 4 incisors around 22 days of age and 8 incisors at 45 days of age. The temporal order of deciduous canine and first premolar eruption is irregular. In general, males erupt deciduous canines and first deciduous premolars around 72 days after birth. Females erupt deciduous canines and first deciduous premolars correspondingly around 75 and 78 days of age.

The second premolar tooth of the mandible begins to appear in cynomolgus monkeys at the fourth month of life. The average time of tooth eruption in female monkeys is 139 days, the earliest is 105 days, and the latest is 228 days. The corresponding times of maxillary second premolar eruption are 154 days, 120 days, and more than 260 days. The average time of mandibular second molar eruption is 147 days, the earliest is 105 days, and the latest is 245 days. The corresponding times of maxillary second molar eruption were 152 days, 120 days, and greater than 260 days.

Typically, cynomolgus monkeys have full deciduous teeth about 5 months after birth. After that, there is an interval period of 8–20 months, that is, the tooth transition begins from 1 year and 3 months to 2 years old, and the first pair of permanent molars in the lower and upper jaws erupt.

The general rule of teething in deciduous teeth is that the same type of tooth appears almost at the same time on the left and right sides, but sometimes there are slight differences, or the left precedes the right, or the right precedes the left by several days. In addition, for incisors and second molars, the lower jaw usually precedes the upper jaw by several days, whereas for canines and first molars, the upper jaw precedes the lower jaw by several days.

2. *Eruption of dentate order 2-1-2-1.* In the permanent tooth series of cynomolgus monkeys, the mandibular first molar appears first, followed by the maxillary first molar. At the age of 2 years and 6 months, cynomolgus monkeys shed mandibular and maxillary incisors successively and give birth to permanent teeth. Usually, the mandibular incisors erupt 1–2 months before the maxillary incisors. This is the second stage of permanent tooth eruption.

3. *Eruption and three periods of permanent teeth in tooth order 2-1-2-2.* The second molar (M2) in the lower jaw of cynomolgus monkeys usually erupts at about 3.5 years of age. The second molar in the lower jaw erupts 1–2 months earlier than that in the upper jaw, which is the third period of permanent tooth eruption. At this point, the dentition has changed from 2-1-2-1 to 2-1-2-2. The fourth period of permanent tooth eruption is the loss of deciduous canines and premolars to replace permanent teeth, and the duration of this period is longer, and the time sequence of the replacement of canines and premolars to permanent teeth is not obvious. According to Hurme et al., all deciduous teeth are replaced by permanent teeth in female monkeys at about 4 years old, and in male monkeys at about 4 years and 5 months old.

4. *Eruption of the third molar.* After the cynomolgus monkey has all 2-1-2-2 permanent dentitions, the male monkey usually has to stagnate for 20 months, the female monkey has been stagnant for about 30 months before the third molar of the lower jaw begins to appear, and the third molar of the upper jaw is 3–6 months late, or even longer. In this way, the average male monkey is about 6.5 years old to produce a complete set of permanent teeth, while the female monkey is about 7 years old.

4.3 Characteristics of Pubertal Development of Cynomolgus Monkeys

The acquisition of mature reproductive functions is one of the most important and complex series of developmental processes in an organism's lifetime. The development of adolescence is a dynamic process involving the overlap of developmentally related indicators and the balance of physiology, and a high degree of variability can occur at the individual level.

4.3.1 Definitions of Terms

Puberty itself has many factors and interdependent processes and is a long-term process that does not occur at a steady rate. Some people define puberty as the end of the first menstrual period in humans, but important organ systems continue to develop after this time, and the onset of menstruation usually does not coincide with the first ovulation. Moreover, reproductive capacity has not been established in this period. There is some disagreement in the literature between toxicologists and pathologists on how to define and distinguish between puberty and sexual maturation. The Merriam–Webster dictionary defines it as follows.

Puberty ① A state or period marked by the maturation of reproductive organs and the development of secondary sexual characteristics, in which sexual reproduction is possible for the first time. Menstruation is first observed in humans and higher primates. ② The age of puberty in human boys is 13–16 years old, girls are 11–14 years old, and boys are usually 14 years old, and girls are 12 years old.

Sexual maturity: Sufficient maturity or development to produce children (i.e., offspring).

The definitions of puberty and sexual maturity in the US Webster's dictionary create potential confusion in the use of these terms because both include fecundity as a defining feature. The recent definition of puberty may also help to understand the definition of sexual maturity, i.e., "the transition from childhood to adulthood, with the emergence of adult characteristics, secondary sexual characteristics, and reproductive capacity considered to be the end of this period" [19].

The term puberty is considered a period of transition from childhood to adulthood (or immaturity to maturity), and sexual maturity is considered a state in which reproduction can be reliably carried out (implying the establishment of a normal functional ovarian cycle). Of course, it is important to note that not all women maintain a regular cycle all the time, even in adulthood. Thus, in this book, puberty is referred to as beginning at the time of neuroendocrine changes that drive the physiological changes of puberty, ending with the establishment of a functioning ovarian cycle in most females and the completion of physical development of all reproductive tissues.

4.3.2 Female Pubertal Development

A species comparison of key morphological and functional features of the postnatal development of the female reproductive system is shown in Table 4.14 and is outlined in Fig. 4.6. It includes the transition of the female reproductive system from puberty to sexual maturity and all aspects of reproductive decline/menopause.

Such comparisons are challenging because the processes involved and the sequence of events may differ between species [20]. Thus, this book simply uses a general description to assign a particular mean age to an event. Table 4.15 provides a species comparison of the type and time of the female ovarian reproductive cycle.

Table 4.14 Species comparison of endocrinologic, morphologic, and functional events during the postnatal development of the female reproductive system

Index		NHP	Dog	Rat	Human	Other
Puberty						
Neuroendocrine initiation of puberty		20–24 months (Rhesus)	<4 months	Before PND_{20}	10 years	Mouse PND_{15}–PND_{20}
Opening of the vaginal lumen		Prenatal	PND21	PND_{30}–PND_{36} (SD)	Prenatal	Mouse (CD-1) PND_{26}, Rabbit PND_{29}
Ovarian gonadarche: increased estradiol levels		2.5–3 years	7–10 months	–	–	Mouse (C57BL) PND_{28}
HPG axis established, i.e., onset of ovarian cycle		18 months–2.5 years, menarche	12 months	PND_{30} First Estrus	12–14 years, menarche	–
Onset of the ovulatory ovarian cycle, i.e., first ovulation		2.5–4 years	6–14 months	PND_{33}–PND_{46}	6 months after menarche	–
Breast development	Thelarche: beginning of pubertal breast development	Prior to the first menarche (macaques); during estrus of the first cycle	–	PND_{25}	9–12 years	–
	Completion of breast development	–	–	PND_{45}–PND_{55}	15 years	–
Attainment of sexual maturity						
Ability to reliably reproduce the onset of regular ovulatory ovarian cycle		3–5 years	12–24 months	PND_{65}	16–19 years	Minipig 6.5–7.5 months, Rabbit 4–5 months
Onset of reproductive senescence/menopause		20–30 years, menopause	–	Rat: 4–5 months (SD)	50 years, menopause	Mouse >10 months, Rabbit 1–3 years

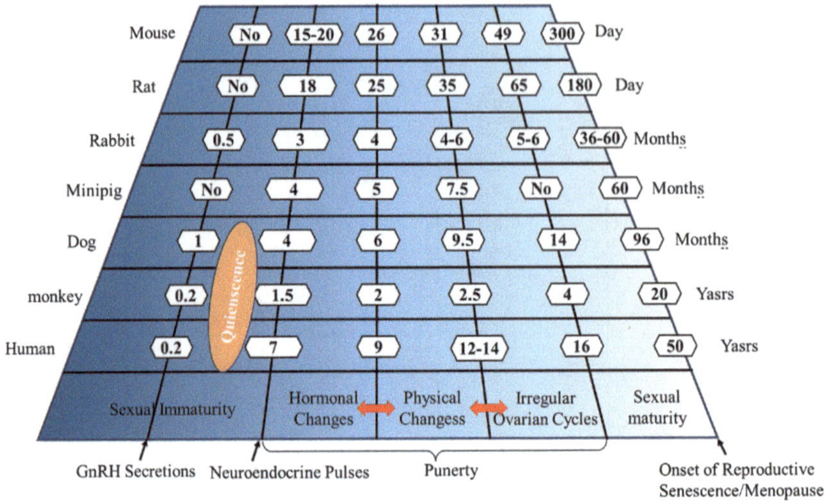

Fig. 4.6 Species comparison of the developmental timing of the female reproductive system

Note: To enable making comparisons across species, specific aspects and milestones of development were defined with more precision than is generally advisable. All comparisons should be considered imprecise, providing only a rough estimate of the order and timing of events. It should be noted that puberty is a continual process and not a series of defined events. Several of these milestone events occur over a span of time and involve overlapping processes. Additionally, there is a disparity between publications, likely due to strain, stock, or inter-animal differences and the methods of detection employed. NO indicates uncertainty.

4.3.3 Endocrinology of Female Reproductive System Development

(1) *Neuroendocrine system in early life and quiescent period.* Initially, the gonadotropin-releasing hormone (GnRH) secretion system develops and is transiently active during specific periods of fetal/neonatal development. In NHP animals, initial secretory activity occurs in early infancy (sometimes referred to as mini-puberty in males) [21]. In contrast to males, the GnRH pulse generator in newborn females is unable to produce GnRH release at the same frequency as in adult monkeys. Although a strong pulsatile pattern is established at the female fetal/neonatal age stage, the pattern is slower.

Thereafter, there is a resting quiescent period in the juvenile period, followed by a restart, marking the onset of puberty, which has been likened to neurobiological braking and release. This stationary phase is less pronounced in female monkeys than in males. Low levels of activity of the GnRH secretion system persist throughout early childhood, although they are not fully understood.

Table 4.15 Species comparison of type and developmental timing of female reproductive ovarian cycles

Species	Cycle type	Cycle length	Age at onset of cycle [parameter]	Age at first ovulation	Age at onset of regular cycles	Cycle detection method
Rat	Polyovulatory estrous cycle	4–5 days	PND_{30}	PND_{33}–PND_{46}	PND_{65}	Cytology of vaginal lavage
Mouse	Polyovulatory estrous cycle	4–5 days	CD-1: PND_{27}	CD-1: PND_{35}	PND_{49}	Cytology of vaginal lavage
Dog	Polyovulatory estrous cycle	5–7 months	$PNM_{6.5–14}$	12 months (8–16 months)		Vulvar: swelling and vaginal bleeding Hormones: Hormones and cytology of vaginal lavage
Minipig	Polyovulatory estrous cycle	21 days	4–6 months	6.5–7.5 months	–	Vaginal smear cytology
NHP	Monovulatory menstrual cycle	28–32 days	18 months	2.5–3 years	3–4 years	Daily vaginal swabs and hormones
Human	Monovulatory menstrual cycle	28 days	12–14 years	6 months after menarche	Within 5 years of menarche	Vaginal bleeding

(2) *Neuroendocrine system in puberty*. The hypothalamus is responsible for the "GnRH pulse generator" that generates intermittent GnRH discharges and is required for the onset of puberty [22]. In nonhuman primates, puberty is a secondary activation of the existing stationary GnRH pulse generator system. Because the synthesis of GnRH neurons is not limited by puberty, endogenous secretion of GnRH occurs much earlier in development. After a period of quiescence, even for several years in nonhuman primates, puberty can be seen as a reactivation of GnRH secretion.

From a neurobiological perspective, puberty has the function of controlling the nervous system changes in the release of GnRH. Puberty is not only a chronological age, but also affects the neurotransmitters and neuroregulatory systems of the GnRH secretion network to transmit information about metabolic status, energy storage, and somatic development. For many species, it also conveys information about the season and social environment [23]. Thus, it is particularly noteworthy that the onset and development of puberty vary considerably between individuals in most species, and in NHP and humans. In addition, further evidence suggests that specific signaling pathways differ between males and females.

Activation of GnRH secretion during puberty requires coordinated activation of synaptic and astroglial regulatory systems. Key to this process is the neuronal system that uses glutamate, transfer proteins, and gamma-aminobutyric acid as neurotransmitters. Astrocytes promote GnRH secretion through pathways initiated by growth factors that act directly or indirectly on GnRH neurons to stimulate neurosecretion. Studies have shown that epigenetic regulation affecting the transcriptional activity of neurons that stimulate GnRH release plays a fundamental role during puberty [24].

(3) *Establishment of hypothalamic–pituitary–ovarian axis during puberty*. At the beginning of puberty in female mammals, the HPG axis is activated, leading to GnRH release. This, in turn, activates LH release and the pituitary gonadotropin surge prior to the first ovulation. In response to gonadotropins, the ovaries begin to produce steroids, which marks the onset of pubertal ovarian maturation. Morohashi et al. described a two-step sexual differentiation process in the female mammalian gonad. The first step, independent of steroids, involves the differentiation of granulosa and thecal cells in the fetal ovary; in the second step, the ovary begins to produce higher concentrations of estradiol (E2), which is essential for the function of the ovary at later stages of maturation, while inducing extra-gonadal tissues, such as internal and external genitalia, brain, muscle, mammary glands and other phenotypes. The onset of gonadal function or ovarian function, marked by the ability of the ovaries to produce E2, is not apparent until puberty. This is in stark contrast to males, whose embryonic gonads produce a fair amount of androgens.

Humans and NHP eventually build a network of negative and positive feedback loops to complete the HPG axis. The onset of the ovarian cycle is accompanied by the establishment of a strong HPG axis and marks the beginning of hormonal regulatory fluctuations that send synchronized signals to endocrine reactive tissues [25]. Typically, several cycles are required before all tissues are synchronized and a normal reproductive cycle pattern is established.

4.3.4 Morphological Studies of the Development of the Female Reproductive System

(1) *Physiological characteristics of puberty*. NHP menarche has been reported to occur between the ages of 2.5 and 3, while reaching a more regular menstrual cycle may not occur until closer to the age of 4 [26]. This pattern is similar to that in humans, where prolonged anovulation is normal after menstrual bleeding [27].

(2) Development of the ovaries after birth.

Follicle maturation: During embryonic development, primordial germ cells migrate from the yolk sac to the gonad crest and populate the gonads. These primordial germ cells become oogonia and begin to cluster in an arrangement called a germ cell nest. After multiple rounds of mitosis, oogonia enter meiosis and primary oocytes arrest at the diploid stage of development [28]. Germ cell nests eventually disassemble and individualize to form primordial follicles.

In neonatal NHP, the ovary consists of dense primordial follicles within the cortex. On closer inspection, the oogonia are still evident, and mitosis can be observed. Oogonia can be observed alone or as part of a germ cell nest. Mitoses of oogonia can still be observed in 6-month-old cynomolgus monkeys and have been reported in 10-month-old rhesus monkeys. Follicular development begins slowly, and antral follicles usually appear by 6 months of age. In nonclinical young animal toxicity studies, many NHP are not fully mature, so many small to medium-sized follicles with varying degrees of atresia are common within the ovary, as well as an inactive endometrium [29]. Knowledge of these normal developmental features is critical when assessing NHP in this age group. In addition, large numbers of follicles are often seen in young macaque ovaries.

As NHP approaches puberty, there is continued follicular development, and because these follicles produce estrogen, rupture and bleeding of endometrial glands and stroma, squamous metaplasia within the cervix, and/or vaginal keratosis are observed microscopically in adolescent animals. Common is a similar pattern of change accompanying the corpus luteum remnant. Although this indicates evidence of at least one ovulation, it does not indicate sexual maturity and more likely reflects the long periods of anovulation described above in all young NHP [30].

In addition, NHP have anovulatory bleeding, so do not confuse endometrial bleeding with menstrual endometrial bleeding. Anovulatory cycles will have an inactive endometrium, with simple glands, and may have varying amounts of superficial bleeding, but most importantly, no new corpus luteum will be generated. In contrast, during menstruation, the endometrium is thick, the glands are complex cystic, bleeding is more pronounced, the stroma is ruptured, and the newly formed corpus luteum is present, and degenerative changes may occur [31]. Because bleeding may be part of an anovulatory cycle, the presence of a clinical bleeding event does not necessarily mean that ovulation has occurred.

(3) *Breast and mammary gland development after birth*. Rhesus monkeys also have unique nipple development, several months earlier than reaching a normal cycle. The mammary gland is a complex secretory organ composed of several different cell

types: epithelial cells that make up the mammary duct network, adipocytes that make up the fat pad, vascular endothelial cells that make up the blood vessels, stromal cells (including fibroblasts), and various immune cells [32].

4.3.5 Functional Aspects of Female Reproductive System Development

(1) *First ovulation*. The first ovulation usually marks the end of ovarian development, as the ovaries should be fully hormonal and have acquired the ability to release oocytes. Technically, the first ovulation can also signal reproductive competence, but reproduction also depends on the maturation of other reproductive tissues for proper implantation and support for pregnancy, so sexual maturity cannot be assumed (or tested) from the first ovulation alone. The only way to detect the age of sexual maturity (defined as reproductive capacity) with confidence is to house males and females in groups and monitor the first pregnancy.

(2) *Achieve normal ovulation cycle*. In most mammalian species, female reproductive functions are cycled periodically. The acquisition of reproductive competence in most females is associated with the first ovulation, which is also the decisive event of sexual maturation, because the first ovulation is usually the initiating event of the female reproductive cycle. However, the early reproductive cycle in females of most species is irregular and requires a period of time between the first ovulation and the establishment of a normal reproductive cycle. The single ovulation menstrual cycle of females is not regular until late puberty, although the first ovulation or menstruation occurs in early puberty. The cynomolgus monkey, which is the standard NHP species for toxicity studies, has a single ovulation cycle. In general, the menstrual cycle is the same as in humans, about 30 days.

4.3.6 Evaluation of Postnatal Reproductive Development of Female Laboratory Animals

(1) *In vivo observations*. Different endpoints are used to assess female reproductive development depending on the species. The menstrual cycle of NHP is easily counted by the detection of daily vaginal swabs. In addition, it is possible to monitor hormones that synchronize with the menstrual cycle; this work is tedious and complex and requires careful study design. In rodent studies, the typical design is to examine functional parameters of F1 generation, such as puberty and fertility, but this is not practical in NHP because sexual maturation takes 3–6 years (cynomolgus monkeys), following F1 to sexual maturity, and the birth of the F2 generation takes 4–8 years.

Sexual development milestones of NHP can be observed from appearance and followed by menarche and reproductive cycle, but there is a disconnection between these milestones. With the onset of menarche, this disconnect becomes more obvious at the age of 2–3 years. However, the first ovulation and regular menstrual cycle often occur months to years later. In nonhuman primates, secondary sexual characteristics include increased nipple volume. As the length of the vagina increases due to vaginal opening (VO), the anogenital distance decreases, and adolescent female monkeys exhibit genital swelling and redness.

(2) *Histological evaluation of reproductive system.* The histological features of adolescent animals are not easy to define, which is related to the overlap of features between immature and mature animals. Key histological features for determining immaturity in female animals include evidence of anovulation and evidence of the absence of the onset of menstrual cycles. Histological features in pubertal animals usually include one or both of the following: evidence of ovulation and/or evidence of the onset of the menstrual cycle [33]. Because of the variability in this age group, coupled with the disconnect between the clinical signs of puberty and the onset of the menstrual cycle, researchers often use the term "peripuberty" to emphasize puberty as a time window rather than an event to avoid confusion over definitions [34]. For example, NHP may have clinical evidence of bleeding and be clinically considered pubertal or even mature, but there may be no evidence of ovulation histologically, and in these cases, the term "peripuberty" seems to bridge these differences.

Key histological features for determining sexual maturation in a given animal include evidence of multiple ovulation and evidence of the current menstrual cycle. It is relatively easy to observe these two criteria in rats, mice, and pigs because once the circulation is established, evidence of circulation is evident. This is different from the situation in NHP, dogs, and rabbits. Because of the relatively high incidence of anovulatory cycles in mature NHP, the evidence for monitoring the menstrual cycle is not always reliable [35]. Although age is not recommended as an independent determinant of sexual maturation, in these anovulatory NHP, age may be useful as part of the evidence to determine whether a given animal is at puberty or sexually mature.

4.3.7 Male Pubertal Development

Male puberty is usually defined by gross anatomical changes alone, such as preputial separation (PPS). However, others may be defined on the basis of histological changes, such as sperm in the epididymis, or hormonal changes [36, 37]. Most importantly, development is an ongoing process and is not considered to be a defined series of events. Because of this, it is difficult to accurately determine the exact timing of the different developmental stages.

Comparisons between species are difficult because different species use different developmental stage protocols. NHP is divided into six developmental stages (Stages 1–6) [38], whereas rats are divided into four stages (from neonatal to peripubertal) and pigs into three stages (immature, peripubertal/transition, and mature). Furthermore, these stage protocols are not specific to any one system and, therefore, may not correspond to gross or microscopic changes in the male reproductive tract. For example, developmental stages in human infancy and childhood are not closely related to testicular morphological changes because the testes are quiescent. Table 4.16 summarizes the major morphological and endocrine events occurring in the various animal species and humans [39].

Table 4.16 Morphologic and endocrinologic timepoints during development of the male reproductive system

Index	Cynomolgus monkeys	Dog	Rat	Human
Gestation length	164 days (cynomolgus); 143–153 days (marmoset)	63 days	21 days	39 weeks
Sex determination	–	35–36 days	GD_{12}	GW_{7}
T production	–	–	Onset $GD_{14.5}$–$GD_{15.5}$, Peaks GD_{18}	Onset GW_{8} begins, Peaks GW_{11}–GW_{14}
LH production starts	–	–	$GD_{17.5}$	GW_{12}
HPG components established	–	–	GD_{19}	GW_{12}
Gonadotropin control over testis established	>GD_{80} (rhesus)	–	PND_{10}	HCG: GW_{7}; LH: >GW_{20}
Gonocyte mitotic hiatus	–	–	Yes, GD_{18}–birth (Up to PND_{3})	No
MPW	GW_{7}–GW_{15} (marmoset); GD_{35}–GD_{90} (cynomolgus)	–	$GD_{15.5}$–$GD_{17.5}$	GW_{9}–GW_{14}
Male:female AGD is maximum	–	–	Birth	GW_{17}–GW_{20}
Testicular descent	At birth	Starts $PND_{3\ or\ 4}$ and is completed 5–6 weeks of age	Phase I: GD_{19} Phase II: PND_{15}	Phase I: GW_{15} Phase II: GW_{25}–GW_{35}
Preputial separation	2.53 years (rhesus)	PND_{51}	43 days	9 months–3 years
MB	–	–	GD_{18}–PND_{10}	Perinatal (specific start/end unknown)
Mini-puberty	<4 months	–	0–6 h	3–6 months
Stages of development	Neonatal (0–1 months) Infantile (1–12 months) Juvenile (12–24 months) Peripubertal (2–5 years)	Neonatal (0–3 weeks) Infantile (3–6 weeks) Juvenile (6–24 weeks) Peripubertal (24–37 weeks)	Neonatal (0–PND_{7}) Infantile (PND_{8}–PND_{20}) Juvenile (PND_{21}–PND_{32}) Peripubertal (PND_{33}–PND_{60})	Neonatal (0–28 days) Infantile (28 days–2 years) Juvenile (2–11 years) Peripubertal (11–14 years)

Table 4.16 (Continued)

Index	Cynomolgus monkeys	Dog	Rat	Human
Burst of spermatogonial/ sertoli cell proliferation	–	18–20 weeks	PND_5–PND_{15}	9–11 years
BTB forms and spermatocyte differentiation begins	–	20 weeks	PND_{18}	12–13 years
Quiescence	4–11 months (marmoset); <38 months (cynomolgus)	3–18 weeks	None	3–9 years
Maturation of the testis	Lobule by lobule	Diffuse	Diffuse	Lobule by lobule
Epididymis–phases of maturation	–	–	Undifferentiation: 0–PND_{14} Differentiation: PND_{15}–PND_{44} Expansion: >PND_{44}	–
Prostate	Secretion starts postnatal	Secretion starts postnatal	Secretion starts PND_{15} Adult histology by PND_{28}	Secretion starts: GW_{15}–GW_{18}

1. *Testis*. The basic sequence of testicular maturation in all mammals, includes (in chronological order) the formation of the spermatic cord containing gonad cells before birth, The transformation of gonadal cells into spermatogonia, a large number of sertoli cells and spermatogonia proliferated, sertoli cell maturation and blood–testis barrier (BTB) formation, spermatocyte development (i.e., meiosis), spermatogenesis (the formation of round and elongated sperm cells). In cynomolgus monkeys, testicular maturation occurs over a period of several months.

In NHP, the testes develop more like humans before and after birth: The same quiescent phase as humans; the testis develops in a lobular pattern similar to that in humans [40]; cell proliferation does not stop during the perinatal period; Gonadal development is dependent on hCG and LH before birth. In rhesus monkeys, GD_{80} testes are under the control of pituitary gonadotrophins.

Weinbauer et al. reported that [41] the developmental stages of cynomolgus monkeys are divided into newborn (0–1 month), infant (1–12 months), juvenile (12–24 months), and adolescent (2–5 years). However, as in humans, these stages are prevalent in multiple organ systems and have no significant correlation with the microscopic development of the testis. It is not possible to correlate these brief developmental stages with microscopic changes in the testis, which are associated with quiescent periods occurring in the early stages and variability between animals. Unlike this temporal staging scheme used in rats and humans, the microscopic evaluation of monkey testicles is based on the scheme of a grade 1 (immature) to grade 6 (adult). In order to compare rats with NHP, Table 4.17 compares the microscopic results of different grades of cynomolgus monkeys with the microscopic results of temporal developmental stages of rats.

There are two points to note in Table 4.17. First, the age of the cynomolgus monkeys does not tell the level or stage of testicular development; second, the period of up to 38 months in NHP (equivalent to neonatal and infancy in rats) may include a quiescent period. There is no literature on the profiles of gonadotropins in cynomolgus monkeys during the first 38 months of life. The quiescent phase of cynomolgus monkeys has not received enough attention. Part of the reason is that most research on cynomolgus monkeys has focused on the timing of sexual maturity [42, 43]. Because the ideal nonclinical toxicity study requires the examination of sexually mature males. As a result, the microscopic details of the neonatal, infantile, or quiescent phases are largely ignored.

There is a wide range of variability in testicular development in cynomolgus monkeys: the testicles of a 4-year-old cynomolgus monkey can be at any stage from grade 1 (immature) to grade 6 (adult). In addition, there is interspecies (rhesus, marmoset, and cynomolgus) and strain variation (Mauritian and Asian cynomolgus). These changes, together with the maturation of one leaflet, may explain the seemingly different reports in the literature regarding the stage and timing of maturation.

In NHP, there is a strong association between body weight and puberty. It has been proven that most cynomolgus monkeys are at puberty if they are over 5 years of age and weigh no less than 5 kg, or if a single testicle weighs more than 8 g (grade 4).

Table 4.17 Comparison of testicular stages used in cynomolgus NHP and rat

Developmental stage(NHP, cynomolgus)and grade scale	Approximate age ofcynomolgus monkey(months)	Characteristic microscopic feature described in the cynomolgus monkey	Equivalent "rat" developmental stage based on these same microscopic features of the testis
Immature, grade 1	0–38	No lumen	Neonatal and infantile
Prepubertal, grade 2	38–43	Lumen and early spermiogenesis	Juvenile
Onset of puberty, grade 3	44–76	Round and elongated spermatids are present	Peripubertal (early)
Puberty, grade 4		Complete spermiogenesis in some tubules and a few to moderate sperm in the epididymides	Peripubertal (late)
Early adult, grade 5		Complete spermiogenesis throughout the testes and abundant sperm in the epididymides	Adult

Smedley et al. [42] reported similar findings that 90% of male cynomolgus monkeys will reach sexual maturity if they weigh at least 5.3 kg and are at least 5.5 years old.

There are some strain differences in the timing of sexual maturation in cynomolgus monkeys. Mauritian cynomolgus monkeys mature sexually about 2 years earlier than macaques from mainland Asia. Mauritian monkeys are larger animals than the cynomolgus monkeys of the Asian continent, and they have larger testicles.

2. *Seminiferous duct.* The seminiferous duct, a continuation of the epididymis, is a muscular conduit responsible for transporting sperm from the epididymis to the ejaculatory duct (Fig. 4.7). It arises from the mesonephric duct (or Wolffian duct), the same origin as the epididymis and seminal vesicles. As with the epididymis and seminal vesicles, testosterone is required for their development, and seminiferous duct agenesis may occur after exposure to antiandrogens such as phthalates or AR antagonists such as flutamide before birth [44].

This schematic shows the embryologic origin and hormonal regulation of male reproductive structures. Mesonephric (Wolffian) duct-derived structures (epididymis, vas deferens, seminal vesicles) depend on fetal Leydig cell-produced testosterone (T) during the MPW. Urogenital sinus-derived structures (prostate, bulbourethral glands, prepuce/penis) rely primarily on dihydrotestosterone (DHT), which also drives fetal nipple regression. Testicular descent involves gubernacular changes; the first transabdominal phase depends on fetal Leydig cell-produced INSL-3.

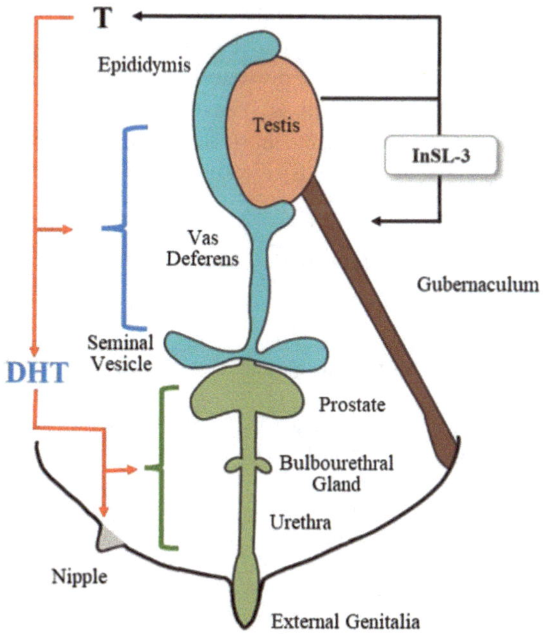

Fig. 4.7 Hormonal control of male reproductive system development

3. *Seminal vesicle.* The development of the seminal vesicles is slightly behind that of the prostate. Seminal vesicles develop from the Wolffian duct and are dependent on the development of testosterone (Fig. 4.7). The seminal vesicle cavity of cynomolgus monkeys is narrow, lined with flat epithelial cells, and the mucosal epithelium of grades 1–3 (immature, prepubertal, and onset of puberty) is simply folded. Only when the animal reaches grade 4 (puberty), the accumulation of secretions in the cavity increases and the epithelial cell layer develops and folds further.

4. *Prostate embryologically.* The prostate develops from the genitourinary sinus of the endoderm (Fig. 4.7). This is in contrast to the seminal vesicles, epididymis, and seminiferous duct, which develop from the Wolffian duct of the mesoderm. This source of the prostate may result in higher morbidity and abnormal growth compared with other tissues in the male reproductive tract. The major androgen responsible for prostate development is dihydrotestosterone. However, testosterone and estrogen also play a role. During early differentiation, stromal cells of the prostate express αER, and the glandular epithelium expresses β-ER [45].

The external gross and microscopic lobulation of the prostate in humans and laboratory animals are different, and Table 4.18 summarizes these anatomical differences.

The cynomolgus monkey prostate is similar to that of humans, but there is no glandular cavity at the immature stage (grade 1), an early glandular cavity forms at the prepubertal stage (grade 2), and a complete glandular cavity forms at the onset of puberty (grade 3). After that, it reaches morphological maturity (grade 4). Near puberty, the weight of the prostate and seminal vesicles surges. Thus, the maturation process of the cynomolgus monkey prostate is more similar to that of humans than in rats, as no prostatic fluid is secreted until after birth.

5. *Bulbourethral gland.* The bulbourethral gland arises from the urogenital sinus and is the same structure that gives rise to the prostate, bladder, and urethra (Fig. 4.7). This gland, also known as the Cowper gland, is a pea-shaped exocrine gland located near the urethra. Its main function is to secrete lubricating mucus. These glands are androgen-dependent tissues that require dihydrotestosterone for development. However, AR

Table 4.18 Comparison of anatomic features of prostate/seminal vesicles

Index	Human/NHP	Rat/mouse	Rabbit	Dog
Prostate	Three zones[a] • One median • Two laterals	Three paired lobes: (six total) • Dorsocranial (coagulating gland) • Ventral lobe • Dorsolateral Ventral	Four lobes: • Dorsocranial • Two laterals • Dorsocaudal	Two paired lobes: (four total) • Dorsocranial • Lateral
Gross lobulation of the prostate	No	Yes (mild)	Yes (mild)	Yes (between lateral lobes)
Seminal vesicle	Yes	Yes	None	None

Note: [a] Prenatally, five anatomical lobes evident in human prior to GW 20, two lobes regress, leaving only three at birth; gland capable of secretion unlike in rat, NHP, and dog where secretions occur postnatally blockers such as flutamide will alter dihydrotestosterone (DHT) mediated growth of the bulbourethral gland, as flutamide does for other DHT-dependent tissues.

6. *Masculinization programming window (MPW).* The MPW is a sensitive period of early prenatal development that initiates and "controls" the proper development and growth of the internal and external male genitalia and the perineum. It is during MPW that disturbed androgen levels will lead to testicular dysgenesis syndrome (TDS), including changes such as penile malformation (i.e., hypospadias), cryptorchidism, smaller testes, decreased sperm volume, smaller penis during puberty, decreased testosterone levels, smaller prostate, decreased AGD, etc. [46].

There is a distinction between sexual differentiation and masculinization. Sexual differentiation occurs prior to masculinization and is the period of recognizable testis formation and fetal sex that can be morphologically distinguished as male. Masculinization refers to the subsequent phenotypic transformation of the fetus (Testis with endocrine function) into a male. Masculinization includes not only the initial degeneration of the Mullerian duct in response to anti-Mullerian hormone, but also the differentiation of the internal (epididymis, seminiferous duct, seminal vesicles, and prostate) and external (penis, scrotum, and perineum) genitalia. Phthalates, pesticides, and therapeutic agents such as steroid hormones, statins, and glitazone may inhibit testosterone production during MPW, resulting in TDS; therefore, MPW has received considerable attention in recent years [47].

Few studies have identified MPW in NHP. In cynomolgus monkeys, seminiferous tubules were formed at GW_{79}, indicating that MPW occurred at or shortly after this period (approx. GW_{89}; 164 days or 5.5 months of gestation). The time point of MPW in cynomolgus monkeys has been confirmed by the study.

7. *External genitalia.* The male external genitalia include the penis and scrotum, and their normal development and growth depend on the appropriate exposure of androgens during MPW, as well as the continued exposure of androgens during puberty. DHT, an androgen produced from testosterone in response to 5α-reductase, is the major androgen controlling external genital differentiation and growth (Fig. 4.7). While a small penis at birth or adolescence may indicate inadequate androgen exposure after MPW, inadequate androgen exposure during MPW has more dire consequences and results in more severe external genital phenotypic changes. During the first to second trimester of NHP pregnancy, the penis develops during MPW. GD_{39-90} is the masculinization time of the Wolffian duct in rhesus monkeys.

The administration of finasteride (an inhibitor that converts testosterone to the key 5α reductase of DHT) will result in a smaller penis and a dysplastic scrotum, suggesting that both testosterone and DHT play key roles in masculinization of the male external genitalia. The administration of flutamide (an AR blocker) in the first trimester (gestational GD_{35-70}) rather than the second trimester (gestational $GD_{115-155}$) has the same effect. Exposed to high doses of testosterone during early pregnancy (GD_{39-90}), female fetuses exhibit complete masculinization at birth. However, female fetuses develop normally when exposed to the same treatment late in pregnancy ($GD_{115-139}$), highlighting the androgen sensitivity of MPW and its influence on external genital development [48].

8. *Testicular descent*. The cryptorchidism is connected to the diaphragm through the cranial suspensory ligament. Ligaments degenerate, with concomitant enlargement of the proper inguinal band (the inguinal scrotal tail ligament that connects the testes to the lower abdomen). As the peritoneum widens, it gradually shortens, allowing the testis to enter the scrotum.

Testicular descent has different control mechanisms, depending on whether it occurs at an earlier abdominal stage or a later inguinal scrotal stage. Transabdominal descent is controlled by InSL3 and androgens produced by fetal interstitial cells (Fig. 4.7). However, the testicular inguinal region requires a thick and less elastic inguinal gland, whereas adjacent organs such as the kidney are allowed to move anteriorly and posteriorly. The inguinal scrotal descent is controlled by androgens and is controlled by the HPG axis. These androgens control the release of calcitonin gene-related peptide through the genitofemoral nerve, which assists the testis in guiding the testis to the scrotum [49].

Either the first or the second stage of testicular descent failure will result in congenital cryptorchidism. Endocrine disturbances during MPW are a cause of cryptorchidism; other causes include primary hormone deficiency, dysfunction of the HPG axis controlling the second descending phase, or possibly due to anatomical defects [50].

As in humans, testicular descent in cynomolgus monkeys occurs before birth at the end of gestation. Soon after birth, however, the testes will rise back into the inguinal canal. At about 3 years of age, the testis descends again, along with an increase in volume.

9. Masculinization of the brain In NHP, brain masculinization occurs late in gestation, but exactly when and for how long is not known.

10. Micropuberty micropuberty (MB) is a period of the neonatal period characterized by transient surges in GnRH, serum LH, and serum testosterone. It is triggered by a sudden decrease in maternal sex hormones, stimulating gonadotropin levels in the newborn. Male fetuses in the third trimester will be exposed to high concentrations of androgens (from the testis) and estrogens (from the placenta). Maternal hormones are suddenly reduced at birth, and the HPG axis of newborns is released under the inhibitory effect of maternal estrogens. Micropuberty is also important for normal spermatogenesis and maturation of the internal and external genitalia.

Micropuberty is found in NHP, where a testosterone surge is evident during the first 4 months of life. Although studies are limited, there is no clear association between this micropuberty and sex-related behavior in rhesus monkeys [51, 52]. However, the hormone surge during micropuberty is important for normal spermatogenesis and testicular development in male monkeys.

11. *Hypothalamic–pituitary–gonadal (HPG) axis*. The HPG axis controls sexual maturation and the transition from juvenile to adult state. The components of the HPG axis include GnRH in the hypothalamic arcuate nucleus, pituitary gonadotropins (LH, FSH, and prolactin), and steroid hormones (mainly androgens) released by the testicular gonadotropin response elements (Leydig cells and Sertoli cells). The basic mechanism of the occurrence of the HPG axis is conserved in most species. HPG is formed before birth but does not mature until the onset of puberty.

The maturation of the HPG axis can be divided into three steps. The first is the formation of its components, which usually occurs before the birth of all species. The second is gonadal-induced masculinization of the brain, during which the hypothalamus is programmed into a male HPG axis with tonic beats; The third is the biochemical/phenotypic maturation of the hypothalamic glial network before puberty.

Maturation of the HPG axis in NHP occurs before the onset of puberty. However, some specific features of the HPG axis and endocrine regulation differ in the marmoset. The pituitary gland of the marmoset does not produce LH, but it produces the β subunit of chorionic gonadotropin (βCG), the only gonadotropin with LH activity in the marmoset [53, 54]. Exogenous GnRH can not increase the level of gonadotropin or testosterone in marmosets. There is no direct correlation between the pituitary BCG vaccine and testosterone level. Testosterone production is apparently regulated by events other than βCG levels; however, sex hormone binding globulin has a lower affinity for testosterone. This low affinity of binding globulins may partly explain the erratic testosterone levels observed in developmental traits of marmosets after birth. Testosterone levels in marmosets are relatively high: usually 20–40 ng/dL, while testosterone levels in Old World monkeys are 3–9 ng/dL and 10 ng/dL in humans. Although the details of the HPG axis of the marmoset are not fully understood, there are high βCG and high testosterone levels at 70 weeks of sexual maturity.

Ethical Approval

This chapter is a review of previously published accounts; as such, no animal or human studies were performed.

References

1. Kang Y (2020) Early embryonic development and disease models in non-human primates. Kunming Univ Sci Technol https://doi.org/10.27200/d.cnki.gkmlu.2020.000323
2. Martin PL, Weinbauer GF (2010) Developmental toxicity testing of biopharmaceuticals in nonhuman primates: previous experience and future directions. Int J Toxicol 29(6):552–568
3. Derelanko MJ, Hollinger MA (2001) Handbook of toxicology. CRC Press
4. Wood SL, Beyer BK, Cappon GD (2003) Species comparison of postnatal CNS development: functional measures. Birth Defects Res B 68(5):391–407
5. Golub MS (1990) Use of monkey neonatal neurobehavioral test batteries in safety testing protocols. Neurotoxicol Teratol 12(5):537–541
6. Golub MS, Eisele JH, Donald JM (1991) Effect of intrapartum meperidine on the behavioral consequences of neonatal oxygen deprivation in rhesus monkey infants. Dev Pharmacol Therap 16:231–240
7. Lemon RN (1999) Neural control of dexterity: what has been achieved?. Exp Brain Res 128(1):6–12
8. Olivier E, Edgley SA, Armand J et al (1997) An electrophysiological study of the postnatal development of the corticospinal system in the macaque monkey. J Neurosci 17(1):267–276
9. Yamaguchi K, Harada S, Kanemaru N et al (2001) Age-related alteration of taste bud distribution in the common marmoset. Chem Senses 26(1):1–6

10. Herschkowitz N, Kagan J, Zilles K (1997) Neurobiological bases of behavioral development in the first year. Neuropediatrics 28(06):296–306
11. Michejda M (1980) Growth standards in the skeletal age of rhesus monkey (*M. mulatta*) chimpanzee (*Pan tryglodytes*) and man. Dev Biol Standard 45:45–50
12. Van Wagenen G, Asling CW (1958) Roentgenographic estimation of bone age in the rhesus monkey (*Macaca mulatta*). Am J Anat 103(2):163–185
13. Fukuda S, Cho F, Honjo S (1978) Bone growth and development of secondary ossification centers of extremities in the cynomolgus monkey (*Macaca fascicularis*). Exp Anim 27(4):387–397
14. Fukuda S, Matsuoka O (1980) Comparative studies on maturation process of secondary ossification centers of long bones in the mouse, rat, dog and monkey. Exp Anim 29(3):317–326
15. McNamara JrJA, Graber LW (1975) Mandibular growth in the rhesus monkey (*Macaca mulatta*). Am J Phys Anthropol 42(1):15–24
16. Turpin DL (1968) Growth and remodeling of the mandible in the *Macaca mulatta* monkey. Am J Orthod 54(4):251–271
17. Zeng Z, Bai S, Chen Y (1984) Relation in the tooth sequence, age and ontogeny of rhesus monkeys (*Macaca mulatta*). Acta Theriol Sin 4(2):81–87
18. Zeng Z, Bai S, Qian R et al (1980) Development of deciduous teeth in rhesus monkeys (*Macaca mulatta*). Chin J Zool 4:1416
19. De Silva NK, Tschirhart J (2016) Puberty-defining normal and understanding abnormal. Curr Treat Opt Pediatr 2(3):121–130
20. Laffan SB, Posobiec LM, Uhl JE et al (2018) Species comparison of postnatal development of the female reproductive system. Birth Defects Res 110(3):163–189
21. Plant TM (2001) Neurobiological bases underlying the control of the onset of puberty in the rhesus monkey: a representative higher primate. Fronti Neuroendocrinol 22(2):107–139
22. Grumbach MM (2002) The neuroendocrinology of human puberty revisited. Hormone Res Paediatr 57(Suppl 2):2–14
23. Ebling FJP (2005) The neuroendocrine timing of puberty. Reproduction 129(6):675–683
24. Morohashi K, Baba T, Tanaka M (2013) Steroid hormones and the development of reproductive organs. Sex Dev 7(1-3):61–79
25. Ojeda SR, Roth C, Mungenast A et al (2006) Neuroendocrine mechanisms controlling female puberty: new approaches, new concepts. Int J Androl 29(1):256–263
26. Weinbauer GF, Niehoff M, Niehaus M et al (2008) Physiology and endocrinology of the ovarian cycle in macaques. Toxicol Pathol 36(7_suppl):7S–23S
27. Weinbauer GF, Fuchs A, Niehaus M et al (2011) The enhanced pre-and postnatal study for nonhuman primates: update and perspectives. Birth Defects Res C 93(4):324–333
28. Wear HM, McPike MJ, Watanabe KH (2016) From primordial germ cells to primordial follicles: a review and visual representation of early ovarian development in mice. J Ovarian Res 9(1):1–11
29. Pepling ME (2012) Follicular assembly: mechanisms of action. Reproduction 143(2):139–149
30. Buse E, Zöller M, Van Esch E (2008) The macaque ovary, with special reference to the cynomolgus macaque (*Macaca fascicularis*). Toxicol Pathol 36(7_suppl):24S–66S
31. Bussiere JL, Moffat G, Zhou L et al (2013) Assessment of menstrual cycle length in cynomolgus monkeys as a female fertility endpoint of a biopharmaceutical in a 6 month toxicity study. Regul Toxicol Pharmacol 66(3):269–278
32. Cline JM, Wood CE (2008) The mammary glands of macaques. Toxicol Pathol 36(7_suppl):130S–141S
33. Vidal JD (2017) The impact of age on the female reproductive system: a pathologist's perspective. Toxicol Pathol 45(1):206–215
34. Golub MS, Hogrefe CE, Germann SL et al (2003) Effects of exogenous estrogenic agents on pubertal growth and reproductive system maturation in female rhesus monkeys. Toxicol Sci 74(1):103–113

35. Halpern WG, Ameri M, Bowman CJ et al (2016) Scientific and regulatory policy committee points to consider review: inclusion of reproductive and pathology end points for assessment of reproductive and developmental toxicity in pharmaceutical drug development. Toxicol Pathol 44(6):789–809
36. Wistuba J, Schrod A, Greve B et al (2003) Organization of seminiferous epithelium in primates: relationship to spermatogenic efficiency, phylogeny, and mating system. Biol Reprod 69(2):582–591
37. Chandolia RK, Luetjens CM, Wistuba J et al (2006) Changes in endocrine profile and reproductive organs during puberty in the male marmoset monkey (*Callithrix jacchus*). Reproduction 132(2):355–363
38. Haruyama E, Suda M, Ayukawa Y et al (2012) Testicular development in cynomolgus monkeys. Toxicol Pathol 40(6):935–942
39. Picut CA, Ziejewski MK, Stanislaus D (2018) Comparative aspects of pre-and postnatal development of the male reproductive system. Birth Defects Res 110(3):190–227
40. Dreef HC, Van Esch E, De Rijk EPCT (2007) Spermatogenesis in the cynomolgus monkey (*Macaca fascicularis*): a practical guide for routine morphological staging. Toxicol Pathol 35(3):395–404
41. Weinbauer GF, Chellman GJ, Rasmussen AD et al (2012) Use of primate pediatric model. Pediatric nonclinical drug testing: pediatric nonclinical drug testing: principles, requirements, and practices, pp 255–279
42. Smedley JV, Bailey SA, Perry RW et al (2002) Methods for predicting sexual maturity in male cynomolgus macaques on the basis of age, body weight, and histologic evaluation of the testes. J Am Assoc Lab Anim Sci 41(5):18–20
43. Luetjens CM, Weinbauer GF (2012) Functional assessment of sexual maturity in male macaques (*Macaca fascicularis*). Regul Toxicol Pharmacol 63(3):391–400
44. Gray JrLE, Furr J, Tatum-Gibbs KR et al (2016) Establishing the "biological relevance" of dipentyl phthalate reductions in fetal rat testosterone production and plasma and testis testosterone levels. Toxicol Sci 149(1):178–191
45. Prins GS, Birch L (1997) Neonatal estrogen exposure up-regulates estrogen receptor expression in the developing and adult rat prostate lobes. Endocrinology 138(5):1801–1809
46. Scott HM, Mason JI, Sharpe RM (2009) Steroidogenesis in the fetal testis and its susceptibility to disruption by exogenous compounds. Endocrine Rev 30(7):883–925
47. Johnson KJ, Heger NE, Boekelheide K (2012) Of mice and men (and rats): phthalate-induced fetal testis endocrine disruption is species-dependent. Toxicol Sci 129(2):235–248
48. Herman RA, Jones B, Mann DR et al (2000) Timing of prenatal androgen exposure: anatomical and endocrine effects on juvenile male and female rhesus monkeys. Hormones Behav 38(1):52–66
49. Hutson JM, Southwell BR, Li R et al (2013) The regulation of testicular descent and the effects of cryptorchidism. Endocrine Rev 34(5):725–752
50. Hutson JM, Li R, Southwell BR et al (2013) Germ cell development in the postnatal testis: the key to prevent malignancy in cryptorchidism?. Front Endocrinol 3:176
51. Hurd PL, Vaillancourt KL, Dinsdale NL (2011) Aggression, digit ratio and variation in androgen receptor and monoamine oxidase a genes in men. Behav Genetics 41(4):543–556
52. Pasterski V, Acerini CL, Dunger DB et al (2015) Postnatal penile growth concurrent with mini-puberty predicts later sex-typed play behavior: evidence for neurobehavioral effects of the postnatal androgen surge in typically developing boys. Hormones Behav 69:98–105
53. Muller T, Simoni M, Pekel E et al (2004) Chorionic gonadotrophin beta subunit mRNA but not luteinising hormone beta subunit mRNA is expressed in the pituitary of the common marmoset (*Callithrix jacchus*). J Mol Endocrinol 32(1):115–128
54. Luetjens CM, Weinbauer GF, Wistuba J (2005) Primate spermatogenesis: new insights into comparative testicular organisation, spermatogenic efficiency and endocrine control. Biol Rev 80(3):475–488

Check for updates

Reproductive System Pathology of Cynomolgus Monkey

5

Yanjun Cui

Abstract

In nonclinical safety assessment studies, animal age determines not only whether the reproductive system is developmentally mature but also the interpretive framework for histopathological findings. In large animals, especially nonhuman primates, individual differences in the timing of sexual maturation can be substantial. If control and treated animals are not adequately matched for age, sexual maturity, or reproductive-cycle status, it becomes difficult for pathologists to distinguish normal development or physiological fluctuations, background findings, and test-article–related reproductive toxicity. This chapter focuses on the cynomolgus monkey (*Macaca fascicularis*), a species commonly used in nonclinical safety evaluation, and systematically describes the normal anatomy and histology of the male and female reproductive systems. It summarizes the morphological features of the ovary, uterus, vagina/vulva, testis, epididymis, vas deferens, prostate, and seminal vesicles across stages of sexual development. The chapter also reviews common spontaneous or background changes in this species. By integrating these findings with reproductive-system changes that may be misinterpreted as test-article related in practice, the chapter further discusses a comprehensive approach to differentiating background lesions from treatment-related alterations based on temporal sequence, dose relationship, sex/organ selectivity, reversibility, concordance with functional endpoints, and class-specific compound knowledge.

Keywords

Reproductive system · Cynomolgus monkey · Nonclinical safety evaluation · Sexual maturity · Normal histology · Pathologic changes

Y. Cui (✉)
Hubei Topgene Biotechnology Co. Ltd., Wuhan, China
e-mail: cuiyanjun@topgenebio.com

L. Zhou and Z. Sun (eds.), *Reproductive and Developmental Toxicology on Macaca Fascicularis*, https://doi.org/10.1007/978-981-92-3834-7_5

In nonclinical safety evaluation studies for drugs, the sexual maturity status of animals can significantly impact the microscopic assessment of the reproductive system, the interpretation of potential lesions related to the test article, and the ultimate evaluation of whether the test article poses a potential risk to humans. However, there has been a lack of consistent standards and uniform recording methods for assessing the sexual maturity of animals in nonclinical drug safety studies. An international working group composed of nonclinical pathologists and toxicologists has published a series of best practice guidelines aimed at establishing expertise in reproductive systems, pathological terminology, and standards for exchanging nonclinical data, which includes best practices for documenting sexual maturity in both rodent and non-rodent species [1].

5.1 Key Recommendations

(1) The primary method for determining sexual maturity is the microscopic evaluation of the reproductive system and tissues; other data, such as age, body weight, daily observations during the in vivo trial phase, genetic origin, gross examination, organ weights, and/or other unconventional techniques (such as semen analysis, testicular volume, estrous/menstrual cycles, and hormone measurements), should also be considered as part of the weight of evidence.
(2) The microscopic observation of sexual maturity in males and females is based on the microscopic examination of the entire reproductive system; the maturity of individual reproductive organs should not be assessed singly. When documenting sexual maturity based on microscopic observations of the reproductive organs in both sexes, it is recommended that for all animals' reproductive system maturity data to be entered into the system, the following terms shall be used: "Reproductive tissue, maturity: immature, pubertal, mature, or indeterminate."
(3) In studies where sexual maturity is recorded based on microscopic observations, summaries or descriptions are generally not required in most of the pathology reports because the documentation of sexual maturity status reflects normal characteristics rather than histopathological diagnoses. However, additional details may be necessary in the results and/or discussion sections of pathology reports to explain any potential impact of the maturity status on the ability to detect and/or interpret potential findings in the reproductive system. Moreover, pathology reports should provide more detailed information regarding the sexual maturity of individual animals and/or groups, including the type of study, species, and animal age.

5.1.1 Additional Considerations for Assessment

(1) In studies requiring the evaluation of animal sexual maturity, sufficient details shall be provided in the study protocol or plan to ensure that the personnel responsible for pathological diagnosis clearly understand how to determine and document sexual maturity.

(2) When a study design includes microscopic evaluation of the reproductive system, study data and/or reports should contain clear information on sexual maturity, such as age/body weight (for rodents and rabbits), confirmation of sexual maturity prior to the start of the study, such as determination through age (for non-rodents) and/or through microscopic assessment (for all species and both sexes, except for female rabbits). Female rabbits are induced to ovulate since they typically lack corpora lutea, making it difficult to establish standards for microscopic detection of sexual maturity. Age and body weight are the only available endpoints for determining sexual maturity in female rabbits.
(3) Although age and/or body weight are suitable criteria for determining sexual maturity in individual animals and/or animals in the dose groups of rodents and rabbits, routine microscopic observations in repeated-dose toxicity studies generally offer little help in assessing sexual maturity of rodents and male rabbits. Microscopic evaluation results can be used as needed (such as in juvenile toxicity studies, early deaths/early termination of dose groups).
(4) In dogs and mini-pigs, age and/or body weight may assist in determining sexual maturity, but the microscopic examination of sexual maturity, depending on the age at study initiation and the timing of dissection, might be more valuable.
(5) In nonhuman primates (NHPs), age and/or body weight alone are usually not reliable indicators of sexual maturity; therefore, when sexually mature animals are required, confirmation of sexual maturity shall be part of the study evaluation and/or part of the microscopic assessment by the study's pathologist.

In most short-term general toxicity studies, non-rodent animals may be a mix of sexually mature, immature, and pubertal states. The process of sexual maturation in NHPs can vary greatly in terms of the age at which it begins and the duration of the process (which can be measured in months or years). Literature reports indicate that the peripubertal stage in cynomolgus monkeys occurs between 2.5 and 5.5 years of age [2]. Due to the relatively long puberty and variable onset in NHPs, age and body weight are not good indicators of sexual maturity status in NHPs. Therefore, the assessment of sexual maturity in NHPs often requires additional study endpoints. Other research parameters include age, weight, semen analysis, testicular weight, testicular volume measurements, semen analysis, and vaginal smears to assess menstrual cycles, as well as hormone measurement as part of pre-study evaluations; during the study, these can serve as experimental endpoints and complement histopathological assessment results as part of microscopic evaluation [3].

5.2 Toxic Pathological Manifestations of the Male Reproductive System

The evaluation of fertility in male animals includes the development, maturation, and release of gametes, sperm composition, mating behavior, and the final fertilization of the ovum; therefore, this type of study can only be conducted in sexually mature animals. Immature testes have incomplete germ cell development, approximately one-tenth the number of interstitial cells and Sertoli cells compared to adult testes, and lack G-protein coupled estrogen receptors around the seminiferous tubules, with limited Sertoli cell response to follicle-stimulating hormone. A significant difference between immature and mature testes is the formation of the blood–testis barrier (also known as the Sertoli cell barrier), formed by tight junctions, adherent junctions, and gap junctions between Sertoli cells. This barrier controls the environment within the seminiferous tubule lumen. Spermatogonia are located outside the barrier, making them more susceptible to substances harmful to spermatocytes and spermatozoa [4].

5.2.1 Anatomical, Physiological, and Histological Observations of the Sexual Maturity Status in Male Animals

The age of animals used for nonclinical safety assessment studies varies widely based on study design, species, type of experiment, and individual development of the

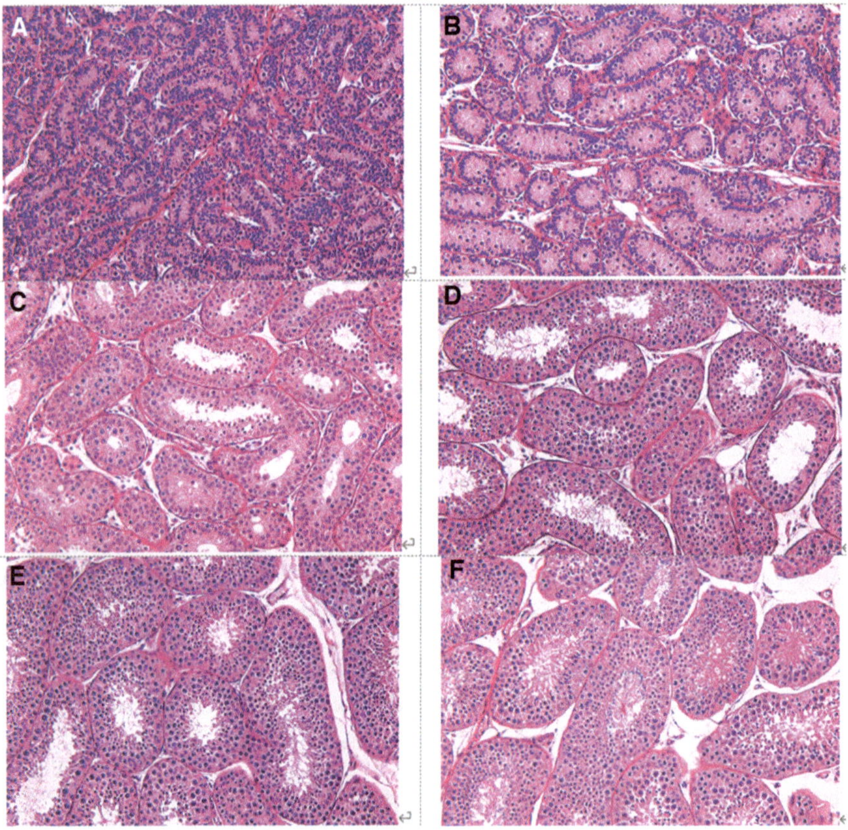

Fig. 5.1 Classification of testicular development in cynomolgus monkeys (HE staining, ×200). Testicular development is divided into six grades based on histological observations. (**A**) Grade 1 (underdeveloped): only Sertoli cells and spermatogonia are visible. (**B**) Grade 2 (prepubertal): lumen formation, round spermatids visible. (**C**) Grade 3 (onset of puberty): 14th step spermatids visible, narrow lumen, sloughing of spermatogenic cells. (**D**) Grade 4 (pubertal): all types of spermatogenic epithelium, narrow seminiferous tubules. (**E**) Grade 5 (early adulthood): fully formed sperm. (**F**) Grade 6 (adulthood): fully formed and active sperm

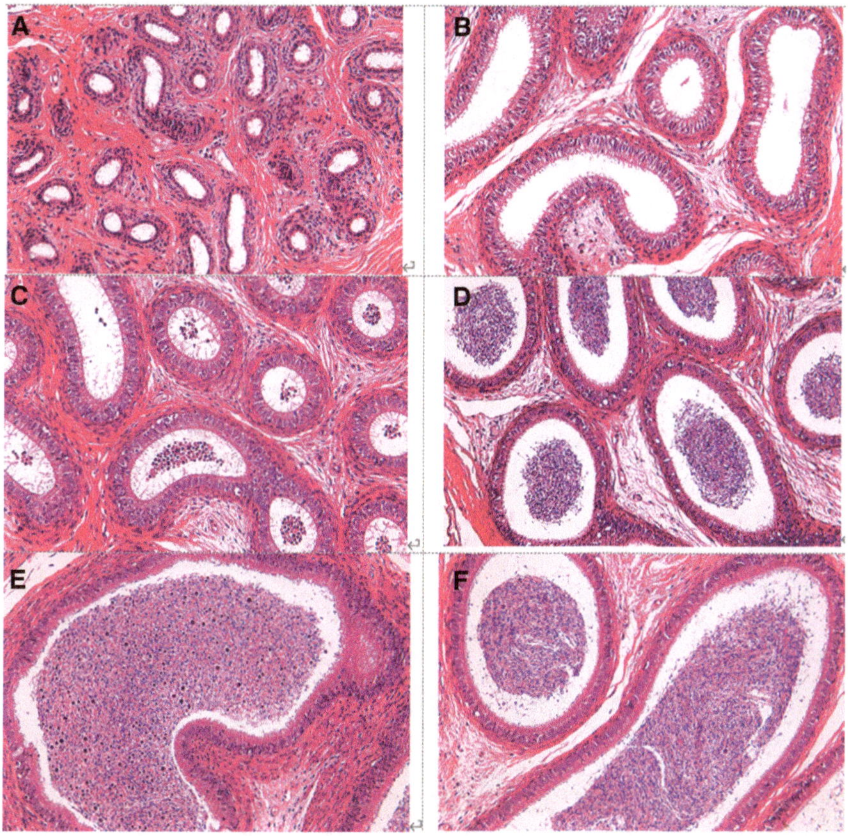

Fig. 5.2 Morphological characteristics of the epididymis in cynomolgus monkeys (HE staining, × 200). According to histological observation, epididymis maturity can be divided into six levels. (**A**) Grade 1 (immature): no sperm and very mild debris. (**B**) Grade 2 (prepubertal): no sperm and very mild debris. (**C**) Grade 3 (onset of puberty): few or small amounts of sperm and moderate debris. (**D**) Grade 4 (pubertal): few to moderate numbers of sperm, significantly reduced debris. (**E**) Grade 5 (early adulthood): moderate or large amounts of sperm. (**F**) Grade 6 (adulthood): large or very large amounts of sperm

animal. In different studies or within a single study, toxicologic pathologists may observe male reproductive systems of varying ages and developmental stages. This variability requires toxicologic pathologists to have an in-depth understanding of the normal anatomy, physiology, and histological characteristics and differences of the male reproductive system across different ages and species. Therefore, familiarity with the various indicators of sexual maturity facilitates accurate and consistent documentation of the sexual maturity status of experimental animals.

Besides the commonly used three-level grading method ("immature," "peripubertal," "mature"), there are also reports dividing the male reproductive system into six grades from "immature" to "mature." The specific histological characteristics are shown in Figs. 5.1–5.4.

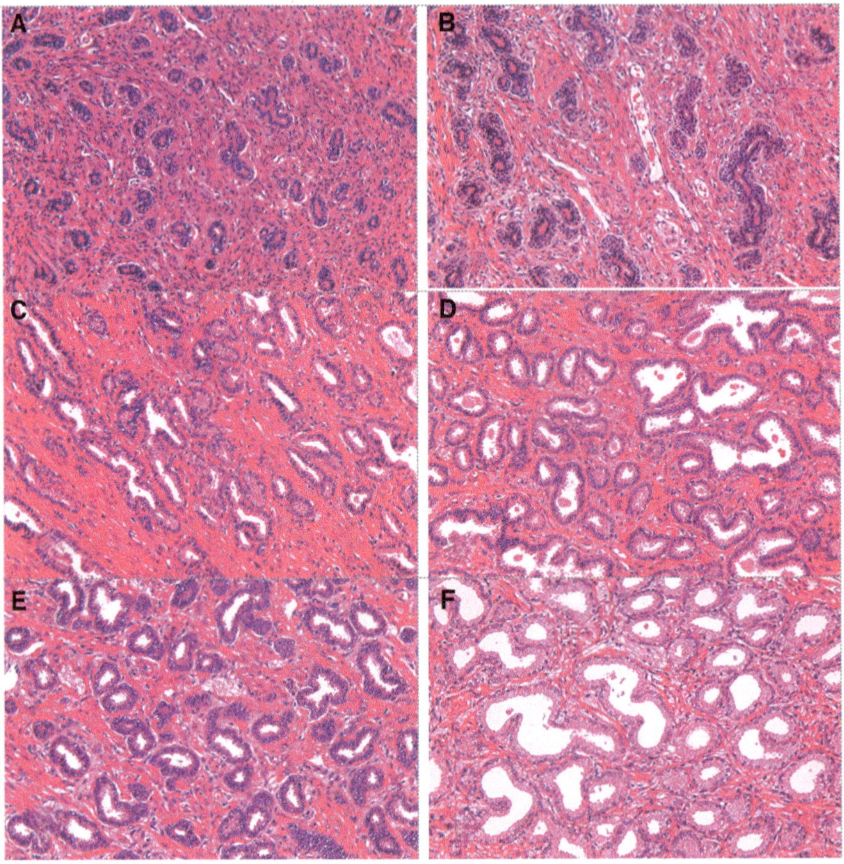

Fig. 5.3 Morphological characteristics of the prostate (HE staining, ×200). According to histological observation, the prostate is divided into six grades. (**A**) Grade 1 (immature). (**B**) Grade 2 (prepubertal). (**C**) Grade 3 (onset of puberty). (**D**) Grade 4 (pubertal). (**E**) Grade 5 (early adulthood). (**F**) Grade 6 (adulthood)

Grade 1 (Immature) and Grade 2 (Prepubertal), no signs of sperm production in the testes, no sperm observed in the epididymis, and little or almost no glandular lumina visible in the prostate. The seminal vesicles show narrow lumina with flat epithelial cells and simple folds of mucosal epithelium.

Grade 3 (Onset of Puberty), the spermatogenic cycle just begins. Seminiferous tubules are small in diameter and few in number, and sections can reveal all types of germ cells and luminal cells, including spermatogonia, spermatocytes, round and elongated spermatids, but very few or no sperm in the epididymis, with more cellular debris, the range of which is larger than other grades, suggesting immature Sertoli cell function.

Grade 4 (Pubertal), almost complete spermatogenesis is observed in the seminiferous tubules. Despite small tubule diameters and low height of spermatid epithelium,

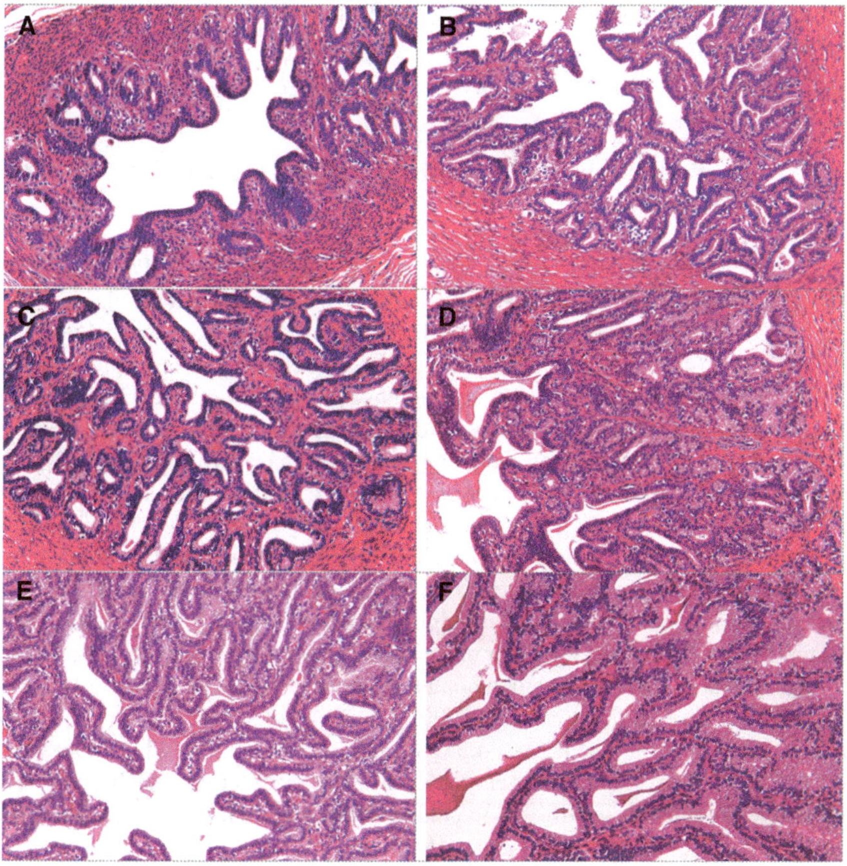

Fig. 5.4 Morphological characteristics of the gland (HE staining, ×200), divided into six grades based on histological observations. (**A**) Grade 1 (immature). (**B**) Grade 2 (prepubertal). (**C**) Grade 3 (onset of puberty). (**D**) Grade 4 (pubertal). (**E**) Grade 5 (early adulthood). (**F**) Grade 6 (adulthood)

sections of seminiferous tubules show a few germ cells and some immature tubules. The sperm numbers in the epididymis range from few to moderate, with less debris than that observed in Grade 3. Thus, toxicological assessment of the testes is feasible in cynomolgus monkeys with this grade of testes.

Grade 5 (Early Adulthood), complete spermatogenesis is visible in seminiferous tubules, and moderate or large amounts of sperm are observed in the epididymis, making this grade suitable for testicular toxicity evaluation.

Grade 6 (Adulthood), complete spermatogenesis is present within seminiferous tubules, and a large amount of sperm is observed in the epididymis, allowing for semen collection for sperm analysis.

Histological examination indicates that prostatic gland lumina are fully formed in Grade 3, with distinctly wide regions. In Grade 1 or 2, the folds of mucosal epithelium in the seminal vesicles become complex, but almost no secretions are observed in the lumina. After testicular maturation, the acini of the seminal vesicles continue to develop.

5.2.2 Age, Body Weight, Reproductive Organ Weights, and Other Assessments

The use of cynomolgus monkeys with "an age of at least 4 years and a weight of at least 4 kg" has been proposed as a broad standard for evaluating testicular toxicity. However, this standard is now considered insufficient. In monkeys aged 4 years or weighing 4 kg (4.00–4.99 kg), testicular grades range from 1 to 6. Approximately 37% of monkeys older than 4 years and weighing 4 kg (4.00–4.99 kg) have 50% of individuals with a testicular maturity grade of 4 or higher. Approximately 63% of 4-year-old cynomolgus monkeys weighing around 4 kg have 35% of individuals with a testicular maturity grade of 3 or lower. About 96% of animals older than 5 years and weighing more than 5 kg have a testicular maturity grade of 4 or higher. Based on current assessments, evaluations of testicular toxicity in animals shall be designed for those aged 5 years or older or weighing more than 5 kg. Although greater average age and weight tend to correlate with higher testicular maturity grades, there is no linear relationship between testicular maturity and age or weight due to the significant variability of age and body weight among nonhuman primates [5, 6].

Literature suggests that to ensure a 90% probability of sexual maturity, the body weight should generally be at least 4.5 kg or more (5 kg), age should be at least 5.5 years, or testicular volume should exceed 20 mL. However, relying solely on testicular size measurement is insufficient to predict sexual maturity, as genital growth and testicular size are variable. Many animals mature sexually at a younger age without noticeable changes in weight or testicular size. When hormone analysis, such as testosterone concentration, is regarded as a criterion for defining sexual maturity, special and complex sampling schedules must be established to reduce experimental variation and error caused by the synthesis/release of sex hormone pulsing and circadian hormones and multiple peaks of sex hormones during puberty [7].

A retrospective survey found that the presence of sperm in semen samples can confirm complete testicular maturation. This test collected semen samples from 956 untreated animals, correlating the presence of sperm in semen samples with the mature testicular histology of each animal at the study end. Although some animals had no sperm in their semen samples, about 75% showed mature spermatogenesis upon subsequent histological examination. Therefore, a semen sample containing sperm provides definitive evidence of mature spermatogenesis and can serve as an assessment indicator of sexual maturity for the species [8] (Tables 5.1 and 5.2).

In male animals, it is crucial to identify different cell morphologies within seminiferous tubules that constitute the spermatogenic cycle to diagnose conditions like missing cell populations, retention of spermatocytes, or inappropriate appearance of spermatocytes. Another challenge concerning male animals is to identify immaturity and diagnose immaturity and degenerative lesions, particularly in dogs and nonhuman primates. Prepubertal and peripubertal monkeys exhibit extensive degeneration and sloughing of germ cells in the testes and epididymal duct lumina. Sometimes, focal areas within immature testes may show complete spermatogenesis in seminiferous tubules. Immature or pubertal testes may also be associated with absent or reduced sperm in the epididymis. The secretory activity and size of the seminal vesicles and prostate depend on the monkey's maturity status. Preservation of testes by using the correct fixatives helps with the staging of spermatogenesis. Bouin's solution or modified Davidson's fluid can display cellular details well and reduce artifacts, and can replace 10% neutral buffered formalin as the routine fixative for testes. Resin-embedded sections are superior to conventional paraffin sections in showing cellular structures and can provide high-definition images for detecting early lesions.

ICH S6 (R1) states that when nonhuman primates are the only species relevant for nonclinical safety assessment of biotechnology products, the potential effects on male and female fertility are assessed by assessing the reproductive tract (organ weight and histopathology) through repeated dose toxicity studies using sexually mature NHP lasting at least 3 months. If there are specific reasons of concern based on pharmacological activity or previous findings, the menstrual cycle, sperm count, sperm morphology/motility, and male or female reproductive hormone levels can be evaluated in repeated dose toxicity studies. It is suggested that the sexual maturity of male animals can be demonstrated by the presence of sperm in a semen sample, and the sexual maturity of female animals can be demonstrated by at least two consecutive menstrual cycles. In addition to the default parameters (reproductive organ weight and histopathology), for indirect assessment of sexual fertility, daily vaginal swabs are

Table 5.1 Baseline age and body weight of 956 cynomolgus monkeys with sperm presence or absence in semen samples

Parameter	All animals		Mauritian		Asian (Chinese or Vietnamese)	
	Sperm absent	Sperm present	Sperm absent	Sperm present	Sperm absent	Sperm present
Number of animals (*n*)	230	726	174	505	56	221
Age (years old)						
Number of animals	230	726	174	505	56	221
Mean ± SD	4.1 ± 0.9*	5.2 ± 1.2	3.8 ± 0.6	4.6 ± 0.7	5.1 ± 1.2	6.5 ± 1.3
Range	3.0–7.7	2.6–11.9	3.0–5.8	2.8–7.1	3.2–7.7	3.9–11.9
Median	3.8	5.0	3.7	4.6	4.9	6.3
Body weight (kg)						
Number of animals	222	726	166	505	56	221
Mean ± SD	4.6 ± 1.0	5.8 ± 1.1	4.6 ± 1.1	5.7 ± 0.9	4.4 ± 0.9	6.1 ± 1.3
Range	3.0–7.5	3.2–11.0	3.0–7.5	3.7–8.7	3.1–6.7	3.2–11.0
Median	4.4	5.7	4.5	5.7	4.2	6.0
Age/body weight ratio (median-based)	0.86	0.88	0.82	0.81	1.17	1.5

Table 5.2 Background age and body weight of testicular histological examination of 322 cynomolgus monkeys with sperm presence or absence in semen samples

Absent/presentsperm histology diagnosis	No. of animals(n)	Age (years old)		Body weight (kg)		Duration (months)		Organ weight (g)	
		Baseline	Terminal	Baseline	Terminal	Duration	Range	Testes	Seminal vesicles
Sperm absent									
Mature	95	4.2 ± 1.1	5.0 ± 1.0	4.6 ± 11	5.5 ± 1.1	9.6 ± 5.1	1.0–18.9	29.4 ± 11.5	5.7 ± 3.5
Adolescent-immature	12	3.7 ± 0.5	4.2 ± 0.5	4.3 ± 0.9	4.5 ± 0.8	5.8 ± 2.1	1.6–8.7	7.8 ± 3.4	2.2 ± 0.8
Immature	18	3.7 ± 0.4	3.9 ± 0.4	3.8 ± 0.7	4.1 ± 0.5	3.0 ± 1.7	1.6–7.5	4.0 ± 3.1	1.6 ± 1.3
Sperm present									
Mature	197	5.2 ± 1.1	5.7 ± 1	5.8 ± 1.1	6.0 ± 1.1	6.9 ± 4.9	1.0–43.4	36.2 ± 12.3	9.5 ± 5.6

recommended for female animals, while for male animals, recommendations include blood collection (for reproductive hormone analysis), testicular volume ultrasound, and collection of frozen testicular samples at autopsy, according to regulatory guidelines.

Recommendations regarding the sampling and paraffin embedding of male reproductive organs allow for the differentiation of left and right organs (Fig. 5.5). The histopathological evaluation of the testes shall begin with an assessment of testicular maturity, and the pathology report should include whether the testes examined are mature (Grade 6), adolescent (Grades 2–5), or immature (Grade 1). Histopathological assessment of the spermatogenic tubules of the testis shall be qualitatively evaluated with a thorough knowledge of the spermatogenic cycle. Terms used to describe morphological changes in the testis and epididymis should follow the International Harmonization of Nomenclature and Diagnostic Criteria (INHAND) for rats and mouse, and morphological terms shall be assigned to specific cell populations within the testis (e.g., germ cells, Sertoli cells, and interstitial cells) or specific anatomic regions of the output duct system (e.g., testicular network, output tube, epididymis head, body, tail, and deferent duct). The reproductive system of monkeys aged 3–5 years old is in a period of relatively large histological and morphological differences. It is necessary for pathologists to note that some of these differences are the result of

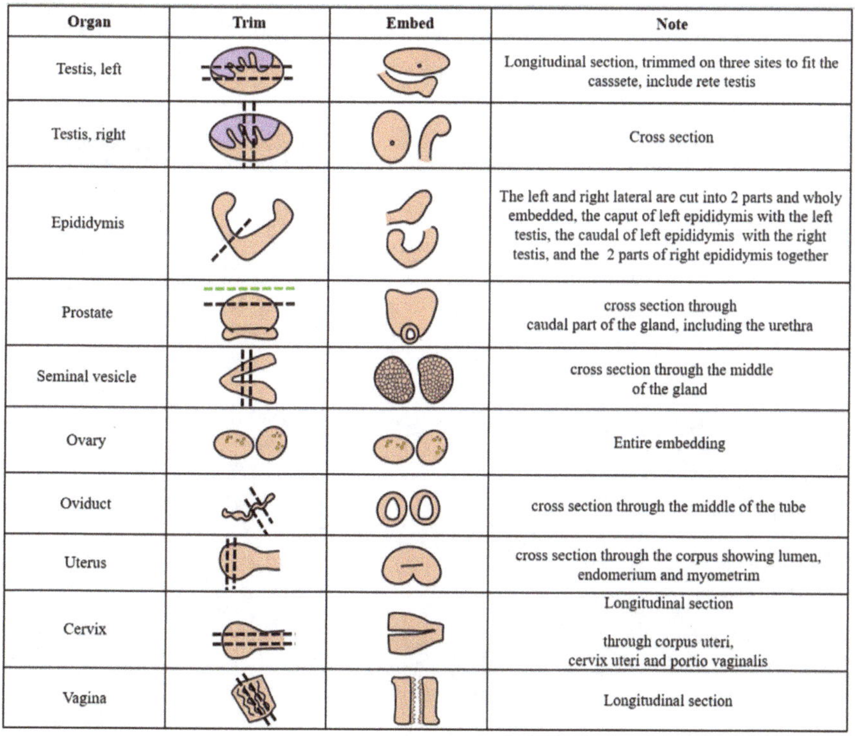

Organ	Trim	Embed	Note
Testis, left			Longitudinal section, trimmed on three sites to fit the casssete, include rete testis
Testis, right			Cross section
Epididymis			The left and right lateral are cut into 2 parts and wholy embedded, the caput of left epididymis with the left testis, the caudal of left epididymis with the right testis, and the 2 parts of right epididymis together
Prostate			cross section through caudal part of the gland, including the urethra
Seminal vesicle			cross section through the middle of the gland
Ovary			Entire embedding
Oviduct			cross section through the middle of the tube
Uterus			cross section through the corpus showing lumen, endomerium and myometrim
Cervix			Longitudinal section through corpus uteri, cervix uteri and portio vaginalis
Vagina			Longitudinal section

Fig. 5.5 Nonhuman primate reproductive organ collection and embedding method reference

normal physiological changes. It is important to be familiar with these normal morphological differences so as not to misdiagnose these changes as pathological changes and recognize the true scope of "normal" [9, 10].

5.2.3 Common Background Changes of the Male Reproductive System in Nonhuman Primates

1. *Immature testis*. This lesion is a common stage of physiological development in nonhuman primates of short-term tests, especially in animals just over 3 years old included in toxicity tests. The entire male reproductive system is immature, the spermatogenic tubule of the testis is small in lumen, and only spermatogonial cells and Sertoli cells can be observed in the epithelium. Some spermatogenic cells degenerate and fall off (Figs. 5.6 and 5.7), or occasionally focal spermatogenic tubules develop before other tubules (Fig. 5.8).
2. *Dysplasia of testicular fibers*. It is an episodic lesion characterized by replacement of the testicular parenchyma by mature collagen (Figs. 5.9 and 5.10). In a retrospective survey, 10.94% of monkeys were found to have this lesion, which ranged in severity from minimal to severe, occurring both unilaterally (38.5%) and bilaterally (61.5%). This lesion occurs regardless of sexual maturity. But when it occurs in mature monkeys, it is usually associated with cystic tubule atrophy of the spermatogenous epithelium. Based on the morphological characteristics and unilateral/bilateral distribution of the lesions, the lesions were considered to be congenital or developmental abnormalities [11].

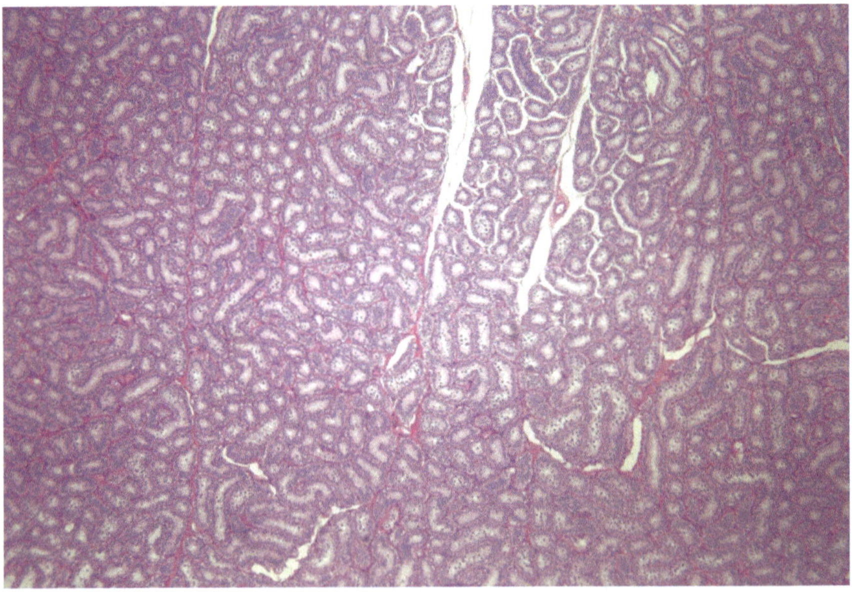

Fig. 5.6 Testicle, immature (HE staining, ×40)

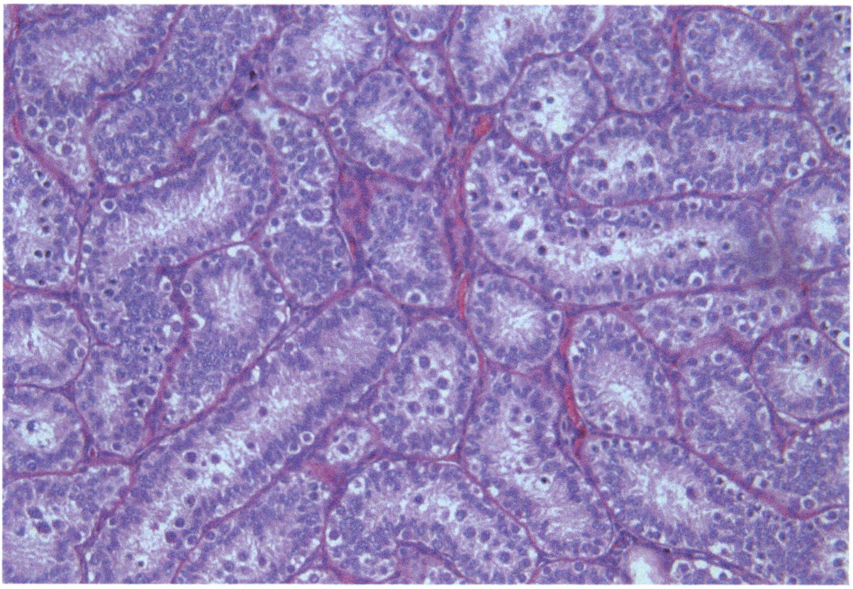

Fig. 5.7 Testicle, immature, spermatogenic tubules with small lumen, covered by spermatocytes and Sertoli cells, and some spermatogenic cells degraded and fell off (arrow) (HE staining, ×200)

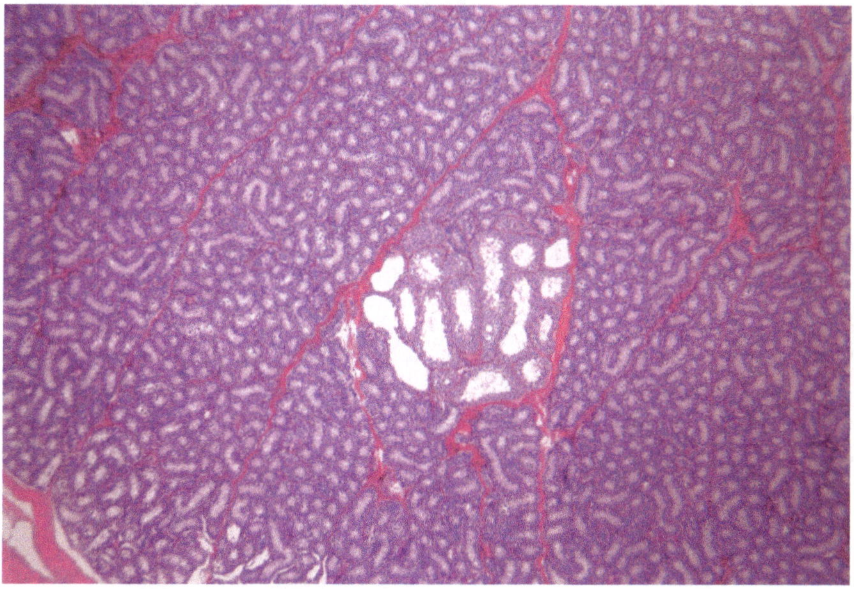

Fig. 5.8 Occasionally, focal seminiferous tubule development prior to other tubules in immature testicular tissue (arrow) (HE staining, ×40)

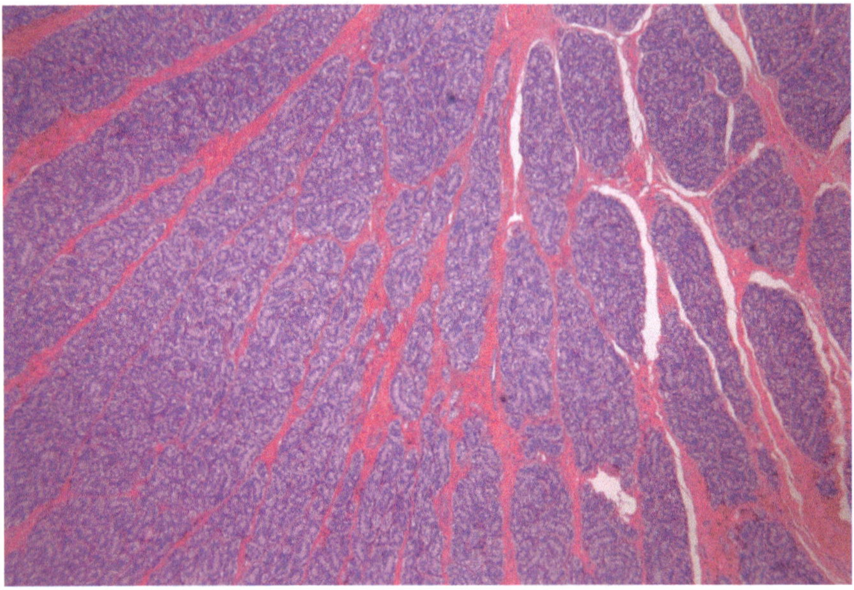

Fig. 5.9 Testicle, fibrous dysplasia (arrow) (HE staining, ×40)

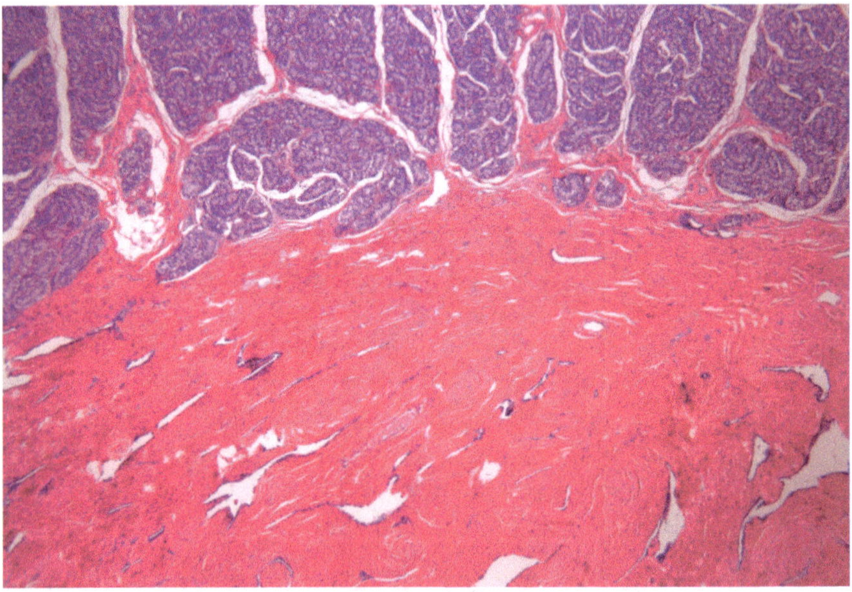

Fig. 5.10 Testicle, fibrous dysplasia (arrow) (HE staining, ×40)

The following five grades shall be divided according to the severity: ① minimal: small lesions, excessive collagen in the testicular reticulum, diaphragm, and/or mediastinum, and 10% of the testicular sections are affected; ② mild: multiple small lesions, excessive collagen in the testicular reticulum, diaphragm, and/or in the mediastinum, 10%–30% of testicular sections are affected. Due to collagen replacement, the number of spermatogenic tubules reduces; ③ moderate: multiple lesions combine, a large amount of collagen in the testicular reticulum, diaphragm, and/or mediastinum. In total, 30%–50% of testicular sections are affected. The testicular sheath is thick. The number of spermatogenic tubules reduces due to collagen replacement; ④ severe: multiple lesions combined. There is a large amount of collagen in the testicular reticulum, diaphragm, and mediastinum. In total, 50%–75% of the testis are affected. The testicular sheath is often thickened, and the number of spermatogenic tubules is significantly reduced due to the replacement of collagen. ⑤ Serious: 75% of the testicular parenchyma is replaced by collagen, affecting the testicular reticulum, diaphragm, and mediastinum, and the number of spermatogenic tubules significantly reduces after collagen replacement.

3. *Immature epididymis*. The male reproductive system is immature, and degenerated and exfoliated spermatogenic cells could be observed in the epididymal tube during prepubertal and peripubertal periods, indicating immature development (Fig. 5.11).

4. Periepididymal inflammatory cell infiltration Focal periepididymal inflammatory cell infiltration, mononuclear (Fig. 5.12).

5. *Granuloma in the interstitial epididymis*. A focal granuloma with mononuclear infiltration was observed in the interstitial epididymis (Fig. 5.13).

6. *Immature prostate and the inflammatory cells infiltrated the interstitial area.* The prostate is scattered in small glandular ducts. The glandular duct epithelium is

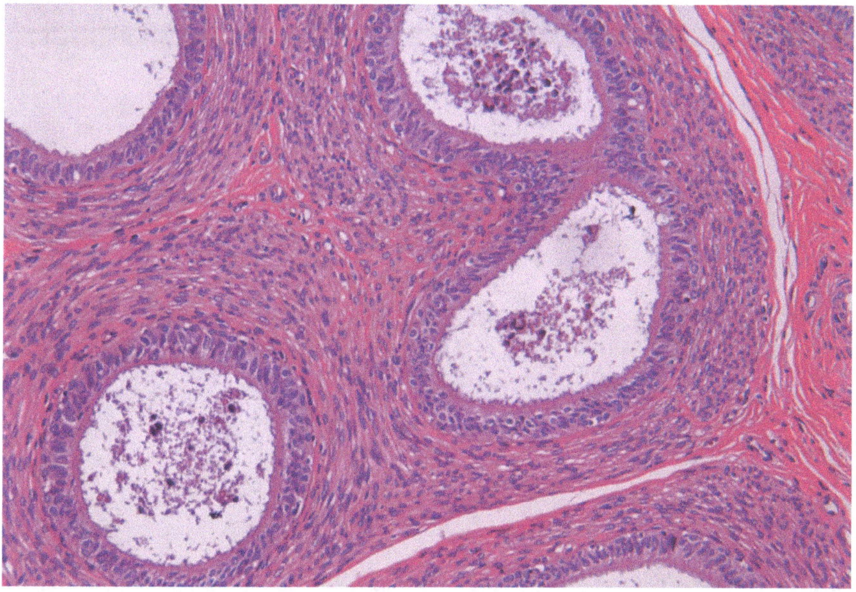

Fig. 5.11 Immature epididymis, early degeneration of sperm cells in the output tubule of the head of the epididymis (arrow) (HE staining, ×200)

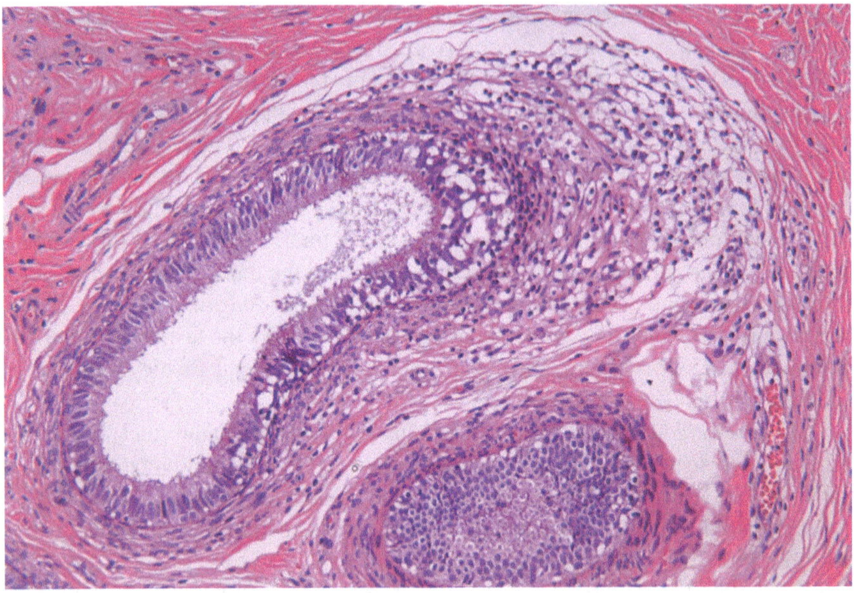

Fig. 5.12 Periepididymal focal inflammatory cell infiltration (arrow), mononuclear cells (HE staining, ×200)

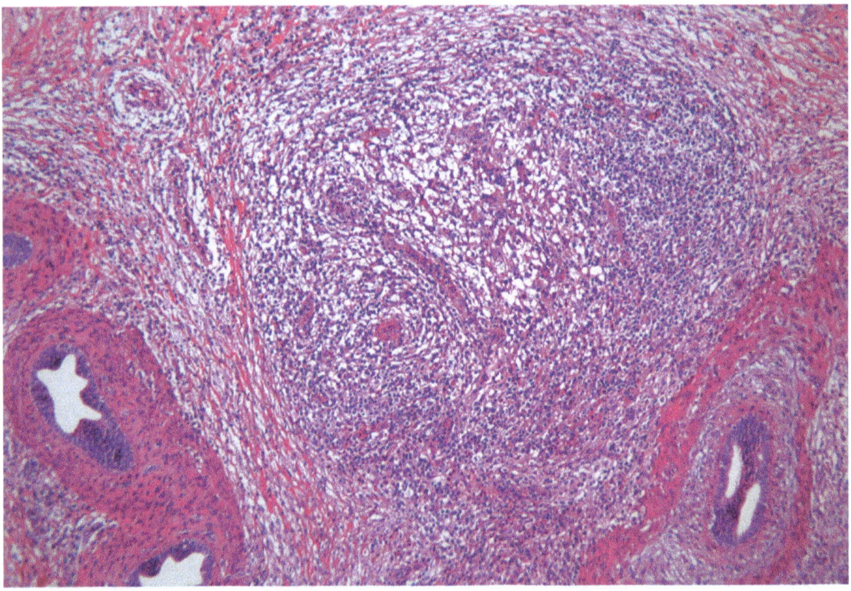

Fig. 5.13 Focal granuloma in the interstitial epididymis with mononuclear cell infiltration (arrow) (HE staining, ×100)

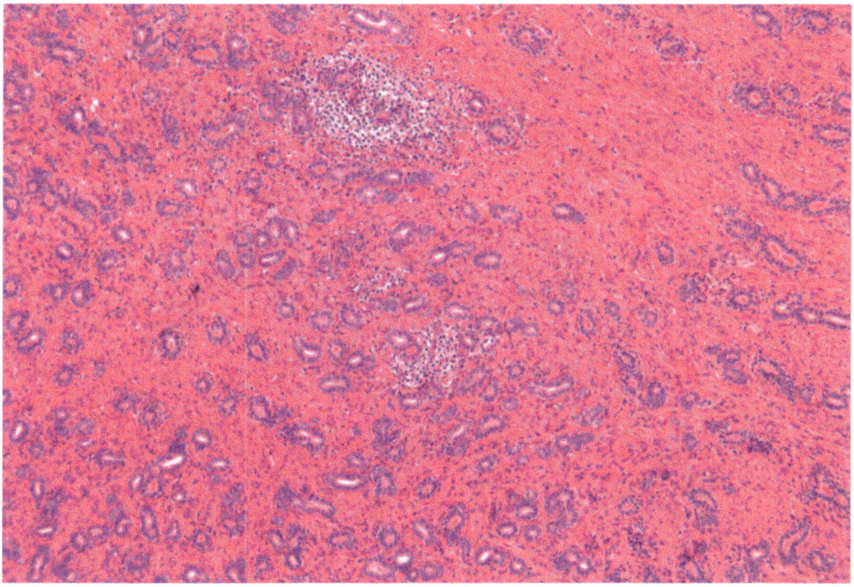

Fig. 5.14 Immature prostate, Interstitial inflammatory cell infiltration (arrow) (HE staining, ×100)

a single layer, with no obvious lumen and no secretion found in the lumen, which is characteristic of the immature male reproductive system. Even in an immature state, the glandular duct of the prostate is surrounded by scattered focal inflammatory cell infiltration, mononuclear (Fig. 5.14).

5.2.4 Artificial Illusion—Spermatogenic Tubule Contraction

When the testis volume is large, the interstitial space of spermatogenic tubules can be widened, and the spermatogenic tubules shrink and become smaller after poor dehydration (Fig. 5.15). Figure 5.16 shows the testis with normal dehydration effect, which needs to be distinguished from true testicular atrophy (reduced lumen diameter, reduced epithelial cell layers, and abnormal arrangement).

5.2.5 Changes in the Reproductive System Caused by Drug Toxicity

1. *Degeneration of the testicular spermatogenic tubule*. After 28-day subcutaneous injection of a small molecule drug for human tumor metastasis (cancer), the histopathological examination of the spermatogenic tubules on both sides of the testis showed

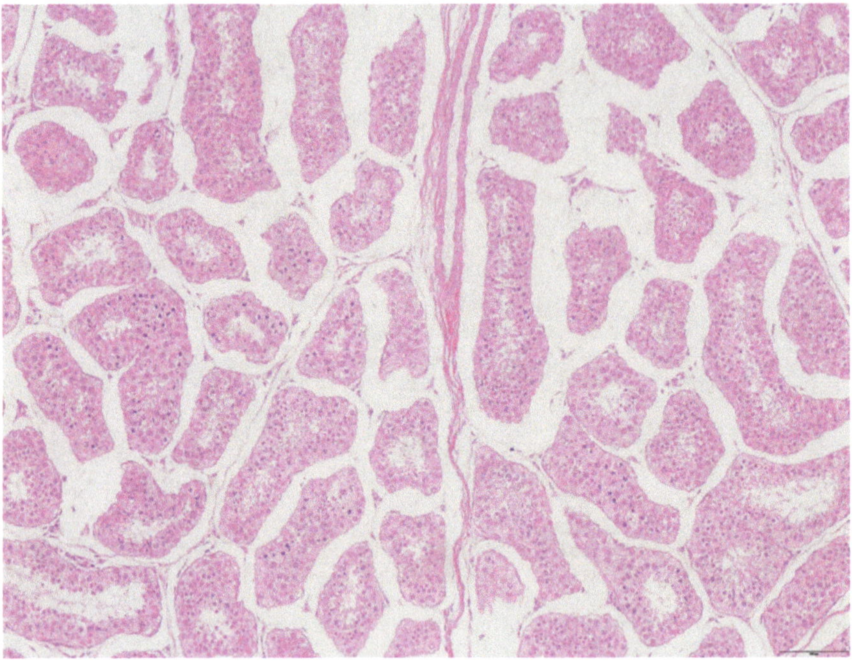

Fig. 5.15 Dosing group, artificial illusion, spermatogenic tubules shrank, and interstitial space widened (HE staining, ×100)

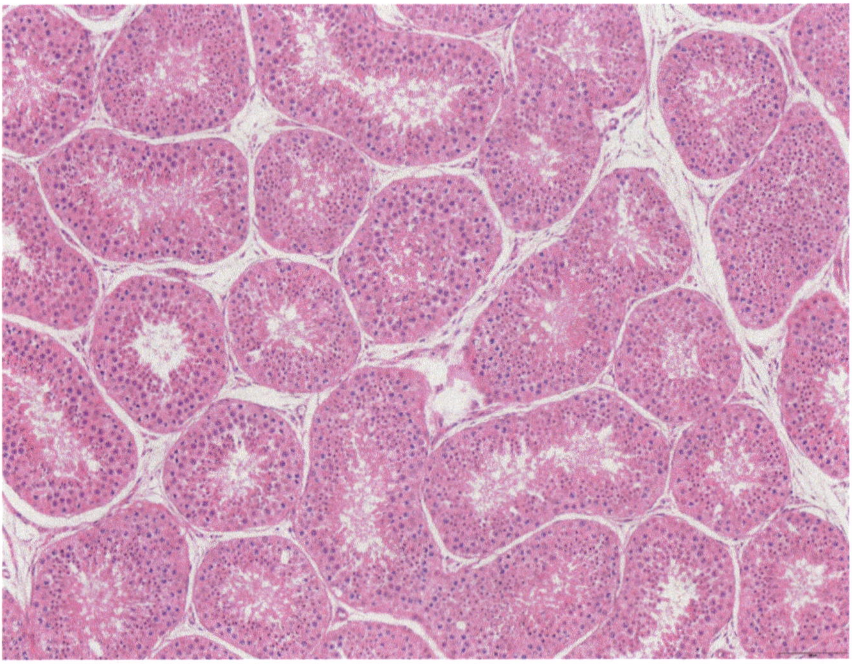

Fig. 5.16 Control group, no abnormal spermatogenic tubules observed (HE staining, ×100)

multinuclear giant cells in a relatively regular arrangement between elongated sperm cells and spermatocytes. Vacuolar degeneration of spermatogenic cells was observed, and the number of germ cell layers in some spermatogenic tubules was reduced. The diseased spermatogenic epithelium was in the early stages of the spermatogenic cycle (Figs. 5.17–5.24).

Spermatocyte swelling is a common background lesion in dogs, with up to 93% of cases in beagles aged 6–36 months, as reported. The lesions are usually mild. Each testicle has only a few tubules. Swollen spermatocytes are considered secondary spermatocytes. They do not undergo a second spermatocyte meiosis and survive to a later stage. When the lesion is less severe, the diagnostic term for spermatocyte swelling is often not clear. However, if this change is a significant feature, a diagnosis of spermatocyte swelling can be given. Swollen spermatocytes are usually distinct from multinucleated giant cells, which are large cells composed of spermatogenic cells (usually round sperm cells) with multiple identical mature reproductive nuclei, may be present in the spermatogenic epithelium, spermatogenic tubule lumen, or epididymis lumen, and often exhibit degeneration or atrophy of the spermatogenic tubule. Since multinucleated giant cells are associated with tubulogenic degeneration, the cells are often considered a component of tubulogenic degeneration and therefore cannot be

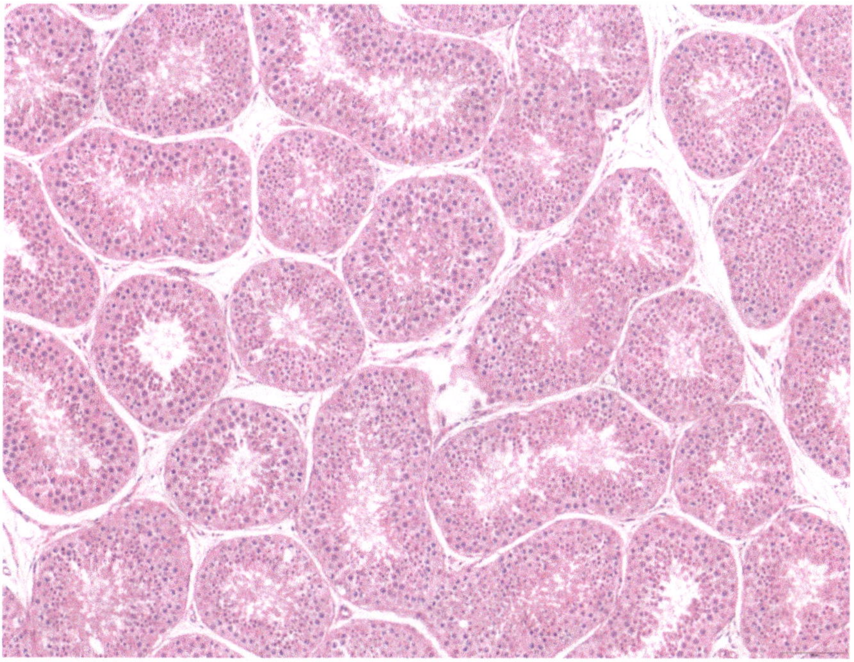

Fig. 5.17 Dosing group, scattered multinucleated giant cells observed in spermatogenic tubules (arrow) (HE staining, ×200)

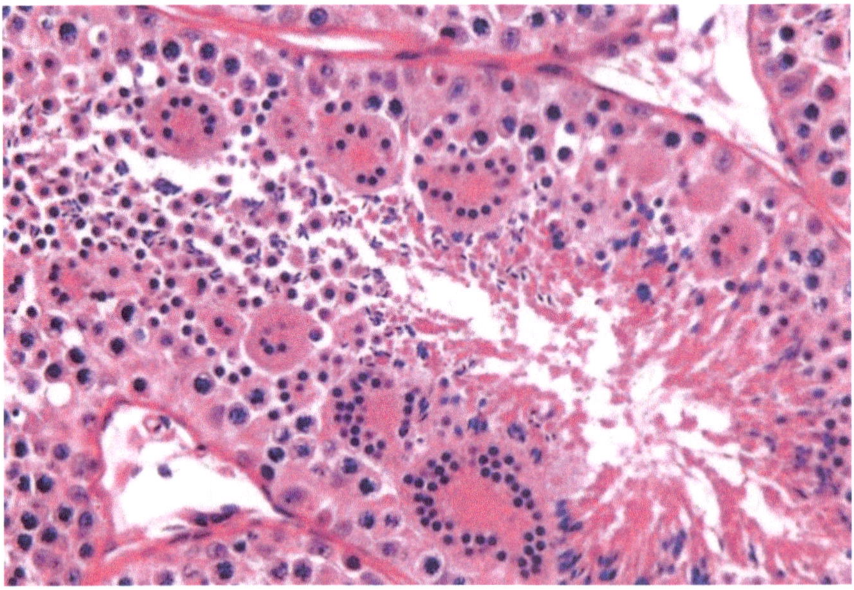

Fig. 5.18 Dosing group, scattered multinuclear giant cells observed in spermatogenic tubules (arrow) (HE staining, ×400)

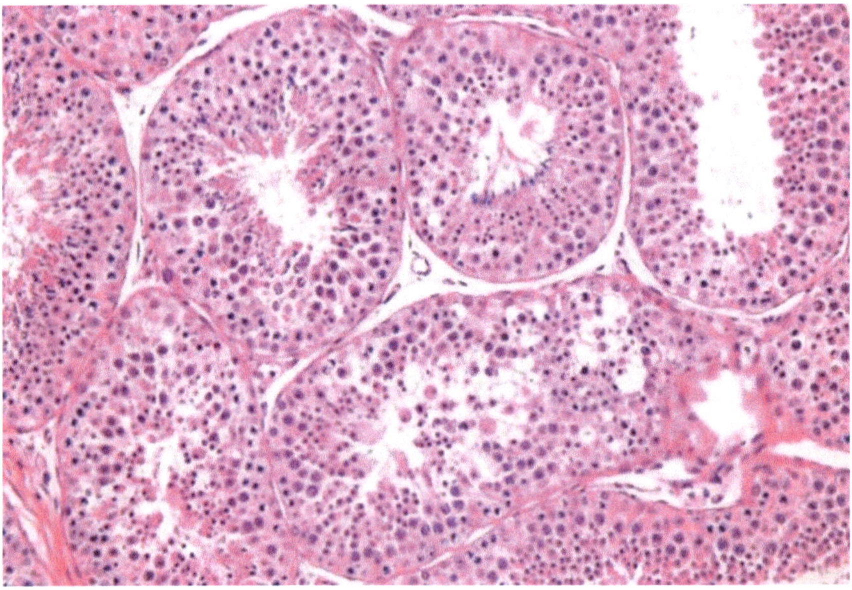

Fig. 5.19 Dosing group, reduced layers of spermatogenic cells in the spermatogenic tubules, scattered and vacuolated (arrow) (HE staining, ×200)

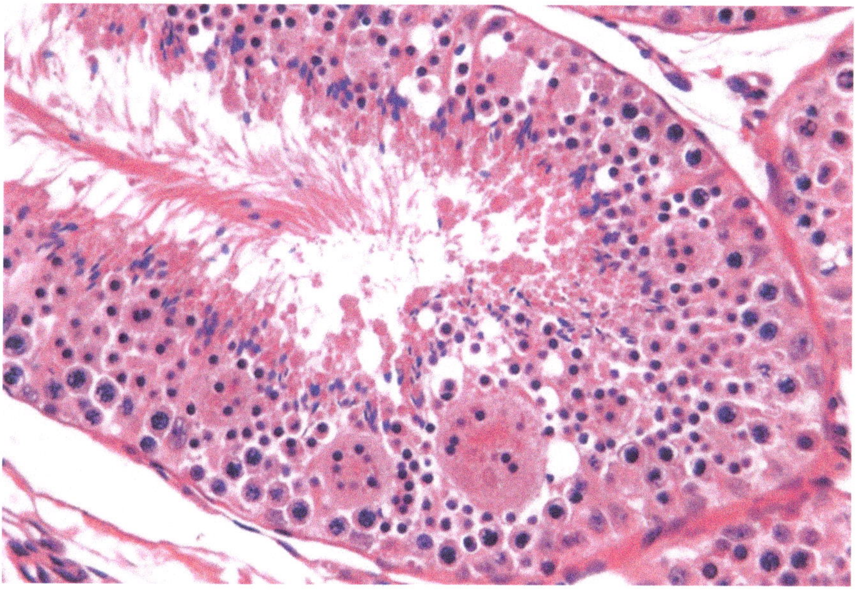

Fig. 5.20 Dosing group, reduced layers of spermatogenic cells in the spermatogenic tubules, scattered and vacuolated (arrow) (HE staining, ×400)

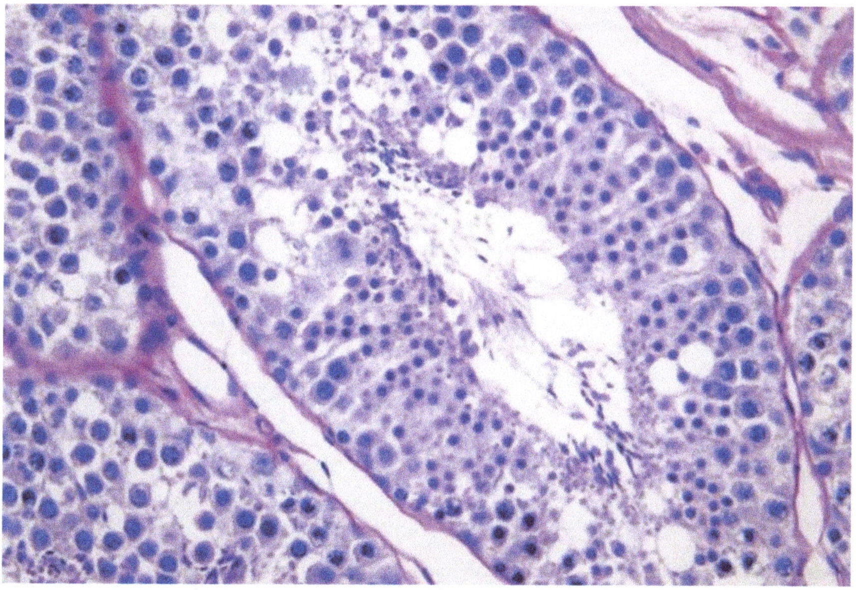

Fig. 5.21 Dosing group, testis, focal degeneration/necrosis of spermatogenic tubules and reduced cell layer, vacuolated (arrow) (PAS staining, ×400)

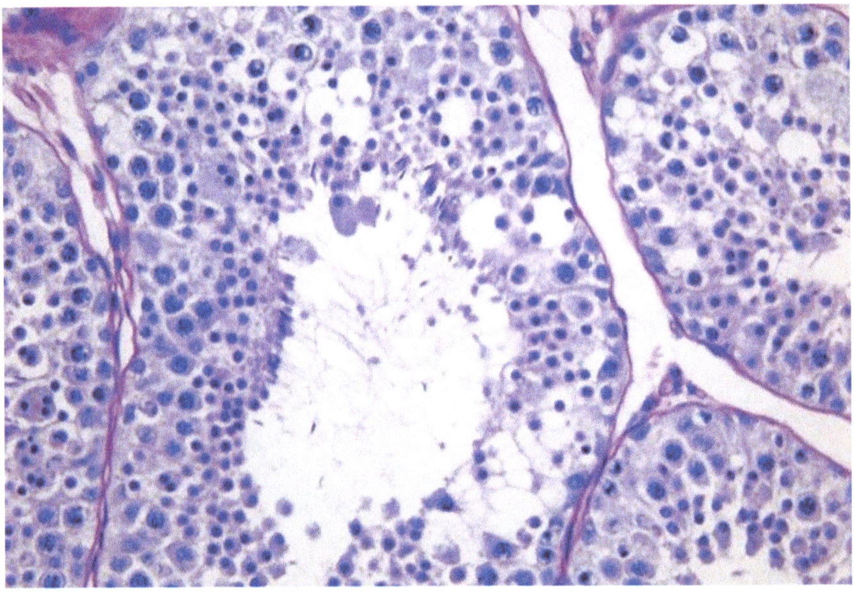

Fig. 5.22 Dosing group, testis, focal degeneration/necrosis of spermatogenic tubules and reduced cell layer, vacuolated (arrow) (PAS staining, ×400)

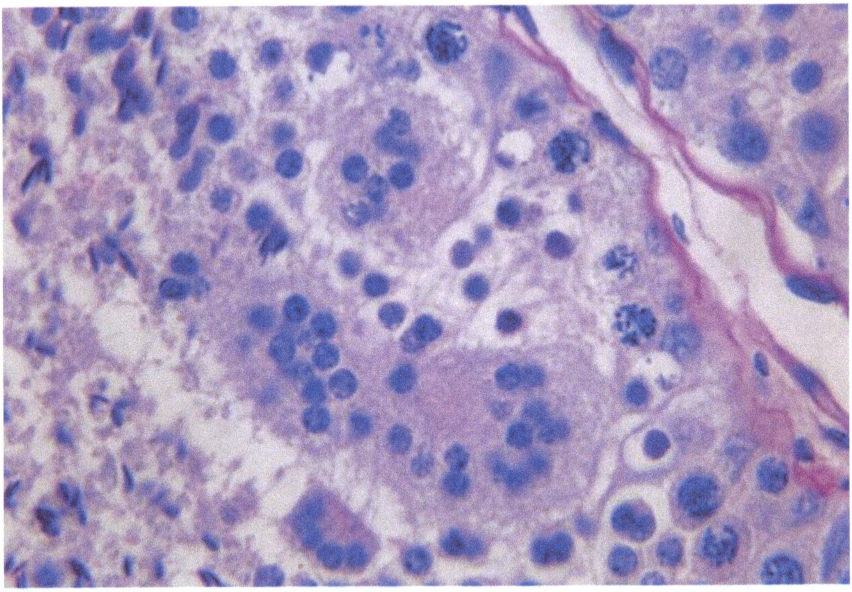

Fig. 5.23 Dosing group, testis, multinuclear giant cells (arrow) were arranged in a relatively regular manner, located between elongated sperm cells and spermatocytes; the focal vacuolar degeneration of spermatogenic cells, combined with a decreased number of germ cell layers. The diseased spermatogenic epithelium was at an early stage of the spermatogenic cycle (PAS staining, ×1000)

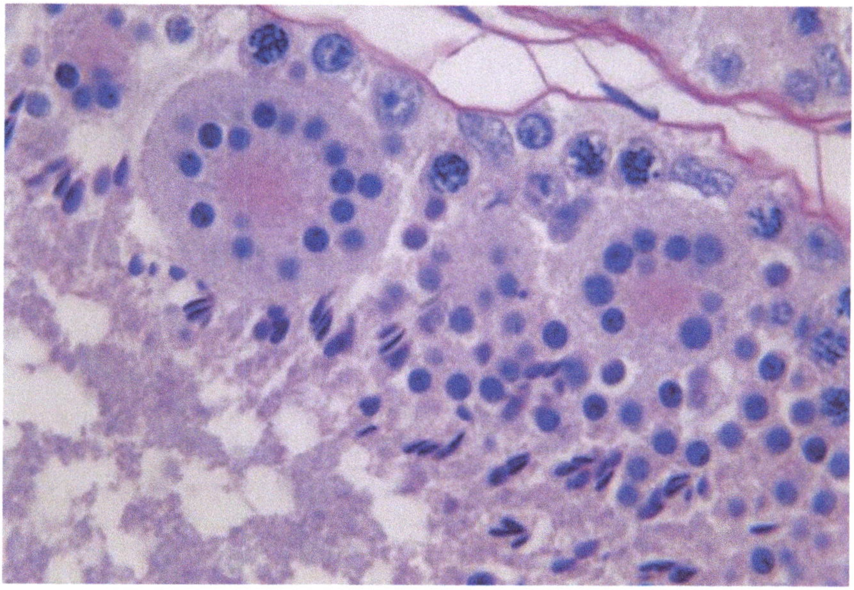

Fig. 5.24 Dosing group, testis, multinuclear giant cells (arrow) were arranged in a relatively regular manner, located between elongated sperm cells and spermatocytes. The diseased spermatogenic epithelium was at an early stage of the spermatogenic cycle (PAS staining, ×1000)

diagnosed separately. However, if they are the only changes, this particular diagnosis is appropriate. Multinucleated giant cells may be more prevalent in immature animals and shall only be recorded when the incidence is significantly greater than that in contemporaneous control animals.

2. *Antibody/protein drugs for testicular vasculitis*. Due to its molecular weight and structural characteristics, unexpected immune reactions caused by its immunogenicity, such as hypersensitivity reactions, can be found in nonclinical safety evaluations. The most common hypersensitivity reactions in animal studies are type I and type III. Type III hypersensitivity reaction, also known as the immune complex type, can be observed in the deposition of an immune complex in the blood vessel wall and the kidney. The formation and deposition of an immune complex in the blood vessel wall mainly occurs in the middle and/or small arteries and/or intima and media of small arteries (less common in small veins/veins) and perivascular interstitium, extracellular area, or macrophage. Blood vessels usually present as vasculitis/perivascular inflammatory changes observed in the kidneys, gastrointestinal tract, testicles, epididymis, heart, and cerebral choroid plexus [12, 13] (Figs. 5.25–5.28).

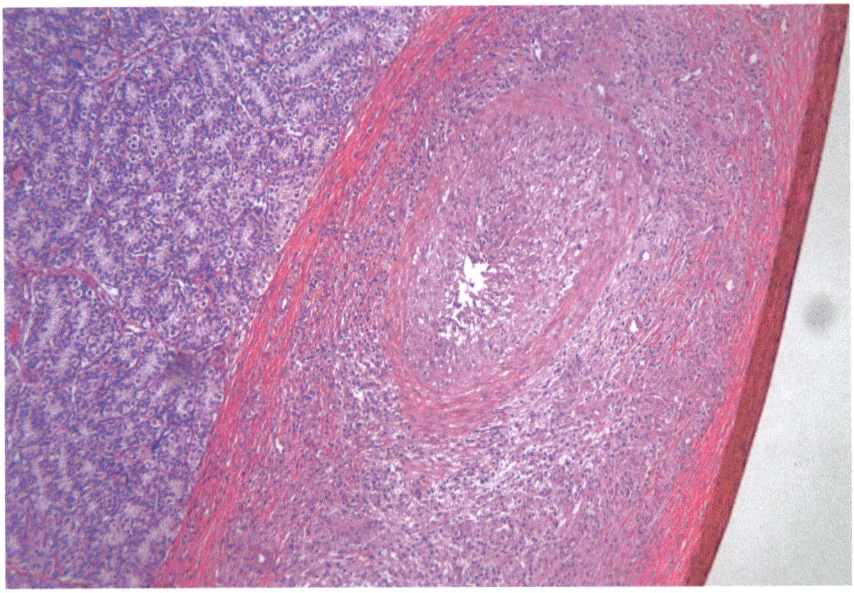

Fig. 5.25 The test article was a monoclonal antibody drug. Dosing group, vasculitis changes, and intimal hyperplasia were observed in the blood vessels of one testicle. A large number of inflammatory cells were infiltrated around the blood vessels (arrow), mainly monomorphic nuclei (HE staining, ×100)

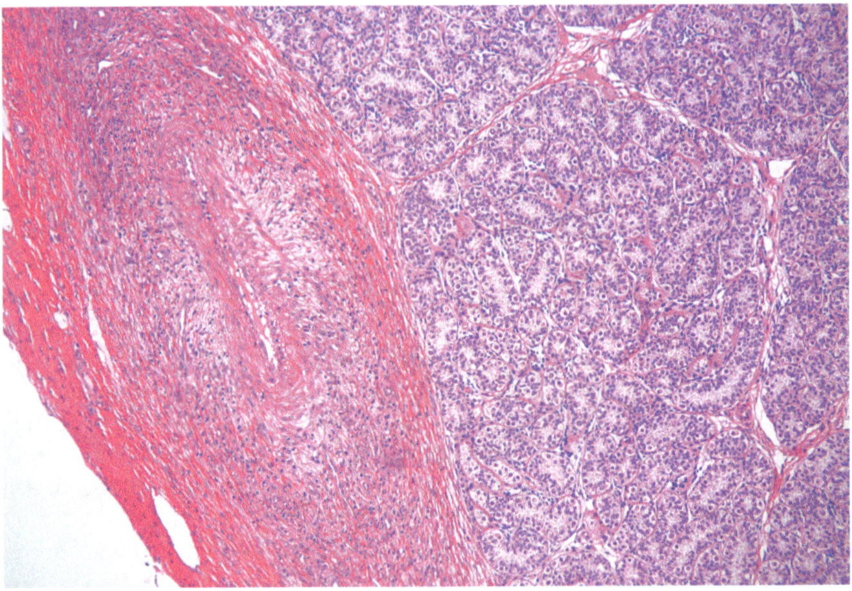

Fig. 5.26 The test article was a monoclonal antibody drug. Dosing group, vasculitis changes, and intimal hyperplasia were observed in the blood vessels of the other testicle. A large number of inflammatory cells were infiltrated around the blood vessels (arrow), mainly monomorphic nuclei (arrow) (HE staining, ×100)

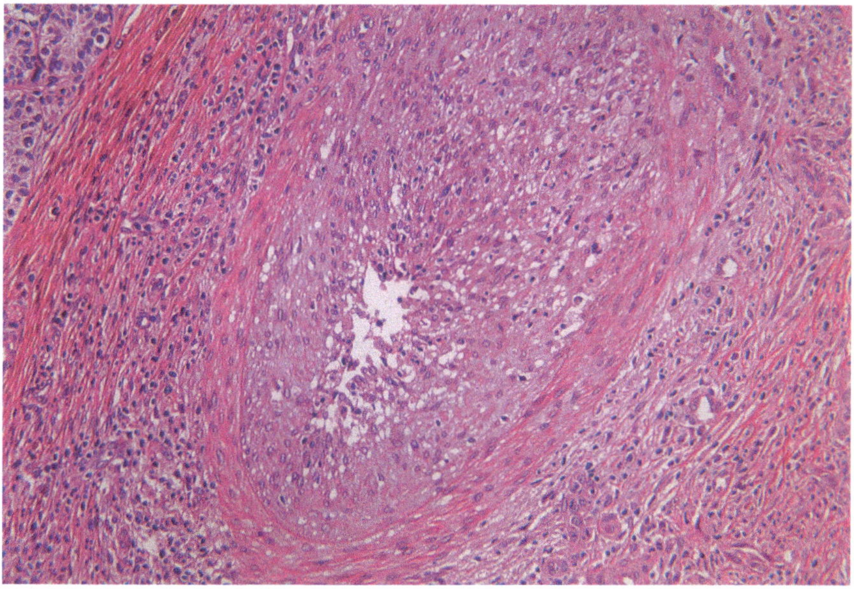

Fig. 5.27 The test article was a monoclonal antibody drug; dosing group, vasculitis changes, and intimal hyperplasia were observed in the blood vessels of one testicle. A large number of inflammatory cells were infiltrated around the blood vessels (arrow), mainly monomorphic nuclei (arrow) (HE staining, ×200)

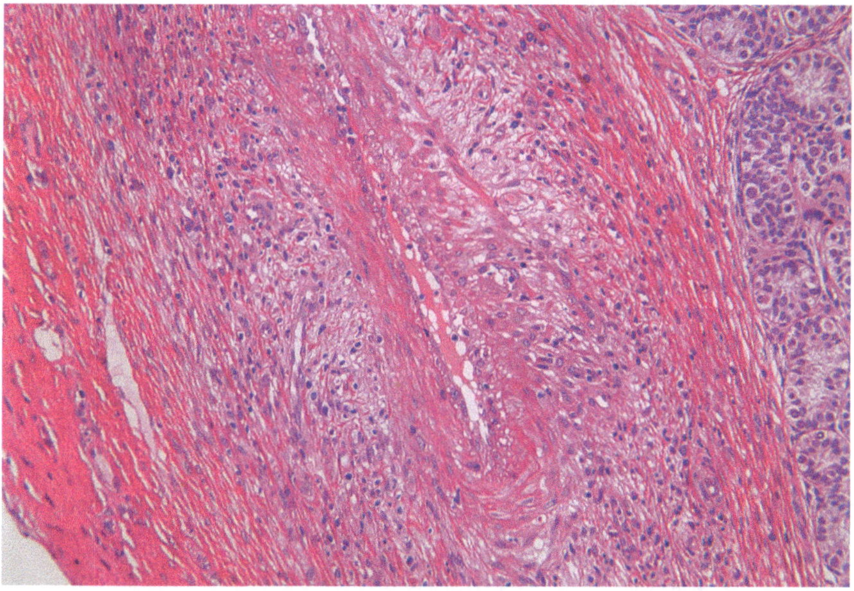

Fig. 5.28 The test article was a monoclonal antibody drug; dosing group, vasculitis changes, and intimal hyperplasia were observed in the blood vessels of the other testicle. A large number of inflammatory cells were infiltrated around the blood vessels (arrow), mainly monomorphic nuclei (arrow) (HE staining, ×200)

5.3 Pathological Manifestations of Toxicity in The Female Reproductive System

The characteristics of immature, adolescent, and mature females of laboratory animals commonly used in nonclinical safety evaluation tests (including rats, mice, dogs, miniature pigs, and nonhuman primates) are summarized in Tables 5.3– 5.5.

The overall duration of the cynomolgus monkey ovary cycle is 30 (±5) days and consists of three major phases: the follicular phase of 12–14 days, the menstrual phase of 3 days, and the luteal phase of 14–16 days. Corresponding to the ovarian cycle, the uterus presents the proliferative phase, the secretory phase, and the resting phase.

The proliferative phase of the uterus is characterized by a gradual increase in mitotic activity in endometrial glandular epithelium and stromal or fibrous cells. During this period, the endometrial glands are relatively sparse and straight, lined with pseudostratified epithelium and a narrow glandular cavity. Endometrial blood vessels are not prominent. After ovulation, the uterus enters the secretory phase, corresponding to the luteal phase of the ovaries. The mitotic activity in the endometrium has reduced. The endometrial glands are lined with medium to tall columnar epithelium, containing subnuclear and subonuclear vesicles filled with glycogen. As the secretory phase develops, the glands become more prominent and tortuous than those in the proliferative phase, with cystic features and wider glandular cavities,

Table 5.3 Microscopic observation characteristics of immature female reproductive system of nonclinical safety evaluation test species

Organ	Rat	Mouse	Dog	Minipig	NHP
Ovary	Small to medium size, degenerative/atretic, and no corpora lutea				
Uterus	Small, with limited glandular development; thin epithelium, compact stroma				
Cervix	Thin, inactive epithelium				Thin inactive epithelium, limited mucous production, boundary epithelium of the squamous column in the cervix
Vagina	Cranial: Inactive epithelium with mucification and luminal debris/ dilation Caudal: Closed, consisting of nonkeratinized squamous epithelium		Thin epithelium, nonkeratinized		
Mammary gland	Branching ducts extending through the mammary fat pad; terminal end buds present		A small duct may be present in the nipple, but no ducts or lobules are present within the fat pad	Ducts present within the mammary fat pad, with limited lobular development	

Table 5.4 Microscopic observation characteristics of the female reproductive system during the peripubertal period in nonclinical safety evaluation test species

Organ	Rat	Mouse	Dog	Minipig	NHP
Ovary	Corpus luteum (current and/or regressing) from at least one cycle		Any evidence of corpus luteum	Corpus luteum (current and/or regressing) from at least one cycle	
Uterus	Evidence of cyclic changes		May see evidence of cyclic changes, but inactive anestrus appearance is difficult to distinguish from immaturity, and the maturity designation should be based on the presence of the corpus luteum	Evidence of cyclic changes	May see evidence of cyclic changes, but anovulatory animals may have an inactive endometrium and maturity designation based on the presence of the corpus luteum
Cervix	Evidence of cyclic changes				The boundary epithelium of the squamous column is everted to the outer opening of the cervix
Vagina	Evidence of cyclic changes				Thickened and heavily keratinized
Mammary gland	Limited mammary gland development in the absence of a pregnancy or pseudopregnancy, and generally not useful for determining sexual maturity		Extensive ductal and lobular development during the first cycle; secretory activity during the luteal phase; the mammary gland is inactive during anestrus, but the presence of abundant mammary tissue is a reliable indicator of maturity in the dog	Lobules with secretory material often present	Ducts and lobules present

especially at the base of the endometrium. During the luteal phase (i.e., the secretory phase), there is a large infiltration of lymphocytes in the endometrium, many of which contain particles. In addition, spiral arteries become extremely prominent in the endometrium, and some areas containing a cross-section of spiral arteries are surrounded by prominent connective tissue. During the menstrual period, the spiral arteries in the upper endometrium contract, resulting in ischemia and loss of the surface layer. Tissue necrosis, bleeding, thrombus, and leukocyte infiltration are the hallmarks of the menstrual period. During this period, blood and necrotic tissue can be found in the cervix and vagina. As the menstrual period nears its end, non-necrotic residual glands in the lower endometrium begin to exhibit proliferative activity, forming a fusion layer on the eroded stromal epithelium, which marks the beginning of the regeneration period. During this period, the matrix below the surface of the endometrium is composed of

Table 5.5 Microscopic observation characteristics of the mature female reproductive system of nonclinical safety evaluation test species

Organ	Rat	Mouse	Rabbit	Dog	Minipig
Ovary	Corpus luteum (current and/or regressing) from multiple cycles		Visible corpus luteum	Corpus luteum (current and/or regressing) from multiple cycles	
Uterus	Evidence of cyclic changes		May see evidence of cyclic changes, but inactive anestrus appearance is difficult to distinguish from immaturity, and the maturity designation should be based on the presence of the corpus luteum	Evidence of cyclic changes	May see evidence of cyclic changes, but anovulatory animals may have an inactive endometrium and maturity designation based on the presence of the corpus luteum
Cervix	Evidence of cyclic changes				Cervical opening, squamo-columnar junction
Vagina	Evidence of cyclic changes				Thickened and heavily keratinized
Mammary gland	Limited mammary gland development in the absence of a pregnancy or pseudopregnancy, and generally not useful for determining sexual maturity		Extensive lobular development is present; secretory activity occurs during the luteal phase; the mammary gland is inactive during anestrus, but the presence of abundant mammary tissue is a reliable indicator of maturity in the dog	Lobules with secretory material are often present	Ducts and lobules present

small and dense basophilic cells. The spiral arteries remain prominent in the basal part but are not observed in the newly formed surface endometrium, while the basal endometrial glands are often in a resting state.

Female nonhuman primates most commonly reach sexual maturity at least 4 years old, with a weight of at least 2.5 kg. But, similar to male nonhuman primates, some uncertainty remains. The duration and regularity of the ovarian cycle in nonhuman female primates are influenced by a large number of confounding factors, of which transport stress is a well-known one. Animals shall be given 3 months to acclimatize before assessing their ovarian cycle. Social living of long-tailed macaques can significantly affect sexual function, and even cause the ovarian cycle to stop or prolong for months. Likely, the test design should include a period of at least 3 months in order for the animals to become familiar with each other.

The most reliable way to confirm the sexual maturity of female macaques is to assess menstrual bleeding, which requires daily collection of vaginal swabs. The marker of sexual maturity is to identify at least 2 days and more of bleeding between two bleedings at an interval of at least 20 days. Simple clinical observation of bleeding is feasible, but less accurate and reliable. It is recommended that the amount of bleeding be assessed by grading the swab, and it is better to collect vaginal swabs daily rather than every 2–3 days. Likely, the assessment of perineal skin swelling and skin redness is not a reliable indicator of continuous monitoring of the ovarian cycle. Monitoring ovarian activity can be achieved by measuring progesterone, 17-estradiol, LH, and FSH concentrations in serum. However, due to the need for frequent blood collection, it is not recommended to rely solely on hormone analysis to assess female sexual maturity.

Puberty in female nonhuman primates occurs at 2.5–4 years old. The reproductive tissue manifestations of female nonhuman primates in immaturity and puberty (but immature): the ovaries are small, with only primitive or primary follicles and stroma. As puberty approaches, the follicles may begin to develop, and sinus chambers may appear, but most of these will show signs of atresia. Uterine contractions, endometrium, and the muscle layer are basophilic and inactive. The inner diameter of the vagina is also small, lined with a thin cuboidal epithelium. The mammary glands of immature nonhuman primates have a ductal primordium that begins to develop before the first menstrual cycle. The dominant tube begins to extend and branch, along with the development of terminal buds that are surrounded by a loose mucoid periglandular matrix. The connective tissue of the mammary glands of nonhuman primates has extensive lobular development during peripuberty, and the growth rate varies significantly among different animals. Pathologists need to recognize that normal pubertal glandular development should not be misdiagnosed as hyperplasia or tumor when comparing different individuals.

5.3.1 Congenital and Genetic Abnormalities of the Female Reproductive System in Nonhuman Primates

1. Both pseudohermaphrodite and true hermaphrodite of hermaphrodite congenital lesions may appear in NHP. True hermaphroditism is characterized by the presence of two gonads, which can be regarded as a testicle on one side and the ovary on the other side (hermaphrodite on different sides); testicle or ovary on one side and testis–ovum on the other (unilateral hermaphroditism), or both-sided testicle and ovary or ovotestis (bilateral hermaphroditism). The ovotestis is a mixed gonad consisting of an underdeveloped central spermatogenic tubule (testis) surrounded by relatively normal ovarian cortical tissue. There may be a testicular net at the porta of the ovotestis. The ovotestis is usually located within the pelvis and may also be located at the head end of the underdeveloped uterus. The relative ratio of testicular to ovarian tissue is usually related to the degree of decline of the ovotestis into the groin, and it is generally believed that the abdominal position of the ovotestis or the secretion of estrogen by the ovarian tissue causes the spermatogenic tubule agenesis of the testis. On chromosomes, true hermaphrodites may be systemic chimeras or chimeras, or pseudohermaphrodites of the XY or XX genotypes. Pseudohermaphrodites have chromosomes and gonads of one sex and also modified tubular organs of the other

sex. Pseudohermaphrodites are classified according to the gonadal tissue present, and are more common in males than females. Female pseudohermaphrodites have ovaries and XX genotypes, with normal but stunted tubular organs and distinctly masculine external genitalia (including enlarged clitoris and mismatched labia similar to prepuce and scrotum). This deficiency may occur spontaneously or may be caused by intrauterine exposure to androgens or androgen-like substances. Endogenous factors include fetal adrenal hyperplasia or the presence of androgen-secreting tumors in the fetus. Male pseudohermaphrodites may have an underdeveloped uterus [13].

2. In the congenital abnormalities of the tubular organs of the female reproductive tract, defects in the normal developmental sequence of the renal ducts may result in congenital abnormalities of the tubular organs of the female reproductive tract, characterized by complete failure of the development of half of the uterus (hemiuterus or unicorned uterus), often accompanied by ipsilateral renal and/or ovarian hypoplasia, or segmental hypoplasia of part of the reproductive tract. The broad ligament on the affected side may contain only dense fibers or fibrous muscle bands. The two caudal ends of the pararenal canal are partially or completely unable to fuse into the normal pyriform (simple) uterus, which may result in uneven division of the uterus (uterine bifida), with possibly two separate horns, the cervix, and even a duplicate anterior vagina under macroscopic observation.

3. *Cystic residue of the mesonephric duct*. Cystic remnants of the medirenal duct may persist after birth as an occasional lesion of NHP called "Morgagni hydatid," which is a vesicular structure attached by a short pedicle near the tubal coat. It is histologically shown as: tall epithelium, cube-like, with a large nucleus and different forms of cilia, similar to the fallopian tube, located on an obscure basement membrane. Without the testicular influence, the mesrenal tubules and tubules usually degenerate, leaving only marks. Cystic remnants of the mesonephric and Wolffian ducts may be present in the mesangium (parafovarium cysts), the mesosalpinx (para-fallopian cysts), or the vaginal wall (Gartner catheter cysts). Mesonephric remnant cysts can be distinguished by shorter, cubic cells that are not ciliated and located on a well-developed basal membrane. Both types of cysts may have smooth muscle infiltration in the cyst wall. Cystic dilation of the cervical glands with mucous contents (Nabothian cysts) may be secondary to inflammation and obstruction.

4. *Turner syndrome*. Turner Syndrome has also been reported in rhesus monkeys and baboons. Ovaries that do not develop properly have historically been called "striated gonads." Oogenesis does not occur normally due to the absence or abnormality of the second X chromosome, which is selectively reactivated in germ cells, and the rate of follicle loss is greatly accelerated. This can lead to premature follicle failure. The resulting ovaries consist of elongated chains of atrophic fibrous connective tissue, which is similar to the ovarian stroma but lacks germ cells and follicular structures. In addition, the uterus and fallopian tubes are clearly stunted, and the animals may be small, always sterile, and usually do not menstruate.

5. *Congenital fused labia*. The congenital fused labia of common marmosets is a recessive defect. The size of the vulvar opening reduces from an average of 6–10 mm to 1.5–2.5 mm and is centered on the urethral opening. The rest of the reproductive tract is normal, with a normal estrus cycle, but the animal remains functionally sterile.

5.3.2 Common Background Changes of the Female Reproductive System in Nonhuman Primates

In general, background lesions are uncommon in adolescent and young adult nonhuman primates in toxicity tests [14, 15].

1. *Ovarian cysts*. Ovarian cysts are common and include cysts that originate from tissue structures adjacent to the ovary, such as embryonic mesonephric duct remnants, enlarged rete ovarii, and cystic follicles or corpus luteum. Cystic structures within the ovary can be classified as follicular cysts, which originate from ovarian follicles, luteal cysts, which originate from the corpus luteum, or inclusive cysts, which originate from the ovarian epithelium.

Follicular cysts develop from secondary follicles that do not ovulate or are not atretic. The adenohypophysis secretes sufficient levels of follicle-stimulating hormone, leading to follicle maturation, but insufficient luteinizing hormone levels lead to ovulation failure or follicular cyst formation. Follicular cysts vary in size and may resemble normal follicles, usually lacking mature oocytes. Follicular cysts are usually larger than normal follicles and are frequently visible to the naked eye. The walls of the follicular cyst are gray with a large amount of serous fluid. The walls of these cysts may consist of several layers of normal-shaped granular cells and may even resemble normal cumulus formation. Larger cysts have thinner walls with thin outer fibrous layers and one to two layers of cubic or flat granular cells. Large cysts may press on adjacent ovaries, and the presence of multiple cysts may displace normal ovarian structures. Follicular cysts can secrete normal or excessive estrogen for a long time, resulting in clinical hyperestrogen. Associated lesions include cystic endometrial hyperplasia, cervical squamous metaplasia, and mammary hyperplasia. Literature shows that two female macaques developed spontaneous mammary and endometrial neoplasia after 12 months of continuous estrus.

Luteal cysts originate in the normal corpus luteum and do not subside. Luteal cysts may resemble the central phase of a newly formed corpus luteum, but the latter loses its central cavity due to the proliferation of granular luteal cells, while the former retains the central fluid-filled sac cavity. Luteal cysts are generally yellow, reflecting their rich lipid content and ability to synthesize sterols. The cell wall consists of several layers of granulocyte lutein cells with large, pleomorphic cytoplasm containing large amounts of eosinophilic substances, surrounded by round to fusiform follicular membrane cells in different quantities from the ovarian stroma with large eosinophilic cytoplasm and few vacuoles. The progesterone secreted by luteal cysts is normal or elevated, and the secreted hormones do not enter the circulation and last for a long time.

Inclusion cysts originate from an ectopic focus or invagination of the surface epithelium of the ovary and may arise after repairing the ovulation hole during ovulation. These cysts vary in size and are visible as a single chamber, consisting of a thin layer of epithelial cells resembling normal ovarian surface epithelium or accompanied by tubal metaplasia (ciliated columnar epithelium) surrounded by a thinner layer of ovarian stroma. Inclusion cysts must be distinguished from follicular cysts and ovarian cystadenomas. The incidence of inclusion cysts increases with age, and sand bodies (lamellar concentric calcification) are visible in the lumens.

2. *Cortical mineral deposition.* Cortical mineral deposition is common in the ovaries of juvenile nonhuman primates and may be a dystrophic mineralization of atretic follicles (Figs. 5.29 and 5.30). Follicles containing multiple oocytes, caused by the epithelial hyperplasia on the surface of the ovary, are also often considered a background change due to.
3. *Uterine surface epithelial bleeding.* The uterine surface epithelial bleeding is a characteristic of the endometrium during menstruation, but it often occurs in peripubertal females who have not ovulated or have not had a regular menstrual cycle. It is irregular bleeding. Irregular endometrial bleeding can be distinguished from true menstruation by the fact that irregular bleeding occurs in the endometrium during the proliferative phase, while normal menstruation occurs in the secretory phase of the endometrial menstrual cycle. In addition, menstruation is complete endometrial shedding, while irregular endometrial bleeding is characterized by surface bleeding with little endometrial shedding or necrosis (Fig. 5.31 and 5.32). When examining the ovaries, it may also provide clues based on the presence of luteal degeneration (menstruating females have luteal degeneration, but prepubertal females do not). Inactive (aperiodic) uterine morphology is often found in nonhuman primates after puberty (that is, the ovaries contain luteal residue) and is the result of an unovulating menstrual cycle. This condition is commonly observed in female monkeys that have just entered puberty, and may also reflect nonspecific stress, such as social stress or stress related to the administration of the test article in toxicity tests.
4. Endometriosis, including the serous membrane and myometrium, is characterized by ectopic endometrial glands and stroma in varying proportions, a relatively

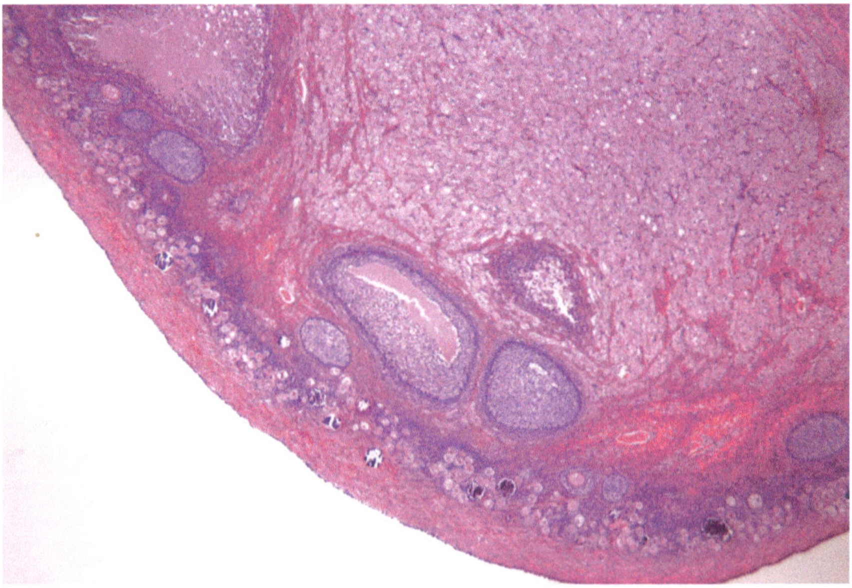

Fig. 5.29 Cynomolgus monkey (3 years old) ovarian cortex is scattered with mineralization (arrow) (HE staining, ×40)

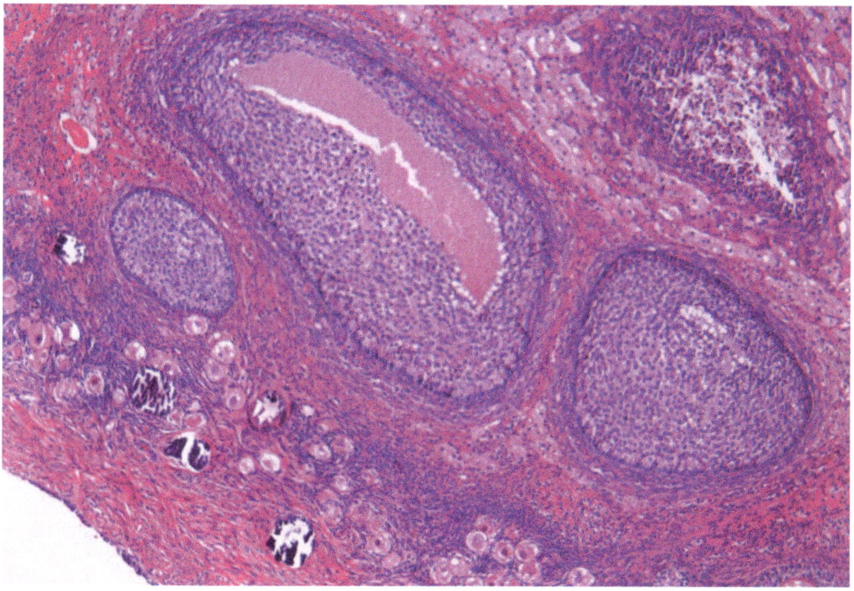

Fig. 5.30 Cynomolgus monkey (3 years old) ovarian cortex is scattered with mineralization (arrow) (HE staining, ×100)

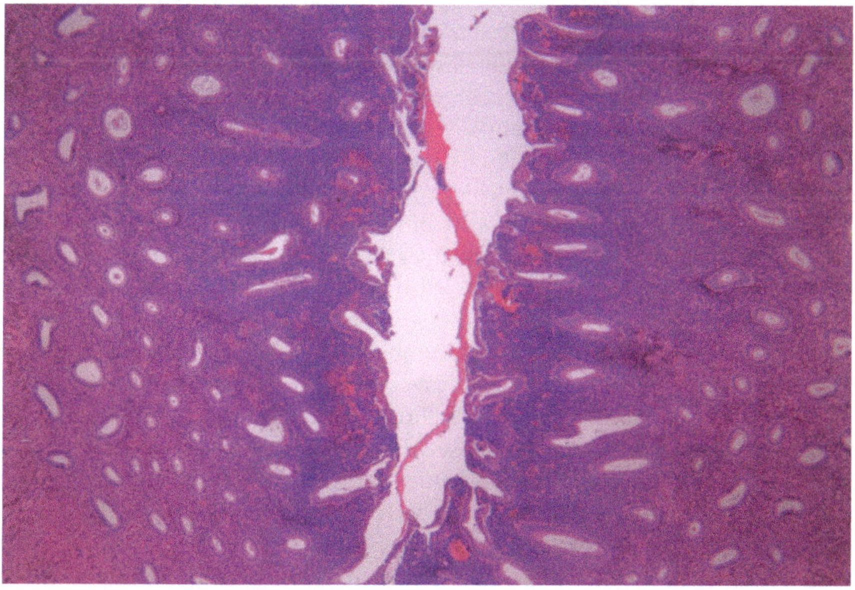

Fig. 5.31 Cynomolgus monkey (3.5 years old) urine surface bleeding (arrow) (HE staining, ×40)

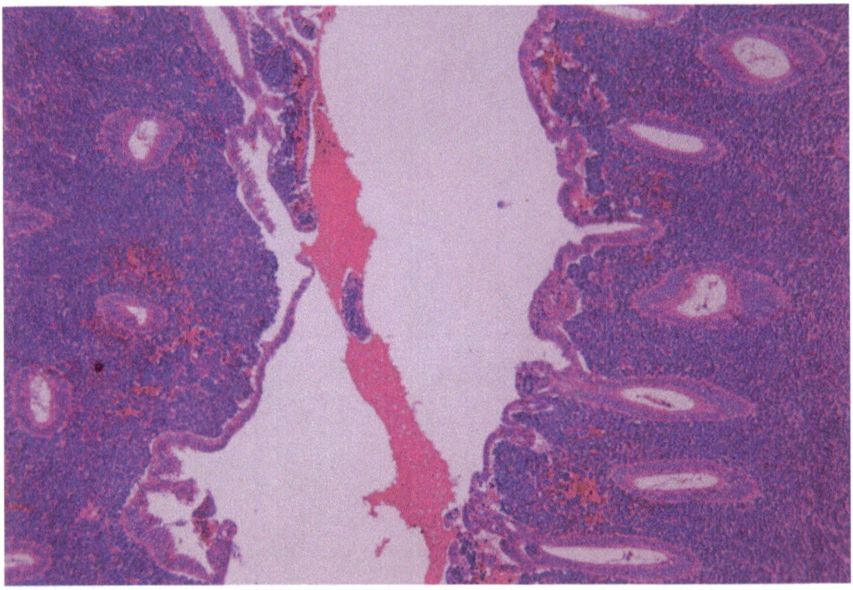

Fig. 5.32 Cynomolgus monkey (3.5 years old) urine surface bleeding (arrow) (HE staining, ×100)

common background lesion in the uterus of nonhuman primates. Adenomyopathy is the presence of well-differentiated endometrial glandular foci and stroma within the endometrium, which may be attached to the lumen surface, suggesting endometrial diverticulosis. Occasionally, adjacent muscle layers may also be hypertrophic. Due to the irregular junction between the endometrium and the myometrium, it is also found that the endometrium is superficially invaginated into the myometrium. In addition, this lesion can be induced in nonhuman primates and some domestic animals by exposure to high levels of estrogen compounds.

Endometriosis occurs spontaneously only in menstruating species (Old World monkeys and apes). Current theories favor retrograde menstruation through the fallopian tubes (Sampson hypothesis), rather than epitheliosis in the mesothelium. Bilateral retrograde menstruation is observed in baboons and human females under laparoscopy. Various studies in humans and animals have shown that there are a large number of immune alterations in individuals with endometriosis lesions, particularly those involved in cell-mediated immunity. In the cases of spontaneous endometriosis, baboons treated with immunosuppressive drugs had accelerated disease progression, compared to untreated spontaneous disease controls. Spontaneous endometriosis has also been reported in cynomolgus monkeys. Endometriosis can also be induced by exposure to ionizing radiation, experimental surgical implants, surgical occlusion of the cervix, or the creation of a uteroabdominal fistula. Other risk factors include advanced age, estradiol implantation, hysterectomy, barrenness, and a history of infertility.

Based on the experimentally induced baboon model, a two-step process for the onset of endometriosis is proposed. The initial stage occurs within 6 months after implantation of ectopic endometrial tissue and depends on the survival and proliferation of estrogen synthesized by the ovaries. Later, aromatase is upregulated in the lesion and may then autonomously synthesize estrogen. Common locations for endometriosis lesions include the dorsal lateral peritoneum located between the ventral side of the uterine body and the dorsal side of the colon and rectum, lateral edges along the uterine body and fallopian tubes, and the serous surface of the pelvic and abdominal cavity. The "metastases" of this lesion to the diaphragm, liver, intestine, mesentery, and pelvic lymph nodes have been occasionally reported. The lesion may also be present in the umbilical cord or be a scar left by abdominal surgery. The distribution and severity of endometriosis lesions can be scored according to the classification of the American Fertility Society Classification (1985). In general, the lesions are white, yellowish, red, dark purple, or brown raised plaques, miliary lesions, vesicles, or gelatinous or sac-like structures. Congestive cysts are known as "chocolate cysts." The growth of endometrial solid tissue without cyst formation is called an endometriosis tumor. Different degrees of fibrosis or hemosiderosis can be found. The histological manifestations of the lesions are cubic to low columnar endometrial epithelium with foamy cytoplasm, occasionally periodic PAS positivity, rare cilia supported by stromal cells with sparse cytoplasm, small round nuclei, and deep staining. The epithelium forms a glandular structure, with occasional cysts containing eosinophilic substances, fresh and old bleeding, cell debris, and macrophages. Cysts may contain papillary lobes, usually with extensive angiogenesis and fibrosis in the connective tissue that supports the endometriosis focus. The presence of interstitial endometriosis, where the ectopic endometrial stroma is mixed with bleeding and/or hemosiderin-containing macrophages, may represent an early lesion of endometriosis.

In nonhuman primates with prior reproductive experience, muscular blood vessels show significant widening of the media due to deposition of eosinophilic transparent substances similar to amyloid. The lumen of the affected vessel is often occluded. This change is the result of the invasion of the trophoblast into the uterus during pregnancy. Female monkeys that had never given birth did not have these changes.

5. Lymphocyte aggregation of vaginal and cervical mucosa, lymphoid follicles, and infiltrated inflammatory cells is unequal in number. The vaginal and cervical mucosa often presents lymphocyte aggregation and lymphoid follicles with varying numbers of infiltrated inflammatory cells (Figs. 5.33 and 5.34). The presence of chronic mononuclear cell infiltration in the vagina and uterus is a normal background finding.

The incidence of such infiltration is higher in the vagina (34%–80%) than in the uterus (9%). Trichomonas vaginalis is a cause of NHP vaginitis. Acute and chronic inflammatory infiltrations may occur in the cervix, occasionally concurrently. Acute cervicitis is often accompanied by suppurative mucous exudation, while subacute to chronic inflammation may be confined to the squamo-columnar junction or squamous metaplasia.

6. *Pigmentation of vaginal muscular layer*. Diffuse deposition of brown pigment in the interstitium is observed in the muscular layer of the vagina, which may be hemosiderin or malariin and can be identified by Prussian blue staining (Figs. 5.35 and 5.36).

7. *Cervical mucosal cyst*. Muco-filled cysts can be found on the mucosa of the cervix surface. The epithelium of the cysts can be a single cube or flat epithelium containing mucus, and usually has a low incidence.

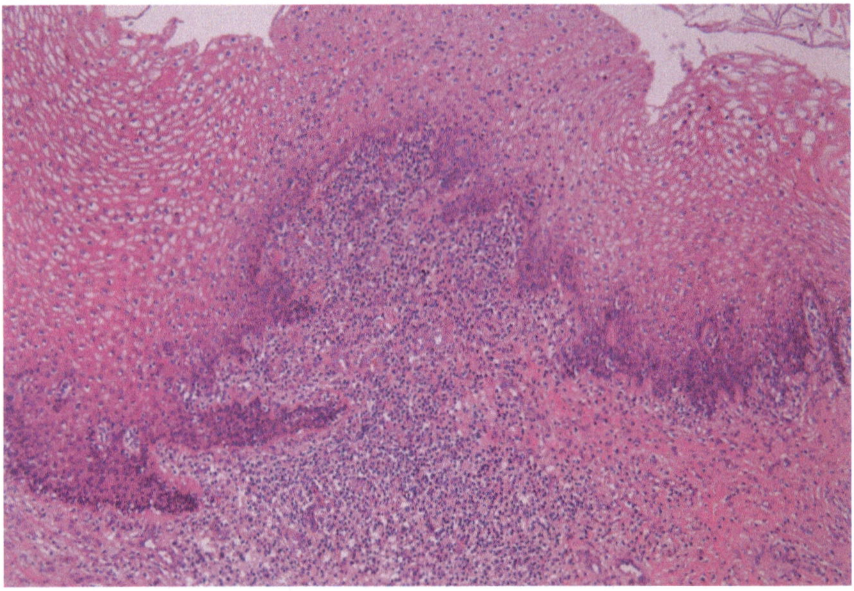

Fig. 5.33 Cynomolgus monkey (3.5 years old). The vaginal submucosa is infiltrated by scattered inflammatory cells (arrow), mainly mononuclear (HE staining, ×100)

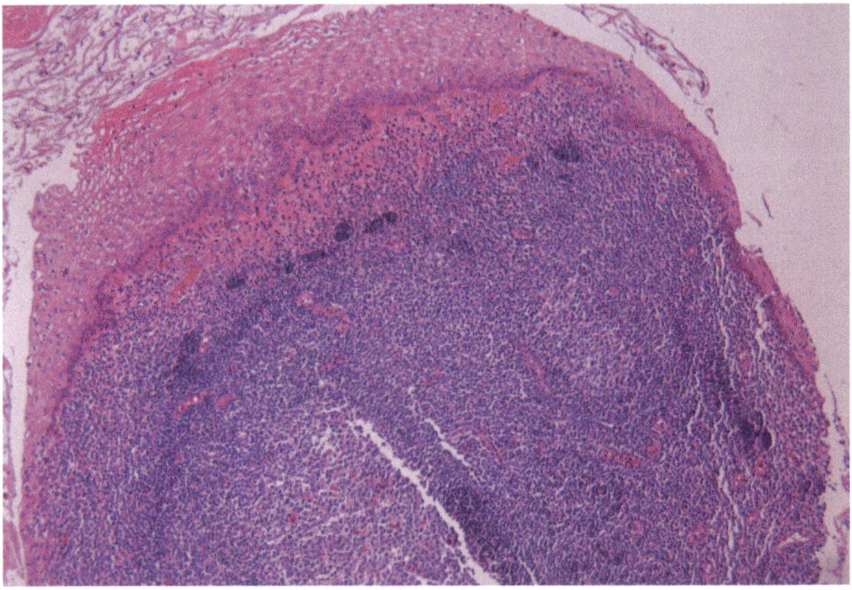

Fig. 5.34 Cynomolgus monkey (3.5 years old). Lymphoid follicles can be observed in the vaginal submucosa (arrow) (HE staining, ×100)

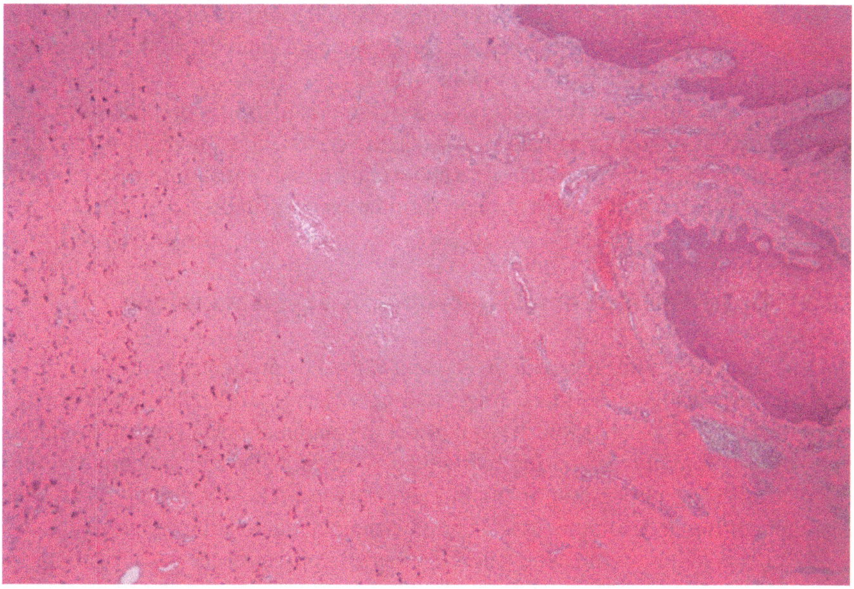

Fig. 5.35 Cynomolgus monkey (3.5 years old). Pigmentation of vaginal muscular layer (arrow) (HE staining, ×40)

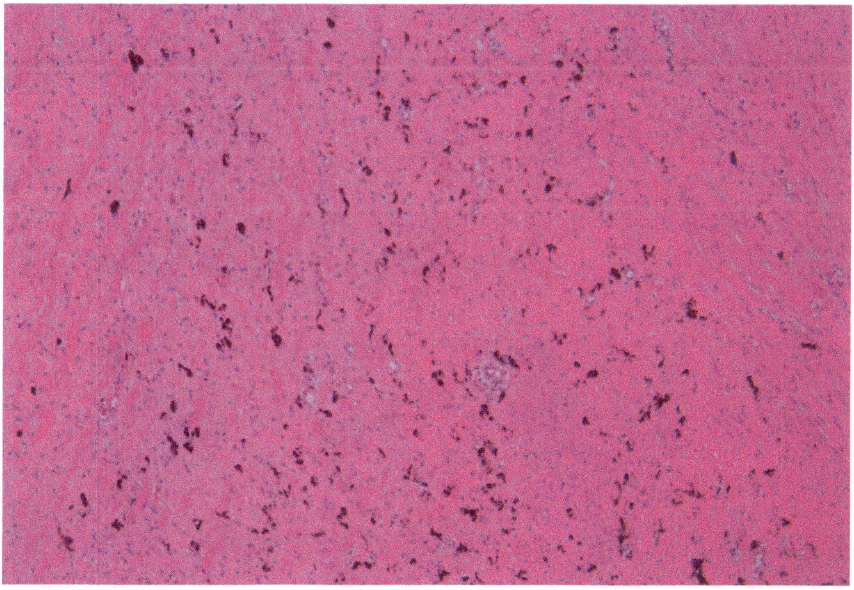

Fig. 5.36 Cynomolgus monkey (3.5 years old). Pigmentation of vaginal muscular layer (arrow) (HE staining, ×100)

Cervical mucous cyst. The mucous membrane on the surface of the cervix is filled with a mucous cyst; the cyst epithelium can be a single cuboidal or flat epithelium, containing mucous, with a usually low incidence.

8. Squamous metaplasia of cervical glands is a common finding in prepubertal or peripubertal female nonhuman primates and is due to a dominant hormonal state (estrogen excess) and should not be considered an abnormal finding. Squamous metaplasia can also occur under the influence of chronic stimulation or (usually excessive) estrogen.

5.3.3 Drug-Related Female Reproductive System Lesions

The lesions of the female reproductive system caused by drugs are relatively rare, but hormones, especially sex hormone drugs, can cause changes in the female reproductive organs. Figures 5.37–5.40 show the changes of the mammary gland and uterus during repeated drug toxicity test, performed in the chief editor Zhou Li's laboratory, for a long-acting progesterone drug in nonhuman primates, which is mainly manifested as mammary tissue development and endometrial decidualization reaction [16–18].

The effects of long-term, noncyclical exposure to progesterone or estrogen (physiological or supraphysiological doses) have been well characterized in macaques, which is usually accomplished by ovariectomy and then treatment with exogenous

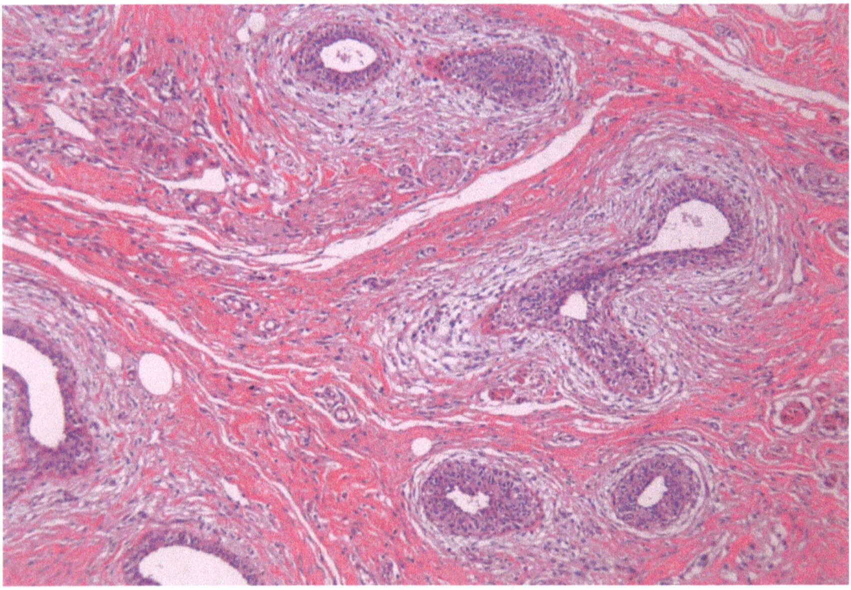

Fig. 5.37 Rhesus monkey (3 years old). Breast tissue development, loose around the glandular duct, likely edema, likely fibroblast/myoepithelial proliferation (arrow), caused by a progesterone drug (similar forms can also be found in normal animal development, and attention shall be paid to the comprehensive judgment of animal age and morbidity) (HE staining, ×100)

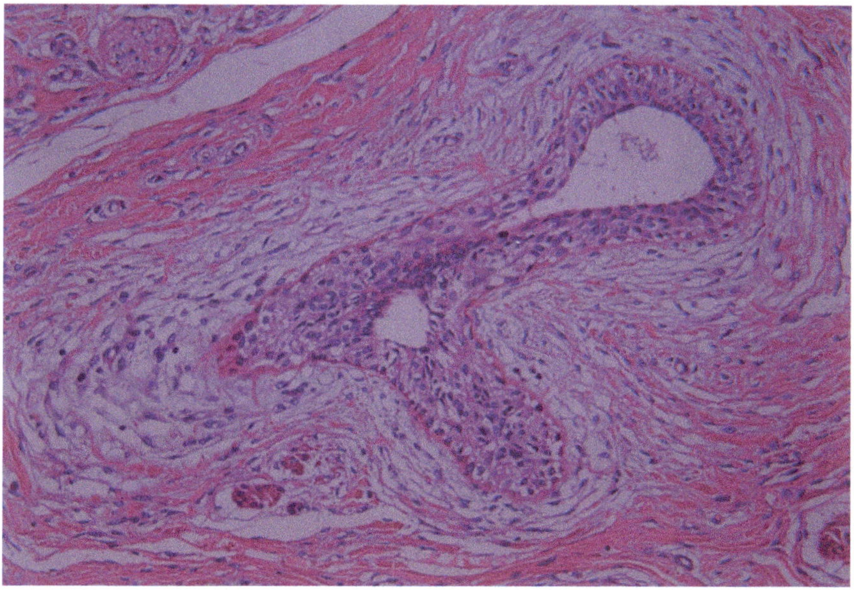

Fig. 5.38 Rhesus monkey (3 years old). Mammary tissue development (arrow), caused by a progesterone drug (similar forms can also be found in normal animal development, and attention shall be paid to the comprehensive judgment of animal age and morbidity) (HE staining, ×200)

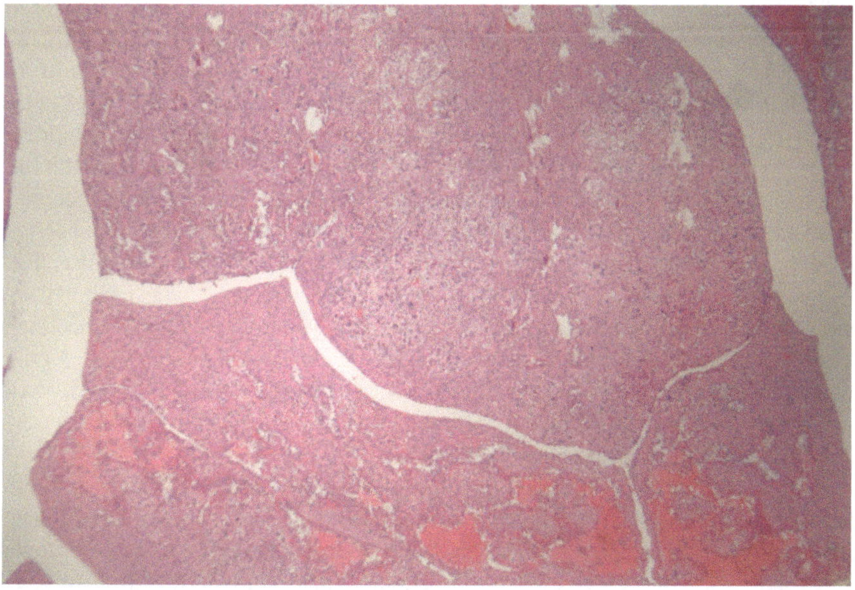

Fig. 5.39 Rhesus monkey (3 years old). Endometrial bleeding and necrosis (arrow), like menstrual cycle change, caused by a progesterone drug (HE staining, ×40)

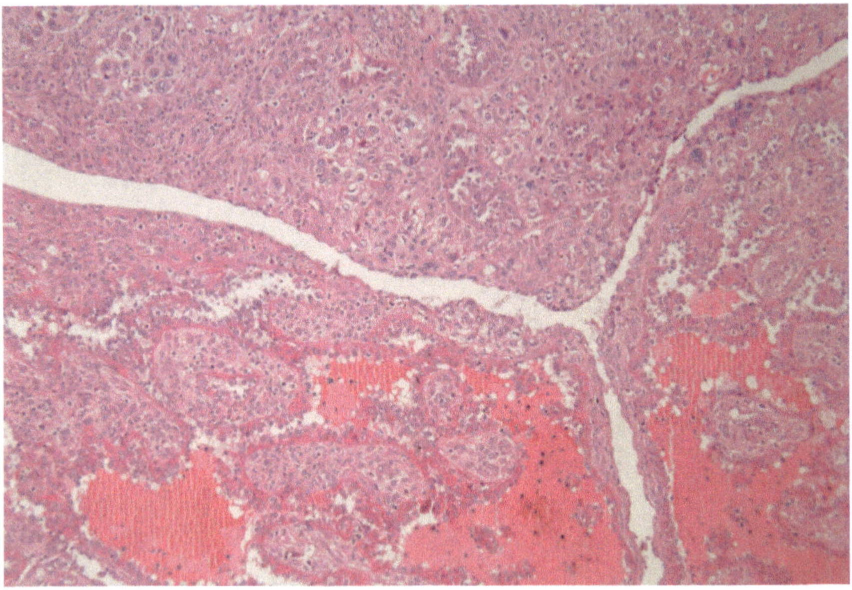

Fig. 5.40 Rhesus monkey (3 years old). Endometrial bleeding and necrosis (arrow), like menstrual cycle change, caused by a progesterone drug (HE staining, ×100)

steroids. The oophorectomy makes the endometrial glands atrophic, showing thin and dense interstitial cells and short, narrow, straight glands. The cervical epithelium is in infancy, and the glandular epithelium and surface epithelium have only one layer of fusiform cells. High levels of estrogen lead to glandular curl and distortion, epithelial hyperplasia, increased mitosis, decreased cytoplasmic ratio, epithelial false stratification, and varying degrees of endometrial hyperplasia, including typical cystic hyperplasia. Estrogen has also been linked to adenomyopathy and endometrial polyps. Under the influence of estrogen, the uterine interstitium becomes edematous and hyperplastic, mitosis increases, and the muscle layer may become hypertrophic. NHP shows a relatively large proportion of interstitial hyperplasia compared to human females. There may be squamous metaplasia in the endometrium and cervix. Cervical interstitium shows hypertrophy, edema, and glands secrete a lot of mucus, with rich blood vessels. During the estrogenic phase of the ovarian cycle, the vaginal mucosa has significant hyperkeratosis, especially in Old World monkeys, which may become apparent with age or excessive estrogenic therapy. The labia often show thickening and edema.

For squirrel monkeys that had been given diethylstilbestrol (DES, a synthetic estrogen) for a long time, seven out of ten animals given the drug developed malignant mesothelioma from the serous membrane of the uterus. The combination of estrogen and progesterone causes hyperplasia of mammary gland epithelium. Estrogens given after ionizing radiation have also been reported to act as cocarcinogens or accelerators, while estrogens alone have not been shown to develop tumors. Progesterone administration resulted in increased complexity and curvature of the endometrial glands, increased secretory activity, and characteristic perinuclear vacuolation of the epithelium.

5.3.4 Proliferation and Neoplastic Lesions of the Female Reproductive System in Nonhuman Primates

Nonhuman primates also have similar diseases of female reproductive tract tumors, similar to proliferative and neoplastic lesions, although they appear to be less common than their human counterparts under superficial examination. In one study, female genital tract tumors accounted for about 15% of all tumors in NHP and 5%–10% of all malignancies. While benign uterine leiomyomas are relatively common, all other reproductive tract tumors are quite rare. The study was based on zoo reports and retrospective autopsy analyses by research institutions, most of which examined young animals. More complete studies involving older animals have shown that the incidence of tumors in NHP is similar, although the incidence of different types of tumors generally differs from the incidence in humans, possibly due to epidemiological factors. The increase in tumor lesions in animals aged 11–20 years, and the apparent increase in tumor lesions in animals over 20 years, are comparable to the incidence of tumors in humans. The incidence of ductal carcinoma of the mammary gland in aged rhesus monkeys was 4.5%, the incidence of cervical cancer was 2.3%, and the incidence of ovarian cancer was 0.6%. Most tumor reports of NHP come from rhesus monkeys and cynomolgus monkeys. There is an interesting difference between New and Old World nonhuman primates. Tumors of Old World nonhuman primates are more likely to occur in the female reproductive tract tubular organs, while, where the tumors of New World nonhuman primates are more likely to occur in the gonads [19].

1. *Cervical cancer.* Cervical tumors of NHP are relatively rare compared to humans. Although cervical cancer is the most common gynecological malignancy worldwide, NHP is rarely reported. Human cervical cancer is closely associated with human papillomavirus (HPV) infection, mainly HPV16 and HPV18. By serological testing, far more nonhuman primates are positive for macaque papillomavirus (RhPV) than RhPV DNA, suggesting that infections are more common and widespread in nonhuman primates than lesions in humans. Hertig et al. found cervical dysplasia in 11 out of 78 captured wild female cynomolgus macaques. Wood et al. (2004) identified cervical lesions in 20 (5.2%) of 385 female cynomolgus macaques. All female cynomolgus monkeys were immunohistochemically positive for papillomavirus antigen, with a mean age of 18.6 years old. Of the 20 cases, 14 were cervical intraepithelial neoplasia (CIN), and 2 were CIN- II , Cin-III and epidermoid carcinoma. Five of the 20 animals also had condyloma acuminatum or genital warts. The lesions included papillary, exophytic lesions with fibrous blood vessels as the core, acanthodilation with nucleophil proliferation, variable mononuclear inflammation, and little or no basal expansion. This lesion is associated with human benign papillomavirus (HPV6 or HPV11) infection.

Low-grade cervical lesions include squamous metaplasia of the cervical glands or Abnormal epithelial hyperplasia in the outer cervical epithelium. In Wood et al.'s study, CIN grade II and above involved the cervical transition zone, while grade I lesions (also known as vaginal intraepithelial neoplasia or VIN) occurred in the vagina, fornix, outside the cervix, or in the transition zone. Mild or moderate dysplasia, comparable to cervical intraepithelial neoplasia I or II in human classification, includes nuclear enlargement, nuclear atypia, and nuclear hyperstaining. The presence of mastoid cells is highly associated with HPV. Mastoid cells are surface or intermediate mature squamous cells with perinuclear cytoplasmic vacuoles, dense and irregularly stained peripheral cytoplasm, large, round, and finely punctured nuclei, which can be binucleated or multinucleated. Atypical cells are confined to the basal layer of CIN, whereas CIN II has a more extensive atypia, maintaining sustained cell differentiation toward the lumen surface despite abnormalities. Basal cell expansion is less than one-third of the total epithelial thickness in CIN I and 1/3–2/3 in CIN II. Severe atypical hyperplasia is comparable to carcinoma in situ or CIN III, characterized by cell atypia, loss of maturation from the basal layer to the superficial layer, and increased basal mitosis rate. Intraepithelial lesions of HPV infection can be found with a colposcope. A 3% acetic acid solution is applied to the cervix to give the lesion a typical shiny white color. The Papanicolaou smear is also suitable for NHP and uses a similar grading standard. Since the differentiation of surface epithelial cells stops, the shed cytology is characterized by a decrease in cytoplasm, an increase in the nucleocytoplasm ratio, and changes in the nucleus, hyperpigmentation, and proliferation of nucleophilic cells.

Invasive cervical cancer reported in NHP includes epidermoid carcinoma and adenosquamous carcinoma. Both CIN and invasive carcinoma originate from the cervical adenosquamous metaplasia focus. The CIN grading system indicates that there is a development trend from moderate atypical hyperplasia to CIN and then to invasive carcinoma. Not all lesions progress, and the risk of cancer is proportional to how atypical it is. Epidermoid carcinoma is essentially a squamous cell carcinoma of the cervix. There are varying degrees of keratosis and keratosis bead formation, occasional cyst formation, and cavitation. Subtypes include keratosis, large cell non-keratosis, and small cell. The tumor may be exogenous, ulcerative, or infiltrated. Severe non-menstrual vaginal bleeding is usually caused by the invasion or erosion of blood vessels. Because of the better prognosis, the minimally invasive epidermoid carcinoma with the invasion depth of less than 3 mm into the basement membrane is classified separately. There are reports of its metastasis to local lymph nodes and lungs. Adenosquamous carcinoma shows a mixed pattern of squamous and cervical glandular differentiation. Human adenosquamous carcinoma usually has a worse prognosis than epidermoid carcinoma because they are poorly differentiated tumor and usually appears at a later stage.

2. *Uterine body tumor*. The most common tumor in the female reproductive tract of NHP is leiomyoma. Benign smooth muscle tumors of the uterine body can show as single or multiple nodular, firm, grayish–white fleshy masses that are elevated on the section surface. They can grow to a large size and occasionally undergo red degeneration, becoming soft, cystic, and hemorrhagic. Histologically, the tumors consist of

hypertrophic smooth muscle cells with nodular, compressive, and expansive proliferation, and have pale fibrillar eosinophilic cytoplasm and are arranged in interlacing bundles and spirals. It may be difficult to distinguish well-differentiated leiomyomas from the normal aging myometrium without examining the tumor margins. Tumor α smooth muscle actin (αSMA) and Desmin positive. It has been reported that in diseased NHP animals, leiomyomas occur simultaneously with endometriosis, and these two lesions also frequently occur in humans. Human leiomyomas are usually estrogen-responsive, increasing in size during pregnancy and regressing after menopause. Leiomyomas can exhibit significant atypia and giant cells, but are not malignant. Leiomyosarcomas can metastasize but have minimal atypia. For humans, the mitotic rate in the proliferative area is considered the most useful diagnostic criterion for malignant tumors. Tumors with fewer than five mitoses per ten high-power fields (HPF, 400×) are almost benign, and malignant transformation is considered extremely rare. Even if well-differentiated, tumors with more than ten mitoses per ten HPF are considered malignant. These tumors usually show typical malignant features such as cellularity, necrosis, multinucleated giant cells, nuclear pleomorphism, and hyperchromatism. Tumors with five to nine mitoses per ten HPF are considered borderline. There has been a report of a well-differentiated Rhesus monkey leiomyosarcoma with a moderate mitotic rate (0–2/HPF), but it was classified as malignant due to its infiltrative growth pattern within the uterine body and cervix. There was also a case of a well-differentiated Rhesus monkey uterine sarcoma (possibly a leiomyosarcoma) with peritoneal infiltration and omental metastasis, but it consisted of morphologically benign spindle-shaped cells with a low mitotic rate. Leiomyosarcomas are more likely to recur locally or metastasize to the draining lymph nodes rather than metastasize distantly. A case of clear cell epithelioid leiomyosarcoma (malignant leiomyoblastoma) in the uterus of a macaque has been reported. The tumor consisted of poorly differentiated round cells arranged in cords and solid clusters on a fine fibrovascular stroma. The tumor grew infiltratively with rare mitotic figures. The cells had a moderate amount of pale eosinophilic fibrillar cytoplasm, clear cell boundaries, nuclei ranging in size from round to indented, chromatin in vesicular to peripheral clumps, and small one to two nucleoli. Multinucleated giant cells were visible, and tumor cells invaded blood vessels. Immunohistochemistry of tumor cells showed positive Desmin and αSMA, and negative pan-cytokeratin.

Tumors of the endometrium may originate from the glandular epithelium or connective tissue stroma. These tumors may occur in the endometrium and rarely occur in the ectopic focus of endometriosis. Epithelial lesions range from hyperplasia to neoplasia to malignancy. Endometrial hyperplasia refers to the hyperplasia of endometrial glands and stroma, which is usually affected by hormones. In Old World monkeys, endometrial hyperplasia is associated with persistent estrogen imbalances, while New World monkeys, especially squirrel monkeys, may exhibit exuberant endometrial hyperplasia under the influence of progesterone. In humans and NHP, the severity of endometrial hyperplasia is usually related to the duration of exposure rather than the dose, and can be classified as mild, moderate (adenoma), or severe. The hyperplastic endometrium thickens from a normal thickness of about 1–17 mm and may appear flat, curled, or polypoid. In contrast, in proliferative lesions, endometrial adenomatous polyps are characterized by the endometrial stroma forming a dense fibrous stromal core, with abundant extracellular matrix and large, thick-walled blood vessels, while in proliferative lesions, there is abundant intracellular matrix and large vesicular nuclei. The proliferative glands are usually round, showing cystic dilation, hence the common name "cystic endometriosis." The epithelium ranges from simple columnar (mild or moderate) to pseudolamellar or lamellar (atypical) columnar, with the presence of glycogen-rich perinuclear vesicles when associated with estrogen. Perinuclear vacuolation is observed only in the endometrium after ovulation in females and is associated with progesterone, but it may occur before ovulation in macaques. The epithelium rarely exhibits squamous or tubular metaplasia. The cavity is empty or filled with amorphous protein secretions. The interstitium is diffusely cellular, with uniform distribution of small blood vessels and varying degrees of nuclear density. Interstitial hyperplasia includes hyperplasia and hypertrophy of interstitial components. Immunohistochemistry shows positive CD10 in endometrial stromal cells. The mitosis rate is low, and adenomyopathy may be present. With increasing severity, the incidence of clear fluid-filled cysts and interstitial hyperplasia decreases, while the proportion of glandular hyperplasia increases. In adenomatous hyperplasia, the glands are tightly packed with little interstitium. Atypical features include nucleus crowding, accumulation, increased staining and pleomorphism, loss of cell polarity, heteronucleosis, change in cytoplasmic staining from amphophilic to eosinophilic, irregular glands, dense glands arranged back to back, and sparse but dense interstitial. In humans, early nontypical changes are reversible, and the degree of atypia appears to be proportional to the risk of adenocarcinoma occurrence. The endometrial adenocarcinoma retains the cytological features of atypical hyperplasia with a superimposed pattern change. A sessile, polypoid mass or diffuse infiltrating muscle layer can be observed with the naked eye. The glands become complex, disordered, and bifurcated, and may appear solid or sieve-shaped. Intraglandular bridging is common in malignancies and may have extensive exophytic papillary alterations containing hypertrophic smooth muscle cells, mixed fibrous connective tissue, and blood vessels. Subserous capillary dilatation, myofibrosis, and endometrial atrophy.

3. *Ovarian tumors*. NHP ovarian tumors that have been reported include epidermal and stromal (cystadenoma, cystadenocarcinoma, papillary serous adenocarcinoma, papilloma, papillary serous adenocarcinoma endometrioid, and serous cystadenofibroma), sex cord and mesenchymal tumor (granuloma and granulosa cell tumor, luteoma), germ cells (choriocarcinoma, germ dysplasia, teratoma, and dermoid cysts), and ovarian stromal tumors (cavernous hemangioma and ovarian sarcoma). Papillary serous cystadenoma with dermoid cysts (benign cystic teratoma) in unilateral ovaries, cystadenocarcinoma with granulosa cell tumor, and contralateral ovarian choriocarcinoma, teratoma, and ovarian hamartoma have also been reported in nonhuman primates. The overall incidence of ovarian and uterine tumors accounts for 7%–15% of all tumors, of which about 20% are malignant. There are significant differences between human and NHP in the cell origin and malignancy proportion of ovarian tumors. Human tumors of epithelial (body cavity) origin make up the majority, accounting for 65%–70% of ovarian tumors, 90% of which are malignant. This is followed by germ cell tumors

(15%–20%, of which 3%–5% are malignant), sex cord stromal tumors (5%–10%, 2%–3% are malignant), and tumors of other origin (5%, of which 5% are malignant). In NHP, 38% of ovarian tumors originate from the sex cord stroma (17% malignant), 25% from germ cells (10% malignant), 23% from the epidermis (39% malignant), and 14% from other tissues (91% malignant).

Sex cord stromal tumor originates from the ovarian stromal that develops from the sex cord of the primordial gonad. Granulosa cell tumors vary in size from solid to cystic and are generally white to brownish yellow to brown, depending on lipid content. Granular cells are large, polyhedral, with clear cell boundaries, clear cytoplasm or eosinophilic cells, arranged in anastomotic cords and sheets. The diagnosis of granulosa cell tumor is characterized by the presence of light-colored tumor cells surrounding the central eosinophilic protein material (CallExner bodies similar to follicles), possibly with varying numbers of luteinized cells. Granulosa cell tumors produce estrogen and rarely androgens. Malignant granulosa cell tumors often occur in combination with other germ cell tumors.

Tumors of the ovarian surface epithelium originate from the coelomic mesothelium and show "Müllerian" differentiation into fallopian tube (serous), endometrial (endometrioid), or endocervical (mucinous) epithelium. These tumors can consist of varying amounts of solid, cystic, and fibrous components. In humans, the increase in malignancy is directly proportional to the amount of solid epithelial growth (including papillary projections, thickened cyst wall, or necrosis of solid tissue). Serous cystic tumors are composed of one or several fibrous-walled cysts. Benign tumors have smooth and shiny walls without epithelial thickening or small papillary projections. Malignant tumors contain increased papillary or solid tissue and can show capsular fixation. The cyst walls are lined with tall columnar ciliated epithelium, visible micropapillae can be observed, and the cysts are filled with clear serous fluid. There is an increase in the complexity of the stromal papillae, stratification of atypical epithelium, an increased mitotic rate, and stromal infiltration. Malignant tumors can spread across the coelomic cavity into the peritoneum, resulting in abdominal carcinomatosis. Psammoma bodies (laminated concentric calcifications) are occasionally encountered in serous tumors. Solid adenocarcinomas are composed of anaplastic cuboidal epithelial cells arranged in sheets, nests, or complex acinar structures formed by numerous closely packed papillary projections. Endometrioid tumors are generally solid and cystic and histologically show tubular glandular and arborescent papillary hyperplasia, similar to endometrial glands, and occasionally have foci of squamous metaplasia. Endometrioid carcinomas in baboons and humans are associated with endometriosis. Although endometrioid carcinomas may originate from foci of endometriosis, most are thought to result from neoplastic transformation of the surface epithelium. Mucinous tumors usually have more cysts of varying sizes, and the cysts are filled with mucus. The tumor walls are lined with tall columnar non-ciliated epithelium with basal nuclei and apical mucin droplets, and without cilia. Malignant tumors show stratification, increased complexity, or loss of glandular structure, solid growth, cellular atypia, necrosis, and stromal infiltration. Stromal infiltration is difficult to determine. In humans, atypical epithelial cells less than four cell layers thick are borderline lesions, while atypical epithelial cells with four or more layers are considered malignant. Cystadenofibromas may be serous, mucinous, or endometrioid and are characterized by an increase in the fibrous stroma of the uterine cavity wall. Despite hematogenous or lymphatic metastasis, surface epithelial tumors can grow to a large size before diagnosis and can spread into the abdomen through coelomic spread.

4. *Breast tumors*. Breast tumors in Old World monkeys are relatively rare, while in humans, breast cancer is the most common malignant tumor in women and the leading cause of cancer deaths. Breast tumors can be classified into a micropapillary pattern that consists of disorganized bulbous luminal epithelial projections without fibrovascular cores and usually form complex intraductal patterns. Other types include papillary and solid types, with the latter having pale cytoplasm and clear cell boundaries. The typical cell morphology is cuboidal to columnar, with abundant basophilia, typical vacuolated cytoplasm, and large, round, basal hyperchromatic nuclei. Infiltrated ductal carcinomas usually show more cellular pleomorphism and are often accompanied by significant fibrosis (desmoplastic reaction or desmoplasia). Other manifestations include calcification, psammoma bodies, squamous metaplasia, and extensive necrosis. Tumors may be locally invasive and most commonly metastasize to local lymph nodes, lungs, and liver, but metastasis to the adrenal glands, brain, coronary arteries, skin, mesentery, kidneys, ovaries, colon, pancreas, perineural areas, and eyes has also been reported. Lobular carcinoma in situ and invasive lobular carcinoma are rare lesions and are usually discovered incidentally. Typical lobular hyperplasia tends to occur in nulliparous, non-pregnant females who have not received exogenous hormonal treatment. The hyperplastic acini are composed of regular, well-differentiated lobules of cells, and the hyperplastic cells do not fill or expand more than half of the acini of the lobules. Atypical hyperplasia has been observed in rhesus monkeys, with multiple firm subcutaneous nodules in the breast area, some of which regress over time. Histologically, there are hyperplastic acinar cells in the lobules surrounded by fibrous connective tissue. The acini may be solid or may contain amorphous eosinophilic secretory material. Basal cells are distributed along the basement membrane, are relatively evenly distributed in layers, have small, round nuclei with clear nucleoli, and have abundant fine granular eosinophilic or lightly stained vacuoles in the cytoplasm. The intralobular ducts are normal. Lobular carcinoma is of the acinar type, with solid hyperplasia, uniform cells of small to medium-sized round nuclei with orthochromatic chromatin, and the acini are completely filled, expanded, and distorted. There is little or no atypia, nuclear pleomorphism, mitotic figures, and necrosis. The expression of E-cadherin decreases in lobular tumors. Fibroadenomas are benign proliferations of breast ductal epithelium surrounded by a large amount of concentrically proliferating connective tissue, and the stroma may be edematous. Estrogen steroids, growth hormone, and insulin-like growth factor, although not necessarily inducing breast tumors, seem to promote the occurrence of breast tumors.

5.4 Morphological Characteristics, Anatomical and Histological Structure, and Common Abnormalities of Nonhuman Primate Placentas

In the process of life's conception, from a tiny fertilized egg to a vibrant fetus, the placenta is an indispensable "behind-the-scenes engineer." This special organ, existing only during gestation, is not only the physiological basis for maintaining fetal survival but also symbolizes the most intimate "life connection" between the mother and the new life. It connects to the maternal uterus on one end and anchors the fetus through the umbilical cord on the other, using a unique "semipermeable membrane" structure to build a "life channel" for material exchange between the mother and fetus. Simultaneously, the placenta plays a dual role as both an "immune barrier" and an "endocrine gland": it can block the invasion of certain pathogens while allowing maternal antibodies to pass through, thus establishing an innate immune defense for the fetus; it also secretes hormones such as progestogens and human chorionic gonadotropin, acting like "signal switches" to regulate the state of the maternal uterus and ensure a stable pregnancy [20].

The human placenta, morphologically, is a hemochorial placenta, discoid in shape, with its fetal villi anchored in the basal plate of the maternal endometrium and surrounded by the maternal hemal cavity. The villous interstitium contains a complex branched vascular system consisting of villous capillaries, intermediate villous capillaries, and terminal villous capillaries. However, this specific type of placenta is not present in most laboratory animals. Therefore, researchers must carefully select laboratory animals based on the research objectives of the planned study and the dimensions of placental function they wish to be "most similar" to the human placenta. The similarities and differences in reproduction, placental characteristics, and immunological characteristics of different species are shown in Table 5.6. The ideal animal model should meet the following conditions: small size, short reproductive cycle, and close resemblance to the human placenta in terms of external placental morphology, maternal–fetal interface, and trophoblast invasion.

The cynomolgus monkey (*Macaca fascicularis*) is a nonhuman primate laboratory animal with highly human-like histological and physiological characteristics. Due to its close evolutionary relationship with humans and similar physiology (including reproductive physiology), it is increasingly considered the most suitable human model in toxicology research. The cynomolgus monkey has a hemochorial placenta, similar in morphology to the human placenta, and its placental histology and physiology are similar to those of humans. This is also true for the rhesus monkey (*Macaca mulatta*); however, the seasonal interruption of its reproductive cycle limits its use in reproductive toxicity studies. Other nonhuman primates used for laboratory research include baboons, vervet monkeys, and common marmosets, all of which exhibit reproductive physiology characteristics different from humans. Therefore, the cynomolgus monkey has become the most commonly used nonhuman primate model in reproductive

Table 5.6 Reproductive, placental, and maternal–fetal immunological characteristics of different animal species

Human	Human	Cynomolgus Monkey	Rodent (Mouse)
General characteristics			
Evolutionary distance from humans	–	31 million years	65–75 million years
Chromosomal homology with humans (%)	46 (100%)	42 (93%)	40 (97.5%)
Date of delivery	Day 266	Days 160–165	Day 20
Endometrial physiological characteristics	Decidual	Decidual	Non-decidual
Embryo implantation	Deep interstitial implantation	Superficial, incomplete implantation	Superficial, complete implantation
Time of maternal–fetal circulatory connection initiation	Day 63	Day 50	Day 16
Placental classification	Discoid, chorioallantoic, multilobed, monochorionic monoamniotic	Bilobed, chorioallantoic, multilobed, monochorionic monoamniotic	Yolk sac discoid, labyrinthine, hemochorial, cuboidal
Morphophysiological characteristics			
Time of maternal–fetal blood circulation initiation	Week 6 (clear fluid) Week 8 (blood)	Week 3	Day 1
Vascular trophoblast invasion	Extensive invasion into one-third of the myometrium	Limited decidual invasion	No data
Placental plate	Chorionic plate: small; villous lobules: small and flat	Chorionic plate: small; villous lobules: small to large; chorionic plates: large	No data
Decidua–trophoblast junction	Cell intermingling (interstitial trophoblast cells)	Minimal intermingling	Giant cells in contact with the decidua (equivalent to extravillous trophoblast cells)
B-cell production	B cell precursors: Week 7	Day 85	Low numbers of B cells at birth (Day 17)
T cell production	T cell precursors: Week 9	Days 60–70	–
Natural killer cell receptor phenotype	pNK: $CD56^{+}$, CD16dim uNK: $CD56^{-}$, $CD16^{+}$	$CD16^{+}$	Ly49 expression (via breast milk supply)

Human	Human	Cynomolgus Monkey	Rodent (Mouse)
Natural killer cell receptor family	KIRs expression	KIRs expression	Absent (via breast milk supply)
Neonatal immunocompetence	Present	Present	Absent (via breast milk supply)
Molecular physiological characteristics			
MicroRNA	MicroRNA cluster on chromosome 19	Present	Sfmbt2 microRNA cluster on chromosome 17
Transforming growth factor beta 2-related inhibitory activity	Lower in decidual leukocytes than in humans	Higher in decidual leukocytes than in mice	–
Chorionic gonadotropin	Highly glycosylated, predominantly hexose	Primate-specific	None
Gene cluster	Presence of placental lactogen/growth hormone and galectin gene clusters	Primate-specific	Presence of prolactin-related genes (23 genes, 1 gene unexpressed in humans)
Glycoprotein A	Expressed	Expressed	Not expressed
Placental estrogen synthetase (aromatase)	Present	Present	Absent
Placental progesterone production capacity	High	High	Limited
Fetal IgG receptor expression	Weeks 18–25 (maximum at Week 33)	From Days 85–100 onwards	From Days 11–12 onwards
Percentage of fetal IgG levels at birth relative to adult IgG levels	130%–200%	80%–100%	~1%
IgG transport receptor (FcRn)	Transport sites/cells: Syncytiotrophoblast brush border to fetal vascular endothelium, from Week 18 onwards; IgG1 ≈ IgG4 > IgG3 > IgG2, only IgG can be transcytosed; FcRn is also continuously expressed in placental endothelium, macrophages, and intestines	Transport sites/cells: Syncytiotrophoblast brush border to fetal vascular endothelium, IgG1 ≈ IgG4 > IgG3 > IgG2, high affinity for human IgG; expresses intestinal FcRn throughout life, similar to humans	Transport sites/cells: Mainly yolk sac endoderm, very few in placental syncytiotrophoblast; IgG2a/2b > IgG1; low IgG levels before birth, large amounts of maternal IgG absorbed by intestinal FcRn after birth, broader intestinal binding spectrum

toxicology research. It should be noted that in reproductive toxicity studies, much attention is paid to the mother and fetus, while relatively little attention is given to the examination, morphological analysis, immunological role of the placenta, and the effects of drugs on it. This chapter will describe placental morphology and anatomical and histological structure in nonhuman primates and briefly introduce the developmental process of the cynomolgus monkey placenta, as well as the differences in structure and immune function compared with humans [20, 21].

5.4.1 Morphological Characteristics and Anatomical and Histological Structure

1. *Morphological characteristics of nonhuman primate placentas.* Two "extreme" types of placentas exist in nonhuman primates. Many reproductive biologists are familiar with the discoid, usually villous, hemochorial placenta of most Haplorhini primates (e.g., humans, macaques: rhesus monkeys, cynomolgus monkeys, and apes). On the other hand, the placentas of most strepsirrhine primates (e.g., thick-tailed bushbabies, lorises, and lemurs) are diffuse, villous, and have an epitheliochorial structure. Many strepsirrhines have coarse placental villi that are usually unbranched and interdigitated with the endometrial crypts. In early gestation, trophoblast cells are columnar, but the blood–placental barrier thins significantly as gestation progresses. Indented regions at the tips of the villi appear to be involved in the absorption of histiotrophic nutrients. Accessory placental structures called chorionic vesicles are present. These cup-shaped specializations develop opposite the openings of the uterine glands and are active in absorption and secretion. In addition, most strepsirrhines have a large yolk sac early in pregnancy, a transient choriovitelline placenta, and many have a large allantois. In strepsirrhines, amnion forms via folding. In contrast, most haplorhine primates have a discoid, villous, hemochorial chorioallantoic placenta. Placental villi are covered by a layer of syncytiotrophoblast, which plays an active role in maternal–fetal substance transport and hormone synthesis. In some haplorhines, the extravillous trophoblast invades deeply into the endometrium and the spiral arteries that supply blood to the placenta. Other fetal membranes include: (1) the non-villous chorion (smooth chorion); there is evidence that the trophoblast of the smooth chorion has absorptive and synthetic functions; (2) the yolk sac, which is unusual in that it forms a secondary yolk sac. The yolk sac has synthetic and absorptive functions in early pregnancy; (3) the amnion; the amnion in haplorhines forms via cavitation. Further subdivided, New World monkeys (a group of primates located in Central and South America, i.e., the New World, belonging to Platyrrhini) also differ from apes and Old World monkeys (macaques, baboons, golden monkeys, etc.): New World monkey placentas are "pseudolabyrinthine" and seem to lack extravillous trophoblast (EVT) cells, which are crucial for placental invasion and maternal–fetal vascular remodeling. Old World monkeys (e.g., macaques) have a similar pattern of trophoblast invasion of the spiral arteries of the decidua basalis to humans, although the degree of interstitial EVT invasion into the decidual tissue is very limited.

1. *Anatomical and histological structure of the macaque placenta*

The placentas of cynomolgus and rhesus monkeys are typically bilobed (Fig. 5.41, left), with the two lobes situated on the anterior and posterior walls of the uterus. Each lobe contains several fairly distinct cotyledons, which are aggregations of adjacent stem villi and their branches. Compared to the stem villi of the human placenta, the stem villi of these two species are relatively more numerous and less extensively branched. Each cotyledon is supplied with maternal blood by a single endometrial spiral artery, which enters near the center of the maternal surface of the cotyledon.

Fetal tissues (chorion and fetus: gray) are surrounded by maternal tissues (endometrium/decidua: yellow; myometrium: pink). The chorionic cavity is filled with maternal blood (red). Villous lobules/stems/villi float in the maternal blood.

The cynomolgus monkey placenta is hemochorial, very similar to the human placenta. The amniotic cavity and fetus are encased by fetal membranes, which consist of the chorion and amnion, surrounded by maternal endometrium/decidua. The embryo is connected to the placenta via the umbilical cord. The side of the placenta facing the embryo is called the chorionic plate (fetal side), while the side attached to the decidua is called the basal plate (maternal side). The placental tissue between these two plates is filled with villi, and maternal blood fills the intervillous space. The intervillous space is a large cavity located between the chorionic plate and the basal plate, filled with maternal blood, and is the core site of maternal–fetal exchange. The chorionic plate faces the fetal side, originates from fetal tissue, and is the "starting point" of the fetal villous trees. The basal plate faces the maternal side and is composed of both maternal and fetal tissues. It serves as the "anchor point" for the fetal villous trees. Fetal villous trees extend from the chorionic plate into the intervillous space, with their distal ends (tips) anchoring to the basal plate, forming a "three-dimensional network" structure. This structure greatly increases the contact area between fetal tissue and maternal blood, providing the basis for nutrient transport and waste removal [22–24].

Primary villi originate from the chorionic plate and anchor in the decidua (Fig. 5.41, right). During gestation, villous branching gradually increases. In cynomolgus monkeys, the intervillous space is filled with maternal blood from the third week of gestation. The entire villus is covered by a specialized epithelial layer—the

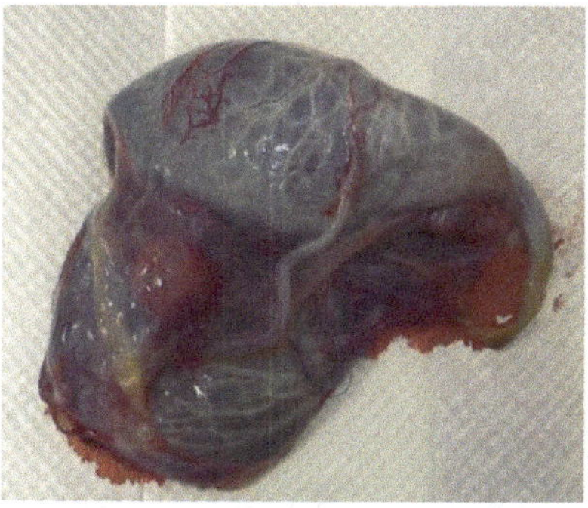

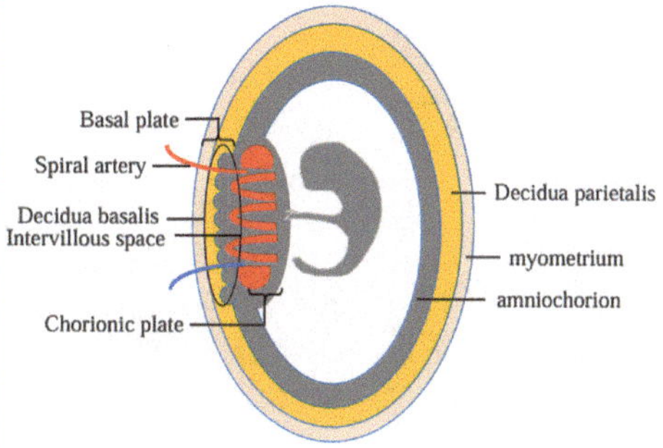

Fig. 5.41 Gross observation (left) and basic structural diagram (right) of the nonhuman primate placenta

syncytiotrophoblast (trophoblast cells can be broadly classified as cytotrophoblast, syncytiotrophoblast, or extravillous trophoblast). The distribution of extravillous trophoblast (EVT) cells in cynomolgus monkey and human placentas exhibits significant differences: cynomolgus monkey EVT cells are distributed in a continuous, dense, and distinct layer clearly separated from the maternal endometrium (decidual tissue); human EVT cells, however, are highly interwoven and fused with decidual cells, without obvious layering. This difference suggests that the placental invasion mechanisms and maternal–fetal immune regulation patterns may have subtle distinctions between cynomolgus monkeys and humans, which should be noted in experimental research (Fig. 5.42).

The fetus is encased within the amniotic sac, which is closely connected to the chorion. The yolk sac degenerates toward the end of the first trimester of gestation. The fetal side of the placenta is easily identifiable by its smooth surface and large blood vessels. The chorion contains a small number of mesenchymal cells within a loose fibrous connective tissue matrix and is traversed by interspersed paired arteries and veins. These vascular pairs branch to form a complex, lobulated villous network with attachment points on both the fetal side (chorionic plate, Fig. 5.43) and the maternal side (Fig. 5.44, trophoblast and decidua). Stem villi originating from the chorionic plate branch progressively into terminal villi, with the vascular smooth muscle gradually diminishing and ultimately disappearing. Villi are composed of fetal blood vessels, perivascular mesenchymal cells, cytotrophoblast epithelial cells, and large, multinucleated syncytiotrophoblast cells (Fig. 5.45). Directly lining the intervillous space (the maternal blood contact side), the fetal tissue surface is covered by two layers of trophoblastic epithelium with different functions: the syncytiotrophoblast layer, whose outer layer is a multinucleated syncytial

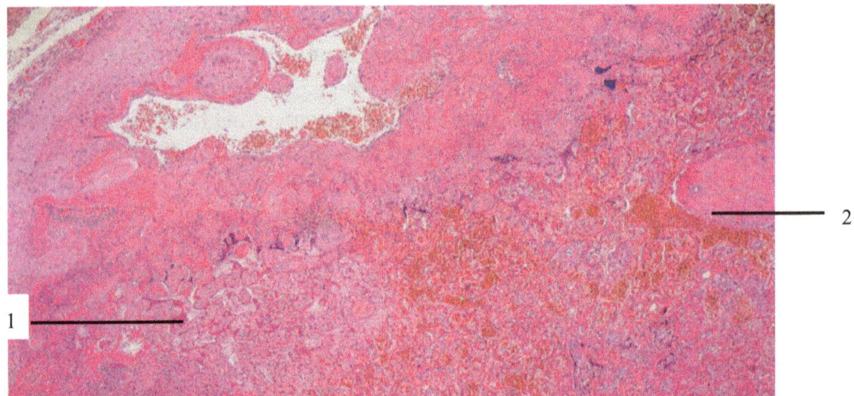

Fig. 5.42 Cynomolgus monkey placenta, hemochorial, filled with villi (1). Maternal blood fills the intervillous space (2). HE stain, ×40. (Photo from this laboratory)

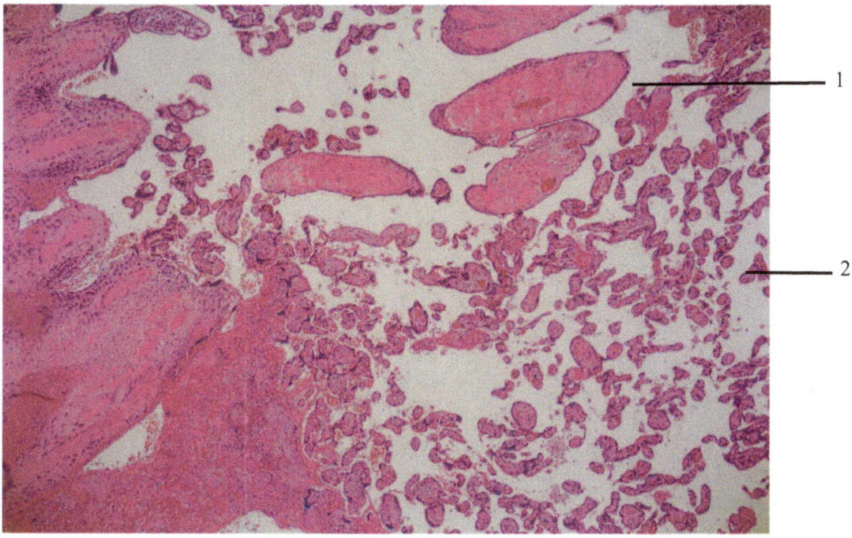

Fig. 5.43 Cynomolgus monkey placenta, fetal side. Stem villi (1) originating from the chorionic plate branch into terminal villi (2). Vascular smooth muscle gradually decreases until it disappears. HE stain, ×40. (Photo from this laboratory)

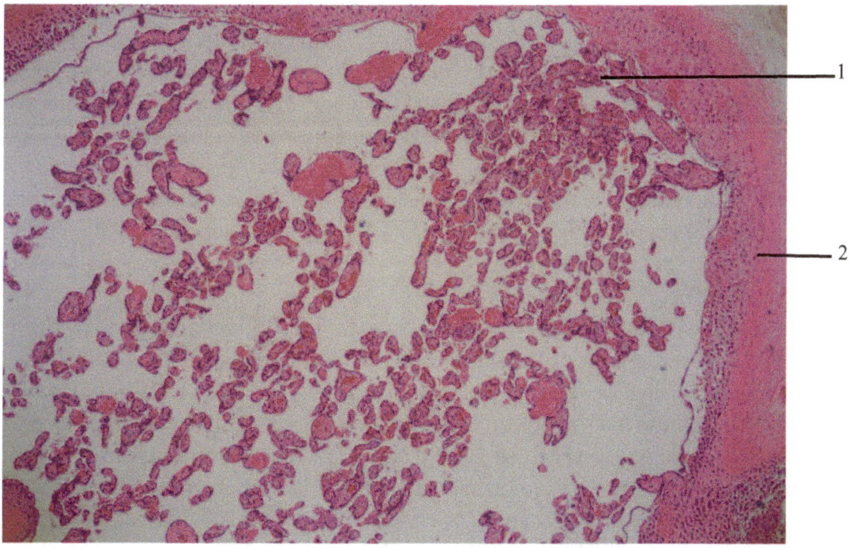

Fig. 5.44 Cynomolgus monkey placenta, maternal side. Trophoblast (1) and decidua (2) are visible. HE stain, ×40. (Photo from this laboratory)

cell layer without cell boundaries, and is the "functional interface" for maternal–fetal exchange (such as gas, nutrient, and hormone transport); the cytotrophoblast layer is located below the syncytiotrophoblast layer. It is a single layer of cuboidal cells with

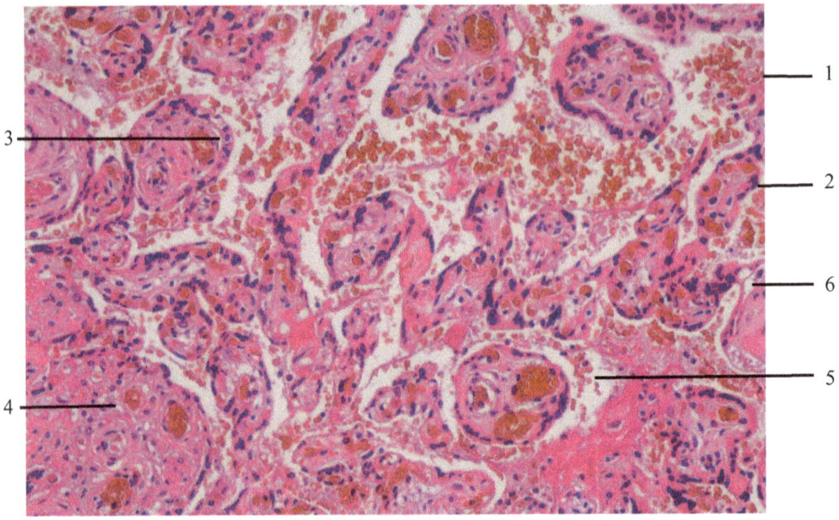

Fig. 5.45 Cynomolgus monkey placenta, chorionic structure. 1. Maternal blood sinus, 2. Villi, 3. Fetal blood vessels. Villi are composed of fetal blood vessels, perivascular mesenchymal cells (4), cytotrophoblast epithelial cells (5), and large multinucleated syncytiotrophoblast cells (6). HE stain, ×200. (Photo from this laboratory)

high proliferative capacity, which can continuously differentiate and replenish the outer syncytiotrophoblast layer (because the syncytiotrophoblast layer has no division ability and needs to rely on the cytotrophoblast layer for renewal). Fetal trophoblast cells also invade the endometrium, surrounding and infiltrating the walls of maternal endometrial blood vessels; these cells are called extravillous trophoblast cells. Whether syncytiotrophoblast, cytotrophoblast, or extravillous trophoblast, all can be clearly identified by histochemical staining for cytokeratin 18 (CK18, a characteristic skeletal protein of epithelial cells, including trophoblast cells, which can serve as an "identity tag" for trophoblast cells) or other specific markers.

The non-discoid, membranous part of the placenta lacks villi and is covered by a layer of trophoblastic epithelium. Normal noncellular components of the placenta include intervillous and intravillous placental fibrinoid deposits, composed of fibrin, laminin, and other extracellular matrix molecules, and multifocal mineralization of the placental villi (Fig. 5.46). Coagulation necrosis at the placental margin at term is a normal finding.

Beneath the placenta, endometrial glands are dilated and sparse; beneath the membranous portion of the placenta, the endometrial glands are dilated by fluid and lined by a single layer of cuboidal epithelium (Figs. 5.47–5.49), surrounded by plump decidual cells. Throughout the gravid endometrium, decidual cells derived from the stroma are abundant, as are granular endometrial lymphocytes. Postpartum uterus: due to the effect of oxytocin, the myometrial fibers are in a contracted state, the transverse diameter of the muscle fibers is small, and the myometrium is rich in spiral arteries. Histological changes undergo "involution–regeneration–remodeling." The acute involution phase generally lasts from 0 to 3 days postpartum, characterized by persistent

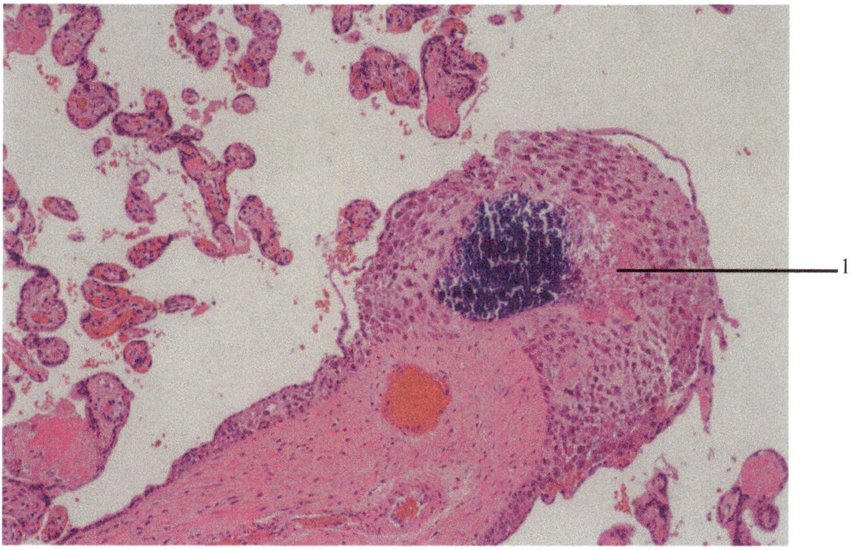

Fig. 5.46 Cynomolgus monkey placenta. Mineralization (1) is visible within the villi. HE stain, × 100. (Photo from this laboratory)

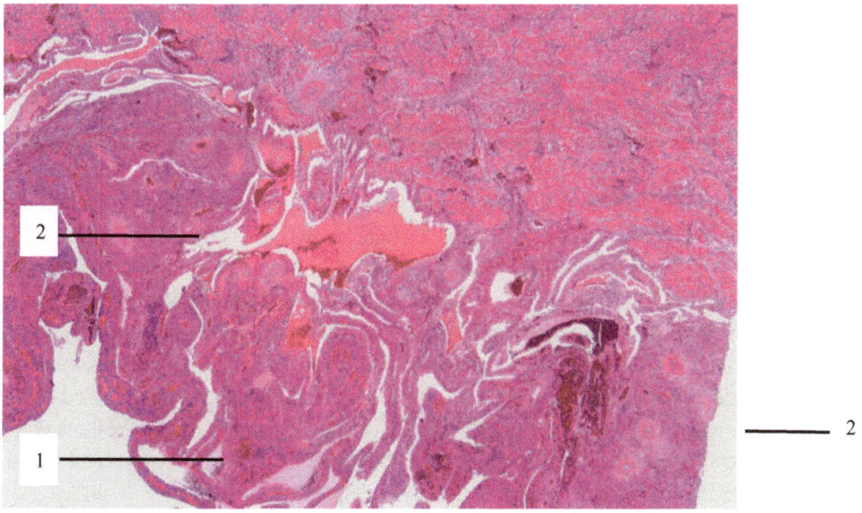

Fig. 5.47 Postpartum cynomolgus monkey, endometrial glands (1) dilated with fluid, lined by a single layer of cuboidal epithelium, scattered spiral arteries (2) are visible, HE stain, ×20 (photo from this laboratory).

myometrial contractions and the formation of lochia from the residual chorionic villi fragments and necrotic decidua on the surface of the uterine cavity. The proliferative regeneration phase lasts from 4 to 14 days postpartum, during which the stromal cells

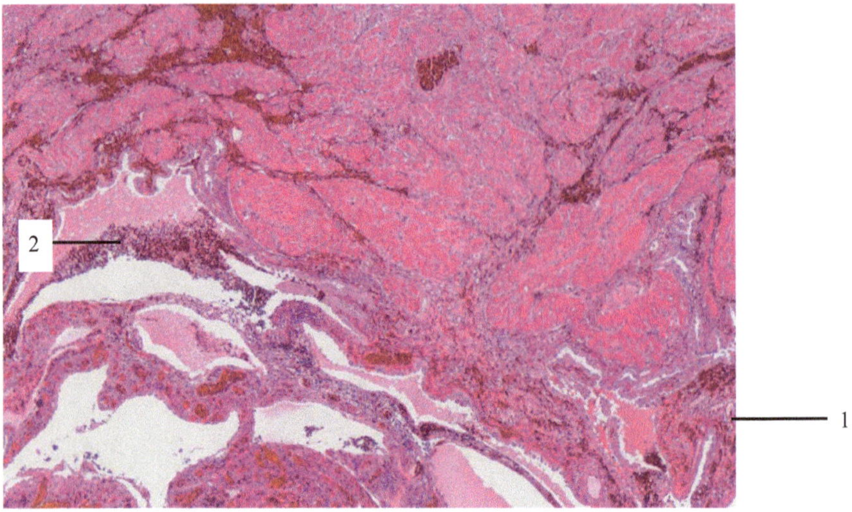

Fig. 5.48 Postpartum cynomolgus monkey, dilated endometrial glands (1), obvious congestion (2), HE stain, ×40. (Photo from this laboratory)

of the basal layer of the endometrium proliferate, migrate upwards, and reconstruct the functional layer. Myocyte cytoplasm is eosinophilic. Functional recovery is typically completed in about 6 weeks. The spiral arteries that dilated during pregnancy gradually close, degenerate, and their lumens narrow after childbirth. Local ischemia promotes autolysis and volume reduction of uterine muscle cells. The muscle fibers in the uterine myometrium gradually atrophy, leading to a decrease in overall volume, and the myometrial thickness returns to the nonpregnant state.

The fetal side of the placenta usually shows a centrally located umbilical cord. Similar to human umbilical cord vessels, it typically contains two arteries and one vein (Figs. 5.49–5.51). It is an important model for studying fetal development and placental function. The umbilical arteries carry fetal blood to the placenta for gas and nutrient exchange, while the umbilical vein returns oxygenated and nutrient-rich blood from the placenta to the fetus. HE staining reveals clear vascular structures within the cynomolgus monkey umbilical cord, surrounded by Wharton's jelly. The umbilical arteries, carrying deoxygenated blood and metabolic waste, appear darker in color during in vivo observation and have thick walls with a well-developed muscular layer. The umbilical vein, containing oxygenated blood, appears lighter in color with thinner, more elastic walls (Fig. 5.52).

5.4.2 Morphological and Immunological Characteristics of the Cynomolgus Monkey Placenta at GD50 Compared to the Human Placenta

During gestation, the placenta is the interface between maternal and fetal allograft (fetal) heterologous proteins, and thus plays an important immunological role. Direct

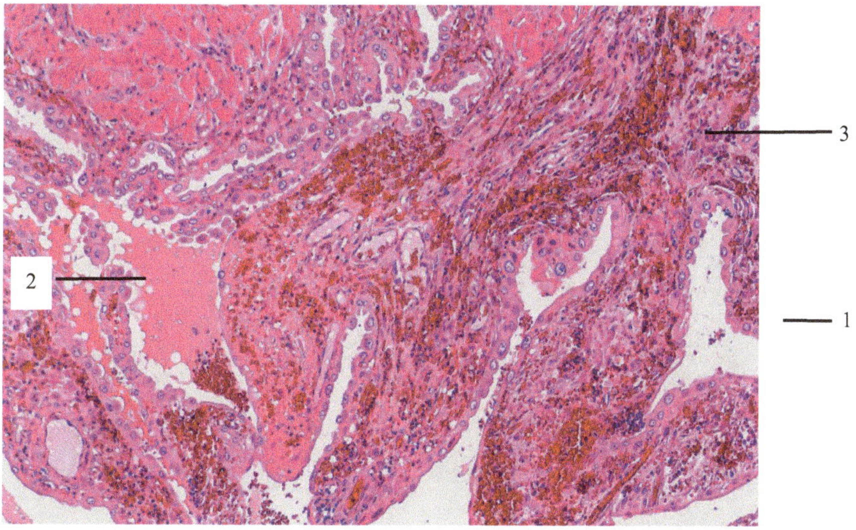

Fig. 5.49 Postpartum cynomolgus monkey, endometrial glands lined by a single layer of cuboidal epithelium (1), dilated with fluid (2), obvious congestion (3), HE stain, ×100. (Photo from this laboratory)

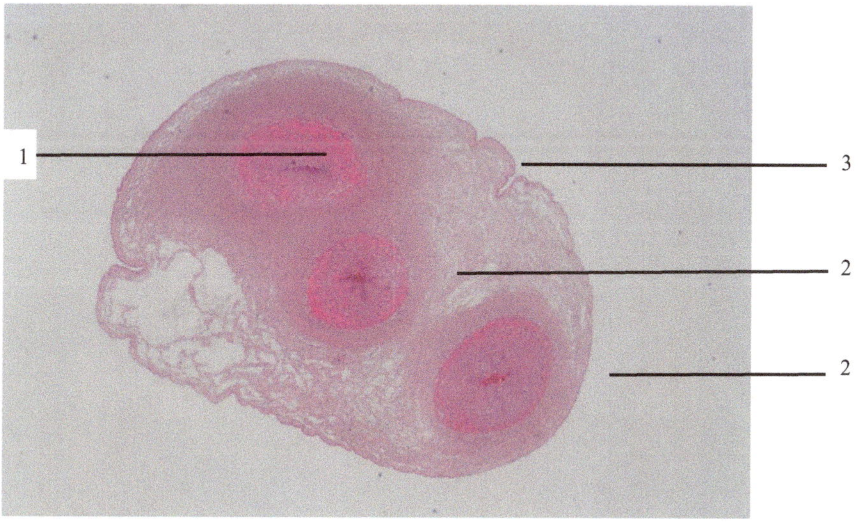

Fig. 5.50 Cynomolgus monkey, umbilical cord, containing three vessels, one vein (1), two arteries (2), abundant Wharton's jelly (3) surrounding the vessels, HE stain, ×20. (Photo from this laboratory)

maternal–fetal contact occurs at five interfaces: syncytiotrophoblast in contact with maternal blood in the intervillous space; interstitial extravillous trophoblast in contact with various maternal cells in the decidua, and some with cells in the myometrium;

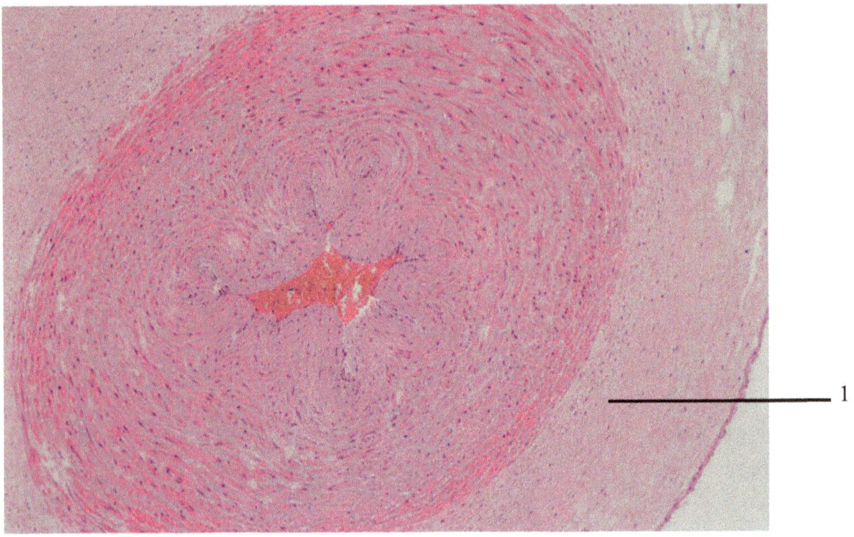

Fig. 5.51 Cynomolgus monkey, umbilical cord, umbilical artery (1), thick vascular wall, well-developed myometrium, small lumen, HE stain, ×100. (Photo from this laboratory)

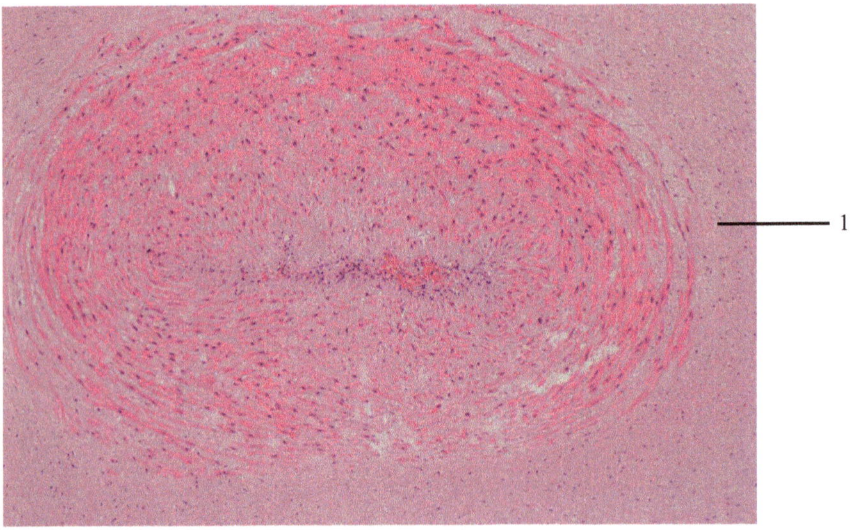

Fig. 5.52 Cynomolgus monkey, umbilical cord, umbilical vein (1), thin vascular wall, large lumen, HE stain, ×100. (Photo from this laboratory)

chorion in contact with the parietal decidua; endovascular trophoblast replacing the endothelium of the decidual spiral arteries and thus in contact with the perfusing maternal blood; and extracellular vesicles derived from the syncytiotrophoblast in contact with maternal blood and endothelial cells in the maternal circulation [23].

Within the placenta, bacteria, foreign (heterologous) proteins, and proteins that may be introduced in toxicology research or by medication are prevented from entering the fetus, while the maternal immune system is "primed" to accept non-maternal proteins from the fetus. Both fetal immune protection and maternal immune tolerance to the fetus require effective mechanisms to prevent maternal–fetal immune conflict and maintain the balance between the mother and the fetus. Because the placenta possesses this immune organ function, it requires special attention in toxicology research.

Research on cynomolgus monkey placentas often focuses on two key developmental stages: the early developmental stage at gestational day 50 (GD50, embryo–fetal transition period), and the late developmental stage near parturition at gestational day 150 (GD150; the mean gestational period for cynomolgus monkeys is 160–165 days).

In cynomolgus monkey placentas at GD_{50}, the intervillous space is large, villi are immature, lacking vascularization and differentiated immune cells; at GD_{80-100}, villous branching and vascularization increase; at GD_{150}, villi are highly branched with mature vascularization, and the interstitium contains various immune cells [24, 25].

5.4.2.1 Morphology of Cynomolgus Monkey Placenta at GD_{50}

Fetal tissues (chorion, villi, and extravillous trophoblast): At GD_{50}, the chorionic plate is composed of a loose connective tissue matrix, lined by a simple squamous epithelium towards the amniotic cavity and by a multinucleated syncytiotrophoblast towards the intervillous space. This connective tissue extends into the stem of the main villous trunks. Fetal umbilical vessels enter the connective tissue of the chorionic plate without significant branching and do not extend into the main villous trunks. At both GD_{52} and GD_{150}, vimentin and actin are expressed in the chorion and chorionic arteries, but cytokeratin is not observed until GD_{150}. Desmin is present at GD_{52}, but is highly expressed in myofibroblasts starting at GD_{100}. In the villous interstitium, histological staining for desmin is negative, indicating that vascularization is not yet fully established, but vimentin expression indicates the presence of mesenchymal cell clusters, and these areas may be potential sites for microvessel formation. The lack of vascularization and macrophages in first-trimester samples suggests the presence of secondary (intermediate or immature) villi branching from the primary villous stem. These characteristics are immunologically significant, as they indicate that at GD_{50}, the villi lack fetal blood perfusion, mature maternal–fetal metabolic exchange, and mature maternal–fetal immune interaction [26].

The first maternal–fetal interface: The syncytiotrophoblast covering the chorion is the maternal–fetal interface with key immunological implications. The syncytial layer does not proliferate, but is supplied by highly proliferative (Ki67-positive) sub-syncytiotrophoblast cells.

The second maternal–fetal interface: Represented by the extravillous trophoblast, which is in direct contact with the decidua. Extravillous trophoblast cells are highly proliferative. In terminal villi, extravillous trophoblast cells appear to proliferate, while those in the extravillous trophoblast region near the decidua do not.

Extravillous trophoblast cells can be clearly identified by the expression of cytokeratin 18 or glycogen-specific PAS staining. Glycogen is particularly abundant in the inner (proximal) extravillous trophoblast adjacent to the intervillous space, and is weakly expressed in the outer (distal) layer adjacent to decidual stromal cells. The extravillous trophoblast–decidua interface in the cynomolgus monkey is clearly discernible, with minimal intermingling of cells (i.e., interstitial trophoblast cells); whereas in humans, extensive intermingling of these cells is evident, which represents one of the major interspecies differences in placental morphology (see Table 5.6 for details). In the human first-trimester placenta, an additional area of extravillous trophoblast cells is found within the chorionic plate; this area is not observed in the cynomolgus monkey at GD_{50} but is evident at GD_{100} and beyond.

The third immune-related maternal–fetal interface: represented by endovascular extravillous trophoblast cells integrated into and replacing the spiral artery endothelium. In humans, extravillous trophoblast cells can often be found in the spiral artery endothelium, decidual stroma, and even the myometrium (confirmed by the expression of cytokeratin 7, 8, and 18). In cynomolgus monkeys at GD_{50}, this phenomenon can also be observed in invasive trophoblast cells (extravillous trophoblast) covering the decidual endothelium (glands and arteries), through the expression of cytokeratin 18. While deep invasion of the myometrium in the decidua has been reported in early pregnancy in rhesus monkeys, it is rare in cynomolgus monkeys.

5.4.2.2 Morphological Changes of the Placenta at GD_{150} (Preppartum)

Further differentiated fetal tissues (chorionic plate, villi, and extravillous trophoblast): In cynomolgus monkeys and humans, a key criterion for placental morphological maturation is the transformation of secondary villi into tertiary villi through cell differentiation, vascularization, and syncytiotrophoblast changes. This process progresses well at GD_{85-100} and gradually slows down before delivery. The cynomolgus monkey placenta at GD_{100} typically exhibits the three-layered barrier between fetal and maternal blood common to primates (including humans): villous endothelium, interstitium, and syncytiotrophoblast. With morphological maturation, such as villous vascularization, the shortening of the distance between maternal and fetal blood likely facilitates transplacental exchange (e.g., the exchange of IgG from the maternal to the fetal circulation). At GD_{85}, the villous interstitium still contains a small but increasing number of macrophages (CD68+), T cells (CD3), and individual B cells (CD20). Syncytial knots, shed from the syncytiotrophoblast, are observed in the maternal blood of the intervillous space. The extravillous trophoblast (chorionic extravillous trophoblast cells) on the chorionic plate and the extravillous trophoblast on the basal plate are moderately increased in thickness; however, the extravillous trophoblast cells are not intermingled with adjacent decidua and chorionic stroma. The amount of syncytiotrophoblast damage and intravillous or Langhans' fibrinoid "repair reaction" gradually increases over gestation.

Further differentiated maternal tissues (decidua and intervillous space blood): Information on the maternal–fetal extravillous trophoblast–decidua interface in cynomolgus monkeys is limited, while this interface in humans has been extensively studied [27].

5.4.2.3 Structural and Immunological Differences Between Cynomolgus Monkey and Human Placentas

Due to the biological and evolutionary distances between species, caution is needed when interpreting observations of immune-related physiology and molecular expression in different placental species. Human and cynomolgus monkey placentas share similarities and differences in structure, immune cell distribution, and expression of immune-related molecules. Understanding these similarities and differences is crucial for using cynomolgus monkeys as a model to study human placental-related physiological and pathological processes [28].

① **Similarities**

Similar placental structure: all are hemochorial placentas, composed of fetal membranes, umbilical cord, placental plate, and villi; the material exchange between mother and fetus relies only on three physical barriers on the fetal side, namely the trophoblast layer, the mid-layer interstitial tissue, and the endothelial cell layer. The trophoblast layer is composed of a single layer of syncytiotrophoblast cells. During placental formation, all undergo a process from early embryonic development to the formation of a placenta with specific structure and function, and the placenta is mainly composed of cytotrophoblast, syncytiotrophoblast, and extravillous trophoblast cells.

Similar expression of immune-related molecules: Both express immune-related molecules such as HLA-G (Mafa-AG in cynomolgus monkeys), FAS/FAS-L, IDO, progesterone, and annexin II. Additionally, these molecules play similar roles in maintaining maternal–fetal immune balance. For example, HLA-G is involved in immune evasion mechanisms, and FAS/FAS-L participates in regulating immune cell activity to protect the placenta from maternal immune attack.

Similar IgG transport mechanisms: Both mediate maternal–fetal IgG transport through the FcRn receptor, which is mainly expressed in syncytiotrophoblast cells in the hemochorial placenta, located on the endosomal membrane, and its binding to IgG is pH-dependent.

Expression and Function of Immune Tolerance Molecules

Progesterone: Present throughout gestation, it is initially produced by the corpus luteum and later synthesized by the placenta after GD_{50}. It can regulate immunity and affect the fetal adrenal glands and myometrium.

Annexin II: Widely present, it has immunosuppressive and allograft-protective functions. It is expressed in various cells at GD_{50} and disappears in the villous interstitium at GD_{150}.

HLA molecules: HLA-DR is widely stained in placental villous tissue at GD_{50} and disappears at GD_{100}. HLA-G is expressed in maternal decidual cells at GD_{50} and later in the syncytiotrophoblast and extravillous trophoblast; it can suppress maternal immune responses.

FAS–FAS ligand (FAS-L): Present at GD_{50}, it is expressed in the syncytiotrophoblast, extravillous trophoblast, and some immune cells. It can inhibit lymphocyte activity.

IDO: It may exhibit nonspecific staining at GD_{50} and is highly expressed in fetal capillary endothelial cells at GD_{150}, possibly regulating placental vasodilation and cell proliferation.

② **Differences**

Placental structural differences: Human extravillous trophoblast penetrates the decidua and invades the myometrium, while cynomolgus monkey extravillous trophoblast only invades the decidua. The human placental trophoblast penetrates approximately 1/3 of the myometrium, while in cynomolgus monkeys, only superficial invasion is observed, with a significantly shallower placental implantation depth than in humans. Human extravillous trophoblast invades the chorionic plate to form a fusion zone in early pregnancy, while this zone appears in cynomolgus monkeys at GD_{100}. The number of interstitial extravillous trophoblasts is higher in human placentas compared to cynomolgus monkeys.

Difference in time of immune cell appearance: T and B cells appear earlier in human placentas than in cynomolgus monkey placentas. Blood perfusion in the intervillous space of the cynomolgus monkey placenta begins early in gestation (around gestational week 3), whereas complete perfusion of the human placental intervillous space typically occurs around gestational week 13.

Differences in immune-related molecule expression: HLA-G expression location and timing differ between the placentas of the two species. For example, in cynomolgus monkeys, a large number of decidual cells express HLA-G at GD_{50}, after which expression becomes more specific in cell layers such as syncytiotrophoblast and EVT; human HLA-G expression location and cell type also have their own characteristics at different gestational periods. The cynomolgus monkey placenta lacks progesterone receptors at GD_{50}, with significant expression only appearing at GD_{100}, which differs from the human placenta in the timing and pattern of progesterone receptor expression.

Fetal IgG concentration differences: Before birth, human fetal IgG concentration can reach 130%–200% of the maternal concentration, while in monkey fetuses, it is only 80%–120%, similar to the maternal level.

5.4.3 Development of the Nonhuman Primate Placenta Characteristics

A study by G. van Wagenen and H. R. Catchpole systematically analyzed the developmental characteristics of the fetus and placenta in 343 pregnancies of known conception dates in normal rhesus monkeys, from gestational day 40 to full term. The results showed that the mean gestational period of 225 live birth pregnancies was 168 ± 7 days (range: 140–195 days); fetal weight increased almost linearly from GD90 to GD160, briefly decreased after full-term birth at GD168 and then resumed growth; crown–rump length showed negatively accelerated growth after GD100; placental weight increased linearly overall with an upward inflection point starting from GD160, and the placenta–fetal weight ratio decreased from 10:1 in early pregnancy to 1:4 at full term, with the retained placenta showing no further weight gain/loss after fetal removal; in addition, umbilical cord length increased with gestational weeks, but individual variation was large (e.g. 1.9 cm at GD40 to GD49, 24.3 cm at GD180 to GD189), and amniotic fluid volume increased significantly from GD60 to GD90 (e.g.,

7.8 mL at GD40 to GD49, 104.3 mL at GD90 to GD99). The study also compared data from previous literature, providing key references for rhesus monkey development.

Placental area and volume: Volume is estimated as "total area × maximum thickness of each placental lobe". After GD160, volume increases faster than area, and placental volume increases significantly with extended gestational cycles (possibly due to placental aging). The placenta-to-fetal weight ratio is extremely high in early pregnancy (before GD45), reaching 10:1 (placental weight is ten times the fetal weight); the ratio decreases to 1:1 (placental weight is equal to the fetal weight) between GD75 and GD85; after GD100, it continues to decline, reaching 1:4 (placental weight is 1/4 of the fetal weight) between GD160 and GD169 (full term); after GD170, it slightly increases to 1:3.45, presumably related to late-stage placental edema. This trend reflects the shift in placental function from "rapid development in early pregnancy to support fetal initiation" to "stable supply for fetal weight gain in late pregnancy."

Studies have shown that after fetal removal at GD70–160, the placenta can remain in the maternal body for months (up to 3 months) without gaining or losing weight; "back-calculating" the weight of the spontaneously expelled placenta to the date of fetal removal reveals data that perfectly aligns with the normal placental growth curve. This finding suggests that the fetus directly regulates placental growth, and in the absence of fetal signals, placental growth ceases at the stage of fetal removal.

5.4.4 Gross Abnormalities of Nonhuman Primate Placentas

The normal rhesus monkey placenta is monodiscoid in 18%–20% of cases and has two distinct discs in the remaining 80%. When two discs are present, the primary disc, which is the umbilical cord insertion site, is usually larger. However, the weight ratio between the two discs varies considerably. In very few placentas (less than 1%), the secondary disc may be larger than the primary disc. The umbilical cord usually inserts centrally into the primary disc. However, similar to humans, variations in insertion, such as eccentric and partial velamentous insertion, can occur.

In most captive rhesus monkeys, the fetal surface of the placenta appears relatively flat, with indistinct lobular divisions. Furthermore, the placental parenchyma of these animals exhibits an intense violet color. There is less variation in pattern and color in the placentas of captive animals. It is noteworthy that placentas from animals bred and delivered in free-ranging or wild states differ substantially from those of animals bred and gestated in single cages. The fetal surface of the placenta in wild-gestated animals exhibits a distinct lobular pattern, contrasting sharply with the typically flat placental appearance of captive animals. Furthermore, its placental parenchyma is light brown rather than violet. This placenta is considerably thinner but has a larger surface area than that of captively bred and raised animals [29].

Just as gestation in the wild state is associated with a different gross appearance of the placenta, it also has important implications for the development of the fetus. The fetal weight in free-ranging animals seems to be greater than that of captive pregnancies. The cause of the noticeable differences in the gross morphology of the placenta and fetal birth weight between the two situations is unclear at present. The two situations are associated with major lifestyle differences; captive animals have far less locomotion and physical activity than free-ranging animals. There are also differences in diet. Although not yet thoroughly investigated, significant endocrine differences may exist between wild, free-ranging animals and captive animals, possibly due to the degree of stress experienced in their daily lives. Long-term confinement in cages and daily forced contact with humans can cause significant stress responses in monkeys.

In addition to differences in gross placental appearance based on lifestyle (free-ranging versus captive: relatively stress-free versus stressed), some placental morphological variations unrelated to known fetal abnormalities can occur, such as abnormal placental fusion, which can result in a monodiscoid placenta with an abnormal appearance or an increased number of placentas.

Circumvallate placentas and marginal placentas occur with particularly high frequency in monodiscoid placentas. Furthermore, in such cases, the umbilical cord insertion is typically eccentric; although circumvallate bidiscoid placentas do occur, their frequency is much lower than expected, considering the prevalence of bidiscoid placentas in the overall monkey population.

The reason for the higher-than-expected frequency of circumvallate placentas within the monkey population remains unclear and may be related to surgical procedures. However, circumvallate placentas have also been repeatedly observed in monkeys that have not undergone surgery. Placenta previa is observed in nonhuman primates, but in most cases, the placental location superior to the cervical os is an incidental finding. Diagnosis or confirmation of placenta previa can be made based on gross observation of the placenta, revealing a characteristic conical or circumvallate abnormality, or through the occurrence of significant vaginal bleeding in late gestation [30].

5.4.5 Common Histological Abnormalities of Nonhuman Primate Placentas

Research on histological abnormalities in nonhuman primate placentas is of great significance for understanding placental pathologies and pregnancy complications. However, there is currently limited research in this area, and literature searches reveal some pathological changes such as inflammation, tumors, implantation abnormalities, and infections, as shown in Table 5.7 [31–40].

Table 5.7 Anatomical and histological characteristics and common pathological changes of nonhuman primate placentas

Placenta	Nonhuman primates
Gross anatomical observation	75% are bidiscoid, 25% are monodiscoid. The fetal surface of the placenta is smooth, with large blood vessels arranged radially. The maternal surface is dark red, brittle, and irregularly divided into lobules by maternal tissue septa.
Developmental characteristics	The mean placental weight is 135 ± 32 g, and the mean fetal weight is 480 ± 78 g. Formulas for calculating expected placental weight given gestational day (GD) or fetal weight (BW) are $PW = 1.3\,(GD) - 65.9$ or $PW = 0.29\,(BW) - 0.12$, respectively

Placenta	Nonhuman primates
Histological characteristics	The fetus is encased within the amniotic sac, which is closely connected to the chorion. The yolk sac degenerates toward the end of the first trimester. The fetal surface of the placenta is easily recognizable by its smooth surface and large blood vessels. The chorion contains a small number of mesenchymal cells within a loose fibrous connective tissue matrix and is traversed by interspersed paired arteries and veins. These vessel pairs branch to form a complex, lobulated villous network with attachment points on the fetal side (chorionic plate) and maternal side (trophoblastic shell and decidua). Villi are comprised of fetal blood vessels, perivascular mesenchymal cells, cytotrophoblast epithelial cells, and large, multinucleated syncytiotrophoblast cells. The deep margin of the placenta is delineated by a layer of trophoblast cells known as the trophoblastic shell. Fetal trophoblast cells also invade the endometrium, surrounding and infiltrating the walls of maternal endometrial blood vessels; these cells are called extravillous trophoblast cells. The non-discoid, membranous part of the placenta lacks villi and is covered by a layer of trophoblastic epithelium. Normal acellular components of the placenta include intervillous and intravillous placental fibrinoid deposits, which are composed of fibrin, laminin, and other extracellular matrix molecules, and multifocal mineralization of the placental villi. Coagulation necrosis at the placental margin at term is a normal finding. Beneath the placenta, the endometrial glands are dilated and sparse; beneath the membranous portion of the placenta, the endometrial glands are dilated by fluid and lined by a single layer of cuboidal epithelium, surrounded by plump decidual cells. Throughout the gravid endometrium, decidual cells derived from the stroma are abundant, as are granular endometrial lymphocytes.
Differences from the human placenta	The macaque placenta is similar in gross morphology to the human placenta, with the difference that most macaque pregnancies result in two placentas
Common pathological changes	Mineralization: Multifocally present within villi of the normal placenta Fibrin deposits: Commonly present within and around villi of the normal placenta Marginal coagulative necrosis: Commonly present in full-term placentas Epithelial plaque reaction: A pseudoplacental epithelial lesion occurring during the luteal phase Circumvallate placenta: A constrictive, fibrous malformation at the placental margin, usually asymptomatic Placental number and lobation variations: Approximately 70% of placentas are bidiscoid Infarction: Marginal infarctions are normal at full term Suppurative placentitis: Most commonly caused by Listeria monocytogenes Retained placenta: Usually fatal if untreated Tumors: Choriocarcinoma and trophoblastic tumors; most commonly found in the ovaries
Cases of drug-induced placental pathology	Currently available drug toxicology data (e.g., Trastuzumab, Mepolizumab (IL-5 mAb), NNC0113-0217 (GLP-1R agonist)) show no significant changes in placental weight or gross morphology, with fetal toxicity mainly manifesting as stillbirth/growth restriction.

Ethical approval

This chapter is a review of previously published accounts; as such, no animal or human studies were performed.

References

1. Vidal JD, Colman K, Bhaskaran M et al (2021) Scientific and regulatory policy committee best practices: documentation of sexual maturity by microscopic evaluation in nonclinical safety studies. Toxicol Pathol 49(5):977–989
2. Fortman JD, Hewett TA, Bennett BT (2002) The laboratory nonhuman primate. 2nd edn. CRC Press: New York, Boca Raton, p 198
3. Bluemel J, Korte S, Schenck E, Weinbauer G (2015) The nonhuman primate in nonclinical drug development and safety. Assessment. Elsevier Academic Press, London, 252 p
4. Mecklenburg L, Luetjens CM, Weinbauer GF (2019) Toxicologic pathology forum: opinion on sexual maturity and fertility assessment in long-tailed macaques (*Macaca fascicularis*) in nonclinical safety studies. Toxicol Pathol 47(4):444–460
5. Lanning LL, Creasy DM, Chapin RE (2002) Recommended approaches for the evaluation of testicular and epididymal toxicity. Toxicol Pathol 30(4):507–520
6. Martin PL, Weinbauer GF (2010) Developmental toxicity testing of biopharmaceuticals in nonhuman primates: previous experience and future directions. Int J Toxicol 29(6): 552-568
7. Haruyama E, Suda M, Akukawa Y (2012) Testicular development in cynomolgus monkeys. Toxicol Pathol 40:935–942
8. Haruyama E, Akukawa Y, Kamura K (2012) Morphometric examination for development of reproductive organs in male cynomolgus monkeys. Toxicol Pathol 40:918–925
9. Luetjens CM, Weinbauer GF (2012) Functional assessment of sexual maturity in male macaques (*Macaca fascicularis*). Regul Toxicol Pharmacol 63:391–400
10. Rocca M, Morford LL, Blanset DL et al (2018) Applying a weight of evidence approach to the evaluation of developmental toxicity of biopharmaceuticals. Regul Toxicol Pharmacol 98:69–79
11. Pereira Bacares ME, Vemireddi V, Creasy D (2017) Testicular fibrous hypoplasia in cynomolgus monkeys (*Macaca fascicularis*): an incidental, congenital lesion. Toxicol Pathol 45(4):536–543
12. Ramaswamy S, Walker WH, Aliberti P et al (2017) The testicular transcriptome associated with spermatogonia differentiation initiated by gonadotrophin stimulation in the juvenile rhesus monkey (*Macaca mulatta*). Hum Reprod 32(10):2086–2100
13. Martin PL, Weinbauer GF (2010) Developmental toxicity testing of biopharmaceuticals in nonhuman primates: previous experience and future directions. Int J Toxicol 29(6):552–568
14. Cline M, Wood CE, Vidal. JD (2008) Selected background findings and interpretation of common lesions in the female reproductive system in macaques. Toxicol Pathol 36:142S–163S
15. Reindel JF, Gough AW, Pilcher GD et al (2001) Systemic proliferative changes and clinical signs in cynomolgus monkeys administered a recombinant derivative of human epidermal growth factor. Toxicol Pathol 29(2):159–173
16. Appt S, Kaplan J, Clarkson T et al (2006) Destruction of primordial ovarian follicles in adult cynomolgus macaques after exposure to 4-vinylcyclohexene diepoxide: a nonhuman primate model of the menopausal transition. Fertil Steril 86(4):1210–1216
17. Takayama S, Renwick AG, Johansson SL et al (2000) Long-term toxicity and carcinogenicity study of cyclamate in nonhuman primates. Toxicol Sci 53(1):33–39
18. Taketa Y, Horie K, Goto T et al (2018) Histopathologic characterization of mifepristone-induced ovarian toxicity in cynomolgus monkeys. Toxicol Pathol 46(3):283–289

19. Cooper TK, Gabrielson KL (2007) Spontaneous lesions in the reproductive tract and mammary gland of female non-human primates. Birth Defects Res 80:149–170
20. Furukawa S, Kuroda Y, Sugiyama A (2014) A comparison of the histological structure of the placenta in experimental animals. J Toxicol Pathol 27(1):11–18
21. Van Wagenen G, Catchpole HR, Negri J, Butzko D (1965) Growth of the fetus and placenta of the monkey (*Macaca mulatta*). Am J Phys Anthropol 23(1):23–33
22. Buse E, Häeger J-D, Svensson-Arvelund J (2014) The placenta in toxicology. Part I: animal models in toxicology: placental morphology and tolerance molecules in the cynomolgus monkey (*Macaca fascicularis*). J Toxicol Pathol 42(2):314–326
23. Svensson-Arvelund J, Ernerudh J, Buse E, Cline JM (2014) The placenta in toxicology. Part II. J Toxicol Pathol 42(2):327–338
24. Mark Cline J, Dixon D, Ernerudh J (2014) The placenta in toxicology. Part III: pathologic assessment of the placenta. J Toxicol Pathol 42(2):339–344
25. King BF (1993) Development and structure of the placenta and fetal membranes of nonhuman primates. J Exp Zool 266(6):528–540
26. King BF, Mais JJ (1982) Developmental changes in rhesus monkey placental villi and cell columns. Anat Embryol 165(3):361–376
27. Buse E, Markert UR (2019) The immunology of the macaque placenta: a detailed analysis and critical comparison with the human placenta. Crit Rev Clin Lab Sci 56(2):118–145
28. Chucri TM, Monteiro JM, Lima AR, et al. (2010) A review of immune transfer by the placenta. J Reprod Immunol 87:14–20
29. Woodling BA, Kroener JM, Puffer HW et al (1976) Gross examination of the placenta. Clin Obstet Gynecol 19(1):21–44
30. Myers RE (1972) The gross pathology of the rhesus monkey placenta. J Reprod Med 9(4):171–198
31. Myers RE (1972) The pathology of the rhesus monkey placenta. Acta Endocrinol Suppl 166:221–257
32. Appt S, Kaplan J, Clarkson T et al (2006) Destruction of primordial ovarian follicles in adult cynomolgus macaques after exposure to 4-vinylcyclohexene diepoxide: a nonhuman primate model of the menopausal transition. Fertil Steril 86(4):1210–1216
33. Bourque AC, Singh A, Lakhanpa LN et al (1995) Ultrastructural-changes in ovarian follicles of monkeys administered hexachlorobenzene. Am J Vet Res 56(12):1677–1680
34. Bowman CJ, Breslin WJ, Connor AV et al (2013) Placental transfer of Fc-containing biopharmaceuticals across species, an industry survey analysis. Birth Defects Res 98(6):459–485
35. Breider MA, Ulloa HM, Pegg DG et al (1998) Nitro-imidazole radiosensitizer-induced toxicity in cynomolgus monkeys. Toxicol Pathol 26(5):651–656
36. Catlin NR, Mitchell AZ, Potchoiba MJ et al (2020) Placental transfer of 125 iodinated humanized immunoglobulin G2Δa in the cynomolgus monkey. Birth Defects Res 112(1):105–117
37. Enright BP, Compton DR, Collins N et al (2009) Comparative effects of interferon alpha-2b and pegylated interferon alpha-2b on menstrual cycles and ovarian hormones in cynomolgus monkeys. Birth Defects Res 86(1):29–39
38. Ishida K, Werner JA, Lafleur M et al (2021) Phosphatidylinositol 3-kinase δ-specific inhibitor-induced changes in the ovary and testis in the Sprague Dawley rat and cynomolgus monkey. Int J Toxicol 40(4):344–354
39. Prell RA, Dybdal N, Arima A et al (2018) Placental and fetal effects of onartuzumab, a Met/HGF signaling antagonist, when administered to pregnant cynomolgus monkeys. Toxicol Sci 165(1):186–197
40. Wang H, Schuetz C, Arima A et al (2016) Assessment of placental transfer and the effect on embryo-fetal development of a humanized monoclonal antibody targeting lymphotoxin-alpha in non-human primates. Reprod Toxicol 63:82–95

6 Pharmacokinetics and Toxicokinetics in the Reproductive Toxicity Studies

Xu Xu and Li Xingxia

Abstract

Pharmacokinetic (PK) and toxicokinetic (TK) studies in the reproductive system aim to elucidate the dynamic changes of drugs in complex biological matrices such as reproductive organs, embryos, fetuses, and milk. These studies not only provide key data for interpreting reproductive toxicity test results but also offer indispensable references for clinical drug risk assessment, particularly regarding potential hazards to women of childbearing potential and fetuses. However, the physiological complexity of the reproductive system, exemplified by the blood–testis barrier, placental barrier, and blood-milk barrier, makes it difficult to predict the penetration, distribution, and accumulation characteristics of drugs across these specialized barriers. Furthermore, the physiological state of pregnant and lactating animals (e.g., increased blood volume, hormonal changes) can significantly alter drug kinetic behavior, leading to marked differences compared to nonpregnant or male animals. Currently, PK/TK research on macromolecular drugs (e.g., monoclonal antibodies) in the reproductive system still faces challenges, including animal species selection (e.g., the necessity of nonhuman primates), validation of analytical methods in complex matrices (e.g., amniotic fluid, tissue homogenates), and the interference of immunogenicity with the evaluation of antibody drug exposure levels. Therefore, systematically conducting PK/TK studies in the reproductive system and establishing reliable analytical methods hold significant scientific importance and clinical value for comprehensively understanding the mechanisms of drug reproductive toxicity and optimizing nonclinical safety evaluation strategies.

X. Xu · L. Xingxia
Hubei Topgene Biotechnology Co. Ltd., Hubei, China
e-mail: xuxu@topgenebio.com

L. Zhou and Z. Sun (eds.), *Reproductive and Developmental Toxicology on Macaca Fascicularis*, https://doi.org/10.1007/978-981-92-3834-7_6

Keywords

Pharmacokinetics · Toxicokinetics · Analytical method validation · Anti-drug antibodies

6.1 Pharmacokinetics and Toxicokinetics of Small-Molecule Drugs in the Reproductive System

Pharmacokinetics (PK) mainly studies the dynamic change laws of drugs in the body under clinical administration dosage, providing a theoretical basis for clinical research and the use of new drugs, and the formulation of reasonable dosing plans. Toxicokinetics (TK) is an interdisciplinary subject combining pharmacokinetics and toxicology. It quantitatively studies the processes and characteristics of the absorption, distribution, metabolism, and excretion of drugs in animals at doss higher than clinical administration dosage by using the principles and methods of pharmacokinetics, and then explores the laws of the occurrence and development of drug toxicity.

The purpose of pharmacokinetics research is to reveal the dynamic change laws of drugs in the body, obtain the basic kinetic parameters of drugs, and clarify the processes and characteristics of the absorption, distribution, metabolism, and excretion of drugs in the body. The purpose of toxicokinetics research is to obtain the extent and duration of systemic exposure of test articles at different dose levels in toxicity tests and predict the potential risks when test articles are exposed in humans. Its research focus is to explain the results of toxicity tests and predict human safety, rather than simply describing the characteristics of the basic kinetic parameters of test articles. Toxicokinetics tests are usually carried out simultaneously with repeated-dose toxicity tests and are often referred to as concomitant toxicokinetics tests.

The main differences between PK and TK are as follows: ① The results of pharmacokinetics mainly describe the basic metabolic kinetic characteristics of drugs, while the results of toxicokinetics are used to explain the results of toxicity tests. ② The doses in pharmacokinetics are often effective doses, that is, the metabolic laws of drugs in the body are studied under therapeutic dose conditions; the doses in toxicokinetics are much higher than the effective doses and/or clinical doses, and most of them are repeated dosing. ③ Pharmacokinetics tests are usually carried out separately, while toxicokinetics tests are usually carried out concomitantly with toxicity tests.

The main connections between PK and TK are as follows: ① The requirements for analytical methods are the same (good specificity and high sensitivity). ② The results of pharmacokinetics tests can provide a reference for the setting of sampling time points in toxicokinetics. ③ The results of tissue distribution in pharmacokinetics research can provide a reference for the evaluation of toxic target organs. ④ The results of biotransformation research can provide a reference for the selection of animal species in toxicity tests.

6.1.1 Characteristics of Reproductive Toxicity: Toxicokinetics Research

Developmental and reproductive toxicity (DART) refers to the adverse effects of exogenous substances on the reproductive functions of parental generations, such as germ cells, conception, pregnancy, childbirth, and lactation, as well as the adverse effects on the development of offspring embryos and fetuses and postnatal development.

The DART research toxicity mainly includes studies on fertility and early embryonic development (FEED), embryo–fetal development (EFD), and prenatal and postnatal development (PPND), etc., and reproductive toxicity toxicokinetics research can be carried out synchronously in the above studies.

The main purpose of reproductive toxicity toxicokinetics research is to analyze the results of reproductive toxicity tests and help determine whether different doses at different stages in reproductive toxicity tests have achieved sufficient exposure. The possible differences in kinetic characteristics between pregnant and nonpregnant animals, as well as the differences in kinetic processes between female animals during pregnancy and lactation and normal animals, shall be considered.

The combination of reproductive toxicity tests and toxicokinetics analysis also helps to make scientific and reasonable comparisons among different toxicology test results through exposure levels and provides a reference for the risk assessment of clinical drug use. The toxicokinetics data can come not only from the plasma exposure levels of parental animals but also from the tissues or body fluids of reproductive organs (such as testes, semen, and milk) and data on offspring embryos/fetuses. The focus is to evaluate whether drugs and/or metabolites can pass through the blood–testis barrier, placental barrier, and blood–milk barrier. In male fertility and early embryonic development toxicity tests, common biological samples for detecting the concentration of toxic drugs are plasma, testicular tissue, and semen of male animals, with the focus on analyzing the ability of drugs to penetrate the blood–testis barrier.

The male reproductive system may be damaged by interference from external chemical substances, including damage to the testes, epididymis, sperm production and quality, and hormone secretion. Drug-induced male reproductive toxicity mainly refers to the damage caused by drugs to the male reproductive system (testes, epididymis, etc.) and reproductive functions, generally including organic changes in reproductive organs, a decrease in sperm quantity and quality, changes in sexual behavior, a reduction in fertility, and abnormal secretion of sex hormones, as well as the developmental toxicity of embryos and fetuses caused by the transmission of sperm genetic material and/or vaginal intake of semen.

For drugs with potential developmental toxicity in animals or humans, the determination of the drug content in semen helps to quantitatively estimate the possible exposure level reaching the conceptus (embryo/fetus). The exposure level of the conceptus can be estimated by the following hypothetical model (taking small-molecule drugs as an example). Suppose: the volume of semen ejaculated is 5 mL, the drug concentration in semen = the maximum drug concentration in plasma (C_{max}), 100% of the drug is taken in the vagina, and the blood volume of females is set at 5000 mL, and 100% drug can pass through the placental barrier. Then the exposure level of the conceptus = $C_{max} \times 5\ \text{mL} \times 100\%/5000\ \text{mL} \times 100\%$, that is, the exposure level of the conceptus calculated based on the maximum possibility. If this exposure level is more than ten times lower than the no-observed-adverse-effect level (NOAEL) dose for developmental toxicity, further assessment of the risk of male-mediated developmental toxicity may not be required; if the exposure level is relatively high, risk control strategies (such as contraception) shall be considered.

Toxicokinetic data can be obtained from all animals in reproductive toxicity tests or from some of them. Toxicokinetic data should include data on fetuses/young offspring to evaluate whether the test article and/or its metabolites can pass through the placental barrier and/or be secreted in milk.

Generally speaking, it is preferable to conduct reproductive toxicity assessments of a clinical drug candidate in relevant species. Reproductive toxicity evaluations should only be carried out in pharmacologically relevant species. When a clinical drug candidate has pharmacological activities in both rodents and rabbits, two species shall be used for embryo–fetal development tests, unless embryonic lethality or teratogenicity has been confirmed in one species. When nonhuman NHP are the only relevant species, developmental toxicity tests should only be conducted in NHP. When a clinical drug candidate has pharmacological activities only in NHP, conducting tests on the clinical drug candidate in NHP is the preferred approach. If sufficient scientific justifications can be provided, alternative models can be used to replace NHP [1].

6.1.2 General Principles of Reproductive Toxicity Assessment Strategies

To determine the assessment strategy, the necessity to conduct reproductive toxicity tests shall be determined first for each different reproductive stage and its most appropriate tests. The factors to be considered include: ① the target patients and the duration of administration; ② the known pharmacological properties of the compound; ③ the known toxicity of the compound; ④ any existing information for the impact on reproductive risk targets (such as human and animal genetics, or class effects); ⑤ alternative test data that can be used to identify hazards and/or risks, etc. The timing of reproductive toxicity tests is also an important part of the overall strategy.

The evaluation of male and female fertility through comprehensive standard histopathological examinations of testes and ovaries in repeated-dose toxicity tests with appropriate dosing durations (usually in rodents) is considered to be as sensitive as fertility tests in detecting toxic reactions in female and male reproductive organs. Male fertility tests shall be completed before the start of large-scale or long-term clinical tests (such as Phase III tests).

The purpose of the FEED test is to detect the interference caused by the drug from before mating until mating and implantation in males and/or females. Fertility tests are usually conducted in rodents or rabbits. In nonrodent animals (such as dogs and NHP), mating assessment is usually not feasible. If NHP is the only pharmacologically relevant species (such as many monoclonal antibodies), histopathological examinations of reproductive tissues in repeated-dose toxicity tests with a dosing duration of at least 3 months can be used as an alternative method for fertility assessment. This method should include detailed and comprehensive histopathological examinations of the reproductive organs of female and male animals [2].

There are many differences between biotechnological drugs and small-molecule drugs, such as in species specificity, drug metabolism, and distribution.

6.1.3 Dose Selection for Reproductive Toxicity Tests Accompanied by Toxicokinetics Tests

Dose selection is an important aspect in reproductive and developmental toxicology studies. For reproductive toxicity tests accompanied by toxicokinetics in rodents and rabbits, satellite groups are usually designed, and the doses are consistent with those of the main test groups. For reproductive toxicity tests accompanied by toxicokinetics in NHP, satellite groups are usually not necessary. One of the key issues in the design of toxicity tests is dose design. Appropriate doses can be selected based on all existing research data (such as pharmacology, acute toxicity, dose range-finding tests, and pharmacokinetic studies) [3]. Repeated-dose toxicity tests with a duration of 2–4 weeks have dosing periods that are quite close to those designed for various stages of reproductive toxicity studies and can be used as a reference for dose selection. If the above research data are insufficient, it is recommended to conduct preliminary tests, also known as dose range-finding (DRF) tests. On the basis of the preliminary tests, the dosing doses for the low, medium, and high dose groups shall be confirmed. The low dose is equivalent to several times the pharmacodynamic dose in animals or the clinically used dose. In principle, the high dose should cause obvious toxic reactions in animals. The medium dose shall be set between the high dose and the low dose in combination with the mechanism and characteristics of toxicity to investigate the dose–response relationship of toxicity (Fig. 6.1).

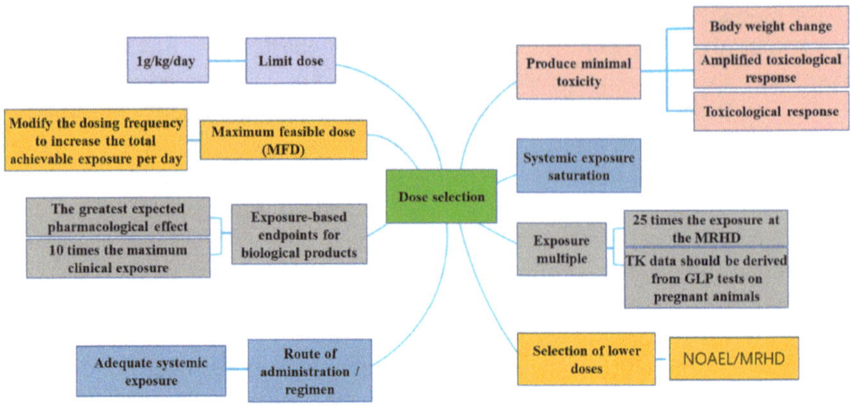

Fig. 6.1 Dose selection in toxicity tests

The setting of sampling time points: Sampling time points should have a sufficient frequency to ensure that the systemic exposure of the drug can be accurately reflected. To obtain a complete blood drug concentration–time curve after dosing, the design of sampling time points should take into account the absorption phase, equilibrium phase (near the peak concentration), and elimination phase of the drug. Generally, at least two to three sampling points are required in the absorption phase. For drugs administered extravascularly with rapid absorption, efforts shall be made to avoid the first point being the peak concentration (C_{max}). At least three sampling points are needed near C_{max}, and four to six sampling points are required in the elimination phase. The entire sampling time should last at least until three to five half-lives or until the blood drug concentration is 1/10–1/20 of C_{max}.

6.1.4 Bioanalytical Methods and Their Validation

The validation of bioanalytical methods aims to prove that the adopted bioanalytical methods are suitable for the intended purposes. The determination of the concentrations of chemical drugs, biological drugs, and their metabolites in biological matrices is an important part of the drug development process. The research results are helpful in supporting regulatory decisions related to drug safety and efficacy. Therefore, the bioanalytical methods used must be fully characterized, appropriately validated, and documented to ensure reliable data for supporting regulatory decisions.

The purpose of developing bioanalytical methods is to determine the design, operating conditions, limitations, and applicability of the methods to achieve the intended purposes and ensure that the analytical methods can be used for validation.

Method development involves clarifying the processes and conditions related to the quantitative detection of the analyte, including the full characterization of the following elements: standards/controls, key reagents, calibration curves, quality control samples (QC), selectivity and specificity, sensitivity, accuracy, precision, recovery rate, and analyte stability, etc. The development of bioanalytical methods does not require the preservation of a large number of records or annotations. Once the method development is completed, it needs to undergo method validation to prove that the method is suitable for the analysis of research samples.

To ensure the acceptability of analytical performance and the reliability of analytical results, bioanalytical methods must be validated. Bioanalytical methods are a series of operational steps used to determine the concentrations of analytes in biological samples. When establishing quantitative analysis methods for analytes in clinical and key nonclinical studies, comprehensive validation of bioanalytical methods shall be carried out. When using literature-reported analytical methods and commercial kits for the analysis of biological samples in the process of drug research and development, complete validation should also be conducted.

The complete method validation of chromatographic analysis methods should include the following contents: selectivity, specificity, matrix effect, calibration curve (response function), range [lower limit of quantification (LLOQ) to upper limit of quantification (ULOQ)], accuracy, precision, carryover, dilution reliability, stability, and injection reproducibility.

Unless otherwise stated, the method validation of ligand-binding assays (LBA) should include the following contents: specificity, selectivity, calibration curve (response function), range (LLOQ to ULOQ), accuracy, precision, carryover, dilution linearity, and stability. If suitable research samples are available, parallelism investigations should also be carried out when necessary.

The various evaluations carried out during method validation shall be related to the analysis workflow of the research samples. The matrices used for the validation of analytical methods (including anticoagulants and additives) shall be the same as those of the research samples. If it is difficult to obtain the same matrix as that of the research samples (such as rare matrices like tissues, cerebrospinal fluid, and bile) or when detecting free drugs, alternative matrices can be used to conduct analytical method validation. It is generally believed that differences in matrices within the same species (such as age, race, and sex) will not affect method validation.

The following is a case study on the bioanalytical methods for cyclophosphamide and thalidomide, which are commonly used as positive drugs in reproductive toxicity tests accompanied by toxicokinetics studies in cynomolgus monkeys. Here, this study is taken as an example to discuss the establishment and validation of relevant analytical methods [4].

Case: Bioanalytical methods and their validation for cyclophosphamide and thalidomide as commonly used positive drugs in reproductive toxicity tests accompanied by toxicokinetics studies in cynomolgus monkey.

6.2 Information on Control Articles and Internal Standards

1. Control Article 1
   (1) Name: Cyclophosphamide.
   (2) Lot No.: 100234201604.

(3) Specification: 100 mg/vial.
(4) Content: 95.3%.
(5) Expiration date: Valid until the notice of discontinuation is issued by the National Institutes for Food and Drug Control.
(6) Storage conditions: Protected from light, sealed. Store under refrigeration at 2°C–8°C.
(7) Stability: Stable under storage conditions and within expiration date.
(8) Source: National Institutes for Food and Drug Control.

2. Control Article 2
   (1) Name: Thalidomide.
   (2) Lot No.: 100504201102.
   (3) Specification: 100 mg/vial.
   (4) Purity: 100.0%.
   (5) Expiration date: Valid until the notice of discontinuation is issued by the National Institutes for Food and Drug Control.
   (6) Storage conditions: Protected from light, sealed.
   (7) Stability: Stable under storage conditions and within expiration date.
   (8) Source: National Institutes for Food and Drug Control.

3. Internal Standard
   (1) Name: Tolbutamide.
   (2) Lot No.: K2125618.
   (3) Specification: 1 g/vial.
   (4) Purity: 99%.
   (5) Storage condition: Store at −20°C.
   (6) Source: Aladdin.

6.3 Detection Conditions

6.3.1 Chromatographic Conditions

(1) Cyclophosphamide: The instruments used were an LC30AD infusion pump and a SIL30AC automatic sampler. The chromatographic column was ACQUITY UPLC BEH C18 (2.1 mm × 100 mm, 1.7 μm); the flow rate was 0.30 mL/min, injection volume 1.00 μL, needle wash mode: Before and after aspiration.

(2) Thalidomide: The instrument was the ExionLC system. The chromatographic column was ACQUITY UPLC BEH C18 (2.1 mm × 100 mm, 1.7 μm); the flow rate was 0.30 mL/min, injection volume 1.00 μL, with gradient elution of the mobile phase.

(3) Elution conditions are shown in Tables 6.1 and 6.2.

Table 6.1 Mobile phase elution conditions (cyclophosphamide)

Time (min)	A (aqueous solution containing 0.1% formic acid)	B (Carbinol)
0.01	45	55
2.00	2	98
3.00	2	98
3.01	45	55
4.30	45	55

Table 6.2 Mobile phase elution conditions (thalidomide)

Time (min)	A (aqueous solution containing 0.1% formic acid)	B (Methanol solution)
0.00	45	55
1.80	10	90
3.00	10	90
3.01	45	55
4.50	45	55

(1) Instrument (Cyclophosphamide): The Qtrap 5500 mass spectrometer from ×× Company, equipped with a Turbo Spray ion source, adopting an electrospray ionization (ESI), and operating in the positive ion scanning mode.

(2) Instrument (Thalidomide): The Qtrap 5500+ mass spectrometer from ×× Company, equipped with a Turbo Spray ion source, adopting an electrospray ionization (ESI), and operating in the positive ion scanning mode.

(3) Detection mode (Cyclophosphamide): Multiple reaction monitoring (MRM); ion source (GS1) at 50.0 psi; ion source gas (GS2) at 50.0 psi; curtain gas (CUR) at 30.0 psi; collision cell gas (CAD) set as medium, the source temperature was 550°C, and the ion spray voltage (IS) was 5500 V; the data acquisition time was 4.30 min.

(4) Detection mode (Thalidomide): Multiple reaction monitoring (MRM); ion source (GS1) at 60.0 psi; ion source gas (GS2) at 60.0 psi; curtain gas (CUR) at 45.0 psi; collision cell gas (CAD) set as 9, the source temperature was 600°C, and the ion spray voltage (IS) was 5500 V; the data acquisition time was 4.50 min.

(5) The main mass spectrometry parameters are shown in Table 6.3.

6.4 Solution Preparation

6.4.1 Preparation of Stock Solutions

(1) Cyclophosphamide stock solutions: Precisely weigh two portions of the cyclophosphamide control article and place them into glass bottles, respectively. Add a certain volume of methanol to dissolve them, and then continue to add methanol

Table 6.3 Main mass spectrometry parameters of the analytes and internal standards

Compoundtype	Compoundname	Monitoring-ion pair(MRM)	Dwell time(ms)	DP(V)	CE(V)	EP(V)	CXP(V)
Analyte	Cyclophosphamide (CP)	261.2/139.9	200	100	30	10	15
Internal standard	Metobutamide	271/155.1	200	100	30	10	15
Analyte	Thalidomide	259.1/140.1	100	80	30	10	15
Internal standard	Metobutamide	271.0/155.1	100	80	15	10	15

to prepare cyclophosphamide stock solutions with a concentration of 1.00 mg/mL, respectively (Stock A and Stock B).

(2) Thalidomide stock solutions: Precisely weigh two portions of the thalidomide control article and place them into glass bottles, respectively. Add a certain volume of acetonitrile to dissolve them, and then continue to add acetonitrile to prepare thalidomide stock solutions with a concentration of 1.00 mg/mL, respectively (Stock A and Stock B).

(3) Tolbutamide stock solution (internal standard): Precisely weigh a certain amount of the tolbutamide control article and place it into a glass bottle. Add a certain volume of methanol, and then continue to add methanol to prepare an internal standard stock solution (IS stock) with a concentration of 1.00 mg/mL.

6.4.2 Preparation of Experimental Solutions

(1) Mobile phase A: (aqueous solution containing 0.1% formic acid): Pipette 1 mL of formic acid into a liquid chromatography vial, add 1000 mL of water, and mix well to prepare an aqueous solution containing 0.1% formic acid.

(2) Mobile phase B (methanol).

(3) Needle wash solution: The needle wash solution used in the cyclophosphamide detection method is a 50% methanol aqueous solution(pipette 500 mL of methanol into a liquid chromatography vial, add 500 mL of water to prepare a 50% methanol aqueous solution for needle washing); the needle wash solution used in the thalidomide detection method was a 50% acetonitrile aqueous solution(pipette 500 mL of acetonitrile into a liquid chromatography vial, add 500 mL of water to prepare a 50% acetonitrile aqueous solution for needle washing).

(4) Diluent: The diluent used in the cyclophosphamide detection method was a 50% methanol aqueous solution (pipette 500 mL of methanol into a liquid chromatography vial, add 500 mL of water to prepare a 50% methanol aqueous solution); the diluent used in the thalidomide detection method was a 50% acetonitrile aqueous solution (pipette 100 mL of acetonitrile into a liquid chromatography vial, add 100 mL of water to prepare a 50% acetonitrile aqueous solution).

(5) Internal standard working solution (ISWS): Pipette a certain amount of IS stock and use a 50% methanol aqueous solution to prepare an internal standard solution with a concentration of 1000 ng/mL. Storage condition: 2°C–8°C.

6.4.3 Preparation of Standard Curve Samples and Quality Control Sample Standard Curve Samples and Quality Control Samples

(1) Use cyclophosphamide stock A, cyclophosphamide stock B, thalidomide stock A, and thalidomide stock B to prepare standard curve working solutions and quality control working solutions, respectively. The concentrations of the cyclophosphamide standard curve working solutions were 200, 180, 100, 30, 10, 2, 0.4, and 0.2 μg/mL.

The concentrations of the thalidomide standard curve working solutions were 200, 180, 120, 60, 20, 8, 2, and 1 μg/mL. The concentrations of the cyclophosphamide quality control working solutions were 160, 16, 0.6, and 0.2 μg/mL, and the diluted quality control concentration was 400 μg/mL. The concentrations of the thalidomide quality control working solutions were 160, 24, 3, and 1 μg/mL, and the concentration of the diluted quality control working solution was 400 μg/mL. The dilution steps for the standard curve working solutions and quality control working solutions are shown in Tables 6.4 and 6.5.

(2) Take a certain volume of the working solutions and add them to a certain volume of blank matrix (20-fold dilution) to prepare standard curve samples and quality control samples. The preparation steps for the standard curve samples and quality control samples are shown in Tables 6.6 and 6.7.

6.5 Sample Processing Methods

(1) Cyclophosphamide: Take 60 μL of the sample and place it in a centrifuge tube. Add 60 μL of the internal standard working solution, and then add 480 μL of methanol. Vortex and mix evenly. Centrifuge at 10,000 × *g* at 4°C for 10 min. Take 150 μL of the supernatant and place it in a 96-well plate. Add 150 μL of an aqueous solution, mix evenly, and then inject for determination. The injection volume is 1 μL.

(2) Thalidomide: Take 40 μL of the sample and place it in a centrifuge tube. Add 40 μL of the internal standard working solution, and then add 320 μL of methanol.

Table 6.4 Preparation information of cyclophosphamide working solutions

Source solution	Source solution conc.(μg/mL)	Source solution volume(μL)	Diluent volume(μL)	Final volume(μL)	Final conc.(μg/mL)	Solution name
Stock A	1000	200	800	1000	200	WS-C1
Stock A	1000	180	820	1000	180	WS-C2
Stock A	1000	100	900	1000	100	WS-C3
Stock A	1000	30	970	1000	30.0	WS-C4
WS-C3	100	100	900	1000	10.0	WS-C5
WS-C3	100	20	980	1000	2.00	WS-C6
WS-C5	10.0	40	960	1000	0.400	WS-C7
WS-C5	10.0	20	980	1000	0.200	WS-C8
Stock B	1000	200	300	500	400	WS-DQC
Stock B	1000	160	840	1000	160	WS-HQC
WS-HQC	160	100	900	1000	16.0	WS-MQC
WS-MQC	16.0	30	770	800	0.600	WS-LQC
WS-MQC	16.0	10	790	800	0.200	WS-LLOQ

Note: The diluent used in the dilution process was a 50% methanol aqueous solution; if necessary, the actual diluent used can be adjusted according to the proportion

Table 6.5 Preparation information of thalidomide working solutions

Source solution	Source solution conc.(μg/mL)	Source solution volume(μL)	Diluent volume(μL)	Final volume(μL)	Final conc.(μg/mL)	Solution name
Stock-A	1000	400	1600	2000	200	WS-C1
Stock-A	1000	180	820	1000	180	WS-C2
Stock-A	1000	120	880	1000	120	WS-C3
WS-C1	200	300	700	1000	60.0	WS-C4
WS-C1	200	100	900	1000	20.0	WS-C5
WS-C1	200	40	960	1000	8.00	WS-C6
WS-C5	20.0	100	900	1000	2.00	WS-C7
WS-C5	20.0	100	1900	1000	1.00	WS-C8
Stock-B	1000	400	600	1000	400	WS-DQC
Stock-B	1000	160	840	1000	160	WS-HQC
WS-HQC	160	150	850	1000	24.0	WS-MQC
WS-MQC	24.0	125	875	1000	3.00	WS-LQC
WS-MQC	24.0	40	920	960	1.00	WS-LLOQ

Note: The diluent used in the dilution process was a 50% acetonitrile aqueous solution; if necessary, the actual diluent used could be adjusted according to the proportion

Table 6.6 Preparation information of cyclophosphamide standard curve samples and quality control samples

Source solution	Source solution conc.(μg/mL)	Source solution volume (μL)	Diluent volume (μL)	Final volume(μL)	Final conc.(ng/mL)	Name
WS-C1	200	3	57	60	10,000	C1
WS-C2	180	3	57	60	9000	C2
WS-C3	100	3	57	60	5000	C3
WS-C4	30.0	3	57	60	1500	C4
WS-C5	10.0	3	57	60	500	C5
WS-C6	2.00	3	57	60	100	C6
WS-C7	0.400	3	57	60	20.0	C7
WS-C8	0.200	3	57	60	10.0	C8
WS-DQC	400	3	57	60	20,000	DQC
WS-HQC	160	3	57	60	8000	HQC
WS-MQC	16.0	3	57	60	800	MQC
WS-LQC	0.600	3	57	60	30.0	LQC
WS-LLOQ	0.200	3	57	60	10.0	LLOQ

Note: The diluent used in the dilution process was the blank plasma of cynomolgus monkeys; if necessary, the actual diluent used could be adjusted according to the proportion

Table 6.7 Preparation information of thalidomide standard curve samples and quality control samples

Source solution	Source solution conc.(μg/mL)	Source solution volume (μL)	Diluent volume (μL)	Final volume(μL)	Final conc.(ng/mL)	Name
WS-C1	200	3	57	60	10,000	C1
WS-C2	180	3	57	60	9000	C2
WS-C3	120	3	57	60	6000	C3
WS-C4	60.0	3	57	60	3000	C4
WS-C5	20.0	3	57	60	1000	C5
WS-C6	8.00	3	57	60	400	C6
WS-C7	2.00	3	57	60	100	C7
WS-C8	1.00	3	57	60	50.0	C8
WS-DQC	400	3	57	60	20,000	DQC
DQC	20000	6	54	60	2000	DQC/d10
WS-HQC	160	3	57	60	8000	HQC
WS-MQC	24.0	3	57	60	1200	MQC
WS-LQC	3.00	3	57	60	150	LQC
WS-LLOQ	1.00	3	57	60	50.0	LLOQ

Note: The diluent used in the dilution process is the blank plasma of cynomolgus monkeys; if necessary, the actual diluent used could be adjusted according to the proportion

Vortex and mix evenly. Centrifuge at 10,000 × *g* and 4°C for 10 min. Take 150 μL of the supernatant and place it in a 96-well plate. Add 150 μL of an aqueous solution, mix evenly, and then inject for determination. The injection volume is 1 μL.

6.6 Method Validation

6.6.1 Inspection of Stock Solutions

(1) Take an appropriate amount of cyclophosphamide stock A and stock B, dilute them to the same concentration level with a 50% methanol aqueous solution, and then inject for detection. Compare the differences between the two stock solutions by checking the peak areas of the analytes in the two stock solutions.

(2) Take an appropriate amount of thalidomide stock A and stock B, dilute them to the same concentration level with a 50% acetonitrile aqueous solution, and then inject for detection. Compare the differences between the two stock solutions by checking the peak areas of the analytes in the two stock solutions.

(3) Acceptance criteria: The RSD of the peak area of the analyte in each stock solution should be ≤10.00%. If the percentage difference in the mean peak area of the analyte in the two stock solutions is within the range of ±5.00%, the preparation of the stock solutions should be considered accurate.

6.6.2 Selectivity and Specificity

(1) Double blank matrix samples (without the analyte and internal standard): Take 60 μL/40 μL(60 μL for cyclophosphamide and 40 μL for thalidomide) of blank plasma from different donors. Replace the internal standard working solution with an equal volume of methanol, and prepare the other samples using the same method as the sample processing method.

(2) Matrix samples at the lower limit of quantification: Prepare an analyte sample at the concentration level of the lower limit of quantification and process it according to the sample processing method.

(3) Matrix samples at the upper limit of quantification containing only the analyte: Prepare a sample at the ULOQ concentration level and process it according to the sample processing method.

(4) Matrix samples containing only the internal standard (without the analyte): Prepare a single blank sample containing only the internal standard.

(5) Acceptance criteria: For any interference observable in the retention time region of the analyte and generated by the matrix or internal standard, the response of the interference peak should be $\leq$20.00% of the response of the analyte peak at the LLOQ; for any interference observable in the retention time region of the internal standard and generated by the matrix or analyte, the response of the interference peak should be $\leq$5.00% of the response of the internal standard peak at the LLOQ.

6.6.3 System Suitability

(1) Preparation of system suitability samples: Prepare system suitability samples at the lower limit of quantification level. Inject six replicates before submitting the formal analytical run to evaluate the system suitability. System suitability verification is required before carrying out each analytical run. If there was no interruption in injection between subsequent runs and the analytical run, no additional system suitability verification was required.

(2) Acceptance criteria: The RSD of the retention time of the analyte and the internal standard should be $\leq$5.00%, and the RSD of the ratio of the peak area of the analyte to that of the internal standard should be $\leq$20.00%.

6.6.4 Standard Curve

(1) Preparation of standard curve samples: Prepare the standard curve working solutions of cyclophosphamide according to Table 6.4, prepare the standard curve working solutions of thalidomide according to Table 6.5, prepare the cyclophosphamide standard curve samples according to Table 6.6, prepare the thalidomide standard curve samples according to Table 6.7, and then process them according to the sample processing method.

(2) Acceptance criteria: Perform linear regression on the theoretical concentration and the actual response value. Use the least squares method to conduct linear fitting for the points on the standard curve, with a weighting factor of $1/X^2$. The relative error (RE) of the calibration standards should be within the range of ±15.00%, and the RE of the lower limit of quantification should be within the range of ±20.00%. At least 75% of the calibration standards and at least six calibration standards in total should meet the above criteria. The correlation coefficient (R^2) of the standard curve should be greater than or equal to 0.980.

6.6.5 System Carryover

(1) Take 60 μL/40 μL (60 μL for cyclophosphamide and 40 μL for thalidomide) of blank plasma and process them according to the sample processing method (replace the internal standard working solution with an equal volume of methanol) to obtain double blank samples. Inject a ULOQ sample and then inject at least one double blank sample to evaluate the carryover.

(2) Acceptance criteria: The response of the analyte peak area in the double blank samples should be ≤20.00% of the response of the analyte peak area at the lower limit of quantification, and the response of the internal standard peak area should be ≤5.00% of the response of the internal standard peak area at the lower limit of quantification.

6.6.6 Accuracy and Precision

(1) Preparation of accuracy and precision quality control samples: Prepare cyclophosphamide quality control working solutions according to Table 6.4, prepare thalidomide quality control working solutions according to Table 6.5, freshly prepare cyclophosphamide accuracy and precision samples (LLOQ, LQC, MQC, and HQC) according to Table 6.6, freshly prepare thalidomide accuracy and precision samples (LLOQ, LQC, MQC, and HQC) according to Table 6.7, and then process them according to the sample processing method. Each concentration level was processed in parallel for six replicates. This verification should be carried out for at least three runs and completed in at least 2 days.

(2) Acceptance criteria: The RE of the intra-run and inter-run LQC, MQC, and HQC should be within the range of ±15.00%, and the RE of LLOQ should be within the range of ±20.00%; the RSD of the measured concentrations of intra-run and inter-run LQC, MQC, and HQC should be ≤15.00%, and the RSD of the measured concentration of LLOQ should be ≤20.00%. There should be at least 5 valid values for the quality control samples at each concentration in each analytical run.

6.6.7 Dilution Reliability

(1) Take 3 μL of the diluted quality control working solution (WSDQC) and add it to 57 μL of blank matrix. Vortex and mix evenly to prepare diluted quality control samples. Take 6 μL of the diluted quality control samples, add them to 54 μL of blank SD rat plasma (tenfold dilution), vortex and mix evenly, and then process them according to the sample processing method. Process six replicates in parallel.

(2) Acceptance criteria: The RE of DQC should be within the range of ±15.00%, and the RSD of the measured concentration should be ≤15.00%. There should be at least five valid values.

6.6.8 Matrix Effect

(1) Preparation of solution samples: Take 57 μL of water, add 300 μL of methanol precipitant, vortex, and mix evenly. Centrifuge at 10,000 × *g* and 4°C for 10 min. Add 3 μL of the working solution (WSHQC and WSLQC), add 60 μL of the internal standard working solution, vortex and mix evenly. Centrifuge at 10,000 × *g* and 4°C for 5 min. Take 150 μL of the supernatant and place it in a 96-well deep-well plate. Add 150 μL of water, mix evenly, and then inject for determination. Process six replicates in parallel at each concentration level.

(2) Preparation of matrix samples: Take 57 μL of blank plasma (blank plasma from six sources), add 300 μL of methanol precipitant, vortex, and mix evenly. Centrifuge at 10,000 × *g* and 4°C for 10 min. Add 3 μL of the working solution (WSHQC and WSLQC), add 60 μL of the internal standard working solution, vortex and mix evenly. Centrifuge at 10,000 × *g* and 4°C for 5 min. Take 150 μL of the supernatant and place it in a 96-well deep-well plate. Add 150 μL of water, mix evenly, and then inject for determination. Process six replicates in parallel at each concentration level.

(3) Calculate the matrix factor of each analyte and internal standard by calculating the ratio of the peak area in the presence of the matrix (obtained by extracting the blank matrix and adding the analyte and internal standard) to the corresponding peak area without the matrix (pure solution of the analyte and internal standard). Calculate the internal standard-normalized matrix factor by dividing the matrix factor of the analyte by the matrix factor of the internal standard.

(4) Acceptance criteria: The RSD of the matrix factor calculated from six runs of the matrix at each concentration level should be ≤15.00%, and the RSD of the internal standard-normalized matrix factor calculated at each concentration level should be ≤15.00%.

6.6.9 Hemolysis Effect

(1) Preparation of hemolytic plasma: Take a certain amount of frozen whole blood from SD rats. After natural thawing at room temperature, vortex and mix it evenly.

Then centrifuge it at 4°C and 1800×g for 10 min. Take 5% of the supernatant and add it to 95% of blank SD rat plasma to obtain 5% hemolytic plasma.

(2) Preparation of hemolysis samples: Add low and high-concentration quality control working solutions (working solution:hemolysis matrix = 1:19) into 5% hemolytic plasma to prepare hemolysis effect samples (HemLQC/HQC). Process them according to the sample processing method, with six parallel samples processed for each concentration level.

(3) Acceptance criteria: The RE of the samples used for evaluating the hemolysis effect should be within the range of ±15%. The relative standard deviation (RSD) of the measured concentrations should be ≤15.00%, with at least five valid values for each concentration.

6.6.10 Recovery Rate

(1) Preparation of extraction recovery samples: Take 3 μL of quality control sample working solutions (WSHQC, WSMQC, and WSLQC), respectively, and add them to 57 μL of blank matrix. Then, process them according to the sample processing method, with six parallel samples processed for each concentration level.

(2) Preparation of extraction recovery reference samples: Take 57 μL of blank plasma (mixed blank plasma), add 300 μL of methanol precipitant, vortex, and mix evenly. Then centrifuge it at 4°C and 10,000×g for 10 min. Add 3 μL of working solutions (WSHQC, WSMQC, and WSLQC), add 60 μL of internal standard working solution, vortex and mix evenly. Then centrifuge it at 4°C and 10,000×g for 5 min. Take 150 μL of the supernatant and put it into a 96-well deep-well plate. Add 150 μL of water, mix evenly, and then conduct sample injection and determination, with six parallel samples processed for each concentration level.

(3) Evaluate the recovery rates of the analytes and internal standards by comparing the average peak area responses of the extraction recovery samples with those of the extraction recovery reference samples.

(4) Acceptance criteria: The RSD of the extraction recovery rates of the analytes and internal standards for each concentration level should be ≤15.00%. The RSD of the average extraction recovery rates of the analytes and internal standards among different concentration levels should be ≤15.00%.

6.6.11 Stability

(1) Short-term stability of stock solutions: Aliquot a certain amount of stock A, place it at room temperature for a certain period of time (at least 20 h). Then, together with stock A directly taken out from the 4°C refrigerator, dilute them to the same concentration level with the diluent and then conduct sample injection and detection. Calculate the percentage difference in the average peak area between the stability samples and the stability control samples. The calculation formula was: percentage difference in the average peak area = (average peak area of stability samples − average

peak area of stability control samples)/average peak area of stability control samples × 100%. Acceptance criteria: The RSD of the peak area of the analyte in each solution should be ≤10.00%. If the percentage difference in the average peak area between the stability samples and the stability control samples was within the range of ±10.00%, it was considered that the stock solution was stable when placed at room temperature for a short term.

(2) Long-term stability of stock solutions (placed in a 4°C refrigerator): Take stock A that has been placed in a 4°C refrigerator for a certain period of time (at least 15 days) and, together with freshly prepared stock A, dilute them to the same concentration level with the diluent and then conduct sample injection and detection. Calculate the percentage difference in the average peak area between the stability samples and the stability control samples. Acceptance criteria: The RSD of the peak area of the analyte in each solution should be ≤10.00%. If the percentage difference in the average peak area between the stability samples and the stability control samples was within the range of ±10.00%, it was considered that the stock solution was stable when placed in a 4°C refrigerator for a long term.

(3) Short-term stability of working solutions: Place WSC8 and WSC1 working solutions at room temperature for a certain period of time (at least 20 h). Then, together with WSC8 and WSC1 taken out from the 4°C refrigerator, dilute them to the same concentration level with the diluent, and then conduct sample injection and detection. Calculate the percentage difference in the average peak area between the stability samples and the stability control samples. Acceptance criteria: The RSD of the peak area of the analyte in each solution should be ≤10.00%. If the percentage difference in the average peak area between the stability samples and the stability control samples was within the range of ±10.00%, it was considered that the working solutions were stable when placed at room temperature for a short term.

(4) Long-term stability of working solutions (placed in a 4°C refrigerator): Place WSC8 and WSC1 working solutions in a 4°C refrigerator for a certain period of time (at least 15 days). Then, together with freshly prepared WSC8 and WSC1 working solutions, dilute them to the same concentration level with the diluent and then conduct sample injection and detection. Calculate the percentage difference in the average peak area between the stability samples and the stability control samples. Acceptance criteria: The RSD of the peak area of the analyte in each solution should be ≤10.00%. If the percentage difference in the average peak area between the stability samples and the stability control samples is within the range of ±10.00%, it is considered that the working solutions are stable when placed at 4°C for a long term.

(5) Short-term stability of matrix samples: Take the prepared low concentration and high concentration quality control samples and place them at room temperature or in an ice bath (cyclophosphamide at room temperature, thalidomide in an ice bath) for a certain period of time (at least 6 h). Then, process them according to the sample processing method, with six parallel samples processed for each concentration level. Acceptance criteria: The RE of the samples used for stability investigation should be within the range of ±15.00%. The RSD of the measured concentrations should be ≤ 15.00%, with at least five valid values for each concentration.

(6) Freeze–thaw stability of matrix samples (at least four cycles): Take the prepared low concentration and high concentration quality control samples, store and freeze them at −80°C (completely frozen). After the samples are naturally thawed at room temperature, freeze them again at −80°C. The thawing time should be at least 15 min (the first time should be >30 min). Repeat the freeze–thaw cycle at least three times, with each cycle at least 12 h (the first time should be at least 24 h). After the samples are thawed in the 4th cycle, process them according to the sample processing method, with six parallel samples processed for each concentration level. Acceptance criteria: The RE of the samples used for stability investigation should be within the range of ± 15.00%. The RSD of the measured concentrations should be ≤15.00%, with at least five valid values for each concentration.

(7) Long-term stability of matrix samples (stored in a −80°C refrigerator): Take the prepared low concentration and high concentration quality control samples and store them in a −80°C refrigerator for a certain period of time (at least 15 days, covering the time range from sample collection to detection). Then, process them according to the sample processing method, with six parallel samples processed for each concentration level. Acceptance criteria: The RE of the samples used for stability investigation should be within the range of ±15.00%. The RSD of the measured concentrations should be ≤15.00%, with at least five valid values for each concentration.

(8) Stability of sample collection (whole blood stability): Add low concentration and high concentration quality control working solutions to fresh whole blood to prepare whole blood samples (working solution:fresh whole blood = 1:19). Incubate them at 37°C for 30 min and then divide them into three parts. One part was immediately centrifuged (at 1800 × *g* for 10 min), and the plasma was taken as the control sample for whole blood stability investigation. The other two parts were placed on wet ice for 1 and 2 h, respectively, and then centrifuged (at 1800 × *g* for 10 min), and the plasma was taken as the stability investigation samples. Process the control samples and the stability investigation samples according to the sample processing method, with six parallel samples processed for each concentration level. Acceptance criteria: Compared with the average peak area of the control samples, the RE of the peak area of the stability investigation samples should be within the range of ±15.00%. The RSD of the peak area of the samples for each concentration level should be ≤15.00%, with at least five valid values for each concentration.

(9) Stability of post-preparation samples (placed in the environment of an autosampler): Place the accepted analytical runs in the environment of an autosampler for a certain period of time (at least 20 h). Then use the freshly prepared standard curve to conduct quantitative analysis on the low concentration and high concentration quality control samples in the above analytical runs. Acceptance criteria: The RE of the samples used for stability investigation should be within the range of ±15.00%. The RSD of the measured concentrations should be ≤15.00%, with at least five valid values for each concentration.

6.6.12 Maximum Sample Capacity of Analytical Runs

(1) Resubmit the accepted precision and accuracy analytical runs. After injecting all the standard curve samples of the analytical runs, repeatedly submit the LQC (low quality control), MQC (medium quality control), and HQC (high quality control) samples of the analytical run to fill up to the expected maximum sample capacity of a single analytical run in the analysis of test samples. The analytical run capacity refers to the total number of injections of quality control samples in the analytical run.

(2) Acceptance criteria: In the analytical run, at least 67% of the quality control samples, and the RE of at least 50% of the quality control samples for each concentration level should be within the range of ±15.00%.

6.6.13 Acceptance Criteria for Analytical Runs

The RE of the calibration standards should be within the range of ±15.00%, and the RE of the LLOQ should be within the range of ±20.00%. At least 75% and at least six calibration standards should meet this criterion. At least 67% of the quality control samples, and the RE of at least 50% of the quality control samples for each concentration level should within the range of ±15.00% (the items that did not require back-calculation of concentration for calculation did not apply to this criterion; for the runs of accuracy and precision investigations, it was necessary to meet the acceptance criteria of the corresponding quality control samples for accuracy and precision).

6.7 Results of Methodological Validation

The test results of all validation items met the acceptance criteria. The results of methodological validation can be found in Tables 6.8 and 6.9, and the chromatogram results corresponding to each validation item can be found in Figs. 6.2–6.25.

6.8 Conclusion

In this study, the bioanalytical method validation for the determination of the concentrations of cyclophosphamide and thalidomide in the plasma of cynomolgus monkeys was completed using the LC–MS/MS method. The linearity range of the method for detecting cyclophosphamide was 10–10,000 ng/mL, and that for detecting thalidomide was 50–10,000 ng/mL. The comprehensive validation was performed for the stock solution examination of the analytes (cyclophosphamide and thalidomide), the short-term and long-term stabilities of working solutions, system suitability, selectivity, matrix effect, recovery rate, carryover, standard curve, intra-run and inter-run accuracy and precision, dilution reliability, short-term and long-term stabilities of analytes in the matrix, whole blood stability, post-preparation sample stability, and

Table 6.8 Summary of cyclophosphamide validation results

Investigation items	Test results	Acceptance criteria	Result/ evaluation
Stock solution examination	RSD was ≤2.54%; the percentage difference of the means was within the range of −0.58% to 0.52%	RSD should be ≤10.00%; the mean percentage difference should be within the range of ±5.00%	Met acceptance criteria
Selectivity and specificity	The interference peak of the blank matrix at the peak position of the analyte cyclophosphamide was ≤4.48%, the blank matrix had no interference peak at the peak position of the internal standard, and the analyte at the peak position of the internal standard and the internal standard at the peak position of the analyte did not interfere with each other	For any observable interference within the retention time zone of the analyte cyclophosphamide, which was generated by the matrix or internal standard, the response of the interference peak should be ≤ 20.00% of the peak response of the analyte at LLOQ; for any observable interference within the retention time zone of the internal standard, which was generated by the matrix or analyte, the response of the interference peak should be ≤5.00% of the peak response of the internal standard at the LLOQ.	Met acceptance criteria
System suitability	The RSD of the retention time of the analyte was ≤0.32%, the RSD of the retention time of the internal standard was ≤0.25%, and the RSD of the ratio of the peak areas of the analyte and the internal standard was ≤3.37%	The RSD of the retention time of the analyte and the internal standard should be ≤5.00%, and the RSD of the peak area ratio of the analyte to the internal standard should be ≤20.00%	Met acceptance criteria
Standard curve	The RE of the eight nonzero calibration standards was within the range of −9.83% to 13.90%, R^2 was ≥0.9920	Except for the LLOQ, the accuracy of other calibration samples should be within 85.00%–115.00%, and the accuracy of the LLOQ should be within 80.00%–120.00%. At least 75% and at least six calibration samples at different concentrations should meet the criteria, and R^2 should be ≥0.9800	Met acceptance criteria
Intra-run precision and accuracy	The RE of LLOQ was within the range of −10.31% to −1.46%, the precision RSD was ≤ 5.42%, the RE of LQC, MQC, and HQC was within the range of −8.68% to 2.20%, the precision RSD was ≤ 4.33%	The RE should be within the range of −15.00% to 15.00%, and the RSD should be ≤15.00%; the RE of the LLOQ should be within the range of −20.00% to 20.00%, and the RSD should be ≤20.00%	Met acceptance criteria

Investigation items	Test results	Acceptance criteria	Result/ evaluation
Inter-run precision and accuracy	The RE of LLOQ was −6.45%, the precision RSD was 5.85%, the RE of LQC, MQC, and HQC was within the range of −6.06% to −0.29%, the precision RSD was ≤4.70%	The RE should be within the range of −15.00% to 15.00%, and the RSD should be ≤15.00%; the RE of the LLOQ should be within the range of −20.00% to 20.00%, and the RSD should be ≤20.00%	Met acceptance criteria
System residue	The response of the analyte in the blank samples was ≤4.63% of the response of the analyte at LLOQ, and there was no residue of the internal standard	The response of the analyte in the double blank samples should be ≤ 20.00% of the response of the analyte at the LLOQ, and the response of the internal standard should be ≤5.00% of the response of the internal standard at the LLOQ	Met acceptance criteria
Dilution reliability	RSD was 3.70%, RE was −8.72%	The RSD should be ≤15.00%, and the RE should be within the range of ± 15.00%	Met acceptance criteria
Matrix effect	The RSD of the matrix factor calculated from six runs of matrices at each concentration level was ≤2.34%; the RSD of the IS-normalized matrix factor at each concentration was ≤ 3.31%	The RSD of the matrix factor calculated from six runs of matrices at each concentration level should be ≤15.00%, and the RSD of the IS-normalized matrix factor calculated at each concentration level should be ≤15.00%	Met acceptance criteria
Recovery	The RSD of recovery at each concentration was ≤7.49%; mean extraction recovery was 86.25%, RSD was 7.71%; Mean recovery of internal standard was 91.02%, RSD was 9.10%	RSD should be ≤15.00%	Met acceptance criteria
Hemolytic effect	The RSD of the 5% hemolytic matrix samples was ≤3.13%; RE was within the range of −3.67% to 0.96%	RSD should be ≤15.00%; mean RE should be ±15.00%	Met acceptance criteria
Stock solution short-term stability	The RSD of the peak area after being placed at room temperature for 24 h was ≤1.31%, and the percentage difference of the mean peak area was −4.73%	RSD should be ≤10.00%, and the mean percentage difference should be within ±10.00%	Met acceptance criteria

Investigation items	Test results	Acceptance criteria	Result/ evaluation
Stock solution long-term stability	The RSD of the peak area of the stock solution placed in a refrigerator at 4°C for 20 days was ≤1.88%, and the percentage difference of the mean peak area was −0.31%	RSD should be ≤10.00%, and the mean percentage difference should be within ±10.00%	Met acceptance criteria
Working solution short-term stability	The RSD of the peak area after being placed at room temperature for 24 h was ≤6.07%, and the percentage difference of the mean values was within the range of 0.84%–3.50%	RSD should be ≤10.00%, and the mean percentage difference should be within±10.00%	Met acceptance criteria
Working solution for long-term stability	The RSD of the peak area of the working solution placed in a refrigerator at 4°C for 20 days was ≤3.63%, and the percentage difference of the means was within the range of −0.80%–1.46%	RSD should be ≤10.00%, and the mean percentage difference should be within ±10.00%	Met acceptance criteria
Matrix sample short-term stability	The RSD of the matrix samples placed at room temperature for 96 h was ≤2.03%, and the RE was within the range of 0.47%–1.33%. The RSD of the matrix samples placed at room temperature for 6 h was ≤1.92%, and the RE was within the range of 1.07%–13.59%	RSD should be ≤15.00%, mean RE should be ±15.00%	Met acceptance criteria
Matrix sample freeze–thaw stability	The RSD of the matrix samples after four freeze–thaw cycles from 80°C to room temperature was ≤ 2.01%, and the RE was within the range of 2.05%–9.74%	RSD should be ≤15.00%, mean RE should be ±15.00%	Met acceptance criteria
Matrix sample long-term stability	The RSD of the matrix samples placed at −80°C for 20 days was ≤2.07%, the RE was within the range of 1.60%–3.53%	RSD should be ≤15.00%, mean RE should be ±15.00%	Met acceptance criteria

Investigation items	Test results	Acceptance criteria	Result/ evaluation
Whole blood stability	The RSD of the whole blood stability test samples placed in an ice bath for 1 and 2 h was ≤2.15%, and the RE between the peak area of the stability test samples and that of the control samples was within the range of −3.27% to 0.43%	The RSD should be ≤15.00%, and the RE of the peak area of the stability test sample to the peak area of the control sample should be within the range of ±15.00%	Met acceptance criteria
Sample stability after preparation	The RSD of the samples placed in the autosampler for 48 h was ≤3.05%; RE was within the range of −13.75% to −13.21%	RSD should be ≤15.00%; mean RE should be ±15.00%	Met acceptance criteria
Analytic run maximum capacity	In the analysis run of 108 needle quality control samples, the sample accuracy deviation was within the range of −11.21% to 4.34%	In the analytical run, at least 67% of the quality control samples, and at least 50% of the quality control samples at each concentration level should have an RE within the range of ±15.00%	Met acceptance criteria

Table 6.9 Summary of thalidomide validation results

Investigation items	Test results	Acceptance criteria	Result/ evaluation
Stock solution examination	RSD ≤3.15%; the mean percentage difference was within the range of −1.13% to 0.72%	RSD should be ≤10.00%; the mean percentage difference should be within the range of ±5.00%	Met acceptance criteria
Selectivity and specificity	The interference peak of the blank matrix at the peak of the analyte cyclophosphamide was ≤0.00%. Blank matrix had no interference peak at the internal standard peak, and the analyte at the internal standard peak and the internal standard at the analyte peak did not interfere with each other	For any observable interference in the retention time zone of the analyte cyclophosphamide, which was generated by the matrix or internal standard, the response of the interference peak should be ≤20.00% of the peak response of the analyte at LLOQ; for any observable interference in the retention time zone of the internal standard, which was generated by the matrix or analyte, the response of the interference peak should be ≤5.00% of the peak response of the internal standard at the LLOQ	Met acceptance criteria
System suitability	The RSD of the analyte retention time was ≤0.65%, the RSD of the internal standard retention time was ≤0.25%, and the RSD of the peak area ratio of the analyte to the internal standard was ≤5.94%	The RSD of the retention time of the analyte and the internal standard should be ≤5.00%, and the RSD of the peak area ratio of the analyte to the internal standard should be ≤20.00%	Met acceptance criteria
Standard curve	The RE of eight nonzero calibration samples were within the range of −13.81% to 14.10%, and R^2 was ≥0.9934	Except for the LLOQ, the accuracy of other calibration samples should be within 85.00%–115.00%, and the accuracy of the LLOQ should be within 80.00%–120.00%. At least 75% and at least six concentration calibration samples should meet the criteria, and R^2 should ≥0.9800	Met acceptance criteria
Intra-run precision and accuracy	The RE of LLOQ was within the range of −2.86% to 5.32%, and the precision RSD was ≤8.76%; the RE of LQC, MQC, and HQC was within the range of −4.53% to 6.67%, and the precision RSD was ≤8.85%	The RE should be within the range of −15.00% to 15.00%, and the RSD should be ≤15.00%; the RE of the LLOQ should be within the range of −20.00% to 20.00%, and the RSD should be ≤20.00%	Met acceptance criteria
Inter-run precision and accuracy	The RE of LLOQ was 1.78%, and the RSD was 7.31%; the RE of LQC, MQC, and HQC was within the range of −2.63% to 2.36%, and the precision RSD was ≤6.45%	The RE should be within the range of −15.00% to 15.00%, and the RSD should be ≤15.00%; the RE of the LLOQ should be within the range of −20.00% to 20.00%, and the RSD should be ≤20.00%	Met acceptance criteria

Investigation items	Test results	Acceptance criteria	Result/ evaluation
System residue	The analyte response in the blank sample was ≤0.00% of the LLOQ analyte response, and there was no residue of the internal standard	The response of the analyte in the double blank samples should be ≤20.00% of the response of the analyte at the LLOQ, and the response of the internal standard should be ≤5.00% of the response of the internal standard at the LLOQ	Met acceptance criteria
Dilution reliability	RSD was 4.07%, RE was 2.86%	RSD should be ≤15.00%, RE should be within ±15.00%	Met acceptance criteria
Matrix effect	The RSD of the matrix factor calculated from six runs of matrices at each concentration level was ≤6.35%; the RSD of the IS-normalized matrix factor at each concentration was ≤6.87%	The RSD of the matrix factor calculated from 6 runs of matrices at each concentration level should be ≤15.00%, and the RSD of the IS-normalized matrix factor calculated at each concentration level should be ≤15.00%	Met acceptance criteria
Recovery	The RSD of the recovery at each concentration was ≤ 5.46%; the mean extraction recovery was 97.45%, and the RSD was 5.25%; the mean recovery of the internal standard was 97.33%, and the RSD was 5.59%	RSD should be ≤15.00%	Met acceptance criteria
Hemolytic effect	The RSD of the 5% hemolytic matrix sample was ≤6.55%; the RE was within the range of −1.70% to −1.02%	RSD should be ≤15.00%; mean RE should be ±15.00%	Met acceptance criteria
Stock solution short-term stability	The RSD of the peak area after being placed at room temperature for 24 h was ≤3.11%, and the percentage difference of the peak area mean was 1.28%	RSD should be ≤10.00%, and the mean percentage difference should be within ±10.00%	Met acceptance criteria
Stock solution long-term stability	The RSD of the peak area of the stock solution placed in a 4°C refrigerator for 30 days was ≤1.71%, and the percentage difference of the peak area mean was −1.80%	RSD should be ≤10.00%, and the mean percentage difference should be within ±10.00%	Met acceptance criteria
Working solution short-term stability	The RSD of the peak area after being placed at room temperature for 24 h was ≤2.57%, and the mean percentage difference was within the range of −5.94% to −3.11%	RSD should be ≤10.00%, and the mean percentage difference should be within ±10.00%	Met acceptance criteria
Working solution for long-term stability	The RSD of the peak area of the working solution placed in a 4°C refrigerator for 30 days was ≤1.42%, and the mean percentage difference was within the range of −0.14% to 0.50%	RSD should be ≤10.00%, and the mean percentage difference should be within ±10.00%	Met acceptance criteria

Investigation items	Test results	Acceptance criteria	Result/evaluation
Matrix sample short-term stability	The RSD of the matrix sample placed in an ice bath for 6 h was ≤4.66%, and the RE was within the range of −2.06% to 4.33%	RSD should be ≤15.00%, mean RE should be ±15.00%	Met acceptance criteria
Matrix sample freeze–thaw stability	The RSD of the matrix sample after four freeze–thaw cycles from 80°C to room temperature was ≤4.44%, and the RE was within the range of −4.45% to −4.44%	RSD should be ≤15.00%, mean RE should be ±15.00%	Met acceptance criteria
Matrix sample long-term stability	The RSD of the matrix sample placed at −80°C for 30 days was ≤4.80%, and the RE was within the range of 4.68%–7.31%	RSD should be ≤15.00%, mean RE should be ±15.00%	Met acceptance criteria
Whole blood stability	The RSD of the whole blood stability test samples placed in an ice bath for 1 and 2 h was ≤3.46%, and the RE of the peak area of the stability test sample to the peak area of the control sample was within the range of −10.03% to 3.63%	RSD should be ≤15.00%, and the RE of the peak area of the stability test sample to the peak area of the control sample should be within the range of ±15.00%	Met acceptance criteria
Sample stability after preparation	The RSD of samples placed in the autosampler for 48 h was ≤3.13%; the RE was within the range of 6.06%–13.96%	RSD should be ≤15.00%; mean RE should be ±15.00%	Met acceptance criteria
Analytic run maximum capacity	Among the 108 needle quality control samples in the analytical run, the sample accuracy deviation was within the range of −11.39% to 9.02%	In the analytical run, at least 67% of the quality control samples, and at least 50% of the quality control samples at each concentration level, should have an RE within the range of ± 15.00%	Met acceptance criteria

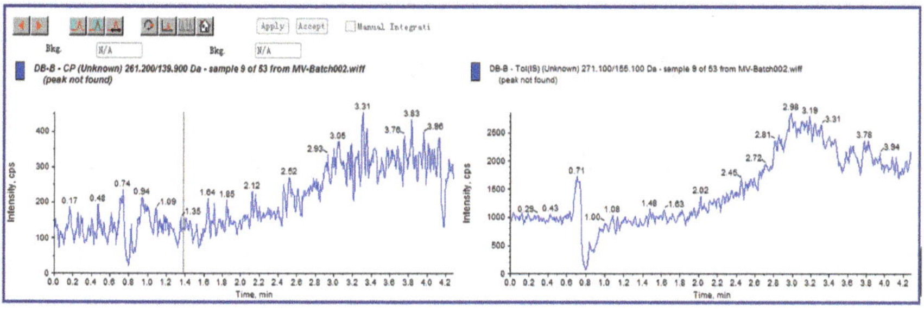

Fig. 6.2 Chromatogram of double blanks from six sources of cyclophosphamide (analytical run name MVBatch002, sample name DBB)

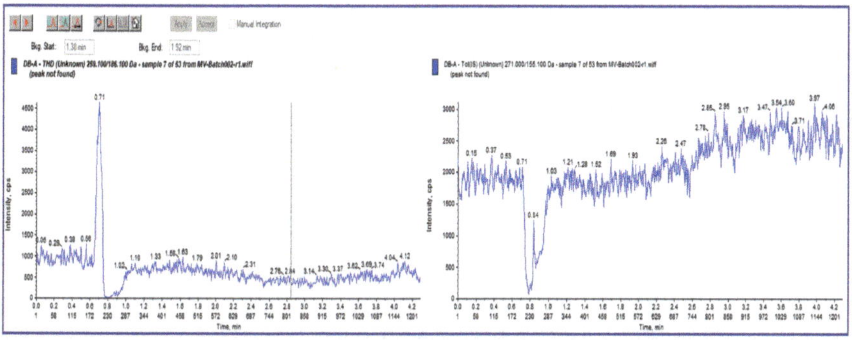

Fig. 6.3 Chromatogram of double blanks from six sources of thalidomide (analytical run name MVBatch008, sample name DBA)

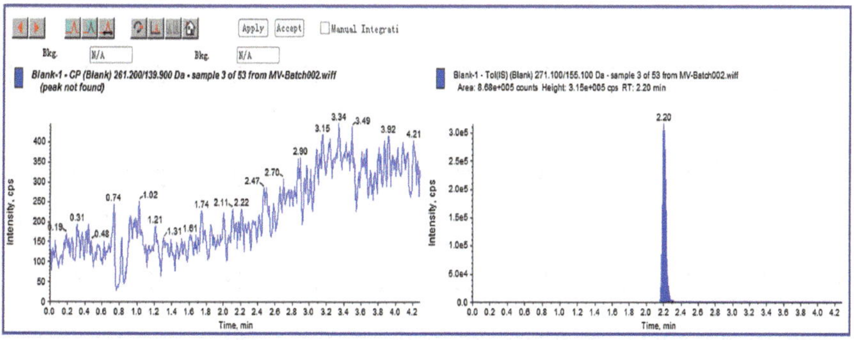

Fig. 6.4 Chromatogram of single blank of cyclophosphamide (analytical run name MVBatch002, sample name Blank1)

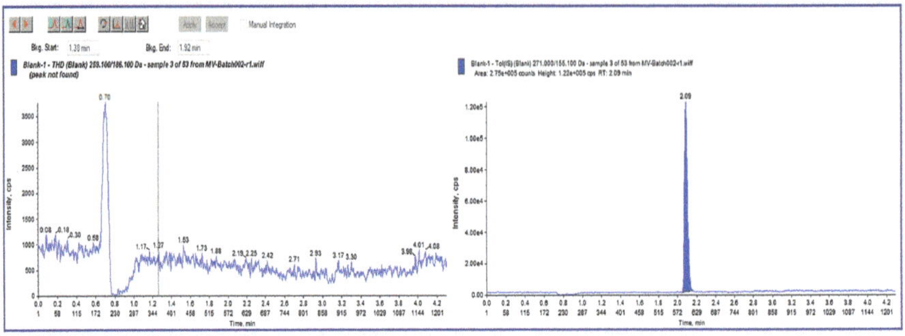

Fig. 6.5 Chromatogram of Single Blank of Thalidomide (Analytical run name MVBatch002, Sample name Blank1)

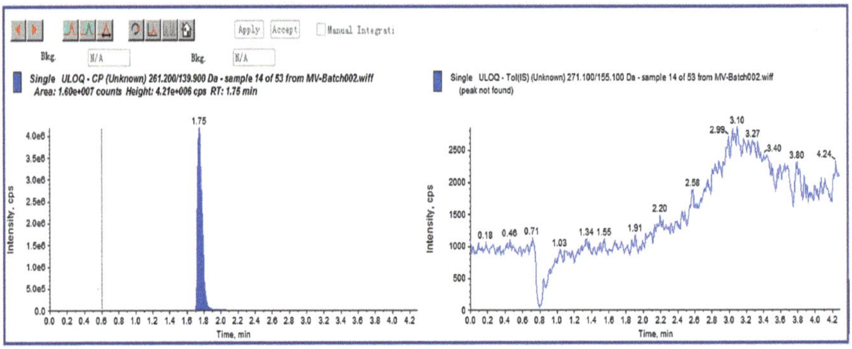

Fig. 6.6 Chromatogram of upper limit of quantification of cyclophosphamide without internal standard (analytical run name MVBatch002, sample name Single ULOQ)

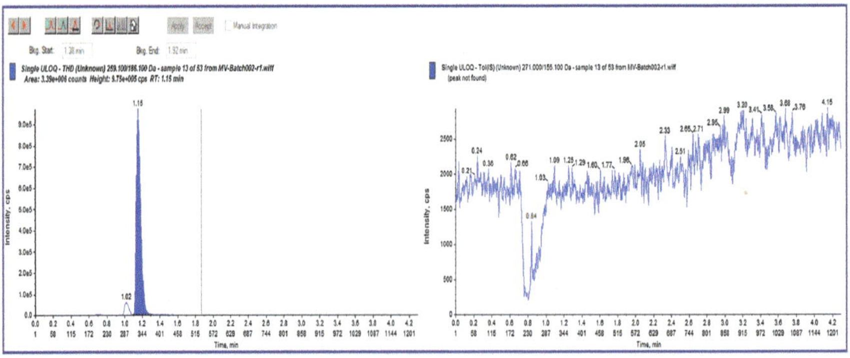

Fig. 6.7 Chromatogram of upper limit of quantification of thalidomide without internal standard (analytical run name MVBatch002, sample name Single ULOQ)

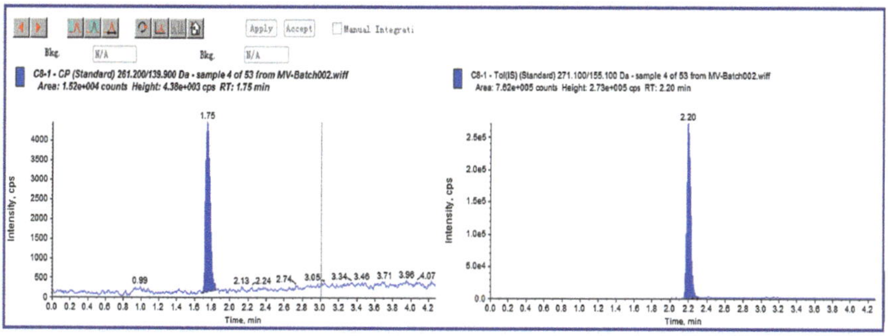

Fig. 6.8 Chromatogram of the lower limit of quantification of cyclophosphamide (analytical run name MVBatch002, sample name C81)

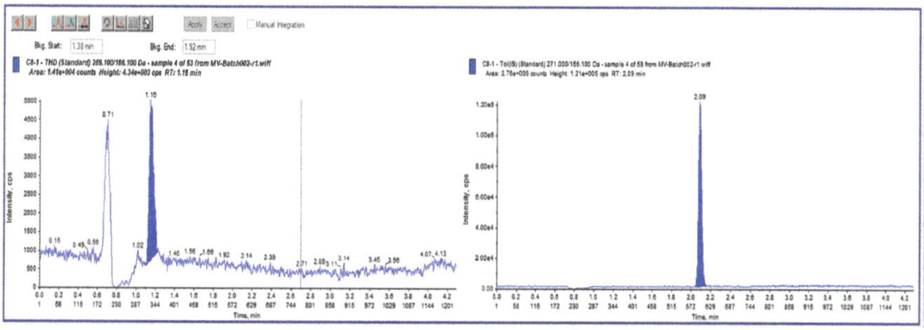

Fig. 6.9 Chromatogram of the lower limit of quantification of thalidomide (analytical run name MVBatch002, sample name C81)

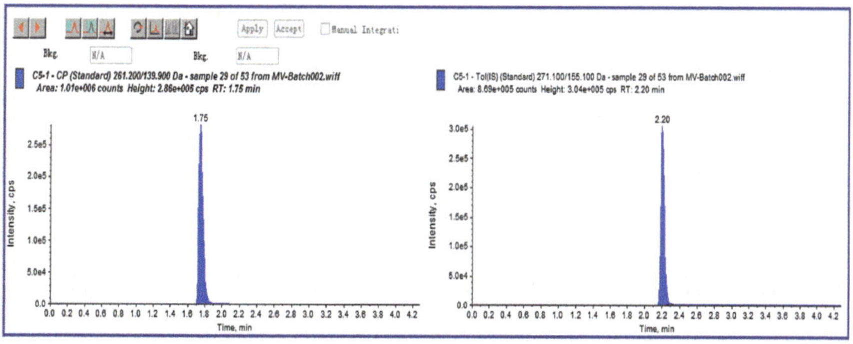

Fig. 6.10 Representative chromatogram of cyclophosphamide standard curve (analytical run name MVBatch002, sample name C51)

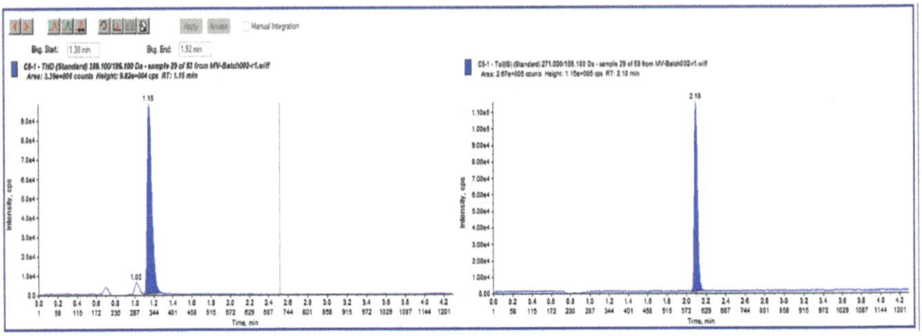

Fig. 6.11 Representative chromatogram of thalidomide standard curve (analytical run name MVBatch002, sample name C51)

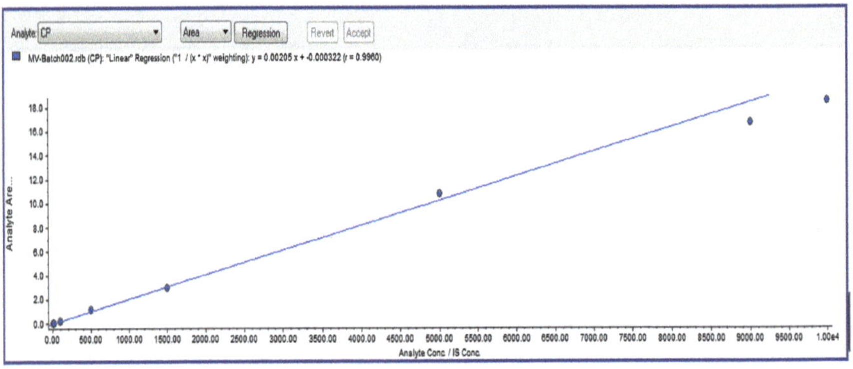

Fig. 6.12 Representative chromatogram of cyclophosphamide linearity (analytical run name MVBatch002)

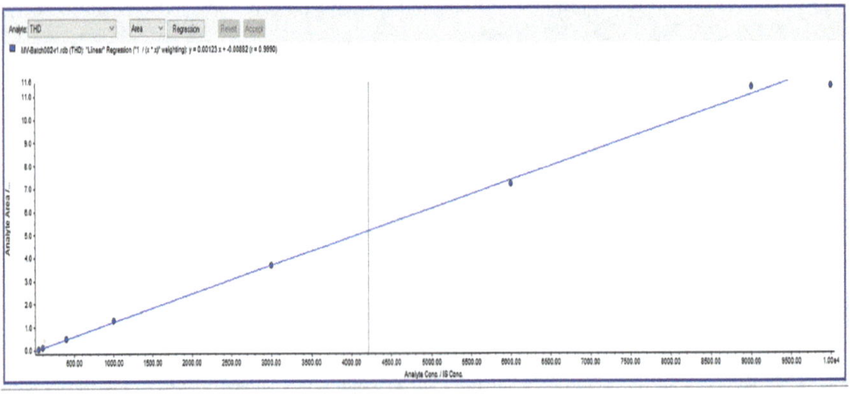

Fig. 6.13 Representative chromatogram of thalidomide linearity (analytical run name MVBatch002)

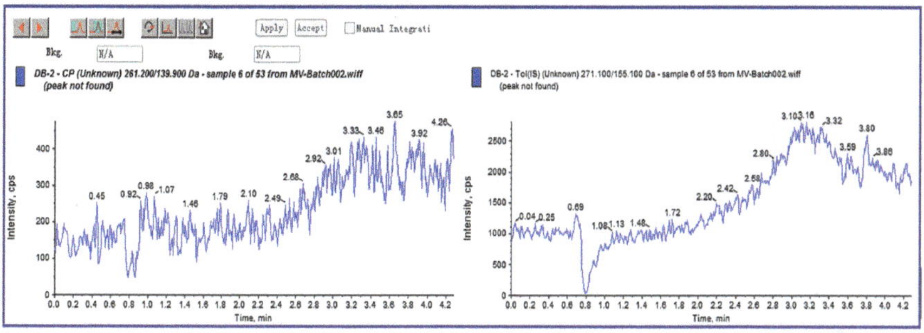

Fig. 6.14 Double blank chromatogram of the first needle after the upper limit of quantification of cyclophosphamide (analytical run name MVBatch002, sample name DB2)

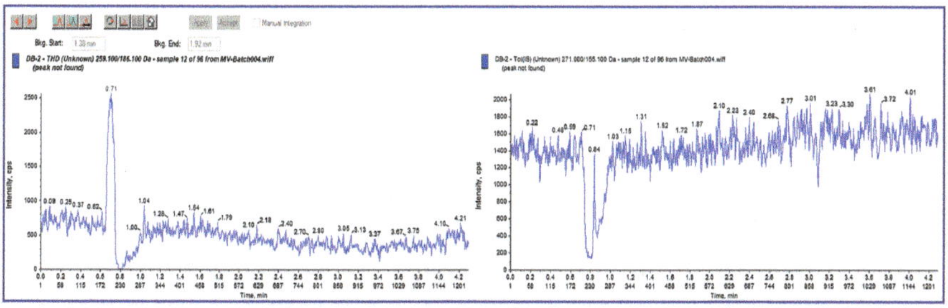

Fig. 6.15 Double blank chromatogram of the first needle after the upper limit of quantification of thalidomide (analytical run name MVBatch004, sample name DB2)

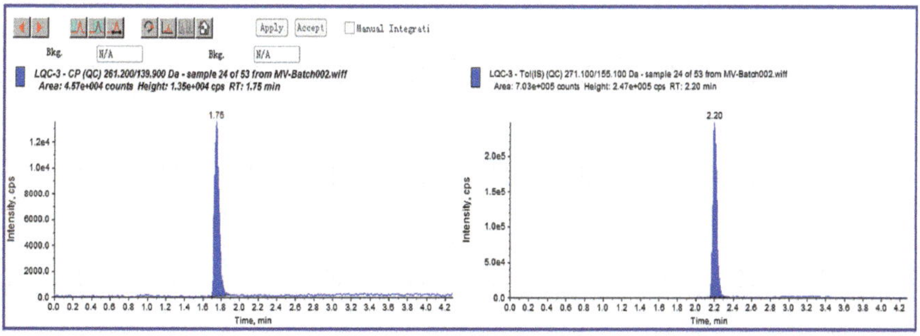

Fig. 6.16 Representative chromatogram of cyclophosphamide quality control (analytical run name MVBatch002, sample name LQC3)

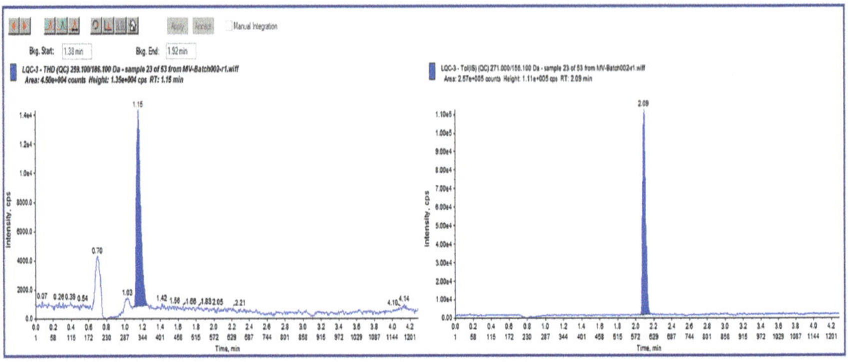

Fig. 6.17 Representative chromatogram of thalidomide quality control (analytical run name MVBatch002, sample name LQC3)

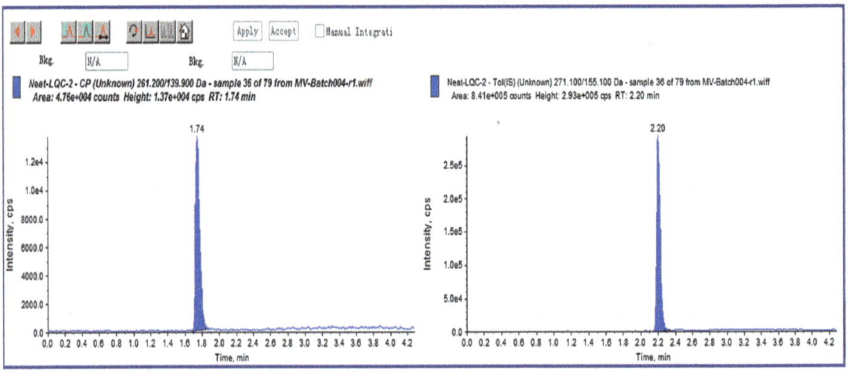

Fig. 6.18 Chromatogram of the analytes in pure solution for cyclophosphamide matrix effect (analytical run name MVBatch004r1, sample name NeatLQC2)

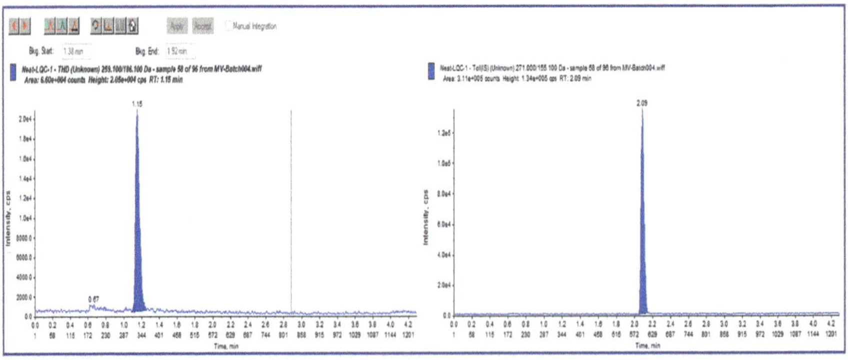

Fig. 6.19 Chromatogram of the analytes in pure solution for cyclophosphamide matrix effect (analytical run name MVBatch004, sample name NeatLQC1)

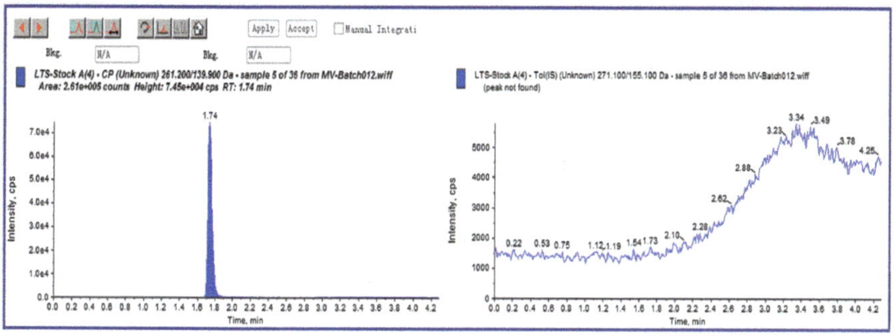

Fig. 6.20 Chromatogram of the long-term stability of cyclophosphamide stock solution [analytical run name MVBatch012, sample name LTSStock A (4)]

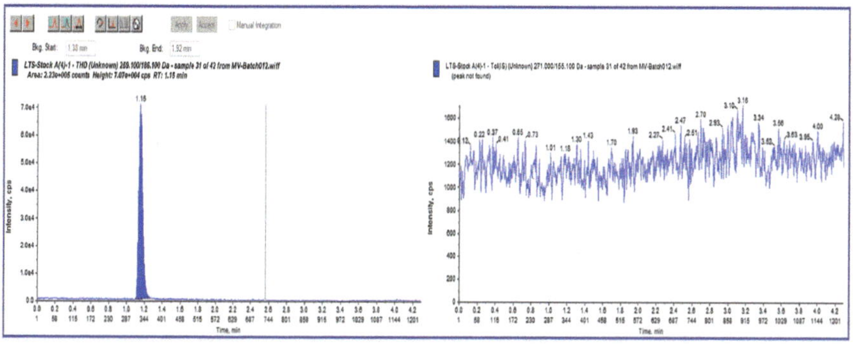

Fig. 6.21 Chromatogram of the long-term stability of thalidomide stock solution [analytical run name MVBatch012, sample name LTSStock A (4)1]

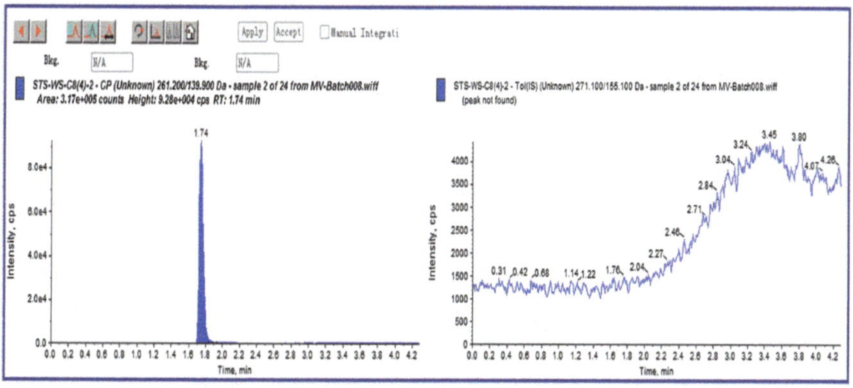

Fig. 6.22 Chromatogram of the short-term stability of cyclophosphamide working solution [analytical run name MVBatch008, sample name STSWSC8 (4)2]

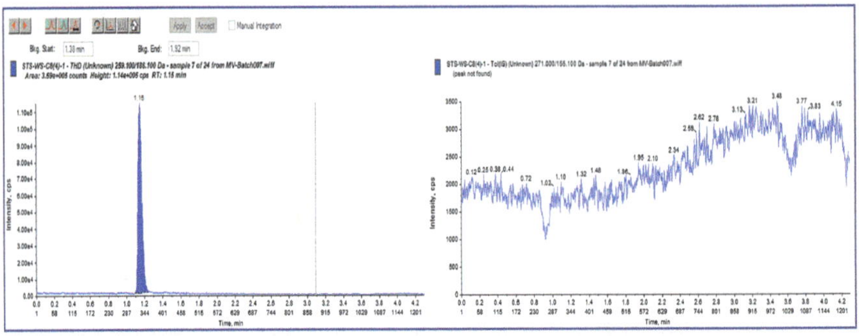

Fig. 6.23 Chromatogram of the short-term stability of thalidomide working solution [analytical run name MVBatch007, sample name STSWSC8 (4)1]

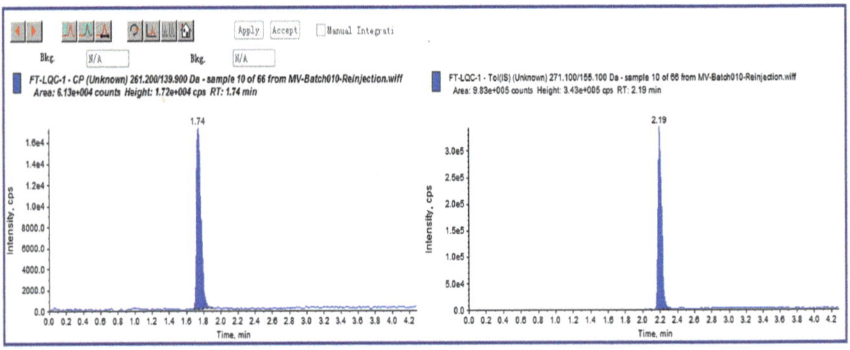

Fig. 6.24 Chromatogram of the freeze–thaw stability of cyclophosphamide (analytical run name MVBatch010Reinjection, sample name FTLQC1)

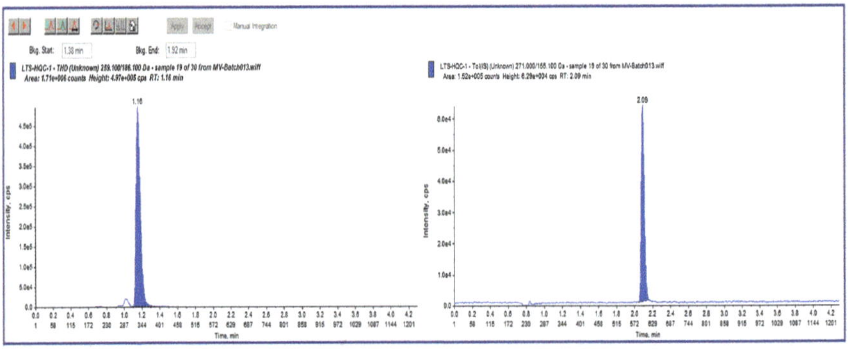

Fig. 6.25 Chromatogram of the freeze–thaw stability of thalidomide (analytical run name MVBatch010Reinjection, sample name FTLQC1)

Table 6.10 Toxicokinetic parameters of cynomolgus monkeys after subcutaneous injection of 15 mg/kg cyclophosphamide

Animal ID	First			Last		
	T_{max} (h)	C_{max} (ng/mL)	AUC_{0-t} (ng h/mL)	T_{max} (h)	C_{max} (ng/mL)	AUC_{0-t} (ng h/mL)
1	0.5	5338.56	5734.29	0.5	96.25	110.72
11	0.5	4718.23	5681.37	0.5	6381.24	7343.12
13	0.5	3680.36	5147.99	0.5	5866.70	6352.23
14	0.5	4135.71	5042.37	0.5	4837.31	4584.53
17	0.5	3996.56	4557.68	0.5	3348.52	5125.44
19	0.5	5305.08	5390.99	0.5	6179.92	7175.02
21	0.5	5139.33	6092.24	0.5	4635.61	6005.60
24	0.5	4451.37	6967.96	0.5	3222.30	4659.78
27	0.5	6586.33	8065.39	0.5	7248.19	9924.58
34	0.5	6915.77	6025.01	–	–	–
37	0.5	5698.87	7103.94	0.5	5470.97	6034.17
38	0.5	4766.54	5234.75	0.5	4705.24	6095.97
41	0.5	5338.01	6872.01	0.5	6118.04	7504.43
42	0.5	6181.96	8428.45	0	4586.47	7932.44
Total mean	0.5	5160.91	6167.46	0–0.5	4822.83	6065.23
Standard deviation	–	960.02	1161.82	–	1837.59	2307.81

Note: The mean value of the parameter T_{max} was replaced by the interval range value, and "–" indicates inapplicable.

the maximum sample capacity of analytical runs. The validation results showed that the validation results of the analytical method for determining the concentrations of cyclophosphamide and thalidomide in the plasma of cynomolgus monkeys using the LC–MS/MS method all met the acceptance criteria, and this method was applicable to the subsequent analysis of test samples.

The LC–MS/MS method was used to determine the concentrations of thalidomide and cyclophosphamide in the plasma of cynomolgus monkeys after gavage administration of thalidomide and subcutaneous injection of cyclophosphamide, to evaluate the exposure levels and other toxicokinetic characteristics of the test articles in cynomolgus monkeys, so as to provide reference information for interpreting the results of toxicity tests and the risk of drug use in clinical trials.

According to the study protocol, cynomolgus monkeys were divided into three groups, namely the vehicle control group, the cyclophosphamide subcutaneous administration group (with a dosing dose of 15 mg/kg), and the thalidomide gavage administration group (with a dosing dose of 20 mg/kg). Blood samples were not collected for detection in the vehicle control group. Pregnant monkeys started to be dosed on GD_{24}, once a day. Cyclophosphamide was administered continuously for 5 days, and thalidomide was administered continuously for 7 days. For the first and last administrations (D_1 and D_5, D_7), the collection time points were before administration

(0h), 30min, 1h, 1h, 2h, 4h, 8h, and 24h after administration. About 1 mL of blood was collected and placed into heparin sodium blood collection tubes. Plasma was obtained by centrifugation and frozen for storage at −80°C for testing. In this study, the validated LC–MS/MS method was used to detect the concentrations of the collected samples, and the main toxicokinetic parameters of the drugs were calculated using the WinNonlin non-compartmental model (NCA).

After the first administration (GD_{24}) of cyclophosphamide (with a dosage of 15mg/kg), the time to reach the peak blood concentration in cynomolgus monkeys was 0.5h; the peak concentration C_{max} was 5160.91±960.02ng/mL, and AUC_{0-t} was (6167.46±1161.82) hng/mL, respectively. After the last administration (GD_{28}), the time to reach the peak blood concentration in cynomolgus monkeys was 0–0.5h; the peak concentration C_{max} was 4822.83±1837.59ng/mL, and AUC_{0-t} was (6065.23±2307.81) hng/mL, respectively. After the first and last administrations, the toxicokinetic parameters and accumulation results are shown in Tables 6.10 and 6.11, and the concentration–time curves are shown in Fig. 6.26.

After the first administration (GD_{24}) of thalidomide (with a dosage of 20mg/kg), the time to reach the peak blood concentration in cynomolgus monkeys was 4–24h; the peak concentration C_{max} was 1231.86±389.07ng/mL, and AUC_{0-t} was (19601.53±7243.93) hng/mL, respectively. After the last administration (GD_{30}), the time to reach the peak blood concentration in cynomolgus monkeys was 2–24h; the peak concentration C_{max} was 2277.09±826.98ng/mL, and AUC_{0-t} was (37949.53±13612.97) hng/mL, respectively. After the first and last administrations,

Table 6.11 Accumulation in cynomolgus monkeys after continuous subcutaneous injection of 15mg/kg of cyclophosphamide for 5 days (last/first)

Animal ID	First C_{max} (ng/mL)	First AUC_{0-t} (ngh/mL)	Last C_{max} (ng/mL)	Last AUC_{0-t} (ngh/mL)	C_{max} ratio	AUC_{0-t} ratio
1	5338.56	5734.29	96.25	110.72	0.02	0.02
11	4718.23	5681.37	6381.24	7343.12	1.35	1.29
13	3680.36	5147.99	5866.70	6352.23	1.59	1.23
14	4135.71	5042.37	4837.31	4584.53	1.17	0.91
17	3996.56	4557.68	3348.52	5125.44	0.84	1.12
19	5305.08	5390.99	6179.92	7175.02	1.16	1.33
21	5139.33	6092.24	4635.61	6005.60	0.90	0.99
24	4451.37	6967.96	3222.30	4659.78	0.72	0.67
27	6586.33	8065.39	7248.19	9924.58	1.10	1.23
34	6915.77	6025.01	–	–	–	–
37	5698.87	7103.94	5470.97	6034.17	0.96	0.85
38	4766.54	5234.75	4705.24	6095.97	0.99	1.16
41	5338.01	6872.01	6118.04	7504.43	1.15	1.09
42	6181.96	8428.45	4586.47	7932.44	0.74	0.94
Total mean	5160.91	6167.46	4822.83	6065.23	0.98	0.99
Standard deviation	960.02	1161.82	1765.50	2217.27	0.36	0.33

Note: "–" indicates inapplicable

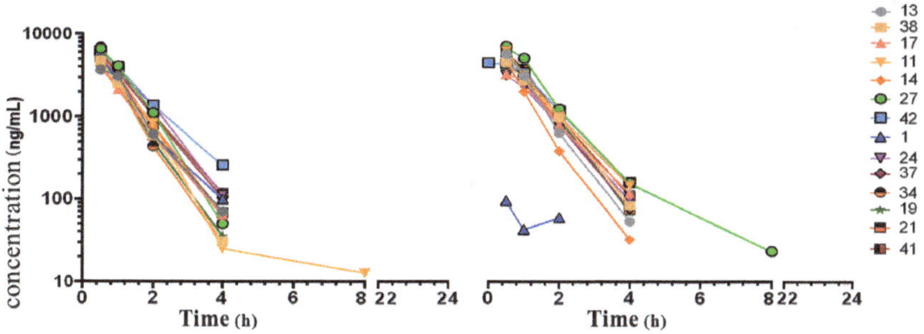

Fig. 6.26 Individual blood concentration–time change curves of cynomolgus monkeys after the first and last administrations of 15 mg/kg cyclophosphamide by subcutaneous injection

Table 6.12 Toxicokinetic parameters of cynomolgus monkeys after gaval administration of 20 mg/kg thalidomide

Animal ID	First			Last		
	T_{max} (h)	C_{max} (ng/mL)	AUC_{0-t} (ng h/mL)	T_{max} (h)	C_{max} (ng/mL)	AUC_{0-t} (ng h/mL)
3	4	1281.79	19,712.65	8	3184.60	53,640.18
4	8	1452.20	27,592.75	8	2093.88	37,123.02
5	24	1128.86	20,656.71	2	1785.51	25,444.63
12	24	1781.98	24,755.47	24	2195.67	28,001.56
18	4	463.25	6989.54	8	3786.92	63,169.17
28	4	1077.37	11,798.73	8	1098.50	24,019.07
29	8	1039.19	16,369.63	8	1827.66	31,808.96
31	8	1671.49	29,478.93	8	2757.83	46,569.48
40	8	1190.61	19,059.35	8	1763.23	31,769.69
Total mean	0.5	1231.86	19,601.53	0–0.5	2277.09	37,949.53
Standard deviation	–	389.07	7243.93	–	826.98	13,612.97

Note: The mean value of the parameter T_{max} was replaced by the interval range value, and "–" indicates inapplicable.

the toxicokinetic parameters and accumulation results are detailed in Tables 6.12 and 6.13, and the concentration–time curves are shown in Fig. 6.27.

In tissue samples, the detection results of the concentrations of cyclophosphamide and thalidomide were all lower than the LLOQ. Reason: The gestation period of animals is about 160 days. Pregnant monkeys started to be dosed on GD_{24}, once a day. Cyclophosphamide was administered continuously for 5 days, and thalidomide was administered continuously for 7 days. The sampling time of various tissues was GD_{150}. Since the animals were not continuously dosed, it was normal that the drug concentrations in the tissues of the reproductive system and fetuses were not detected. Cyclophosphamide and thalidomide were not detected in all tissues.

Table 6.13 Accumulation in cynomolgus monkeys after continuous gaval administration of 20 mg/kg of thalidomide for 7 days (last/ first)

Animal ID	First C_{max} (ng/mL)	First AUC_{0-t} (ng h/mL)	Last C_{max} (ng/mL)	Last AUC_{0-t} (ng h/mL)	C_{max} ratio	AUC_{0-t} ratio
3	1281.79	19,712.65	3184.60	53,640.18	2.48	2.72
4	1452.20	27,592.75	2093.88	37,123.02	1.44	1.35
5	1128.86	20,656.71	1785.51	25,444.63	1.58	1.23
12	1781.98	24,755.47	2195.67	28,001.56	1.23	1.13
18	463.25	6989.54	3786.92	63,169.17	8.17	9.04
28	1077.37	11,798.73	1098.50	24,019.07	1.02	2.04
29	1039.19	16,369.63	1827.66	31,808.96	1.76	1.94
31	1671.49	29,478.93	2757.83	46,569.48	1.65	1.58
40	1190.61	19,059.35	1763.23	31,769.69	1.48	1.67
Total mean	1231.86	19,601.53	2277.09	37,949.53	2.31	2.52
Standard deviation	389.07	7243.93	826.98	13,612.97	2.24	2.49

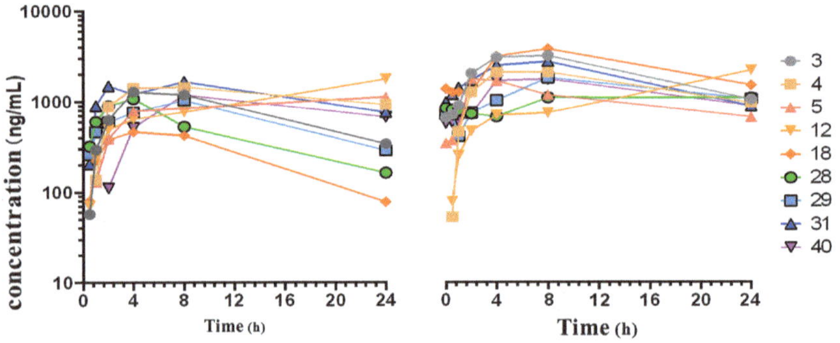

Fig. 6.27 Individual blood concentration–time change curves of cynomolgus monkeys after the first and last administrations of 20 mg/kg thalidomide by gaval administration

6.9 Pharmacokinetics and Toxicokinetics of Macromolecular Drugs in the Reproductive System

Many of the drugs under development are intended for use in infants, women of childbearing potential (WoCBP), men of reproductive age, and infants. Therefore, it is necessary to evaluate whether they affect fertility and/or the early development of offspring, as well as toxicity in juveniles and adolescents. Before starting reproductive toxicity tests, some information on pharmacokinetics has an important guiding role for the selection of animal species, the adjustment of experimental design and dosing regimens, etc [5]. The previous pharmacokinetic information may come from nonpregnant or non-lactating animals. However, pregnant and lactating animals have rapid physiological changes, and their pharmacokinetics may also change [6]. Therefore, in reproductive toxicity studies, reproductive toxicokinetics studies are often carried out simultaneously to obtain the exposure of drugs in the reproductive system, amniotic fluid, milk, and fetuses/infants, and to evaluate the potential teratogenicity of drugs.

The development of biological products has witnessed rapid changes. For many monoclonal antibody drugs, the only pharmacologically relevant animal species is nonhuman primates (NHP) [7]. Among them, cynomolgus monkeys are the nonhuman primates that are more frequently used. Therefore, in reproductive and developmental toxicity studies, cynomolgus monkeys will also be selected as the animal species for reproductive toxicity studies to investigate the potential risks of drugs to embryos and fetuses, whether there is systemic maternal exposure, and whether the molecules can cross the placental barrier and directly contact the embryos [8, 9]. Therefore, the focus of this section is to describe the studies related to the maternal exposure and placental transfer of monoclonal antibodies during the pregnancy of cynomolgus monkeys.

6.9.1 Research Characteristics

When conducting reproductive toxicity tests accompanied by toxicokinetics studies, possible differences in kinetic characteristics between pregnant and nonpregnant animals should be considered. The relationship between pharmacokinetics and toxicokinetics is shown in Fig. 6.28.

In PK and TK (which can be carried out along with single-dose toxicity tests, repeated-dose toxicity tests, genotoxicity tests, reproductive toxicity tests, and carcinogenicity tests) studies, reproductive toxicokinetic data can come from all animals in reproductive toxicity tests or from some animals. Reproductive toxicokinetic data should include fetal/infant data to evaluate whether the test substances and/or their metabolites can pass through the placental barrier and/or be secreted in milk. For a detailed comparison, see Table 6.14.

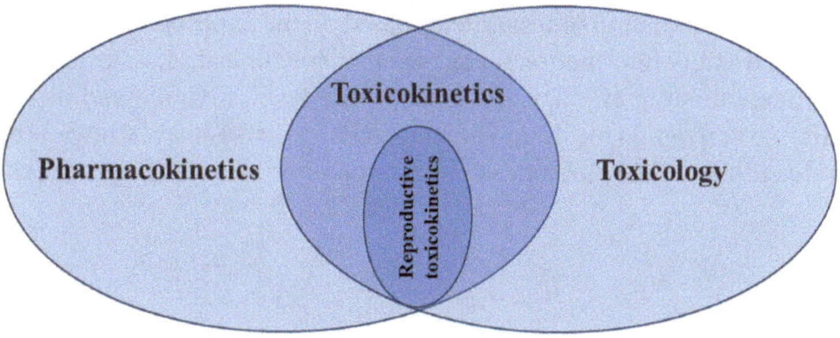

Fig. 6.28 Relationship between pharmacokinetics and toxicokinetics

Table 6.14 Relationship between pharmacokinetics and toxicokinetics

	Toxicokinetics		Pharmacokinetic
	Nonreproductive toxicity studies	Reproductive toxicity study	
Test system	Nonpregnant/non-lactating period	Pregnancy or lactation	Nonpregnant/non-lactating period
Dosage	Higher than the pharmacodynamic or clinical dose	Higher than the pharmacodynamic or clinical dose	Pharmacodynamic dose
Conduct method	Combined with the toxicity study	Combined with the reproductive toxicity test	Separately
Study content	AUC_{0-T}, C_{max}, $C_{(time)}$, and accumulation	T_{max}, C_{max}, AUC, accumulation, reproductive system, amniotic fluid, milk, and fetal/infant drug concentrations	Drug absorption, distribution, metabolism, and excretion, obtained half-life $T_{1/2}$ and other pharmacokinetic parameters
Animal requirement	Analysis by half female and half male	F0 generation females and F1 generation litter/offspring	Analysis by half female and half male
Analysis method	Good specificity	Good specificity. It is necessary to focus on the influence between different types of matrices, and different matrices might be verified separately	Good specificity, high sensitivity

The main value of toxicokinetics research in safety evaluation is reflected in the following aspects:

(1) To elucidate the systemic exposure of test articles and/or their metabolites in toxicity tests and their dose and time relationships with toxic reactions; to evaluate the toxic reactions of test articles and/or their metabolites in different animal species, sexes, ages, and body states (such as pregnancy state); to evaluate the rationality of the selection of animal species and drug regimens in nonclinical toxicity studies [3].

(2) To improve the predictive value of animal toxicity test results for nonclinical safety evaluation. Evaluating the target site toxicity (such as liver or kidney toxicity) caused by the accumulation of test articles based on the exposure level helps to provide quantified safety information for subsequent nonclinical safety evaluation [10].

(3) To integrate drug efficacy and its exposure level, toxicity, and its exposure information so as to guide the design of human trials, such as the starting dose, safety range evaluation, etc., and guide clinical safety monitoring according to the exposure level [11].

6.9.2 Design Key Points of Reproductive Toxicokinetics

The DART for drug safety evaluation aims to evaluate the potential adverse effects of drug treatment on pregnant and developing embryos/fetuses. Adverse effects on development can occur due to the embryos/fetuses being directly exposed to the drugs during development, or indirectly occur due to the toxicity of the mother or placenta. The direct toxic effects of drugs on fetuses mainly depend on the degree of exposure of embryos/fetuses, potential on-target and off-target toxicities, and the duration of continuous exposure during the sensitive period of development. The International Council for Harmonization of Technical Requirements for Pharmaceuticals for Human Use (ICH) S5(R3) describes three in vivo studies that can be used to evaluate the potential effects of pharmaceuticals on reproduction and development, and describes the recommended animal species for each test as follows [1].

(1) Fertility and early embryonic development test (Phase I, FEED Phases A and B). At least one animal species should be used, and rats are recommended.

(2) For the embryo–fetal development test in two species (Phase II, EFD Phases C and D), two animal species are usually employed: one is a rodent, and rats are recommended; the other is a non-rodent, and rabbits are recommended. The rationality of animal selection should be explained.

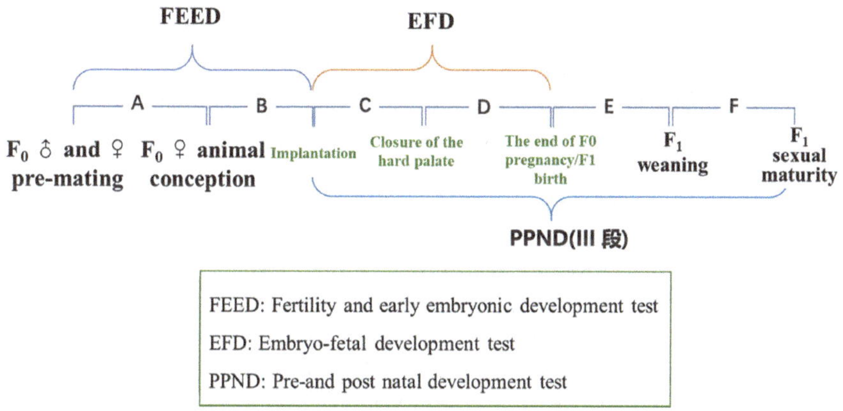

Fig. 6.29 Life cycle of reproductive and developmental toxicity studies. (**A**) From pre-mating to conception (adult male and female reproductive functions, development and maturation of gametes, mating behavior, and fertilization). (**B**) From conception to implantation (adult female reproductive functions, preimplantation development, and implantation). (**C**) From implantation to closure of the hard palate (adult female reproductive functions, embryonic development, major organ formation). (**D**) From closure of the hard palate to the end of pregnancy (adult female reproductive functions, fetal development and growth, and organ development and growth). (**E**) From birth to weaning (parturition and lactation, neonate adaptation to extrauterine life, and preweaning development and growth). (**F**) From weaning to sexual maturity (postweaning development and growth, adaptation to independent life, onset of puberty and attainment of full sexual function, and effects on second generation)

(3) Perinatal development test (Phase III, PPND Phases C–F). At least one animal species should be used, and rats are recommended.

For most drugs, the three-phase study protocol (a commonly used study protocol) is usually appropriate and can identify the reproductive and developmental stages where damage may occur. However, depending on the specific situation of different drugs, other study protocols that can fully reflect the reproductive toxicity of test articles can also be selected, such as a single test design or a two-phase test design, etc. Whichever study protocol is adopted, there should be no interval between each phase of the test (dosing treatment), and each stage of the reproductive process can be directly or indirectly evaluated. The rationality of the selected study protocol should be explained. The general phases for evaluating reproductive toxicity are shown in Fig. 6.29.

According to the *Measures for the Administration of Drug Registration*, drugs can be divided into chemical drugs, biological products, traditional Chinese medicines, and natural medicines. For chemical drugs, traditional Chinese medicines, natural medicines, and some biological products, if they have pharmacological activities in rodents or rabbits, a three-phase test design, DART, is usually adopted, and different combinations of these test design phases can also be made to meet the needs of specific products and reduce the use of animals.

For some biological products, such as monoclonal antibodies, rodents are often not the pharmacologically relevant species. In such cases, the embryo–fetal development assessment can be conducted in a single pharmacologically relevant non-rodent species. ICH M3 allows the use of data from preliminary embryo–fetal development (pEFD) toxicity tests in two species to support the limited inclusion of women with childbearing potential in clinical trials (no more than 150 subjects, with a treatment duration of no more than 3 months) before conducting definitive EFD tests [3]. When nonhuman primates (NHPs, usually cynomolgus monkeys are used in reproductive tests) are the only relevant species, due to the reproductive characteristics of cynomolgus monkeys, it is impossible to conduct mating evaluations for fertility and early embryo development tests. Moreover, since following up on the offspring of cynomolgus monkeys until maturity takes too long, it is also impossible to complete a full perinatal development test. Therefore, for reproductive toxicity tests in cynomolgus monkeys, histopathological examinations of reproductive tissues in repeated-dose toxicity tests with a dosing duration of at least 3 months can be used as an alternative method for fertility assessment. Toxicokinetic studies or studies on the tissue distribution of drugs in the reproductive system can be conducted concomitantly at this phase. Additionally, enhanced perinatal development (ePPND) toxicity tests can be used to replace EFD tests. The DART test designs for different drug types in different species of animals are shown in Table 6.15.

Table 6.15 Toxicity test designs for EFD and PPND in different species of animals

Parameter	pEFD	EFD			PPND	ePPND
	Rodents/rabbit	Rat/mouse	Rabbit	Cynomolgus monkey[a]	Rat	Cynomolgus monkey
GLP state	Selectable[b]	Yes	Yes	Yes	Yes	Yes
Minimum number of pregnant females/group size[c]	6	16	16	16	At least 16 litter	About 16 pregnant females
Number of dose groups	Four (including one control group)	Four (including one control group)	Four (including one control group)	At least two (including one control group)	Four groups (including one control group)	At least two groups (including one control group)
Dosing period	By species	GD6/7–17 (6/7–15)	GD6/7–19	About GD20–at least GD50	From implantation (GD6/7) to lactation (PND20)	From confirmation of pregnancy (about GD20) to parturition
F_0 generation endpoint	By species	GD20/21 (17/18)	GD28/29	GD100	Parturition	Parturition
F_1 generation endpoint	Maternal anatomical time	Maternal anatomical time	Maternal anatomical time	Maternal anatomical time	Sexually mature at 10 weeks of age after mating for male rats; as late as the F2 generation as needed for female rats as needed	At least 1 month of age, depending on the purpose of the evaluation
Drug exposure study	Selectable[b]	TK	TK	TK	TK	When appropriate, F0 generation TK characteristics and/or F0 and F1 generations systemic drug levels should be determined

Parameter	pEFD	EFD			PPND	ePPND
	Rodents/rabbit	Rat/mouse	Rabbit	Cynomolgus monkey[a]	Rat	Cynomolgus monkey
Applicable drug type	Chemical drugs, traditional Chinese medicines (including natural medicines), or biologically active products			Drugs (such as monoclonal antibodies) with only the cynomolgus monkey as a related animal species	Chemical drugs, traditional Chinese medicines (including natural medicines), or biologically active products	Drugs (such as monoclonal antibodies) with only the cynomolgus monkey as a related animal species

[a] If NHP other than cynomolgus monkeys are used, the study design should be adjusted [b] If the pEFD test is used for a delayed deterministic EFD test, the pEFD test should follow the GLP specification. TK data should be collected for pregnant animals, and bone examination should be performed [c] The group size of the EFD test for cynomolgus monkeys should produce a sufficient number of litters so as to assess potential adverse effects on morphological development. The group size in the ePPND studies should ensure the production of a sufficient number of offsprings in order to assess potential adverse effects on pregnancy outcomes, as well as malformations and postnatal development, and to provide opportunities for specific evaluation (e.g., immune system) if necessary. Most ePPND tests require the animals to be within a few months of pregnancy

Table 6.16 Differences between small molecule drugs and macromolecule drugs

Item	Biological products	Chemical medicines
Molecular weight	Large (>1 kDa)	Small (<1 kDa)
Source	Cytosoma	Chemical synthesis
Dosing method	Intravenous, subcutaneous, and intramuscular injections	Oral, intravenous, subcutaneous, and other ways
Drug form	Injection	Solid, injection, suppository, etc.
Molecular interaction with the target	High specificity, simple	Poor specificity, complex
Functional evaluation	Complex	Simple
Physical and chemical properties	The difference in solubility and charged state is large	Good water solubility
Factors affecting pharmacokinetics	FcγR and C1q (ADCC and CDC), nonspecific elimination (FcRn's effect on Ab), isoelectric point, ADA, etc.; Almost no kidney elimination	Liver metabolism (cytochrome P450 enzyme), transporters, etc.; renal and bile excretion
Pharmacokinetic characteristics	Long half-life, up to several days to several weeks, poor tissue permeability, small Vd	Short half-life, generally in min–h, good tissue permeability, large Vd
Linear dynamic characteristics	Nonlinear pharmacokinetic features often appear	Some drugs show nonlinear pharmacokinetic characteristics at high doses
Bioanalytical method	Complex (ELISA, LC–MS/MS, RIA, and other methods)	Specific method, mature method (LC–MS/MS method)
Immunogenicity	Often produce	Almost never produces
Preclinical study	According to the specific case analysis of the mechanism of drug action, the effect of the drug is amplified	Relative modeling
Common reproductive toxic animal species	Nonhuman primates, Rat, Rabbit	Rat, Rabbit
The way to pass the placental barrier	IgG is the only immunoglobulin capable of passing the placental barrier through the active transport process of the FcRn receptor	Passive diffusions

Note: *ADCC* antibody-dependent cell-mediated cytotoxicity, *CDC* complement-dependent cytotoxicity, *ADA* antidrug antibody, *Vd* apparent volume of distribution, *ELISA* enzyme-linked immunosorbent assay, *LCMS* liquid chromatography–mass spectrometry, *RIA* radioimmunoassay, *FcRn* neonatal Fc receptor, *C1q* complement 1q

6.9.3 Evaluation of Reproductive and Developmental Toxicokinetics of Biological Products in Cynomolgus Monkeys

(1) Differences between biological products and small molecule drugs. Biological products are usually also called macromolecular drugs. They are mainly biological drugs produced by genetically modified microorganisms or mammalian cells, including proteins, polypeptides, antibody–drug conjugates, and oligonucleotides. Due to the diversity of biological product drugs, each drug should choose an appropriate evaluation method according to its structure, physical and chemical properties, and pharmacological activities [6]. A common feature of all biological drugs is that their molecular weights are relatively large (1–150 kDa) compared to traditional drugs (200–400 Da). The molecular weight of cytokines is 2–4 kDa, that of enzymes is 6–10 kDa, and that of some polypeptides and oligonucleotides is 2–10 kDa. The molecular weight of monoclonal antibodies (mAbs) is approximately 15 kDa. The relatively large molecular weight of biological products makes them less likely to diffuse across membranes, limiting their distribution in the body. Therefore, their distribution is largely limited to blood volume or the volume of blood and extracellular fluid. The consequence of this limited distribution is that biological drugs do not enter cells, so they do not disrupt intracellular mechanisms, do not interact with DNA or other chromosomal substances, and do not freely cross physiological barriers such as the blood–brain barrier, blood–eye barrier, blood–testis barrier, and placental barrier. Only under specific transmembrane transport mechanisms will macromolecular drugs cross these barriers and enter specific tissues. Common transmembrane mechanisms include antibody transplacental transport mediated by the neonatal Fc receptor (FcRn)

Table 6.17 Classification of monoclonal antibodies

Type	IgG	IgM	IgA	IgD	IgE
Antibody structure	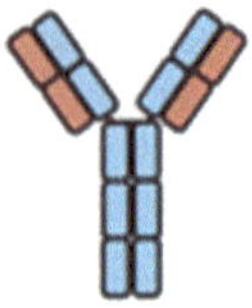	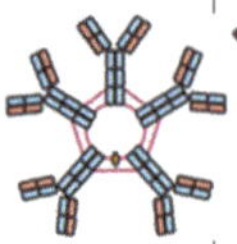	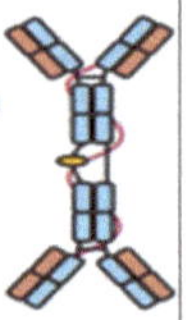	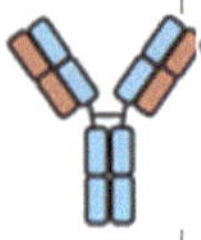	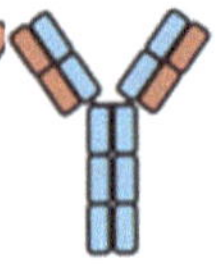
Heavy chain	γchain	μchain	αchain	δchain	ε chain
Molecular weight (kDa)	150	950/1150	160/400	175	190
Serum proportion	70%–75%	10%	10%–20%	<1%	Extremely low
Serum concentration (g/L)	8–16	0.8–1.6	2	0.04	0.0003
Cycle half-life (d)	IgG1/2/4 (18–21) IgG3 (3–7)	5	6	3	2.5
Whether the placental barrier can be passed	Yes	No	No	No	No

in primates and yolk sac and neonatal intestinal transport in rodents [12]. The differences between small molecule drugs and macromolecule drugs are shown Table 6.16.

Although macromolecular drugs (antibodies and non-antibodies) cannot penetrate the placenta through simple free diffusion, a small number of macromolecular drugs may cross the placenta (or other physiological barriers) through the paracellular pathway. As pregnancy progresses, the placenta becomes thinner and more permeable. Therefore, some macromolecular drugs that cannot pass through the placenta in the early stage of pregnancy may slowly pass through the placenta to the offspring in the later stage of pregnancy [13, 14].

(2) Introduction to monoclonal antibodies monoclonal antibody drugs are increasingly being developed for the treatment of cancers, immune system diseases, etc. According to the physical and chemical properties and biological functions of antibodies, antibodies can be divided into five major categories: IgM, IgG, IgA, IgE, and IgD. Among them, IgG is often designed to specifically mimic or inhibit endogenous human proteins involved in the pathogenesis of diseases. The structures, heavy chain types, molecular weights, serum proportions, serum concentrations, and circulating half-lives of various types of antibodies are shown in Table 6.17.

However, among antibody drugs, the IgG type is the only natural drug structural type found in current research that can pass through the placental barrier. The main reason is that the Fc fragment of IgG can pass through the placental barrier by the pathway mediated by FcRn, resulting in the transfer of antibodies. The transfer of antibodies mainly occurs in the second and third trimesters of human pregnancy when FcRn begins to be expressed on the placenta. All antibodies or recombinant proteins with an intact IgG Fc part can be transported through the placenta, while antibody fragments without Fc [Fab, dAb, scFv, $F(ab)'_2$] cannot be transported through the placenta. A similar process of placental transfer of IgG has also been confirmed in humans and NHPs [15].

IgG is the antibody with the highest content in serum and body fluids, accounting for 75%–80% of the total serum antibodies. Human IgG has four subclasses that rank according to their concentrations in serum as IgG1, IgG2, IgG3, and IgG4. The half-life of IgG is 20–23 days. It is the main antibody produced in the secondary immune response and widely distributed in the body, with high affinity and important immune effects, and is the "main force" for the body to resist infections.

IgG1, IgG2, and IgG3 can cross the placental barrier and play an important role in the anti-infection immunity of newborns. IgG1, IgG2, and IgG3 can activate the complement through the classical pathway and can bind to Fc receptors on the surface of macrophages and NK cells to play roles such as opsonization and ADCC. Human IgG1, IgG2, and IgG4 can bind to staphylococcal protein A (SPA) through their Fc segments, which can be used to purify antibodies and for immunodiagnosis. Some autoantibodies, such as anti-thyroglobulin antibodies, antinuclear antibodies, and antibodies that cause type II and type III hypersensitivity reactions, also belong to IgG. The structure of the IgG antibody is shown in Fig. 6.30. Structurally, the antibody can be divided into Fab and Fc segments. The Fab segment is composed of light chains and part of heavy chains, and mainly specifically recognizes relevant antigens and then regulates downstream signaling pathways. The Fc segment is composed of the

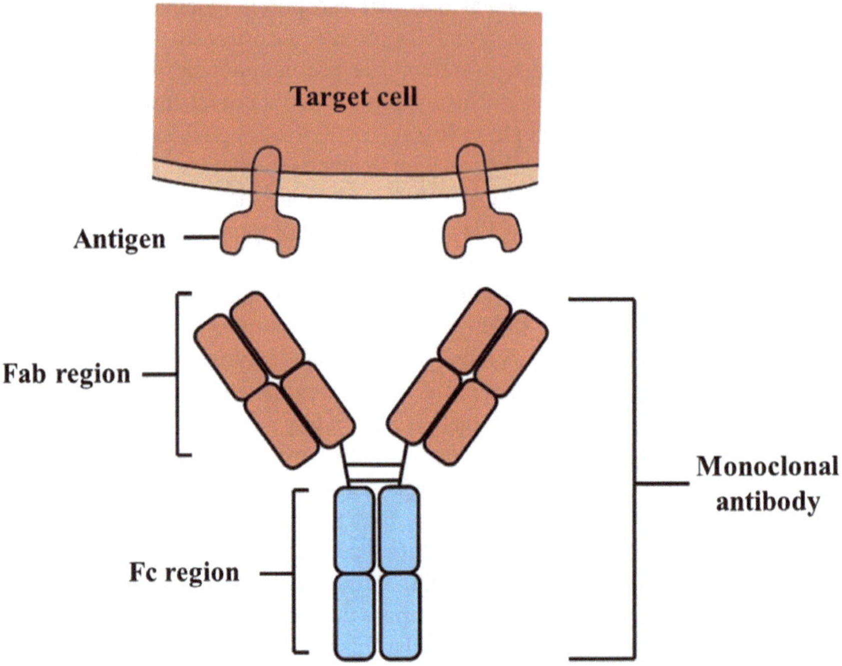

Fig. 6.30 IgG antibody structure

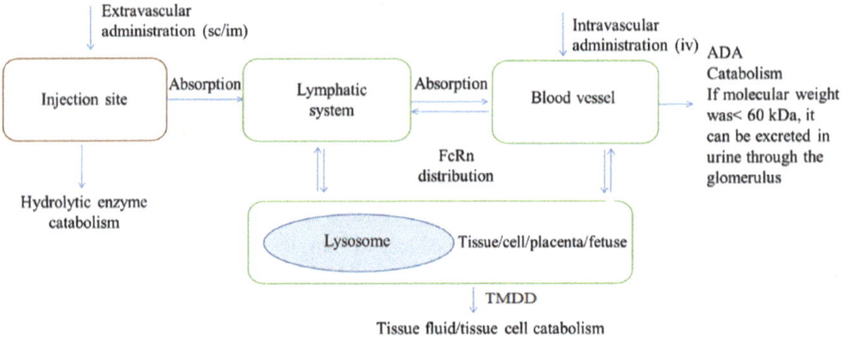

Fig. 6.31 In vivo ADME characteristics of antibody drugs

remaining part of the heavy chains, which can recognize and bind to immune cells (such as natural killer cells, macrophages, and neutrophils) expressing Fc receptors and complement to activate corresponding immune responses, such as antibody-dependent cell-mediated cytotoxicity (ADCC), antibody-dependent cell phagocytosis

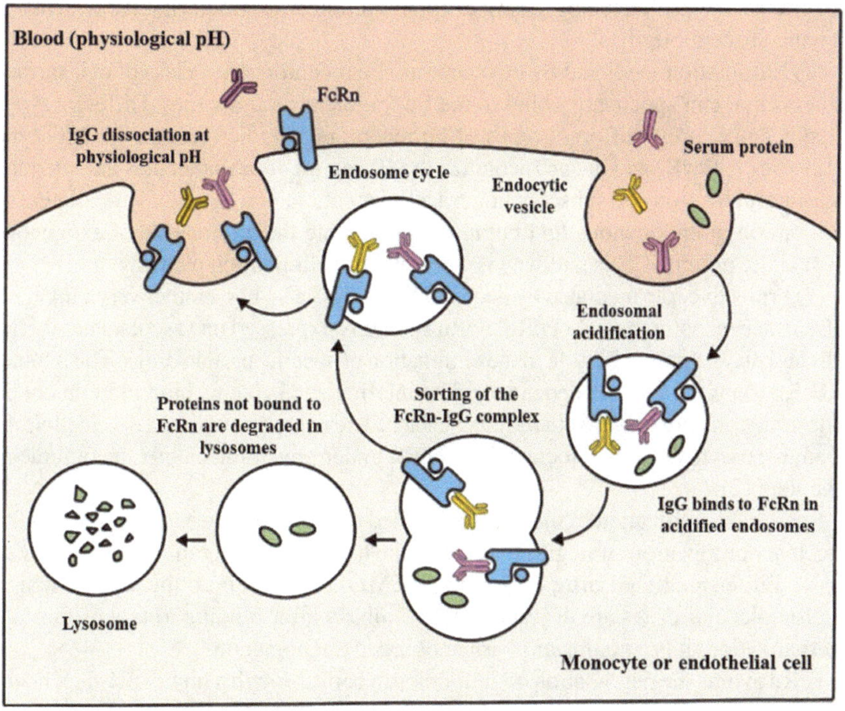

Fig. 6.32 In vivo elimination process of antibody drugs

(ADCP), and complement-dependent cytotoxicity (CDC). The Fc fragment can pass through the placental barrier by the pathway mediated by FcRn.

(3) In vivo ADME characteristics of antibody drugs: ADME is the abbreviation of "absorption, distribution, metabolism, and excretion," representing the process by which the body disposes of drugs after they enter the body. As macromolecular proteins, monoclonal antibody drugs have significant differences in absorption, distribution, metabolism, and excretion in vivo compared to small molecule drugs due to their special structures and physiological properties. The in vivo ADME characteristics of antibody drugs are shown in Fig. 6.31.

(4) In vivo elimination process of antibody drugs: Unlike the classic metabolic process of traditional small molecule drugs mediated by cytochrome P450 enzymes in the liver, antibody drugs cannot be directly metabolized by the liver or kidneys. The in vivo elimination process of antibody drugs is affected by many special factors, such as hydrolysis by proteolytic enzymes, elimination and protection mediated by Fc receptors, target-mediated and antidrug antibody generation, etc. The in vivo elimination process of antibody drugs is shown in Fig. 6.32.

(1) Hydrolysis by proteolytic enzymes: There are various specific and nonspecific proteolytic enzymes in the human body, which play an important role in the metabolism of protein drugs. In the early stage of biological drug research and development, the

half-life can be prolonged by giving enzyme inhibitors or modifying the hydrolysis enzyme-susceptible sites.

(2) Elimination mediated by Fc receptors: Fc receptors are a class of cell surface proteins that can specifically bind to the Fc fragment of antibodies. Different types of cells can express different types of Fc receptors. The Fc receptor for IgG-type antibodies is FcγR, which can recognize the Fc region of biomolecules and mediate their internalization and subsequent intracellular catabolism. It not only mediates the elimination of endogenous IgG but also can mediate the elimination of exogenous therapeutic proteins. This pathway is a nonspecific elimination pathway.

(3) Protective role mediated by neonatal FcRn: IgG also has another very important cell surface receptor, namely FcRn. FcRn is mainly expressed on vascular endothelial cells and plays a protective role in the elimination of specific protein drugs. The binding of FcRn to proteins is pH-dependent. The internalized proteins bind to Fc in acidic endosomes and are recycled to the cell surface. They are then released extracellularly through exocytosis and dissociate from FcRn under physiological pH to continue to function [12].

Reasonable utilization of the FcRn-mediated elimination and evasion is one of the effective optimization strategies to prolong the half-life of macromolecular drugs.

(4) Target-mediated drug disposition (TMDD): It refers to the way in which macromolecular drugs are degraded intracellularly after binding to targets through internalization. It is a nonlinear pharmacokinetic phenomenon.

FcRn avoids the degradation of antibodies in cells through a highly pH-dependent cell recycling mechanism and transports antibodies to the outside of the cells, enabling antibody drugs to maintain a certain blood drug concentration and have a long half-life. After the drug concentration increases, TMDD reaches saturation. At this time, the nontarget-mediated elimination pathways dominate, and the target-mediated nonlinear pathways can be ignored. In nonclinical studies, in order to determine whether an antibody–drug has a TMDD effect, the results can be obtained by performing graphical analysis of the antibody–drug clearance rate or half-life against the dosing dose through in vivo pharmacokinetic (PK) studies with single escalating doses [11].

(5) Elimination mediated by antidrug antibodies (ADA): Macromolecular drugs may cause the body to produce ADA. When ADA binds excessively to monoclonal antibody drugs, immune complexes will be formed, and the disposition of drugs will be accelerated through phagocytosis by cells. The existence of ADA will not only act as a neutralizing antibody to accelerate the clearance rate of antibody drugs and reduce the drug efficacy, but also lead to adverse reactions such as drug allergies in clinical practice. The generation of ADA may cause changes in the PK characteristics of antibody drugs. Especially when combined with target-mediated clearance, the apparent metabolic trend of antibody drugs becomes more difficult to interpret. However, since the detection method for target-mediated elimination is complicated and the detection means for ADA are relatively mature and convenient, in clinical trials, if PK abnormalities are encountered, the fastest troubleshooting plan is to first detect the ADA level in the blood and then consider other potential factors in turn [16].

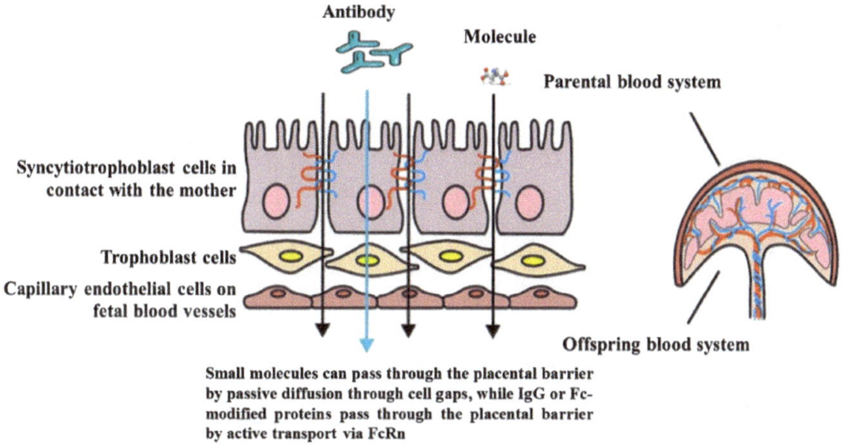

Fig. 6.33 Schematic diagram of placental barrier permeability of various molecules

6.9.4 Studies on the Permeability of the Placental Barrier of IgG Antibodies in Different Animal Species

IgG is the only immunoglobulin capable of passing through the maternal placenta. Because the binding of the Fc fragment of IgG to FcRn is a prerequisite for antibody transport through the placenta, the differences in the affinity of FcRn of different species for antibody drugs' Fc determine the efficiency of passing through the placental barrier in humans and NHPs. A schematic diagram of the placental barrier permeability of various molecules is shown in Fig. 6.33.

In non-rodent animals, the placental transfer of IgG is low during organogenesis, begins to increase in the early and middle stages of pregnancy, and reaches its highest level in the late stage of pregnancy. In rodents, the stage of pregnancy during which IgG undergoes placental transfer in the mother occurs relatively earlier than that in non-rodent animals. After childbirth, IgG is secreted in relatively large amounts in colostrum and in relatively small amounts in mature milk. The placental barrier permeability of 28 antibody drugs in different animal species has been studied, and the summarized results are shown in Table 6.18 [9, 17].

6.9.5 Methodology Validation

The following cases are used to discuss methodology validation [18].

Case 1: Detection of TQ001 and TQ002 Concentrations in Cynomolgus Monkey Serum by ELISA Method.

Table 6.18 Summary of studies on the placental barrier permeability of antibody drugs in different animal species

Number	Animal species	Molecular type	Dosage (mg/kg)	Sample collection time GD	Maternal serum (μg/mL)	Fetal serum (μg/mL)	Fetus/mother
1	Rabbit	IgG4 mAb	30	19[a]	38.25	1.69	0.044
2	Rabbit	IgG1 mAb	50	19[a]	1583	1.04	0.0007
3	Rabbit	IgG4 Fc fusion protein	20	20[a]	586	27	0.046
4	Rabbit	IgG1 Fc fusion protein	30	20[a]	290	3.74	0.013
5	Rabbit	IgG1 mAb	50	28[b]	277	372	1.34
6	Rabbit	IgG1 mAb	0.2	28[b]	0.375	0.244	0.65
7	Rat	IgG4 Fc fusion protein	0.3	21[c]	0.97	0.44	0.69
8	Rat	IgG1 mAb	0.5	21[c]	1.132	1.126	0.99
9	Rat	IgG4 Fc fusion protein	2	21[c]	7.4	10	1.42
10	Rat	IgG1 mAb	2	21[c]	3.357	2.818	0.84
11	Rat	IgG4 Fc fusion protein	20	21[c]	18	34	2.02
12	Rat	IgG1 mAb	20	21[d]	80	76	0.96
13	Rat	IgG4 mAb	30	20[e]	91.5	29.41	0.32
14	Rat	IgG1 mAb	30	20[d]	106.66	15.57	0.15
15	Rat	IgG4 Fc fusion protein	20	18[d]	144	43	0.3
16	Rat	IgG1 mAb	20	18[d]	194	51	0.28
17	Rat	IgG2 mAb	10	21[e]	1.042	1.897	1.82
18	Rat	IgG1 mAb	10	21[c]	6.029	6.072	1.01
19	Cynomolgus monkey	IgG4 mAb	5	140–142	78.7	19.97	0.25
20	Cynomolgus monkey	IgG1 mAb	5	139	27	11.9	0.53
21	Cynomolgus monkey	IgG4 mAb	50	140–142	835.9	153.7	0.18
22	Cynomolgus monkey	IgG1 mAb	50	139	112	68.1	0.61
23	Cynomolgus monkey	IgG2 mAb	12.5	100	203	4.34	0.02
24	Cynomolgus monkey	IgG1 mAb	15	100	20.84	4.93	0.24

Number	Animal species	Molecular type	Dosage (mg/kg)	Sample collection time GD	Maternal serum (μg/mL)	Fetal serum (μ g/mL)	Fetus/mother
25	Cynomolgus monkey	IgG2 mAb	100	100	72.4	21.4	0.3
26	Cynomolgus monkey	IgG1 mAb	100	100	25	14.1	0.56
27	Cynomolgus monkey	IgG1 mAb	75	100	9	5.4	0.69
28	Cynomolgus monkey	IgG1 mAb	75	100	8.2	6.3	0.78

[a] 0–2 days after the last dose [b] 9–10 days after the last dose [c] 5–6 days after the last dose [d] 0–3 days after the last dose [e] 7–9 days after the last dose

Purpose: The study was to validate the established double-antibody sandwich ELISA assay method for detecting two IgG1-type monoclonal antibodies, TQ001 and TQ002, in cynomolgus monkey serum.

Method principle: The double-antibody sandwich ELISA method was used to determine the concentrations of TQ001 and TQ002 in cynomolgus monkey serum, placenta, amniotic fluid, milk, and male reproductive organ tissues. The detection principles of TQ001 and TQ002 were similar. Their respective antigens were used to coat microplates to form solid-phase antibodies, which can bind to TQ001 or TQ002 in the samples. After washing away unbound components, they bound to HRP-labeled goat antihuman IgG antibodies to form antibody-antigen–antibody complexes. After washing, the substrate TMB chromogenic solution was added for color development. TMB converted to blue under the catalysis of HRP enzyme, which was terminated by sulfuric acid, then it converted to yellow. The absorbance value was measured at a wavelength of 450 nm using a multifunctional microplate reader, and the concentration was back-calculated using the software SoftMax Pro 7.1.2 GxP of the multifunctional microplate reader.

6.9.6 Test Article Information

(1) Test Article 1
Identity: TQ001 Injection.
Specification: 150 mg/mL/vial.
Component or concentration: 154.0 mg/mL.
Stability: Stable under storage condition and within expiration date.
Expiration date: xx/xx/xxxx.
Storage conditions: 2°C–8°C, protected from light.
Shipment environment: Cold chain.
(2) Test Article 2
Identity: TQ002 Injection.
Specification: 50 mg/0.5 mL/vial.
Component or concentration: 100 mg/mL (COA concentration).

Table 6.19 Consumables and reagents

Name	Lot No.
Tween-20	21090253
	EZ7890B253
BSA	EZ7890B203/EZ7890C409
PBS powder	16C11B30/17F06A30
TMB chromogenic solution	2021030201
Skim milk powder	J25C03
No RNAase water	AKG1199A
Sulfuric acid	20210107
	20200710
TQ001 antigen	XXX
TQ002 antigen	XXX
Goat antihuman secondary antibody labeled with HRP	26
Human IgG dry powder	20220211
Cynomolgus monkey blank serum	XXXX
Cynomolgus monkey completely hemolyzed matrix	XXXX
Sodium bicarbonate	20200102
Anhydrous sodium carbonate	20210105
Detachable ELISA plate	20019001
Plate sealing film	PETG059F

Table 6.20 Main instruments

Instrument name	Instrument model
Multifunctional microplate reader	SpectraMax M5^{e}
Precision pipette	0.1–2.5, 0.1–10, 2–20, 10–100, 20–200, 30–300, and 100–1000 μL
Freezing refrigerator for medical use	YCD-265
−80°C ultra-low temperature refrigerator	DW-86L626
Vortex mixer	MX-S
Pure water instrument	Direct-Q 8UV
LED digital shaker	SLK-O3000-S
Balance	PR423ZH/E
Incubator	DHP-9052
Plate washer	PW960 Plus

Stability: Stable under storage condition and within expiration date.
Expiration date: xx/xx/xxxx.
Storage conditions: 2°C–8°C, protected from light.
Shipment environment: Cold chain.

6.9.7 Main Instruments and Reagents

(1) Consumables and Reagents Table 6.19.

(2) Main Instruments Table 6.20.

(3) The blank cynomolgus monkey serum matrix was from the blank matrix library of this facility and stored at −70°C for standby use. Before use, the blank serum was equilibrated to room temperature.

6.9.8 Study Method

1. The preparation volumes of various solutions were adjusted according to actual needs and preparation ratios. The preparation table for each validation item is listed using TQ001 as an example.

6.9.8.1 Main Reagents

1) Carbonate buffered saline (CBS): Weigh 0.796 g of anhydrous sodium carbonate and 1.486 g of sodium bicarbonate, add 0.5 L of ultrapure water, and mix evenly.

2) Phosphate-buffered saline (PBS): Take one pack of PBS powder, add 2 L of ultrapure water, and mix evenly.

3) Plate wash solution (PBST): Add 2 mL of Tween 20 to 4 L of PBS solution and mix well.

4) Blocking buffer (5% Skim milk): Weigh 7.504 g of Skim milk, and add it to 150 mL PBS of PBS solution, then vortex and mix well.

5) TQ001 diluent (1% BSA): Weigh 3 g of BSA powder, add it to 300 mL of PBS solution, and mix evenly.

6) TQ002 diluent A (0.5% Skim milk): Weigh 0.505 g of Skim milk and add it to 100 mL of PBS solution, and mix well.

7) TQ002 diluent B (1% BSA): Weigh 0.502 g of BSA and add it to 50 mL of PBS solution, and mix evenly.

8) TQ001 coating buffer: Dilute xxx protein (0.25 mg/mL) to 0.5 μg/mL with CBS solution as the coating working solution.

9) TQ002 coating buffer: Dilute xxx (200 μg/mL) to 0.5 μg/mL with CBS solution as the coating working solution.

10) TQ001 secondary antibody solution: Dilute the HRP-labeled goat antihuman secondary antibody 20,000 times with 1% BSA as the secondary antibody solution.

11) TQ002 secondary antibody solution: Dilute the HRP-labeled goat antihuman secondary antibody 10,000 times with 1% BSA as the secondary antibody solution.

12) Chromogenic solution: The chromogenic solution could be used directly without preparation.

13) Stop Solution (1 mol/L H2SO4): Take 56 mL of 18 mol/L concentrated sulfuric acid, add it to 944 mL of ultrapure water while stirring in a beaker, cool to room temperature, and transfer to a solution bottle.

Table 6.21 TQ001 test article standard curve preparation

Name	Source solution	Source solution volume(μL)	Diluent volume(μL)	Final volume(μL)	Final conc.(ng/mL)
Pre-1	TQ001 stock solution	5	72	77	10,000,000
Pre-2	Pre-1	5	72	77	10,000,000
Pre-3	Pre-2	5	45	50	1,000,000
C01	Pre-2	20	80	100	200,000
C02	C01	30	270	300	20,000
C03	C02	100	100	200	10,000
C04	C03	100	100	200	5000
C05	C04	100	100	200	2500
C06	C05	100	100	200	1250
C07	C06	100	100	200	625
C08	C07	100	100	200	312.5
C09	C08	100	100	200	78.125
Blank	N/A	N/A	100	100	0

14) Human IgG solution: Prepare a 10 mg/mL human IgG solution with human IgG powder using sterile and enzyme-free water for standby use.

15) Blank monkey serum matrix: Mix equal volumes of blank cynomolgus monkey serum from at least ten different sources.

16) 5% Cynomolgus monkey hemolytic matrix: Obtain the completely hemolytic matrix from the matrix library of this facility and dilute the completely hemolytic matrix 20 times with nonhemolytic blank cynomolgus monkey serum to obtain the 5% cynomolgus monkey hemolytic matrix.

6.9.8.2 Standard Curve Samples

1) TQ001: Dilute the test article TQ001 (154 mg/mL) with blank monkey serum to 20,000, 10,000, 5000, 2500, 1250, 625, 312.5, 156.25, 78.13, and 0 ng/mL to prepare standard curve samples, where 20,000 and 78.13 ng/mL were the upper and lower anchor points, respectively. The preparation method of the standard curve of the test article is shown in Table 6.21.

2) TQ002: Dilute the test article TQ002 (100 mg/mL) with the blank monkey serum matrix to 8000, 1600, 800, 400, 200, 100, 50, 25, and 12.5 ng/mL to prepare standard curve samples, where 8000 and 12.5 ng/mL erre the upper and lower anchor points, respectively.

6.9.8.3 Quality Control and Limit of Quantification Samples

1) TQ001: Dilute the test article TQ001 (154 mg/mL) with blank monkey serum to 10,000, 8000, 4000, 400, and 156.25 ng/mL to prepare the ULOQ samples, high, medium, and low concentrations quality control samples (HQC, MQC, and LQC), and the LLOQ samples. The preparation method of the quality control samples of the test article is shown in Table 6.22.

Table 6.22 TQ001 test article quality control sample preparation

Name	Source solution	Source solution volume(μL)	Diluent volume(μL)	Final volume(μL)	Final conc.(ng/mL)
Pre-1	TQ001 stock solution	5	72	77	10,000,000
Pre-2	Pre-1	5	45	50	1,000,000
Pre-3	Pre-2	20	80	100	200,000
ULOQ	Pre-3	20	380	400	10,000
HQC	ULOQ	216	54	270	8000
MQC	HQC	90	90	180	4000
LQC	MQC	20	180	200	400
LLOQ	LQC	60	93.6	154	156.25

Table 6.23 Preparation of TQ001 selectivity samples

Name	Source solution	Source solution volume(μL)	Diluent volume(μL)	Final volume(μL)	Final conc.(ng/mL)
Pre-1	TQ001 stock solution	5	72	77	10,000,000
Pre-2	Pre-1	5	45	50	1,000,000
20× SE-H	Pre-2	30	120	150	200,000
Pre-3	20× SE-H	10	90	100	20,000
20× SE-L	Pre-3	30	162	192	3125
SE-H-serum	20× SE-H	5	95*	100	1000
SE-L-serum	20× SE-L	5	95*	100	31.25

2) TQ002: Dilute the test article TQ002 (100 mg/mL) with blank monkey serum to 1600, 1200, 300, 60, and 25 ng/mL to prepare the ULOQ samples, high, medium, and low concentration quality control samples (HQC, MQC, and LQC), and LLOQ samples.

6.9.8.4 Selectivity Samples

1) TQ001: Dilute the test article TQ001 (154 mg/mL) with blank monkey serum to 200,000 and 3125 ng/mL to prepare 20× SEH and 20× SEL samples. Then, dilute 20× SEH and 20× SEL 20 times with blank monkey serum from ten individuals respectively to obtain the selectivity samples SEH and SEL. The blank monkey serum from ten individuals without the test article was used as the selectivity sample SENC. The preparation method of the selectivity samples of the test article is shown in Table 6.23.

2) TQ002: Dilute the test article TQ002 (100 mg/mL) with the blank monkey serum matrix to 32,000 ng/mL and 500 ng/mL to prepare 20× SEH and 20× SEL samples. Then, dilute 20× SEH and 20× SEL 20 times with blank monkey serum from 10

Table 6.24 Preparation of TQ001 hemolytic samples

Name	Source solution	Source solution volume(μL)	Diluent volume(μL)	Final volume(μL)	Final conc.(ng/mL)
Pre-1	TQ001 stock solution	5	72	77	10,000,000
Pre-2	Pre-1	5	45	50	1,000,000
20× SE-H	Pre-2	30	120	150	200,000
Pre-3	20× SE-H	10	90	100	20,000
20× SE-L	Pre-3	30	162	192	3125

individuals to obtain the selectivity samples SEH (1600 ng/mL) and SEL (25 ng/mL). The blank monkey serum from ten individuals without the control article was used as the blank selectivity sample SENC.

6.9.8.5 Hemolysis Samples

The hemolysis effect should be investigated at the ULOQ, LLOQ, and blank levels.

TQ001/TQ002: Dilute 20 times the 20× SEH and 20× SEL prepared in the selectivity with 5% cynomolgus monkey hemolytic matrix to obtain the hemolysis samples HEH and HEL. The 5% cynomolgus monkey hemolytic matrix without the test article was used as the blank hemolysis sample, HENC, with five replicates of hemolysis samples at each concentration level. The preparation method of the hemolysis samples of the test article is shown in Table 6.24.

6.9.8.6 Specificity Samples

Specificity was investigated at the ULOQ, LLOQ, and blank levels.

1) TQ001: Dilute the interfering article human IgG to 100,000 and 1562.5 ng/mL with blank monkey serum to prepare 10× ULOQ and 10× LLOQ samples as the blank specificity samples SPH and SPL. Use the blank specificity samples SPH and SPL to prepare the test article for the high-concentration specificity samples SPHH and SPLH (at the ULOQ concentration), and then use the blank specificity samples SPH and SPL to dilute the high-concentration specificity samples to low-concentration specificity samples SPHL and SPLL (at the LLOQ concentration), and then measure the high- and low-concentration specificity samples and blank specificity samples, with five replicates of specificity samples at each concentration level. The preparation method of the specificity samples of the test article is shown in Table 6.25.

2) TQ002: The interfering article human IgG solution was diluted with the blank monkey serum matrix to 3200 and 50 ng/mL to prepare 2× ULOQ and 2× LLOQ samples, which were used as blank specificity samples SPH and SPL. The control articlexxx monoclonal antibody injection (100 mg/mL) was prepared into high-concentration quality control specificity samples SPHH and SPLH using the blank specificity samples SPH and SPL. Then, the high-concentration quality control specificity samples were diluted to low-concentration quality control specificity samples SPHL and SPLL using the blank specificity samples SPH and SPL. Subsequently, the high- and low-concentration quality control specificity samples and the blank specificity

Table 6.25 Preparation of TQ001 specificity samples

Name	Source solution	Source solution volume(μL)	Diluent volume*(μL)	Final volume(μL)	Final conc.(ng/mL)
pre-SP-1	TQ001 stock solution	5	72	77	10,000,000
pre-SP-2	pre-SP-1	5	45	50	1,000,000
SP-H-H/ SP-L-H	pre-SP-2	10	90	100	100,000
pre-SP-3	SP-H-H/ SP-L-H	10	30	40	12,500
SP-H-L/ SP-L-L	pre-SP-3	15	45	60	1562.5

Note: *The diluent used for preparing SP-H-H and SP-H-L was SP-H, while the diluent used for preparing SP-L-H and SP-L-L was SP-L

Table 6.26 Preparation of TQ001 dilution linearity and Hook effect samples

Name	Source solution	Source solution volume(μL)	Diluent volume(μL)	Final volume(μL)	Final conc.(ng/mL)
HOOK-1	Test article stock solution	5	72	77	10,000,000
HOOK-2	HOOK-1	40	40	80	5,000,000
pre-DQC-1	HOOK-2	5	120	125	200,000
pre-DQC-2	pre-DQC-1	10	190	200	10,000
DQC-1	pre-DQC-2	60	40	100	6000
DQC-2	DQC-1	20	40	60	2000
DQC-3	DQC-2	20	60	80	500
HOOK-3	DQC-3	5	95	100	25

Note: The dilution multiples used to examine the dilution linearity were the multiples that diluted from HOOK1 to the concentrations of DQC-01, DQC-02, and DQC-03; N/A, no relevant information

samples were simultaneously measured, with five samples in parallel for each condition at each concentration level.

6.9.8.7 Dilution Linearity and Hook Effect

1) TQ001: The test article TQ001 (154 mg/mL) was diluted with the blank monkey serum matrix to 10 and 5 mg/mL as HOOK1 and HOOK2 samples for detection. Then, the HOOK2 sample was diluted with blank monkey serum to 6000, 2000, 500, and 25 ng/mL to prepare DQC01, DQC02, DQC03, and HOOK3, with five replicates in parallel for each dilution factor. HOOK1, HOOK2, and HOOK3 were used for the investigation of the hook effect, and DQC01, DQC02, and DQC03 were used for the investigation of dilution linearity. The preparation method of the dilution linearity and hook effect samples of the test article is shown in Table 6.26.

2) TQ002: The test article TQ002 (100 mg/mL) was diluted with the blank monkey serum matrix to 4 and 0.2 mg/mL as Hook1 and Hook2 samples for detection. Then,

the Hook2 sample was diluted with the blank monkey serum matrix to 1000, 500, 250, and 10 ng/mL to prepare DQC1, DQC2, DQC3, and Hook3, with at least five samples processed in parallel for each dilution factor. Hook1, Hook2, and Hook3 were used for the investigation of the hook effect, and DQC1, DQC2, and DQC3 for the investigation of dilution linearity.

6.9.8.8 Stability Samples

TQ001/TQ002: TQ001/TQ002: The test article was prepared into high and low concentration quality control level samples (STH and STL) as the stability samples of this test. A total of 60 samples were prepared for each concentration. The stability samples were measured immediately after preparation, after being placed at room temperature for 24 h, after being placed at 2°C–8°C for 24 h, after being placed below 70°C for 30 days, 60 days, and 120 days (covering the time range from sample reception to detection), and after being subjected to five cycles of repeated freezing and thawing(during the preparation of freeze–thaw stability samples, they should be thawed at room temperature, placed at room temperature for at least 4 h, frozen for at least 24 h before the first complete thawing, and for each subsequent freeze–thaw cycle, the samples should be frozen for more than 12 h), with four samples at each concentration under each condition.

6.9.8.9 Parallelism Samples

Take respective three authentic samples (C_{max}) of two test articles in the toxicological tests and dilute to the standard curve range with three different dilution factors.

6.9.8.10 Matrix Bridging

During the pharmacokinetic and toxicokinetic studies of reproductive toxicity, to detect drug concentrations in placental, amniotic fluid, milk, and male reproductive organ tissues, matrix bridging verification should be performed in selective validation. If bridging could not be achieved, separate matrix validation should be carried out. If blank matrices were not easily accessible, such as milk, 10% skim milk could be used for alternative validation. Bridging verification for the above tissues was not performed in this method, but this facility had conducted bridging tests between tissue homogenates and serum in other species (rabbits and rats).

6.9.9 Analytical Procedure

6.9.9.1 TQ001

(1) Coating: Add the coating buffer to the microplate at 100 μL/well, seal the plate, and then incubate overnight at 2°C–8°C.

(2) Blocking: Wash the plate five times with PBST buffer at 300 μL/well and pat dry. Add 5% Skim milk blocking buffer at 300 μL/well, seal the plate, and then incubate at 37°C for about 2 h.

(3) Sample addition: Dilute the pending analysis sample 25-fold with 1% BSA. Wash the plate five times with PBST buffer at 300 μL/well and pat dry. Add treated

sample into the ELISA microplate at 100 μL/ well, seal the plate, and incubate at 37°C for about 1 h.

(4) Addition of secondary antibody solution: Discard the liquid in the wells, wash the plate five times with PBST at 300 μL/well, and pat dry. Add secondary antibody solution at 100 μL/well and seal the plate. Incubate at 37°C for about 0.5 h.

(5) Color development: Discard the liquid in the wells, wash the plate five times with PBST at 300 μL/well, and pat dry. Add chromogenic solution at 100 μL/well for color development, protected from light, for 10 ± 5 min at room temperature (depending on the chromogenic result).

(6) Stopping: Add stop solution at 100 μL/well.

(7) Determination: Stop the reaction and measure the OD value at 450 nm within 30 min using a microplate reader.

(8) Result output: The data were fitted into a four-parameter model to plot the standard curve using the concentration as the abscissa and absorbance (OD value) as the ordinate, and the sample concentration was calculated based on the weight factor of $1/x$.

6.9.9.2 TQ002

(1) Coating: Add the coating buffer to the microplate at 100 μL/well, seal the plate, and then incubate overnight at 2°C–8°C.

(2) Blocking: Wash the plate fiove times with PBST buffer at 300 μL/well and pat dry. Add 5% Skim milk blocking buffer at 300 μL/well, seal the plate, and then incubate at 37°C for 2 h.

(3) Sample addition: Dilute the pending analysis sample 25-fold with 0.5% Skim milk. Wash the plate five times with PBST buffer at 300 μL/well and pat dry. Add treated sample into the ELISA microplate at 100 μL/ well, seal the plate, and incubate at 37°C for 2 h.

(4) Addition of secondary antibody solution: Discard the liquid in the wells, wash the plate five times with PBST at 300 μL/well, and pat dry. Add secondary antibody solution at 100 μL/well and seal the plate. Incubate at 37°C for about 0.5 h.

(5) Color development: Discard the liquid in the wells, wash the plate five times with PBST at 300 μL/well, and pat dry. Add chromogenic solution at 100 μL/well for color development, protected from light, for 10 ± 5 min at room temperature (depending on the chromogenic result).

(6) Stopping: Add stop solution at 100 μL/well.

(7) Determination: Stop the reaction and measure the OD value at 450 nm within 30 min using a microplate reader.

(8) Result output: The data were fitted into a four-parameter model to plot the standard curve using the concentration as the abscissa and OD450 value as the ordinate, and the sample concentration was calculated.

6.9.10 Methodology Validation

All samples were duplicated, and the coefficient of variation between the duplicates of the samples was required to be no more than 20.0% (samples with concentrations lower than the lower limit of quantitation were not required).

1. *Calibration curve.* The standard curve takes the concentration as the horizontal coordinate and OD value as the vertical coordinate, and carries out the four-parameter fitting to draw the standard curve. Each analysis batch consists of calibration standards with six concentrations, including LLOQ and ULOQ. Blank samples should not be involved in the calculation of calibration curve parameters. Anchor-point calibration samples whose concentration is higher than ULOQ and lower than LLOQ to improve curve fitting.

At least six separate analysis batches need to be evaluated on different days to examine differences between batches. The standard curve allows for the exclusion of concentration points where errors occur for clear or unknown reasons. After exclusion, the relative error (%RE) [= (measured concentration – nominal concentration)/nominal concentration × 100%] of at least 75% calibration standards with no less than six concentrations should be within ±20.0% (LLOQ and ULOQ are ±25.0%), and the correlation R^2 of the standard curve is greater than 0.95, and the average OD value of the blank sample should be lower than the minimum quantitative limit sample.

Anchor-point calibration samples are outside the quantitative range and may not comply with the above acceptance criteria. The anchor point is used to assist in fitting the standard curve of nonlinear regression. When the standard curve does not meet the acceptable standard, the anchor point can be removed, and when the standard curve meets the acceptable standard, the anchor point can be removed. In addition, the anchor point should not be removed.

2. Precision and accuracy. Accuracy is defined as the relative error (%RE) between the measured and nominal concentration, and precision is defined as the coefficient of variation (%CV). Precision and accuracy shall be examined by two or more persons and in at least six separate analysis batches over two or more days, with each additional person required to conduct at least one analysis batch for precision and accuracy investigation.

Precision and accuracy investigation: Each analysis batch contains at least one standard curve and three sets of quality control samples, in which the standard curve sample is prepared by the control article, and the quality control sample is prepared by the test article. Each set contains five concentrations of quality control samples of LLOQ, LQC, MQC, HQC and ULOQ, of LLOQ, LQC, MQC, HQC and ULOQ, and the measured values are statistically analyzed after testing.

The acceptable criteria are as follows.

Accuracy: The average %RE [(average measured concentration – nominal concentration)/nominal concentration × 100%] of each batch of quality control samples of each concentration does not exceed ±20.0% (ULOQ and LLOQ samples do not exceed ±25.0%).

Intra-batch precision: The %CV of each batch of quality control samples of each concentration shall not exceed 20.0% (ULOQ and LLOQ samples shall not exceed 25.0%).

Inter-batch precision: The %CV of all batches of quality control samples of each concentration shall not exceed 20.0% (ULOQ and LLOQ samples shall not exceed 25.0%).

Total error of method: No more than 30.0% (ULOQ and LLOQ samples shall be no more than 40.0%), the total error of the method is calculated as follows: %RE = (average measured concentration − nominal concentration)/nominal concentration × 100%; total error of method (% TE) = absolute relative error (%) + inter-batch precision (%).

For other validation of methodology and sample determination, an analysis batch was composed of one standard curve, three quality control samples for concentration levels (HQC, MQC, and LQC), two samples for each concentration level, and samples to be tested. The %RE of at least 67% of the quality control samples in each analysis batch should be within ±20.0%. For each concentration, the %RE of at least 50% of the quality control samples should be within ±20.0%.

3. *Selectivity*. The selectivity was examined at the upper limit of quantification (ULOQ) and the lower limit of quantification (LLOQ). For each concentration level, the %RE of the selective samples from at least 80% individual sources should be within ±25.0% (the %RE of the LLOQ samples should be within ±25.0%), and the response of the blank selective samples from at least 80% individual sources should be lower than the response of the LLOQ.

4. *Hemolysis effect*. The hemolysis effect shall be investigated at the ULOQ and LLOQ. At each concentration level, the %RE of at least 80% of individual-derived hemolysis effect samples should be within ±25.0% (the %RE of samples at the LLOQ should be within ±25.0%), and the response of at least 80% of blank hemolytic samples should be lower than the response of LLOQ.

5. *Specificity*. At each concentration level, the %RE of at least 80% of the specific samples should be within ±20.0% (specificity is examined at the ULOQ and LLOQ), and the response of at least 80% of the blank specific samples should be lower than the response of the LLOQ.

6. *Dilution linearity and hook effect*. The OD values of samples HOOK1 and HOOK2 above the ULOQ should be greater than the OD values of the ULOQ of the standard curve. The average %RE of samples within the quantitative range of the standard curve was within ±20.0%, and the %CV of five samples of each dilution did not exceed 20.0%. The OD value of samples below the LLOQ HOOK3 should be less than the OD value of the LLOQ of the standard curve. With the increase of drug concentration, the OD value did not decrease significantly, which was regarded as no prozone effect. With the decrease of drug concentration, the OD value did not increase significantly, which was considered as no postzone effect.

7. *Stability*. For the concentration of stability, there shall be more than 67% stability samples whose %RE of concentration was within ±20.0%, and the average %RE of each concentration shall be no more than ±20.0%.

8. *Parallelism*. The %CV of the concentration of the inter-sample of parallelism serial dilution ≤30.0%.

9. Robustness. Robustness is an indicator of the reliability of an analytical method during normal use and the ability of the analytical method to be unaffected by small changes in its parameters. These changes were evaluated in intra-batch and inter-batch precision and accuracy tests, and the intra-batch and inter-batch precision and accuracy met the acceptance criteria, that is, the method was considered robust in these changes. Robustness tests were carried out for the methodological validation of the three matrix

Table 6.27 Time range for TQ001 robustness investigation

Incubation time	Blocking time	Sample incubation time	Secondary antibody solution incubation time
Minimum time	Incubate at room temperature for 90 min	Incubate at room temperature for 55 min	Incubate at room temperature for 28 min
Maximum time	Incubate at room temperature for 150 min	Incubate at room temperature for 65 min	Incubate at room temperature for 32 min

types. Two analysts conducted two analysis batches with different incubation times. For TQ001 incubation times, see Table 6.27.

6.9.11 Statistical Analysis of Data

The SoftMax Pro 7.1.2GxP, the built-in software of the multimode reader, was used to issue OD value, coefficient of variation between duplicates, and back-calculated concentration of samples. Microsoft Excel was used to organize the data and calculate the relative error and coefficient of variation within and between batches of quality control samples. Three decimal places are reserved for OD value and back-calculated concentration, and one decimal place is reserved for the coefficient of variation and relative error.

6.9.12 Methodology Validation Results

The validation items of TQ001 and TQ002 all include standard curve, precision and accuracy, selectivity, hemolysis effect, specificity, dilution linearity, hook effect, stability, and parallelism, and the test results of each validation investigation item meet the acceptance criteria. The quantitative range of the TQ001 standard curve was 156.25–10000 ng/mL, and the stability samples of TQ001 were stable at room temperature and 2°C–8°C for 24 h, repeated freeze–thaw for five cycles, and below −70°C for 42 days, 69 days, and 134 days. The quantitative range of the TQ002 standard curve was 25–1600 ng/mL. The stability samples of TQ002 were stable at room temperature for 66 h, at 2°C–8°C for 66 h, repeatedly freezing–thawing for five cycles, and at −70°C for 35 days, 65 days, and 295 days. The results showed that the determination of TQ001 and TQ002 in the serum of cynomolgus monkeys by the ELISA method was accurate and reproducible, and the validation of the method met the requirements. For the complete validation results of TQ001, see Table 6.28.

Case 2: Anti-TQ001 and TQ002 antibodies in serum and tissue of cynomolgus monkeys were detected by the ELISA method

Purpose: To validate the established ELISA method for the detection of anti-TQ001 antibody and anti-TQ002 antibody in serum and tissue of cynomolgus monkeys.

Table 6.28 Summary of the verification results of TQ001 drug concentration

Investigation items	Acceptance criteria	Test results		Result evaluation
Standard curve	Standard curve range: 156.25–10,000 ng/mL			Pass
	The %RE of the measured concentrations of calibration standards with no less than six concentrations was within the range of ±20.0% (LLOQ and ULOQ were ±25.0%)	LOQ standards: %RE: −7.3% to 21.5% Calibration standards except LOQ standards: %RE: −7.8% to 16.8%		
	Correlation $R^2 > 0.95$	R^2 of each analytical run was greater than 0.99		
Precision and accuracy	Mean %RE did not exceed ± 20.0% (ULOQ and LLOQ did not exceed ±25.0%) Intra-run %CV did not exceed 20.0% (ULOQ and LLOQ did not exceed 25.0%) Inter-run %CV did not exceed 20.0% (ULOQ and LLOQ did not exceed 25.0%) Total method error: did not exceed 30.0% (ULOQ and LLOQ did not exceed 40.0%)	LLOQ (156.25 ng/mL)	Mean %RE: −1.2% to 18.7% Intra-run %CV: 1.6%–8.3% Inter-run %CV: 7.3% Total method error: 13.7%	Pass
		LQC (400 ng/mL)	Mean %RE: −4.3% to 10.6% Intra-run %CV: 6.0%–7.8% Inter-run %CV: 7.9% Total method error: 10.5%	
		MQC (4000 ng/mL)	Mean %RE: −3.9% to −9.8% Intra-run %CV: 2.6%–11.2% Inter-run %CV: 7.6% Total method error: 7.9%	
		HQC (8000 ng/mL)	Mean %RE: −10.1% to 2.9% Intra-run %CV: 3.7%–9.4% Inter-run %CV: 8.0% Total method error: 12.3%	
		ULOQ (10,000 ng/mL)	Mean %RE: −8.0% to 8.9% Intra-run %CV: 3.0%–9.8% Inter-run %CV: 8.3% Total method error: 10.6%	
Selectivity	SE-NC (0 ng/mL): The response of at least 80% of samples was below that of LLOQ	All samples: The back-calculated concentrations were all below LLOQ	SE-NC (0 ng/mL): The response of at least 80% of samples was below that of LLOQ	Pass
	SE-L (156.25 ng/mL): The %RE of at least 80% of samples did not exceed ± 25.0%	All samples: %RE: −6.9% to 14.2%; %CV was 6.3%	SE-L (156.25 ng/mL): The %RE of at least 80% of samples did not exceed ±25.0%	
	SE-H (10,000 ng/mL): The %RE of at least 80% of samples did not exceed ± 25.0%	All samples: %RE: −18.7% to 4.4%; %CV was 7.4 %	SE-H (10,000 ng/mL): The %RE of at least 80% of samples did not exceed ±25.0%	
Hemolysis effect	HE-NC (0 ng/mL): The response of at least 80% of samples was below that of LLOQ	All samples: The back-calculated concentrations were all below LLOQ		Pass
	HE-L (156.25 ng/mL): The %RE of at least 80% of samples did not exceed ± 25.0%	All samples: %RE: 0.6%–18.5%, %CV was 6.3%		
	HE-H (10,000 ng/mL): The %RE of at least 80% of samples did not exceed ± 25.0%	All samples: %RE: −2.9% to 22.0%, %CV was 9.0%		

continued

Table 6.28 (continued)

Investigation items	Acceptance criteria	Test results	Result evaluation
Specificity	SP-H/SP-L (0 ng/mL): The response of at least 80% of samples was below that of LLOQ	SP-H/SP-L all samples: The back-calculated concentrations were all below LLOQ	Pass
	SP-H-L/SP-L-L (156.25 ng/mL): The %RE of at least 80% of samples did not exceed ± 20.0%	SP-H-L all samples: %RE: 2.0%–11.0%, %CV: 3.2% SP-L-L all samples: %RE: 4.4%–18.7%, %CV: 5.4%	
	SP-H-H/SP-L-H (10000 ng/mL): At least 80% of the %RE did not exceed ±20.0%	SP-H-H all samples: %RE: −10.6% to 2.9%, %CV: 5.9% SP-L-H all samples: %RE: −16.9% to −0.8%, %CV: 6.9%	
Dilution linearity	Mean %RE was less than ± 20.0% %CV was less than 20.0%	6000 ng/mL Mean %RE: 5.4%, %CV: 9.4%	Pass
		2000 ng/mL Mean %RE: −0.4%, %CV: 4.7%	
		500 ng/mL Mean %RE: 4.4%, %CV: 2.6%	
Hook effect	HOOK1 OD value was greater than that of ULOQ	The OD value of HOOK (10 mg/mL) was greater than that of ULOQ	Pass
	HOOK2 OD value was greater than that of ULOQ	The OD value of HOOK2 (5 mg/mL) was greater than that of ULOQ	
	HOOK3 OD value was less than that of LLOQ	The OD value of HOOK3 (25 ng/mL) was greater than that of ULOQ	

continued

Table 6.28 (continued)

Investigation items	Acceptance criteria	Test results		Result evaluation
		Immediate stability	High concentration (8000 ng/mL) quality controls: Sample %RE: −11.6% to 7.0%, Mean %RE: −2.5%; %CV: 9.3% Low concentration (400 ng/mL) quality controls Sample %RE: −4.4% to 13.4%, Mean %RE: 3.6%; %CV: 8.1%	Pass
		RT Stability after storage for 24 h	High concentration (8000 ng/mL) quality controls: Sample %RE: −6.6% to 5.0%, Mean %RE: −1.7%; %CV: 5.1% Low concentration (400 ng/mL) quality controls Sample %RE: 2.1%–10.7%, Mean %RE: 5.8%; %CV: 3.5%	Pass
		Stability after storage for 24 h at 2°C–8°C	High concentration (8000 ng/mL) quality controls: Sample %RE: 1.5%–14.2%, Mean %RE: 9.4%; %CV: 5.1% Low concentration (400 ng/mL) quality controls Sample %RE: 7.4%–11.5%, Mean %RE: 10.0%; %CV: 1.7%	Pass
Stability	The %RE of at least 67% of samples at each concentration did not exceed ±20.0%, and the mean %RE of samples at each concentration did not exceed ±20.0%	Stability after five repeated freezing–thawing cycles under −70°C	High concentration (8000 ng/mL) quality controls: Sample %RE: −9.3% to 11.0%, Mean %RE: 0.4%; %CV: 9.5% Low concentration (400 ng/mL) quality controls Sample %RE: 9.8%–12.7%, Mean %RE: 11.2%; %CV: 1.2%	Pass
		Storage for 42 days under −70°C	High concentration (8000 ng/mL) quality controls: Sample %RE: −3.0% to 13.1%, Mean %RE: 4.2%; %CV: 7.1% Low concentration (400 ng/mL) quality controls Sample %RE: −3.1% to 4.9%, Mean %RE: −0.6%; %CV: 3.8%	Pass
		Storage for 69 days under −70°C	High concentration (8000 ng/mL) quality controls: Sample %RE: −9.4% to 14.9%, Mean %RE: −0.7%; %CV: 10.9% Low concentration (400 ng/mL) quality controls Sample %RE: 2.4%–6.8%, Mean %RE: 4.6%; %CV: 1.7%	Pass
		Storage for 134 days under −70°C	High concentration (8000 ng/mL) quality controls: Sample %RE: −7.4% to 15.7%, Mean %RE: 0.8%; %CV: 10.1% Low concentration (400 ng/mL) quality controls Sample %RE: −16.0% to −0.7%, Mean %RE: −7.6%; %CV: 7.3%	Pass
Parallelism	The %CV of serially diluted samples was ≤30.0%.	%CV between samples: 3.3%–5.7%		Pass

Method and principle: The anti-TQ001 antidrug antibody and anti-TQ002 antidrug antibody in serum, placenta, amniotic fluid, milk, and male reproductive organs of cynomolgus monkeys were determined by bridging ELISA method. The detection principle of TQ001 and TQ002 is similar. The microplates were coated with TQ001 and TQ002, respectively, and the samples were dissociated through a series of acidification pretreatment, washed to remove other components, and then combined with horseradish peroxidase-labeled antibodies. After washing, the substrate TMB coloring solution was added for color development, and TMB was transformed into blue under the catalysis of horseradish peroxidase, and into yellow under the action of sulfuric acid. The absorbance value was measured at 450 nm wavelength by using the SoftMax Pro 7.1.2GxP, built-in software of the multimode reader.

6.9.13 Test Article

6.9.13.1 Test Article 1

Identity: TQ001 injection

Specification: 150 mg/mL each vial
Content or concentration: 154.0 mg/mL
Stability: Stable under storage conditions and within expiration date
Expiration date: xxx/xxx/xxx
Storage condition: 2°C–8°C, protected from light.
Transport environment: Cold chain transportation

6.9.13.2 Test Article 2

Identity: TQ002 injection

Specification: 50 mg/0.5 mL each vial
Content or concentration: 100 mg/mL (concentration in COA)
Stability: Stable under storage conditions and within expiration date
Expiration date: xxx/xxx/xxx
Storage condition: 2°C–8°C, protected from light.
Transport environment: Cold chain transportation

6.9.13.3 TQ001 Positive Antibody

Identity: Rabbit anti-TQ001 polyclonal antibody

Batch number: 20211227
Content or concentration: 0.58 mg/mL
Stability: Stable under storage conditions and within expiration date
Expiration date: xxx/xxx/xxx
Storage condition: −80°C to −20°C
Transport environment: Dry ice transportation

6.9.13.4 TQ002 Positive Antibody

Identity: Rabbit anti-TQ002 polyclonal antibody

Batch number: 20220224

Content or concentration: 0.357 mg/mL
Stability: Stable under storage conditions and within expiration date
Expiration date: xxx/xxx/xxx
Storage condition: −80°C to −20°C
Transport environment: Dry ice transportation

6.9.13.5 Biotin-Labeled TQ001

Identity: BiotinTQ001.
Content or concentration: 1.51 mg/mL.
Stability: Stable under storage conditions and within expiration date
Expiration date February 07, 2023 (tentative).
Storage condition: 2°C–8°C.

6.9.13.6 Biotin-Labeled TQ002

Identity: BiotinTQ002.
Content or concentration: 1.916 mg/mL
Stability: Stable under storage conditions and within expiration date
Expiration date August 18, 2023 (tentative).
Storage condition: 2°C–8°C

6.9.14 Main Instruments and Reagents

1. Reagent and consumables Table 6.29.
2. Main instrument Table 6.30.
3. The blank serum of matrix cynomolgus monkey was obtained from the blank matrix bank of the institution and stored below −70°C for backup. Before using, the blank serum was balanced to room temperature for use.

Table 6.29 Reagents and consumables

Name	Lot No.
Tween 20	EZ7890B253
BSA	EZ7890C409
PBS powder	17H01A30, 17F06A30
TMB chromogenic solution	20220701
HRP-SA	BST17D19B17E88
Sulfuric acid	20211202
1 M Tris–HCl	010722220802
Blank serum	–
Completely hemolytic matrix	–
ELISA coating solution	20220714
Glacial acetic acid	20211214

Table 6.30 Main instruments

Instrument name	Instrument model
Multifunctional microplate reader	SpectraMax M3
Precision pipette	0.1–2.5, 0.5–10, 2–20, 10–100, 20–200, 30–300, 100–1000 μL, and 0.5–5 mL
Graduated cylinder	50 (±0.5), 100 (±1), 250 (±2), and 500 mL (±5 mL)
Dual-temperature refrigerator	YCD-265
Ultra-low temperature refrigerator	DW-86L626
Vortex mixer	MX-S
Palm centrifuge	S1010E/S1010
Ultra-pure water machine	Direct-Q 8UV
LED digital shaker	SLK-O3000-S
Four-unit tray oscillator	BenchMate S4P-D
Electronic balance	PR423ZH/E
Plate washer	405LS
Micro high-speed freezing centrifuge	Sorvall Legend Micro 17R

6.9.15 Test Method

1. The preparation volume of each solution was adjusted according to the actual need and preparation proportion.

2. Main reagent ELISA-coated solution: direct use without preparation.

1 mol/L TrisHCl (pH 8.5): For direct use without preparation.

Phosphate buffer (PBS): Take 1 pack of PBS powder, add 2 L ultrapure water, and mix well.

Plate washing solution (PBST): Add 1 mL Tween 20 to 2 L of PBS solution and mix well.

Blocking buffer (3% BSA): Weigh 3.0 g BSA, add it to 100 mL PBS solution, and mix well.

Diluent (1% BSA): Take 30 mL 3% BSA, add 60 mL ultrapure water, and mix well.

Acidizing solution (0.6 mol/L acetic acid): Take 36 mL acetic acid, add 1008 mL ultrapure water, and mix well.

TQ001 coated solution: Dilute TQ001 (154.0 mg/mL) with ELISA-coated solution to 1 μg/mL.

TQ002 coated working solution: Dilute TQ001 (100.0 mg/mL) with ELISA-coated solution to 5 μg/mL.

Biotin-labeled TQ001 working solution: BiotinTQ001 was diluted 10,000 times with 1% BSA.

Biotin-labeled TQ002 working solution: BiotinTQ002 was diluted 5000 times with 1% BSA.

1% BSATQ001 (20 μg/mL): Dilute TQ001 (154 mg/mL) to 20 μg/mL with 1% BSA.

Biotin-labeled antibody working solution for TQ001 confirmatory analysis: BiotinTQ001 was diluted 10,000 times with 1% BSATQ001 (20 μg/mL).

BiotinTQ002 working solution: BiotinTQ002 was diluted 5000 times with 1% BSA.

Biotin-labeled antibody working solution for TQ002 confirmatory analysis: TQ002 (100 mg/mL) was diluted 5000 times with biotin-labeled antibody working solution to the final concentration of 20 μg/mL.

TQ001 enzyme-labeled antibody working solution: HRPSA (Streptavidin) was diluted 10,000 times with 1% BSA.

TQ002 enzyme-labeled antibody working solution: HRPSA (Streptavidin) was diluted 5000 times with 1% BSA.

TMB chromogen solution: Direct use, no need to prepare.

1 mol/L H_2SO_4: Take 56 mL 18 mol/L concentrated sulfuric acid, add 944 mL ultrapure water while the solution is stirred in a beaker, cool it to room temperature, and transfer it to the solution bottle.

Negative control sample (NC): Take blank cynomolgus monkey serum from at least 10 different sources and mix it in equal volume to obtain a solution.

2% cynomolgus monkey hemolytic matrix: The fully hemolytic plasma is obtained from the matrix bank of the institution, and the fully hemolytic plasma is diluted 50 times with the blank cynomolgus monkey serum without hemolysis, that is, the 2% cynomolgus monkey hemolytic matrix.

3. Serum from 24 blank cynomolgus monkeys was selected as screening cut point (SCP) samples and confirming cut point (CCP) samples, respectively.

4. Sensitivity Sample

(1) TQ001 positive antibody (0.58 mg/mL) was diluted with NC (negative control sample) to 10,000, 5000, 2500, 1250, 625, 312.5, 156.25, 78.13, 39.06, 19.53, and 9.77 ng/mL, and used to prepare sensitivity samples.

(2) TQ002: TQ002 positive antibody (0.357 mg/mL) was diluted with NC to 10,000, 5000, 2500, 1250, 625, 312.5, 156.25, 78.13, 39.06, 19.53, and 9.77 ng/mL, and used to prepare sensitivity samples.

5. Quality Control Sample

(1) TQ001: TQ001 positive antibody (0.58 mg/mL) was diluted with NC to 5000 ng/mL (high concentration positive control, HPC), 1000 ng/mL (medium concentration positive control, MPC), 200 ng/mL (low concentration positive control, LPC). The quality control samples of HPC, MPC, and LPC in the batch of SCP, CCP, and sensitivity calculation were used to investigate the precision and determine the system adaptability.

(2) TQ002: TQ002: Positive antibody (0.357 mg/mL) was diluted with NC to 10,000 (HPC), 1000 (MPC), and 200 ng/mL (LPC). Quality control samples of HPC, MPC, and LPC from all validated analysis batches were used for precision investigation and system suitability determination.

6. Drug Resistance Test Samples

(1) TQ001: TQ001 positive antibody (0.58 mg/mL) was diluted with NC to LPC (200 ng/mL) and HPC (5000 ng/mL) as diluent, and TQ001 (154.0 mg/mL) was diluted in series as resistance samples (abbreviated as DIF1 and DIF2). The diluted concentrations of DIF1 were 2000, 1000, 200, 100, 50, 25, 12.5, and 6.25 μg/mL,

which were used as samples for drug resistance investigation at LPC level. The diluted concentrations of DIF2 were 8000, 4000, 2000, 1000, 200μg/mL, 100, 50, and 25 μ g/mL, and were used as samples for drug resistance investigation at HPC level. Two subpackages were made for each concentration.

(2) TQ002: TQ002 positive antibody (0.357 mg/mL) was diluted with NC to LPC (200 ng/mL) and HPC (10000 ng/mL) as diluent, and TQ002 (100 mg/mL) was diluted in series as resistance samples (abbreviated as DIF1 and DIF2). Among which, the diluted concentrations of DIF1 were 1000, 500, 250, 100, 50, 25, 12.5, and 6.25 μg/ mL, which were used as samples for drug resistance investigation at LPC level. The diluted concentrations of DIF2 were 5000, 2500, 1000, 500, 100, 50, 25, and 12.5 μ g/mL, and were used as samples for drug resistance investigation at HPC level. Two subpackages were made for each concentration.

7. Stability sample: The positive antibodies of TQ001 and TQ002 were diluted with NC to the concentrations of LPC and HPC, respectively, as low- and high-concentration stability samples. Each concentration sample was divided into no fewer than 15 samples. The stability samples were placed at room temperature for no less than 24 h and at 2°C–8°C for no less than 24 h immediately after preparation, respectively, repeated freeze–thaw for three and five cycles (During the preparation of freeze–thaw stability samples, the samples need to be melted at room temperature, and placed at room temperature for not less than 4 h and can be measured after the last melt. Before the first complete melting, the samples need to be frozen at least 24 h below −70°C, and after each freeze–thaw cycle, the samples should be frozen at −70°C for more than 12 h), then the determination were performed. Three samples per concentration per condition ($n = 3$).

8. Selective: Sample TQ001/TQ002: The blank serum of ten different cynomolgus monkeys was selected as the selective blank sample (SNC). The positive antibody was diluted to 10× LPC with blank serum of cynomolgus monkeys, and then the serum of ten different individuals was diluted to 10× LPC to the concentration of LPC to prepare SLPC samples.

9. Hemolysis sample: TQ001/TQ002: Add 2% cynomolgus monkey hemolysis matrix in blank cynomolgus monkey serum to prepare hemolytic negative control samples (HENC), dilute the positive antibody with 2% hemolysis matrix of cynomolgus monkeys to the concentration of LPC, and prepare hemolytic low concentration positive control (HELPC) with five sets of each.

10. Hook effect TQ001/TQ002: TQ001 and TQ002 positive antibodies were diluted to 200 and 100 μg/mL with blank cynomolgus monkey mixed serum matrix, respectively, as Hook1 and Hook2 samples for detection. Hook2 samples were then diluted to 1 ng/mL with blank cynomolgus monkey mixed serum matrix to prepare Hook3, and at least five samples were treated in parallel for each concentration. Hook1 and Hook2 were used to investigate the prozone effect, and Hook3 was used to investigate the postzone effect.

11. Matrix bridging: In the process of immunogenicity studies accompanied by pharmacokinetics and toxicokinetics of reproductive toxicity, when it is necessary to detect antidrug antibodies in the placenta, amniotic fluid, milk, and male reproductive organ tissues, it is best to conduct separate validation of each tissue type to obtain the

screening cut point and confirming cut point of various types of matrix. If the matrix has little influence, matrix bridging validation can also be carried out in selective validation. If the blank matrix is difficult to obtain, such as milk, 10% skim milk can be used in the validation. This method did not carry out the bridge validation of the above tissues, but the bridge test of tissue homogenate and serum, and the bridge test of amniotic fluid, milk, and serum were carried out in other species (rabbits and rats) in the institution.

6.9.16 Analysis Process

6.9.16.1 TQ001

Coating: Add the coated working liquid to the microporous plate, 100 μL/well, seal the plate, and incubate at 2°C–8°C overnight.

Blocking: Wash the plate five times with PBST, 300 μL/well, pat dry, seal with 3% BSA, 300 μL/well, block the plate, incubate at room temperature for about 2 h.

Sample treatment: Appropriate amount of samples were taken, diluted with PBS twice, acidified with 0.6 mol/L acetic acid working solution for five times, and incubated at room temperature for about 1 h.

Adding samples: Wash the plate five times with PBST, 300 μL/well, pat dry, add 100 μL acidified samples into microplates containing 30 μL 1 mol/L Tris buffer, seal the plate, and incubate at room temperature for about 3 h.

Secondary acidification: Wash the plate five times with PBST, 300 μL/well, pat dry, add 0.6 mol/L acetic acid working solution, 150 μL/well, and incubate for about 2 h.

Transfer plate: Add 30 μL 1 mol/L Tris buffer to the new enzyme-labeled plate first, add 100 μL of the sample after secondary acidification to each well, and incubate overnight.

Blocking: Wash the plate five times with PBST, 300 μL/well, pat dry, seal the plates with 3% BSA, 300 μL/well, seal the plate, and incubate at room temperature for about 2 h.

Add biotin-labeled antibodies: Discard the liquid in the well, wash the plate with PBST for five times, 300 μL/well, pat dry. Add biotin-labeled antibody working solution, 100 μL/well (adding biotin-labeled antibody working solution for confirmatory analysis to the confirmatory test), seal the plate, and incubate at room temperature for about 1 h.

Add enzyme-labeled antibodies: Discard the liquid in the well, wash the plate with PBST five times, 300 μL/ hole, pat dry. Add enzyme-labeled antibody working solution, 100 μL/well, and seal the plate. Incubate at room temperature for about 1 h.

Color development: Discard the liquid in the well, wash the plate with PBST five times, 300 μL/well, and pat dry. Add color developing solution 100 μL/ well, and develop color at room temperature without light for 15 ± 5 min, the time was dependent on the color development.

Termination: Add termination solution, 100 μL/well.

Determination: The reaction was terminated, and the OD value at 450 nm was measured on the microplate reader within 30 min.

6.9.16.2 TQ002

Coating: Add the coated working liquid to the microporous plate, 100 μL/well, seal the plate, and incubate at 2°C–8°C overnight.

Blocking: Wash the plate five times with PBST, 300 μL/well, pat dry, seal with 3% BSA, 300 μL/well, block the plate, incubate at room temperature with shaking for 2 h.

Sample treatment: Appropriate amount of samples were taken, diluted with PBS twice, acidified with 0.6 mol/L acetic acid working solution five times, and incubated at room temperature for 1 h.

Adding samples: Wash the plate five times with PBST, 300 μL/well, pat dry, add 100 μL acidified samples to microplates containing 30 μL of 1 mol/L TrisHCl buffer at pH 8.5, seal the plate, and incubate in a room temperature shaker for 3 h.

Secondary acidification: Wash the plate five times with PBST, 300 μL/well, pat dry, add 0.6 mol/L acetic acid working solution, 150 μL/well, and incubate in a room temperature shaker for 2 h.

Transfer plate: Add 30 μL 1 mol/L TrisHCl buffer with pH 8.5 to the new ELISA plate, and then add 100 μL samples after secondary acidification to each well and incubate overnight in a room temperature shaker.

Blocking: Wash the plate five times with PBST, 300 μL/ well, pat dry, seal the plates with 3% BSA, 300 μL/well, seal the plate, and incubate in a room temperature shaker for about 2 h.

Add biotin-labeled antibodies: Discard the liquid in the well, wash the plate with PBST five times, 300 μL/well, pat dry. Add biotin-labeled antibody working solution, 100 μL/well (adding biotin-labeled antibody working solution for confirmatory analysis to confirmatory test), seal the plate, and incubate in a room temperature shaker for about 1 h.

Add enzyme-labeled antibodies: Discard the liquid in the well, wash the plate with PBST five times, 300 μL/well, pat dry. Add enzyme-labeled antibody working solution, 100 μL/well, and seal the plate. Incubate in a room temperature shaker for about 1 h.

Color development: Discard the liquid in the well, wash the plate with PBST for five times, 300 μL/well and pat dry. Add color developing solution 100 μL/well, and develop color at room temperature without light for 15 ± 5 min, the time was dependent on the color development.

Termination: Add termination solution, 100 μL/well.

Determination: The reaction was terminated, and the OD value at 450 nm was measured on the microplate reader within 30 min.

6.9.17 Methodology Validation

All samples shall be duplicated, and the %CV of OD value of LPC, MPC, and HPC duplicates shall not exceed 20% (NC, SCP samples and SNR value below the SCP shall not exceed 30%). If the sample size is exceeded, the sample will be considered invalid and should be excluded during the result analysis. At least two-third NC and quality control samples of each plate are involved in the statistics.

In order to avoid the influence of external environmental factors on the measured values of the analysis batch, all parameters of the OD value calculation method were replaced by SNR in this test method (OD values were still used to calculate NC samples), and the OD value of each plate was determined by the median method, SNR = average OD value (validated sample or sample to be measured)/median OD value (NC).

1. Twenty-four individual samples in 2 analysis batches were conducted, screening and confirming analysis when SCP, TCP, and CCP were involved in SCP and CCP tests, 12 individual samples and three sets of NC, LPC, MPC, and HPC were run in one analysis batch, and screening samples and confirmatory samples are arranged alternately. BiotinTQ001/TQ002 working solution was added to 12 individual samples as unspiked samples, that was, the SCP samples; Confirmatory working fluid was added to 12 individual samples as spiked samples, that was, the CCP samples, while three sets of confirmatory negative control (CNC), confirming low positive control (CLPC), confirming medium positive control (CMPC) and confirming high positive control (CHPC) were conducted confirmatory analysis with confirmatory working fluid.

The cut point evaluation test should be conducted by at least 2 technicians in at least 3 days to complete 12 batches of testing, and the %CV of the NC sample signal value in and between batches should be no more than 30%, and the %CV of the SNR value in and between batches of quality control samples should be no more than 20%. The average inhibition rate of CNC samples was lower than that of the CCP, and the average inhibition rate of quality control samples was higher than that of the CCP. The samples of all blank animals in the qualified analysis batch were counted together.

(1) Exclude outliers: Each blank animal in each analysis batch corresponds to one SCP sample and one CCP sample. Exclude any animal whose coefficient of variation between duplicates exceeds 30%, and allow one-third of the animals in each plate to have a coefficient of variation between duplicates exceeding 30%.

The average method was used to determine the OD value of NC in each analysis batch, and the SNR value of the sample was calculated for Log conversion, and the analytical and biological outliers were excluded.

When outliers were excluded, the data obtained from each blank animal (up to six times) were analyzed using the box diagram of SPSS software. Outliers in SPSS were marked with two symbols: "□;" for extreme outlier ($k = 3$), "○" for mild outlier ($k = 1.5$), and only the analytical outlier marked "□" should be excluded.

When biological outliers were excluded, the abnormal individuals labeled "□" were excluded using the median of each individual and the box diagram of SPSS software.

When the SCP and TCP were determined, the remaining data Log (SNR) with analytical outliers and biological outliers excluded is evaluated by the SW test using SPSS software to determine normal distribution.

If $P > 0.05$ in the SW test, the absolute value of skewness is less than 1, the data will be normally distributed. Log (SCP) = Average + 1.645 SD, Log (TCP) = average + 3.09 SD.

If $P \leq 0.05$ in the SW test, the absolute value of skewness is less than one, which proves that although the data does not belong to the normal distribution, the data is not highly biased and presents a long tail distribution, Log (SCP) = median + 1.645 (1.4826 × MAD), Log (TCP) = median + 3.09 (1.4826 × MAD).

If $P < 0.05$ in the SW test, while the absolute value of skewness is greater than 1, proving that the overall data does not belong to the normal distribution and is severely biased to one side, the Log (SCP) = 95% percentile method is used to calculate the cut point, Log (TCP) = =99.9% percentile method is used to calculate the cut point.

The anti-value of the SCP is the SCP of the test, and the anti-value of the TCP is the TCP of the test.

(2) CCP determination: CCP calculation formula is: inhibition rate % = 100% × (1 − SNR value of spiked sample/SNR value of unspiked sample). The remaining data (inhibition rate), with analysis outliers and individual outliers excluded, were evaluated by the SW test using SPSS software to determine the normal distribution.

If $P > 0.05$ in the SW test, the absolute value of skewness is less than 1, which proves that the data belong to normal distribution, CCP = mean + 2.33 SD.

If $P \leq 0.05$ in the SW test, the absolute value of skewness is less than 1, which proves that the data do not belong to the normal distribution, and the data are not concentrated in the low or high end, CCP = median + 2.33 (1.4826 × MAD).

If $P < 0.05$ in the SW test, and the absolute value of skewness is greater than 1, which proves that the overall data does not belong to the normal distribution and is severely biased to one side, CCP = 99% percentile method.

2. Sensitivity: During the sensitivity determination test, an analysis batch was composed of three sets of NC, LPC, MPC and HPC unspiked samples, 11 sets of sensitivity determination unspiked samples, three sets of CNC, CLPC, CMPC and CHPC spiked samples, and 11 sensitivity-determined samples with drug confirmation. Two or more technicians should run at least three analysis batches, at least two-third sensitivity determination sample above the SCP were involve in statistics (SNR near the SCP must be counted).

The coefficient of variation of the NC sample signal value within and between batches should be no more than 30%, and the coefficient of variation of SNR value within and between batches should be no more than 20%. The average inhibition rate of CNC samples was lower than that of the CCP, and the average inhibition rate of quality control samples was higher than that of the CCP.

In screening sensitivity, sensitivity samples with SNR values on the dilution curve at two points above and below the SCP were performed, and linear fitting was performed; the concentration corresponding to the SCP was calculated by the interpolation method. The confirmation sensitivity was linearly fitted to the sensitivity samples whose inhibition rate was two points above and below the CCP on the dilution curve, and the concentration corresponding to the CCP was calculated by an interpolation method. At least three analysis batches and three sets of sensitivity samples were conducted, at least two-third of the sensitivity should be between one-half and two times of the median sensitivity, if the three sets of sensitivity samples differ greatly, the sensitivity analysis batches should be added until the above requirements were met. The final sensitivity was calculated as follows: Sensitivity = average + t0.05, df × SD, (t0.05 was 95% consistency in the t-test, $df = n$, that is, the number of sensitive samples − 1).

The higher value of screening sensitivity and confirming sensitivity was used as the sensitivity finally reported. If the signal produced without dilution was lower than the SCP/CCP, but reached an acceptable method sensitivity, the sensitivity would be reported as the lowest detection concentration.

3. Precision and system adaptability: During the precision test, six sets of NC, LPC, MPC and HPC were prepared independently, and six sets of NC, LPC, MPC and HPC without adding drugs and six sets of confirming CNC, CLPC, CMPC and CHPC with adding drugs were used to form an analysis batch to investigate the precision, and at least two technicians should run at least three analysis batches for 2 days or more. The coefficient of variation of the NC sample signal value within and between batches should be no more than 30%, and the coefficient of variation of the SNR value of quality control samples within and between batches should be no more than 20%. The average inhibition rate of CNC samples was lower than that of the CCP, and the average inhibition rate of quality control samples was higher than that of the CCP.

Negative quality control (NC) should have an upper limit, and positive quality control should have an upper and lower limit. Quality control samples from all analysis batches of SCP, TCP, and CCP, sensitivity, and precision were used for the calculation of system adaptability, which was calculated as follows:

NC = Mean + $t_{0.01,\,df}$ ×SD; LPC = average (LPC response value) ± $t_{0.005,\,df}$ × SD; MPC = Mean (MPC response value) ± $t_{0.005,\,df}$ × SD; HPC = Mean (HPC response value) ± $t_{0.005,\,df}$ × SD.

After the system adaptability is calculated, the passing criteria for the validation analysis batch and analysis batch of sample testing are as follows: At least 2/3 of the NC and quality control samples in each analysis batch should meet the system adaptability, and the coefficient of variation of the signal value of the NC sample in the batch should not exceed 30%, and the coefficient of variation of the SNR value of the quality control sample in the batch should not exceed 20%.

4. Titer Test For the titer test, three sets of NC, LPC, MPC, and HPC samples, three sets of titer test samples with gradient dilution (first dilute the positive antibody with a blank matrix to a certain concentration, and then double dilute 11 concentrations) are composed of one analysis batch, and at least three analysis batches are run by two or more technicians.

The coefficient of variation of the NC sample signal value within and between batches should be no more than 30%, and the coefficient of variation of the SNR value of quality control samples within and between batches should be no more than 20%. The titer sample with an SNR value greater than TCP meets the SNR value decrease with the decrease of concentration, and the variation coefficient of signal value between duplicates does not exceed 20%, and the titer sample with an SNR value less than TCP meets the variation coefficient between duplicates does not exceed 30%.

5. Drug Resistance The consistency of the two batches of test article was examined in the drug resistance validation of the two analysis batches, and the two batches of test article were investigated at the LPC and the HPC, respectively. Samples with at least 2/3 concentration were included in the statistics (samples with SNR values near the SCP must be counted). The addition of drugs could reduce the signal of positive

antibodies, and the highest drug concentration with an SNR value greater than the SCP was used as the drug tolerance limit.

If the positive antibody is below the level of LPC and HPC, the drug tolerance limit of the two batches of test article is between positive and negative, with a dilution gradient, it will be considered that the interference of the two batches of test article to the test method is consistent.

6. Selectivity Selectivity was examined in one analysis batch, and the difference rate between the selective sample with positive quality control (S-LPC) and the positive quality control (LPC) was calculated [($SNR_{S\text{-}LPC\ sample}$ – mean SNR_{LPC})/mean SNR_{LPC}× 100%]. At least 80% of S-LPC samples had a difference rate of ± 30%, and at least 80% of S-NC were screened as negative.

7. Hemolysis effect Hemolysis effect was investigated in one analysis batch, and the difference rate between the hemolysis sample with positive quality control (HELPC) and the positive quality control (LPC) was calculated [($SNR_{HE\text{-}LPC\ sample}$ – mean SNR_{LPC})/ mean SNR_{LPC}× 100%]. At least 80% of HE-LPC samples had a difference rate of ± 30%, and at least 80% of HE-NC were screened as negative.

8. Hook effect. Hook effect was investigated in one analysis batch, and the mean OD values of Hook1 and Hook2 in the analysis batch should be greater than the mean OD values of HPC, and the mean OD values of Hook3 samples should be lower than the mean OD values of LPC. With the increase of positive antibody concentration, the OD value did not decrease significantly, which was regarded as no prozone effect. With the decrease of drug concentration, the OD value did not increase significantly, which was considered as no postzone effect.

9. Stability The sample is considered stable if the difference rate between 2/3 of the stability sample and the freshly prepared quality control sample [(SNR stability sample – mean SNR immediately)/mean SNR immediately × 100%] is between ± 20%.

6.9.18 Sample Detection

During sample analysis, each batch was accompanied by three sets of NC, LPC, and HPC, and at least 2/3 of the NC and quality control samples passed the system adaptability, and the sample analysis results of the plate were acceptable. The intra-batch and inter-batch variation coefficients of NC sample signal values should be no more than 30%, and the intra-batch and inter-batch variation coefficients of SNR values of quality control samples should be no more than 20%. During confirmatory analysis of samples, the average inhibition rate of CNC samples is less than the CCP, and the average inhibition rate of quality control samples is greater than the CCP.

When the sample to be tested is screened and analyzed, if the SNR value of the sample is less than SCP, the variation coefficient of the signal value of the sample is required to be less than 30%, and the sample will be judged as negative. If the SNR value of the sample is greater than the SCP value, the variation coefficient of the signal value of the sample is required to be less than 20%, and the sample will be judged as positive, and the next confirmatory analysis will be carried out.

In the confirmatory analysis of the sample to be tested, if the inhibition rate of the sample is less than CCP, the variation coefficient of the signal value of the sample is required to be less than 30%, and the sample will be judged as negative. If the inhibition rate of the sample is greater than CCP, the variation coefficient of the signal value of the sample is required to be less than 20%, and the sample will be judged as positive, and the titer analysis will be carried out in the next step.

When conducting titer analysis of the samples to be tested, the titer sample with SNR value greater than TCP should meet the requirement that the SNR value decreases with the decrease of concentration, and the variation coefficient of the signal value between duplicates should not exceed 20%, and the titer sample with SNR value less than TCP should meet the requirement that the variation coefficient between duplicates should not exceed 30%. Using NC as diluent, the sample is diluted two times in a gradient to SNR < TCP. (If the SNR value of the sample screening test is higher than HPC, the sample will be properly diluted with NC and then diluted twice the gradient), If the dilution of the sample does not reach SNR<TCP, the test result will not be accepted, and the sample will be retested.

The titer calculation formula for sample testing is: Titer = Dilution ratio higher than TCP + (Signal value higher than TCP − TCP) × (Dilution ratio lower than TCP − Dilution ratio higher than TCP)/ (Signal value higher than TCP − Signal value lower than TCP).

6.9.19 Statistical Analysis of Data

OD value and coefficient of variation (%CV) were obtained by multimode reader. Excel was used to calculate Log (SNR), mean value, standard deviation (SD), coefficient of variation, etc.

The box diagram of SPSS software was used for analysis and biological outlier elimination, and the SW test was carried out with SPSS software.

The OD value retained four decimal places, the SNR value three decimal places, and the coefficient of variation one decimal place.

6.9.20 Methodological Validation Results

The validation items of TQ001 and TQ002 antidrug antibody detection included SCP and CCP, sensitivity, precision, and system adaptability, drug resistance, selectivity, hemolysis effect, hook effect, drug parallelism, and immediate placement at room temperature for 24 h, placement at 2°C–8°C for 24 h, and repeated freeze–thaw below −70°C for three cycles and five cycles of stability. The test results of each validation investigation were in line with the acceptance criteria.

The SCP of TQ001 was 1.043, TCP was 1.056, and CCP was 8.127%. The screening sensitivity was 10 ng/mL, and the confirming sensitivity was 10 ng/mL. When the positive antibody was 200 ng/mL, the maximum tolerable serum concentration of

TQ001 was 2000μg/mL. When the positive antibody was 5000 ng/mL, the maximum tolerable serum concentration of TQ001 was 8000 μg/mL.

SCP, TCP, and CCP of TQ002 were 1.209%, 1.301%, and 13.859%, respectively. The screening sensitivity was 65 ng/mL, and the confirming sensitivity was 82 ng/mL. When the positive antibody was 200 ng/mL, the maximum tolerated serum concentration of TQ001 was 250 μg/mL. When the positive antibody was 10,000 ng/mL, the maximum tolerated serum concentration of TQ001 was 5000 μg/mL.

The results showed that the bridging ELISA method applied in the determination of antibodies to TQ001 and TQ002 in the serum of cynomolgus monkeys was sensitive, stable, and without matrix effect. The samples were stable immediately placed at room temperature for 24 h, at 2°C–8°C for 24 h, and at −70°C for three and five cycles of repeated freeze–thaw after preparation and could be used for the subsequent detection of TQ001 and TQ002 antidrug antibodies in the serum of cynomolgus monkeys. The complete validation results of TQ001 are shown in Table 6.31.

6.9.21 Pharmacokinetic and Immunogenicity Studies

The pharmacokinetic differences of related antibodies in pregnant and male animals are discussed in the following case.

Case 3: Pharmacokinetics and Immunogenicity Studies of TQ001 and TQ002 Monoclonal Antibodies in Pregnant Cynomolgus Monkeys

Purpose: The purpose of the study was to study the pharmacokinetic characteristics of pregnant animals, detect the concentrations of TQ001 and TQ002 antibodies and the production of antidrug antibodies in the placenta, amniotic fluid, milk, fetal serum and testis, epididymis, seminal vesicle and adrenal tissues of male animals, so as to understand the pharmacokinetic differences of IgG1 antibodies between pregnant and male animals and the distribution of drugs in the male reproductive organs (including the blood–testis barrier), as well as the passage of the placental barrier and blood–milk barrier via the subcutaneous injection of TQ001 and TQ002 monoclonal antibodies in male and pregnant cynomolgus monkeys.

6.9.22 Test Article

6.9.22.1 Test Article 1

Identity: TQ001 injection

Specification: 150 mg/mL each vial

Content or concentration: 154.0 mg/mL

Stability: Stable under storage conditions and within expiration date

Expiration date: xxx/xxx/xxx

Storage condition: 2°C–8°C, away from light

Transport environment: Cold chain transportation

Preparation method: Raw liquid administration with no need for preparation.

Table 6.31 Summary table of TQ001 antidrug antibody verification results and acceptance criteria

Investigation items	Acceptance criteria	Sample names	Test results	Result evaluation
Screening and confirmation (12 analytical runs investigated)	Intra-run and inter-run %CV of OD values were ≤30%	NC samples	Intra-run %CV: 1.5%–11.0% Inter-run %CV: 5.5%	Pass
	Intra-run and inter-run %CV of SNR values were ≤20%	LPC (200 ng/mL)	Intra-run %CV: 0.7%–13.8% Inter-run %CV: 8.1%	
		MPC (1000 ng/mL)	Intra-run %CV: 2.5%–15.9% Inter-run %CV: 8.8%	
		HPC (10,000 ng/mL)	Intra-run %CV: 1.1%–10.6% Inter-run %CV: 7.9%	
	Mean inhibition rate < =CCP	NC samples	Mean inhibition rate <13.859%	
	Mean inhibition rate > CCP	Low, medium, and high concentrations of positive quality control samples	Mean inhibition rate >13.859%	
Sensitivity (three analytical runs investigated)	Intra-run and inter-run %CV of OD values were ≤30%	NC samples	Intra-run %CV: 2.7%–4.9% Inter-run %CV: 4.3%	Pass
	Intra-run and inter-run %CV of SNR values were ≤20%	LPC (200 ng/mL)	Intra-run %CV: 5.6%–7.4% Inter-run %CV: 8.7%	
		MPC (1000 ng/mL)	Intra-run %CV: 2.9%–11.2% Inter-run %CV: 11.7%	
		HPC (10,000 ng/mL)	Intra-run %CV: 1.7%–6.4% Inter-run %CV: 9.1%	
	Mean inhibition rate < CCP	NC samples	Mean inhibition rate <13.859%	
	Mean inhibition rate > CCP	Low, medium, and high concentrations of positive quality control samples	Mean inhibition rate >13.859%	
System suitability (all analytical runs investigated)		NC samples	Mean OD value < 0.0623	
		LPC (200 ng/mL)	Mean SNR value: 1.381–2.067	
		MPC (1000 ng/mL)	Mean SNR value: 3.446–6.184	
		HPC (10,000 ng/mL)	Mean SNR value: 28.388–23.859	

continued

Table 6.31 (continued)

Investigation items	Acceptance criteria	Sample names	Test results	Result evaluation
Titer test (three analytical runs investigated)	Intra-run and inter-run %CV of OD values were ≤30%	NC samples	Intra-run %CV: 6.7%–15.2% Inter-run %CV: 11.4%	Pass
	Intra-run and inter-run %CV of SNR values were ≤20%	LPC (200 ng/mL)	Intra-run %CV: 2.0%–5.0% Inter-run %CV: 3.0%	
		MPC (1000 ng/mL)	Intra-run %CV: 6.0%–9.0% Inter-run %CV: 7.3%	
		HPC (10,000 ng/mL)	Intra-run %CV: 4.3%–9.1% Inter-run %CV: 7.3%	
	Intra-run and inter-run %CV of OD value of NC was ≤30% Intra-run and inter-run %CV of the SNR value of quality control was ≤20% The %CV of the SNR value of the titer sample was greater than the OD value among replicate wells of the SCP was ≤20% The %CV of the SNR value of the titer sample was less than the OD value among replicate wells of the SCP, which was ≤30%	C01 (2500 ng/mL)	Intra-run %CV: 1.9%–7.5% Inter-run %CV: 6.8%	
		C02 (1250 ng/mL)	Intra-run %CV: 3.3%–5.3% Inter-run %CV: 6.4%	
		C03 (625 ng/mL)	Intra-run %CV: 1.8%–6.1% Inter-run %CV: 6.3%	
		C04 (312.5 ng/mL)	Intra-run %CV: 0.8%–2.9% Inter-run %CV: 4.2%	
		C05 (156.25 ng/mL)	Intra-run %CV: 0.6%–1.3% Inter-run %CV: 3.9%	
		C06 (78.13 ng/mL)	Intra-run %CV: 0.9%–2.5% Inter-run %CV: 2.0%	
		C07 (39.06 ng/mL)	Intra-run %CV: 0.8%–3.4% Inter-run %CV: 4.7%	
		C08 (19.53 ng/mL)	Intra-run %CV: 0.6%–1.2% Inter-run %CV: 2.1%	
		C09 (9.77 ng/mL)	Intra-run %CV: 1.8%–4.1% Inter-run %CV: 4.3%	
		C10 (4.88 ng/mL)	Intra-run %CV: 1.0%–1.3% Inter-run %CV: 2.8%	
Hook effect	The OD value of Hook1 should be greater than HPC	The OD value of Hook1 (200,000 ng/mL) was greater than that of HPC		Pass
	The OD value of Hook2 should be greater than HPC	The OD value of Hook2 (100,000 ng/mL) was greater than that of HPC		
	The OD value of Hook3 should be lower than LPC	The OD value of Hook3 (1 ng/mL) was lower than that of LPC		

continued

Table 6.31 (continued)

Investigation items	Acceptance criteria	Sample names	Test results	Result evaluation
Hemolytic effect	At least 80% of the difference rates between HE-LPC and LPC were within the range of ±30%	All samples: HE-LPC difference rate: 4.1%–14.1%		Pass
	At least 80% of HE-NC were screened as negative	All samples: Screened as negative, SNR < SCP		
Selectivity	At least 80% of the difference rates between S-LPC and LPC were within the range of ±30%,	All samples: S-LPC difference rate: −6.0% to 4.4%		Pass
	At least 80% of S-NC were screened as negative	All samples: Screened as negative, SNR < SCP		
Stability	The different rates of 2/3 of the stability samples and those freshly prepared were within the range of ±20%.	2°C–8°C 24 h stability	All samples: 2.5%–11.5%	Pass
		RT 24 h stability	All samples: −4.8% to 16.6%	
		Stability after three repeated freezing–thawing cycles	All samples: −9.7% to 6.3%	
		Stability after five repeated freezing–thawing cycles	All samples: −2.9% to 0.0%	
TQ001 drug resistance"	When positive antibodies were 200 ng/mL, the concentration of the test article TQ001 injection in the highest tolerable serum was 250 μg/mL. When positive antibodies were 10,000 ng/mL, the concentration of the test article TQ001 injection in the highest tolerable serum was 5000 μg/mL.			

6.9.22.2 Test Article 2

Identity: TQ002 injection

Specification: 50 mg/0.5 mL each vial

Content or concentration: 100 mg/mL(COA concentration)

Stability: Stable under storage conditions and within expiration date

Expiration date: xxx/xxx/xxx

Storage condition: 2°C–8°C, away from light

Transport environment: Cold chain transportation

Preparation method: Raw liquid administration with no need for preparation.

6.9.23 Animal Information

(1) Species, strain, and grade: Cynomolgus monkeys, conventional.

(2) Sex and quantity: three pregnant cynomolgus monkeys and three male cynomolgus monkeys.

(3) Body weight and age range: The weight of pregnant cynomolgus monkeys was 3.66–4.94 kg during the gestation period and 3.48–3.68 kg during the lactation period, and they were 4–6 years old. Male cynomolgus monkeys were 2.78–3.70 kg, 3–5 years old.

(4) Animal source: Spare animals of the testing facility that passed the quarantine were applied for the study. The spare animals were purchased from the xxx company.

(5) Laboratory Animal Production Permission No.: SCXK(X)20180006, issued by the Department of Science and Technology of xxx.

(6) Laboratory Animal Use Permission No.: SYXK(X)20210090 issued by the Department of Science and Technology of xxx.

(7) Rationale for selection of study system: Both TQ001 and TQ002 are IgG1 monoclonal antibodies, and the cynomolgus monkey is the only animal species related to the target of the two monoclonal antibody drugs. Cynomolgus monkey was selected for nonclinical safety evaluation of the two drugs, so the cynomolgus monkey was selected as the research species for the pharmacokinetic exploration study of the reproductive system.

(8) Animal identification: Animals were numbered according to the laboratory animal numbering and grouping procedures of the institution, and the animal number corresponded to the ID number of the animal, and each animal had a unique marking number.

(9) Feed and Drinking Water

1) Feed: Cynomolgus monkey maintenance feed was produced by xxx company, batch No. 21128211, 22048211, 22058231, etc. Feed suppliers entrusted a qualified unit to conduct test on feed nutritional components, chemical pollutants and microbial parameters under the parameters specified in GB 14924.32010 and GB 14924.22001, and provided test reports to the facility; the facility entrusted a qualified test unit to conduct annual test on chemical pollutants and microbial parameters and the results met GB 14924.22001; the facility conducted quarterly test on the total number of bacterial colonies under the parameters specified in GB 4789.22022; all the test parameters of the feed met the requirements.

2) Drinking water: The drinking water for laboratory animals was purified by the facility. The facility entrusted a qualified unit to conduct annual tests on microorganisms, chemical contaminants, and toxic substances under the parameters specified in GB 57492006; the facility conducted quarterly tests on the total number of bacterial colonies under the parameters specified in GB 4789.22016; all the test parameters of the drinking water met the requirements.

(10) Animal husbandry conditions and environment: The animals were housed separately in the stainless cages with a size of 900 mm × 1000 mm × 2080 mm in a conventional monkey observation room. Water and feed were provided ad libitum. Room temperature was set at 22.8°C–25.3°C (diurnal temperature range ≤ 4°C), humidity 25.8%–99.9%, air changes ≥8 times/h, working illumination ≥200 Lux, animal illumination 100–200 Lux, 12-h light/12-h darkness, and fresh wind. Except for the humidity, all other parameters met the requirements of GB 149252010.

(11) Animal welfare: All animal welfare involved in this study complied with the Animals Welfare Guidelines of xxx (Guideline No.: GAWxxxx). The management and use of animals during the study were in line with the *Guide for the Care and Use of Laboratory Animals* (2011) and *the Laboratory Animal Management Regulations* revised in 2017 by the State Scientific and Technological Commission. The management, use, and relevant procedures of the animals involved in this study were reviewed and approved by the Institutional Animal Care and Use Committee (IACUC) of xxx, Approval No.: IACUC (Approved)xxxxxxx.

6.9.24 Grouping and Dosage Design

There was a total of six animals, three males and three pregnant animals, and the final test procedure for each animal was slightly different because the pregnancy was ended by natural delivery. At the first dose (D_1), all animals were administered via subcutaneous injection of TQ001 5 mg/kg and TQ002 3 mg/kg simultaneously.

In order to observe placental barrier permeability and ensure a high maternal drug concentration during delivery, 1F01 was administered 5 mg/kg TQ001 and 3 mg/kg TQ002 simultaneously via subcutaneous injection, respectively, on D_{18}, D_{25}, and D_{32} after the first dose.

1M01 was administered 5 mg/kg TQ001 and 3 mg/kg TQ002 simultaneously via subcutaneous injection, respectively on D_{18} and D_{25} after the first dose and was found died on D_{30}.

After the first dose on D_{50} (day 15 after delivery), 2F01 was subcutaneously administered 0.5 mg/kg TQ002. After the first dose on D_{50} (day 5 after delivery), 3F01 was subcutaneously administered 3 mg/kg TQ002.

After the administration on D_1, PK, and ADA blood samples were collected from 2M01 and 3M01, the animals were returned to the animal house. The design and grouping of the tests are shown in Table 6.32 and Fig. 6.34.

6.9.25 Rationale for Dosage Design

TQ001 and TQ002 are biosimilar drugs of two listed IgG1 drugs, respectively. The maximum clinical dose of the marketed control article of TQ001 is 5 mg/kg, and the clinical dose of the marketed control article of TQ002 is 0.833 mg/kg. The nonclinical pharmacokinetic studies of TQ001 and TQ002 in cynomolgus monkeys were set at subcutaneous doses of 3 mg/kg and 10 mg/kg. The doses of TQ001 and TQ002 are 5 and 3 mg/kg, respectively.

6.9.26 PK Sampling Point Setting and Basis

As specified in *Technical Guidance for NonClinical Pharmacokinetic Studies of Chemical Pharmaceuticals*, in order to obtain a complete blood concentration–time curve after administration, the design of sampling time points should take into account the absorption phase, equilibrium phase (near peak concentration), and elimination phase of drugs. The entire sampling time should last for three to five half-lives, or until the blood concentration is 1/10 to 1/20 of C_{max}. In order to ensure the optimal sampling point, it is recommended to conduct a preliminary test before the formal test, and then review and revise the sampling point of the original design according to the results of the preliminary test.

Preliminary test results of TQ001: The blood sampling points designed for a single-dose preliminary pharmacokinetics study of TQ001 in cynomolgus monkey via

Table 6.32 Study design and animal grouping

Animal ID	Test article	Administration time and frequency	Dosage(mg/kg)	Clinical maximum dose multiple	Study phase	Experimental endpoint/ parturition time
1M01	TQ001	$D_1/D_{18}/D_{25}$	5	1	D_1–D_{18} D_{18}–D_{25} D_{25}–D_{30}	Died on D_{30}
	TQ002	$D_1/D_{18}/D_{25}$	3	3.6		
1F01	TQ001	$D_1/D_{18}/D_{25}/D_{32}$	5	1	D_1–D_{18} D_{18}–D_{25} D_{25}–D_{32} D_{25}–D_{42}	Both pregnant monkeys that gave birth and their fetuses died on D_{42}
	TQ002	$D_1/D_{18}/D_{25}/D_{32}$	3	3.6		
2M01/3M02	TQ001	D_1	5	1	D_1–D_{43}	Sampling was completed, and the animals were returned to the animal room
	TQ002	D_1	3	3.6		
2F01	TQ001	D_1	5	1	D_1–D_{43}	Gave birth on D_{35}, the fetus survived. Sampling was completed, and the animals were returned to the animal room
	TQ002	D_1/D_{50}	3/0.5	3.6	D_1–D_{43} D_{50}–D_{67}	
3F01	TQ001	D_1	5	1	D_1–D_{43}	Gave birth on D_{45}; the fetus died. Sampling was completed, and the animals were returned to the animal room
	TQ002	D_1/D_{50}	3/3	3.6	D_1–D_{43} D_{50}–D_{67}	

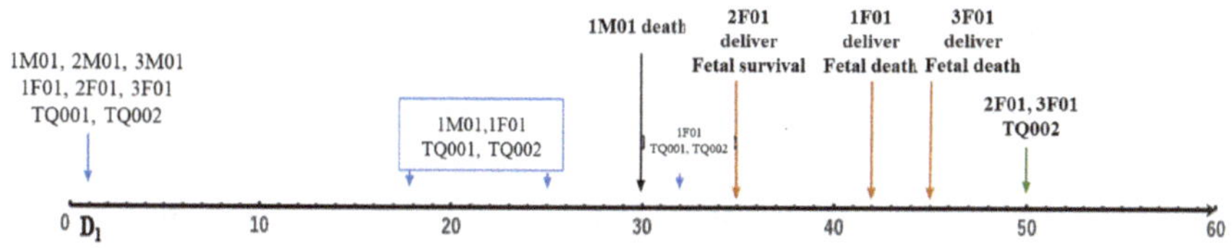

Fig. 6.34 Key time point design for subcutaneous administration of TQ001 and TQ002 in cynomolgus monkeys

subcutaneous injection are as follows: Before administration (0 h), 1 h, 3 h, 6 h, 10 h, 24 h (D_2), 48 h (D_3), 72 h (D_4), 120 h (D_6), 168 h (D_8), 240 h (D_{11}), 336 h (D_{15}), 408 h (D_{18}), 504 h (D_{22}), 576 h (D_{25}), 672 h (D_{29}), 840 h (D_{36}), 1008 h (D_{43}) and 1344 h (D_{57}) post-dose, the T_{max} of the four animals TQ001 (5 and 15 mg/kg) ranged from 10 to 48 h, and the $T_{1/2}$ ranged from 10.45 to 16.76 days.

Preliminary test results of TQ002: The blood sampling points designed for a single-dose preliminary pharmacokinetics study of TQ001 in cynomolgus monkey via subcutaneous injection are as follows: Before administration (0 h), 1 h, 3 h, 6 h, 10 h, 24 h (D_2), 48 h (D_3), 72 h (D_4), 120 h (D_6), 168 h (D_8), 240 h (D_{11}), 336 h (D_{15}), 408 h (D_{18}), 504 h (D_{22}), 576 h (D_{25}), 672 h (D_{29}), 840 h (D_{36}), 1008 h (D_{43}) and 1344 h (D_{57}) post-dose, the measured T_{max} of TQ002 (3 and 10 mg/kg) ranged from 6 to 72 h, and the $T_{1/2}$ of the four animals ranged from 16.02 to 30.87 h, that was, 0.67–1.29 days. The maximum time for which the concentration can be detected at the end was 576 h (D_{25}).

In summary, the sampling time of 2M01, 2F01, 3M01 and 3F01 in all animals after the first dose was before administration (0 h), 1 h, 3 h, 6 h, 10 h, 24 h (D_2), 48 h (D_3), 72 h (D_4), 120 h (D_6), 168 h (D_8), 240 h (D_{11}), 336 h (D_{15}), 408 h (D_{18}), 504 h (D_{22}), 576 h (D_{25}), 672 h (D_{29}), 840 h (D_{36}), and 1008 h (D_{43}) post-dose. To observe the blood–milk barrier, 2F01 was subcutaneously administered 0.5 mg/kg TQ002 on D50 , and 3F01 was subcutaneously administered 3 mg/kg TQ002 on D50. The sampling points of milk and maternal serum were designed as follows: Before the second dose (0 h), 1 h, 6 h, 24 h (D_2), 48 h (D_3), 72 h (D_4), 120 h (D_6), 168 h (D_8), 240 h (D_{11}), 336 h (D_{15}), and 408 h (D_{18}) after the second dose.

The design of blood collection points is shown in Figs. 6.35 and 6.36.

PK blood collection point design: Before the first dose (0 h), 1 h, 4 h, 8 h, 24 h (D_2), 48 h (D_3), 96 h (D_5), 168 h (D_8), 240 h (D_{11}), 336 h (D_{15}), 408 h (D_{18}), 504 h (D_{22}), 672 h (D_{29}), 1008 h (D_{43}) post-dose.

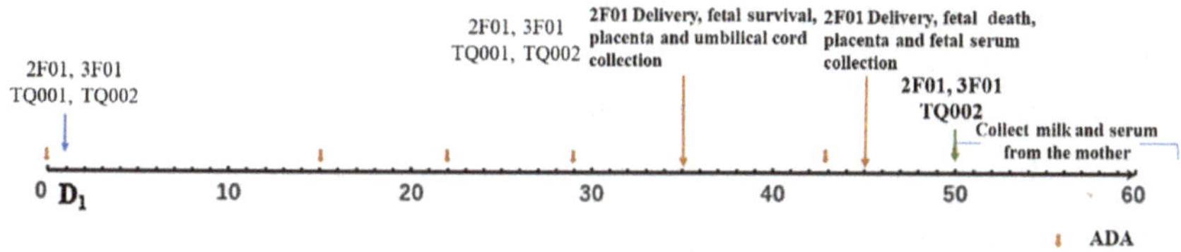

Fig. 6.35 The key sampling point design for subcutaneous administration of TQ001 and TQ002 in cynomolgus monkeys 2F01 and 3F01

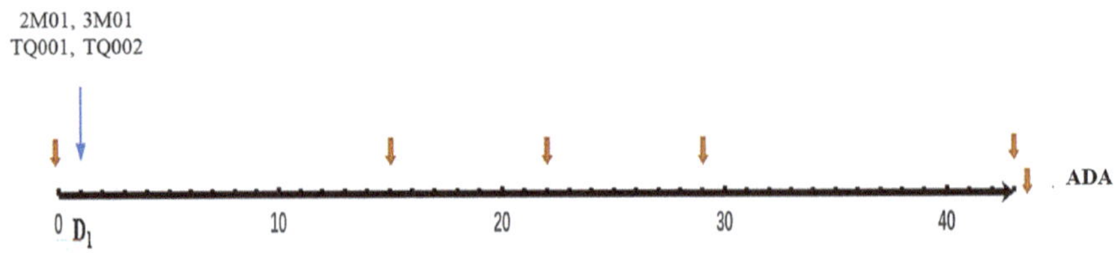

Fig. 6.36 The key sampling point design for subcutaneous administration of TQ001 and TQ002 in cynomolgus monkeys 2M01 and 3M01

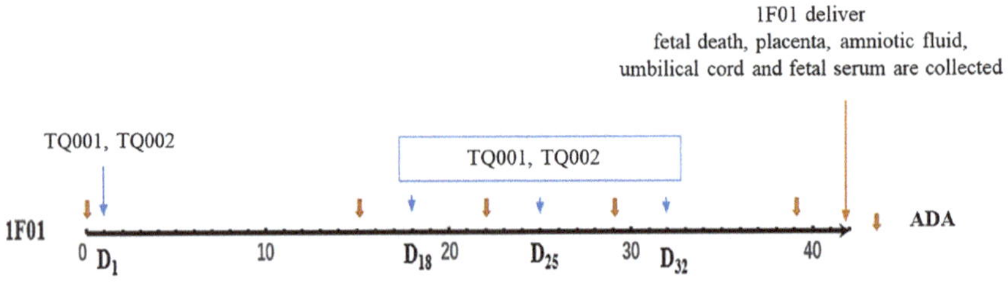

Fig. 6.37 The key sampling point design for subcutaneous administration of TQ001 and TQ002 in cynomolgus monkeys 1F01

Before the second dose (0 h), 1 h, 6 h, 24 h (D_2), 48 h (D_3), 72 h (D_4), 120 h (D_6), 168 h (D_8), 240 h (D_{11}), 336 h (D_{15}), 408 h (D_{18}) after the second dose.

PK blood collection point design: Before administration (0 h), 1 h, 4 h, 8 h, 24 h (D_2), 48 h (D_3), 96 h (D_5), 168 h (D_8), 240 h (D_{11}), 336 h (D_{15}), 408 h (D_{18}), 504 h (D_{22}), 672 h (D_{29}), 1008 h (D_{43}) post-dose.

In order to ensure that the maternal drug concentration was always at a high level during the animal delivery, 1F01 was simultaneously administered TQ001 and TQ002 on D_1, D_{18}, D_{25}, and D_{32}, respectively. The sampling points of 1F01 were: Before the first administration of D_1 (0 h), and 1 h, 4 h, 8 h, 24 h (D_2), 48 h (D_3), 96 h (D_5), 168 h (D_8), 240 h (D_{11}), 336 h (D_{15}), 408 h (D_{18}) post-dose; Before the second administration of D_{18} (0 h), and 1 h, 4 h, 8 h, 24 h (D_2), 72 h (D_4), 120 h (D_6), 168 h (D_8) post-dose; Before the third administration of D_{25} (0 h), and 1 h, 4 h, 8 h, 24 h (D_2), 48 h (D_3), 96 h (D_5), 168 h (D_8) post-dose; Before the fourth administration of D_{32} (0 h), and 1 h, 4 h, 8 h, 24 h (D_2), 48 h (D_3), 96 h (D_5), 168 h (D_8), 240 (D_{11}) post-dose. The design of blood collection points is shown in Fig. 6.37.

1M01 was the parallel control animal of 1F01, and 1M01 was administrated TQ001 and TQ002 simultaneously on D_1, D_{18} and D_{25}, respectively. The sampling points of 1M01 were as follows: Before the first administration of D_1 (0 h), and 1 h, 4 h, 8 h, 24 h(D_2), 48 h(D_3), 96 h(D_5), 168 h(D_8), 240 h(D_{11}),336 h(D_{15}), 408 h(D_{18}) post-dose; Before the second administration of D_{18} (0 h), and 1 h, 4 h, 8 h, 24 h (D_2), 72 h (D_4), 120 h (D_6), 168 h (D_8) post-dose; Before the third administration of D_{25} (0 h), 1 h, 4 h, 8 h, 24 h (D_2), 48 h (D_3), 96 h (D_5), 168 h (D_8) post-dose; Before the fourth administration

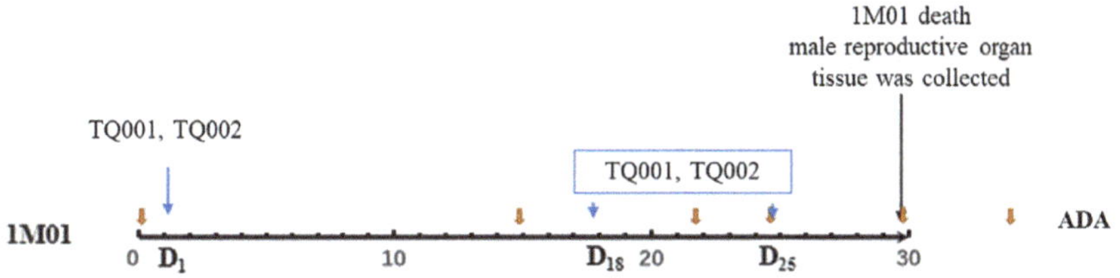

Fig. 6.38 The key sampling point design for subcutaneous administration of TQ001 and TQ002 in cynomolgus monkeys 1M01

of D_{32} (0 h), and 1 h, 4 h, 8 h, 24 h (D_2), 48 h (D_3), 96 h (D_5), 168 h (D_8), 240 (D_{11}) post-dose. The design of blood collection points is shown in Fig. 6.38.

PK blood collection point design: Before the first administration of D_1 (0 h), and 1 h, 4 h, 8 h, 24 h (D_2), 48 h (D_3), 96 h (D_5), 168 h (D_8), 240 h (D_{11}), 336 h (D_{15}), 408 h (D_{18}) post-dose; Before the second administration of D_{18} (0 h), and 1 h, 4 h, 8 h, 24 h (D_2), 72 h (D_4), 120 h (D_6), 168 h (D_8) post-dose; Before the third administration of D_{25} (0 h), and 1 h, 4 h, 8 h, 24 h (D_2), 48 h (D_3), 96 h (D_5), 168 h (D_8) post-dose; Before the fourth administration of D_{32} (0 h), and 1 h, 4 h, 8 h, 24 h (D_2), 48 h (D_3), 96 h (D_5), 168 h (D_8), 240 (D_{11}) post-dose.

PK blood collection point design: Before the first administration of D_1 (0 h), and 1 h, 4 h, 8 h, 24 h(D_2), 48 h(D_3), 96 h(D_5), 168 h(D_8), 240 h(D_{11}),336 h(D_{15}), 408 h(D_{18}) post-dose; Before the second administration of D_{18} (0 h), and 1 h, 4 h, 8 h, 24 h (D_2), 72 h (D_4), 120 h (D_6), 168 h (D_8) post-dose; Before the third administration of D_{25} (0 h), 1 h, 4 h, 8 h, 24 h (D_2), 48 h (D_3), 96 h (D_5), 168 h (D_8) post-dose; Before the fourth administration of D_{32} (0 h), and 1 h, 4 h, 8 h, 24 h (D_2), 48 h (D_3), 96 h (D_5), 168 h (D_8), 240 (D_{11}) post-dose.

Male reproductive organs (testis, epididymis, seminal vesicle, and adrenal gland) and serum were collected from a 1M01 male animal on the day of death, and the tissue distribution of male reproductive organs was observed.

After delivery on D_{42}, placenta, umbilical cord, amniotic fluid, and fetal serum were collected from 1F01. After delivery on D_{35}, the placenta and umbilical cord were collected from 2F01, and maternal and fetal serum were collected on day 5 after delivery. After delivery on D_{45}, placenta and fetal serum were collected from 3F01.

6.9.27 ADA Sampling Point Settings

1M01: Serum (D_{-1}, D_{15}, D_{22}, and D_{25}), tissue homogenate (D_{30}) of testis, epididymis, seminal vesicle, and adrenal gland.

2M01: Serum (D_{-1}, D_{15}, D_{22}, and D_{29}).

3M01: Serum (D_{-1}, D_{15}, D_{22}, and D_{29}).

1F01: Serum (D_{-1}, D_{15}, D_{22} D_{39}, and D_{42}), placenta, amniotic fluid, umbilical cord and fetal serum (D_{42}).

2F01: Serum (D_{-1}, D_{15}, D_{22} D_{29}, D_{40}, and D_{50}), placenta, umbilical cord and fetal serum (D_{40}) and milk (D_{50}).

3F01: Serum (D_{-1}, D_{15}, D_{22} D_{25}, D_{29}, D_{45}, and D_{50}), placenta and fetal serum (D_{45}) and milk (D_{50} and D_{67}).

6.9.28 Administration Method

1. Administration frequency of TQ001: 1M01 ($D_1/D_{18}/D_{25}$), 1F01 ($D_1/D_{18}/D_{25}/D_{32}$), 2M01 (D_1), 2F01 (D_1), 3M01 (D_1) and 3F01 (D_1). TQ002: 1M01 ($D_1/D_{18}/D_{25}$), 1F01 ($D_1/D_{18}/D_{25}/D_{32}$), 2M01 (D_1), 2F01 (D_1/D_{50}), 3M01 (D_1) and 3F01 (D_1/D_{50}).
2. Route of administration: Subcutaneous injection.
3. The dosage of TQ001 was 33.3 μL/kg and TQ002 was 30 μL/kg. The administration was performed in equal concentration and unequal volume via single-point injection. The absolute dose volume of each animal (in mL, two decimal places reserved, 0.01 mL) was calculated from the animal's most recently recorded body weight. The actual dosage volume was extracted according to the syringe scale.

6.9.29 Study Method

1. Animal quarantine. All cynomolgus monkeys need to be quarantined for 15 days after acceptance. The animals entering the test are the animals that have passed the quarantine of the institution, and the female animals are all animals in the middle and late gestation period, GD_{90}–GD_{120}.
2. Adaptive training. All animals began to carry out adaptive training during the adaptive feeding period, and the cynomolgus monkeys were trained to sit in the monkey chair and simulate the operation process. Six animals that passed the training were selected to enter the formal test.
3. General observation Observe at least once a day in the morning or afternoon, and the main observation contents are appearance signs, behavior activities, animal posture, diet, hair, irritation response, glandular secretions, excreta, respiratory status, and death.
4. The dosage volume of each animal was calculated according to the weight of the animal at the last weighing before administration (usually the weight at weighing and grouping the day before administration). The dosage volume was accurate to two decimal places (0.01 mL), and a single point of injection was performed under the skin of both hind limbs of the animal. Before injection, the hind limbs of the animal to be injected were shaved, and the injection site was cleaned with an alcohol cotton ball. And allow to air dry before injection.
5. Serum and tissue samples were collected according to the designed time point. During serum collection, about 1 mL of blood was collected from the limb vein (avoiding the drug administration site), and whole blood was collected into the collection vessels containing coagulant and separation gel. The placenta, umbilical cord, testis, epididymis, seminal vesicle, and adrenal gland were collected. The samples were

rinsed with normal saline and packed into a 2 mL centrifuge tube. Two parts of the tissues were collected, and the tissue samples were weighed. The first part was about 100 mg, and the second was unlimited in weight. The collected tissue samples were temporarily stored in the ultra-low temperature refrigerator at −80°C after being frozen in liquid nitrogen. After the fetus died, after birth, the fetus was necropsied, and 1 mL of whole blood was drawn from the heart and collected into a collection tube containing coagulant and separation gel. The amniotic fluid from the mother was sucked into a 1 mL centrifuge tube with a pipette. Two tubes were collected, and the detection tube was not less than 100 μL. The milk was collected into 1 mL centrifuge tubes; 2 tubes were collected at each time point, and the detection tubes were not less than 100 μL.

6. Sample Processing

(1) Serum: Whole blood was collected into the collection tube and centrifuged at 1800 × *g* for 10 min after blood coagulation. The collected serum was divided into two parts, labeled according to the method of blood sample identification, and placed in the ultra-low temperature refrigerator at −80°C for temporary storage. After sample collection, it should be placed at room temperature for no more than 2 h.

(2) Tissue homogenate: Tissue homogenate was prepared before the test, and the homogenate was added to the sample according to the weight-to-volume ratio (W:V) 1:9 (Homogenate was prepared from sterile PBS, containing PMSF, DTT, and protease inhibitor. Preparation method: Take 100 μL 100 mmol/L PMSF, 10 μL 1 mol/L DTT, and 1 tablet of protease inhibitor, add them into 9.890 mL PBS, mix well, and grind in the frozen grinder (conditions of the frozen grinder are set as follows: Run time is 50 s, interrupt time is 1 s, frequency is set at 60 Hz, temperature is 4°C, and grinding times is ten times). After grinding, centrifuge at 10,000 × *g*, 4°C, for 10 min, transfer the supernatant to the marked centrifuge tube/frozen storage tube (at least three parts, each about 200 μL), and put it into the ultra-low temperature refrigerator at −80°C for temporary storage.

7. Sample Testing The drug concentration and antidrug antibody (ADA) in the samples of cynomolgus monkeys were determined by ELISA. OD values were issued by SoftMax Pro 7.1.2GxP, the built-in software of the multimode reader, and the test results were statistically analyzed by Excel software.

8. Statistic Analysis of Data Prism GraphPad was used to draw the concentration–time curve, and Phoenix WinNonlin 8.3.2 was used to calculate the following pharmacokinetic parameters according to the non-compartmental model: Half-life ($T_{1/2}$), maximum blood concentration (C_{max}), peak time (T_{max}), area under drug time curve (AUC_{0-t} and $AUC_{0-\infty}$), apparent volume of distribution (Vd), clearance rate (Cl), average residence time (MRT_{0-t} and $MRT_{0-\infty}$) and other parameters. $T_{1/2}$, C_{max}, Vd, MRT_{0-t}, and $MRT_{0-\infty}$ retained two decimal places. Cl retained three decimals, AUC_{0-t} and $AUC_{0-\infty}$ retained integers.

T_{max} and C_{max} were directly obtained from the blood concentration–time curve. AUC_{0-t} was calculated by the linear ladder method, and t was the time of the last quantifiable blood concentration. $AUC_{0-\infty} = AUC_{0-t} + C_t/\lambda_z$, C_t was the blood concentration at the last quantifiable time point, λ_z was the end elimination rate constant (Bestfit method); $t_{1/2} = 0.693/\lambda_z$; MRT = AUMC/AUC; $Cl = D/AUC_{0-\infty}$ (*D* was the dosage); $V = Cl \times MRT_{0-\infty}$; $AUC\_\%_{Extrap} = (1 - AUC_{0-t}/AUC_{0-\infty}) \times 100$.

BLQ (below the lower limit of quantitation) was defined before concentration data were imported into WinNonlin 8.3.2 software: BLQ was defined as 0 before the presence of C_{max}, and is defined as missing after the presence of C_{max}. The case of no samples was defined as NS.

Excel was used to sort out the data. Except for the drug concentration data after the first dose, only individual data were listed, and statistical analysis was not carried out due to the small number of animals. The drug concentration and pharmacokinetic parameters after the first dose were analyzed by a *t*-test using Excel software. As discrete data, T_{max} was usually statistically analyzed using a nonparametric test (Wilcoxon method), and $T_{1/2}$ statistics were performed using an independent-samples *t* test.

9. Result

(1) General state observation: 1M01 was found died on D_{30}, while 2M01 and 3M01 were normal. During the delivery of 1F01 on D_{42}, there was massive bleeding, the fetus and the mother were found dead, and no abnormality was observed in the fetus. 2F01 was delivered normally, and the fetus was in a normal state. After 3F01 was delivered at night, a wound in the mouth of the fetus was observed the next day, and the fetus was found to have died, but no deformity was observed. The cause of death could not be determined, whether it was related to drug administration.

(2) TQ001 Drug concentration detection: After all animals were administered 5 mg/kg TQ001 subcutaneously for the first time, the results of drug concentration in the serum of the animals were shown in Table 6.33, and the curve of drug concentration over time was shown in Fig. 6.39. It could be seen that in 1–24 h, the ratio of drug concentration of female animals to that of male animals was less than or equal to 0.5, and the concentration of female animals was lower than that of male animals. To ensure that the maternal drug concentration was always at a high level during delivery, 1F01 was administered TQ001 on D_1, D_{18}, D_{25}, and D_{32}, and 1M01 was the parallel control animal of 1F01, and 1M01 was administered TQ001 on D_1, D_{18}, and D_{25}, respectively. The drug concentration–time curves for 1F01 and 1M01 are shown in Fig. 6.42.

(3) TQ002 Drug concentration detection: After subcutaneous administration of 3 mg/kg TQ002 for the first time in all animals, the results of serum drug concentration were shown in Table 6.34, and the curve of drug concentration over time was shown in Fig. 6.40. After curve fitting the average drug concentration after the first administration of TQ001 and TQ002, the change curve of drug concentration over time is shown in Fig. 6.41. It could be seen that in 1–48 h, the ratio of drug concentration of female animals to that of male animals was less than or equal to 0.5, and the concentration of female animals was lower than that of male animals. To ensure that the maternal drug concentration was always at a high level during delivery, 1F01 was administered TQ002 on D_1, D_{18}, D_{25}, and D_{32}, and 1M01 was the parallel control animal of 1F01, and 1M01 was administrated TQ002 on D_1, D_{18}, and D_{25}, respectively. The drug concentration–time curves for 1F01 and 1M01 are shown in Fig. 6.42.

(4) Pharmacokinetic parameter analysis: After subcutaneous administration of 5 mg/kg TQ001 and 3 mg/kg TQ002 for the first time in all animals, there were no statistically significant differences in the major pharmacokinetic parameters $T_{1/2}$, C_{max}, AUC_{0-t}, $AUC_{0-\infty}$, Vd, Cl, MRT_{0-t} and $MRT_{0-\infty}$ between female animals during gestation and male animals (P>0.05), the ratio was greater than 0.5 and less than 2, no statistical

Table 6.33 Individual drug concentration (ng/mL) in the serum of cynomolgus monkey after subcutaneous injection of TQ001 (5 mg/kg)

Time (h)	1M01	2M01	3M01	1F01	2F01	3F01	Malemean	Femalemean	Female/maleratio	n
0	BLQ	BLQ	BLQ	BLQ	BLQ	BLQ	BLQ	BLQ	–	6
1	254	2131	851	680	406	537	1079	541	0.50	6
4	12,539	29,663	20,897	6958	2792	3608	21033	4453	0.21	6
8	35,713	54,151	47,215	19,223	7677	10,165	45,693	12,355	0.27	6
24	54,758	59,703	55,746	33,483	20,911	19,220	56,736	24,538	0.43	6
48	58,805	61,706	59,962	43,374	32,998	26,541	60,158	34,304	0.57	6
96	54,846	53,526	57,224	55,947	41,440	29,801	55,199	42,396	0.77	6
168	45,693	44,219	32,669	52,017	41,876	28,749	40,860	40,881	1.00	6
240	46,314	40,658	27,153	45,304	33,645	26,011	38,042	34,987	0.92	6
336	38,322	29,647	19,903	35,790	24,300	24,847	29,291	28,312	0.97	6
408		26,632	18,223		19,041	22,490	22,428	20,766	0.93	4
504		21,811	14,789		9880	15,721	18,300	12,801	0.70	4
576		18,529	12,717		5608	12,599	15,623	9104	0.58	4
672	–	14,081	10,169	–	2649	9784	12,125	6217	0.51	4
840		9974	6741		1464	5945	8358	3705	0.44	4
1008		6784	4756		890	3590	5770	2240	0.39	4

Note: –, no relevant data; BLQ, the detected concentration was below LLOQ; The concentration data was back-calculated using the software SoftMax Pro 7.1.2 of the microplate reader, and the concentration values were rounded to integers using Excel software.

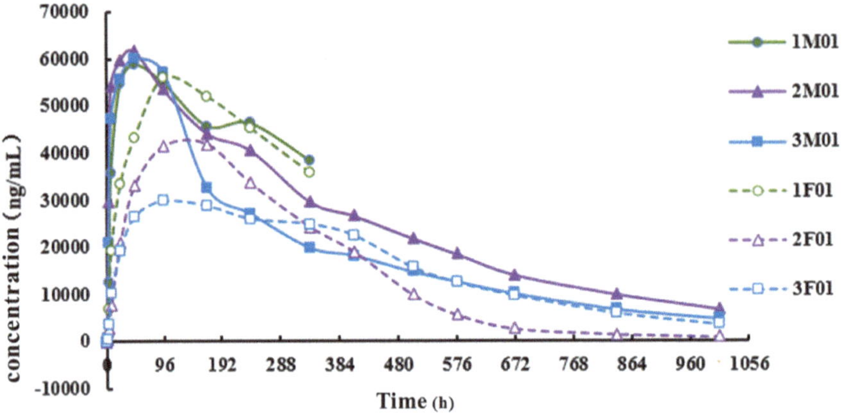

Fig. 6.39 Serum drug concentration–time curve of animals administered TQ001 subcutaneously in cynomolgus monkeys(ng/mL)

difference was found, but the T_{max} of female animals during gestation was greater than that of male animals, and the drug exposure was less than that of male animals. This trend was not observed in nonpregnant females and males (Tables 6.35–6.37).

(5) Drug distribution in male reproductive organs: After the simultaneous administration of 5 mg/kg TQ001 and 3 mg/kg TQ002 on D_1, D_{18}, and D_{25}, respectively, 1M01 was found died on D_{30}. After sampling testis, epididymis, seminal gland, adrenal gland, and serum, the concentration of drugs in the homogenate of male reproductive organs was detected. The results showed that a small amount of the drug was distributed to the male reproductive organs (Table 6.38).

(6) Drug transplacental barrier studies: The placenta, umbilical cord, amniotic fluid, and fetal serum were collected after delivery of 1F01 on D_{42}. The placenta and umbilical cord of the 2F01 were collected after delivery on D_{35}, and maternal and fetal serum were collected on day 5 after delivery. After the birth of 3F01 on D_{45}, the placenta and fetal serum were collected. The results showed that drugs could cross the placental barrier into the placenta, amniotic fluid, and the fetus, but were less distributed in the umbilical cord tissue (Table 6.39).

(7) Studies on blood–milk barrier permeability of drugs: To observe the blood–milk barrier, 2F01 was administered 0.5 mg/kg TQ002 on D_{50} (day 15 after delivery), and 3F01 was administered 3 mg/kg TQ002 on D_{50} (day 5 after delivery). The sampling points of milk and maternal serum were designed as follows: Before the second dose (0 h), 1 h, 6 h, 24 h (D_2), 48 h (D_3), 72 h (D_4), 120 h (D_6), 168 h (D_8), 240 h (D_{11}), 336 h (D_{15}), and 408 h (D_{18}) after the second dose. Drug concentrations in serum and milk of TQ001 and TQ002 female monkeys were measured, and results showed that only a small amount of drugs could cross the blood–milk barrier into mature milk (Table 6.40).

(8) Production of antidrug antibodies against TQ001 and TQ002 in the serum of cynomolgus monkeys: A summary of serum antibody titers against TQ001 and TQ002

Table 6.34 Individual drug concentration in the serum of cynomolgus monkeys after subcutaneous injection of TQ002 (ng/mL)

Time (h)	1M01	2M01	3M01	1F01	2F01	3F01	Malemean	Femalemean	Female/Maleratio	n
0	0	0	0	0	0	0	0	0	–	6
1	2052	1151	1077	311	61	182	1427	185	0.13	6
4	11,211	8365	12,959	1608	727	971	10,845	1102	0.10	6
8	17,187	19,326	20,670	3898	1941	3366	19,061	3068	0.16	6
24	21,398	23,178	20,398	8252	5982	8504	21,658	7579	0.35	6
48	20,402	28,625	21,697	10,735	11,381	12,269	23,575	11,462	0.49	6
96	18,077	24,686	18,487	11,649	15,440	12,215	20,417	13,101	0.64	6
168	16,315	18,774	11,739	12,654	13,489	10,269	15,609	12,137	0.78	6
240	12,759	15,559	9608	10,993	11,321	9296	12,642	10,537	0.83	6
336	9918	9002	7063	7408	8188	7696	8661	7764	0.90	6
408	–	6696	5789	–	6576	5408	6243	5992	0.96	4
504		3325	4671		3912	4657	3998	4285	1.07	4
576		1953	3243		2537	4353	2598	3445	1.33	4
672		890	2709		1526	3317	1800	2422	1.35	4
840		346	1861		796	1889	1104	1343	1.22	4
1008		107	1205		492	768	656	630	0.96	4

Note: –, no relevant data; BLQ, the detected concentration was below LLOQ; The concentration data was back-calculated using the software SoftMax Pro 7.1.2 of the microplate reader, and the concentration values were rounded to integers using Excel software.

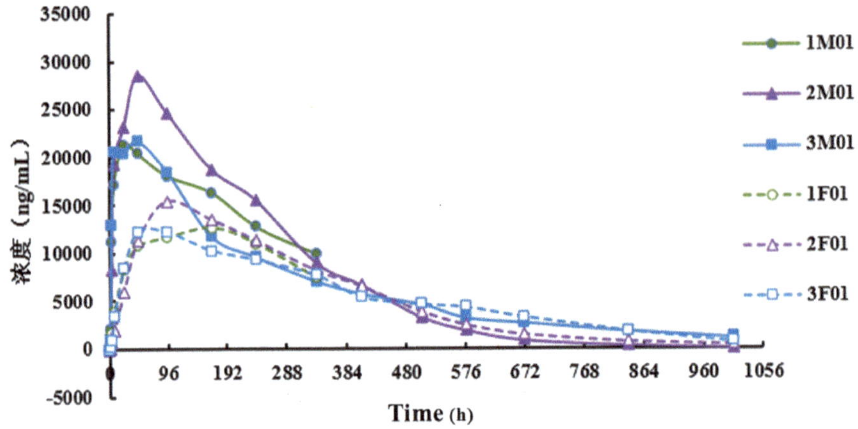

Fig. 6.40 Serum drug concentration–time curve of animals administered TQ002 subcutaneously in cynomolgus monkeys(ng/mL)

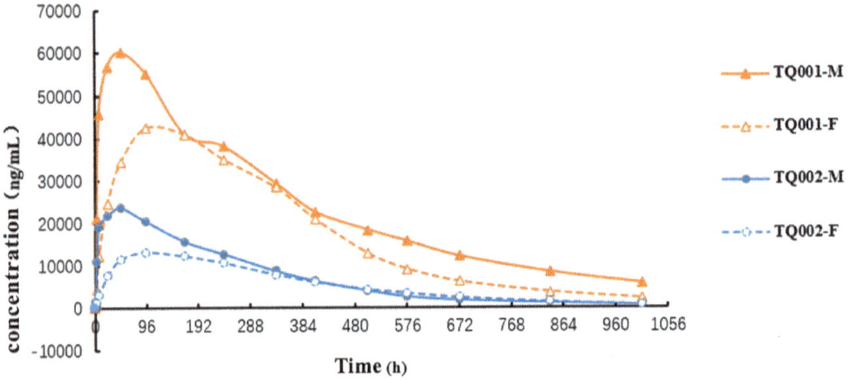

Fig. 6.41 Mean serum drug concentration–time curve of animals administered TQ001 and TQ002 subcutaneously in cynomolgus monkeys(ng/mL)

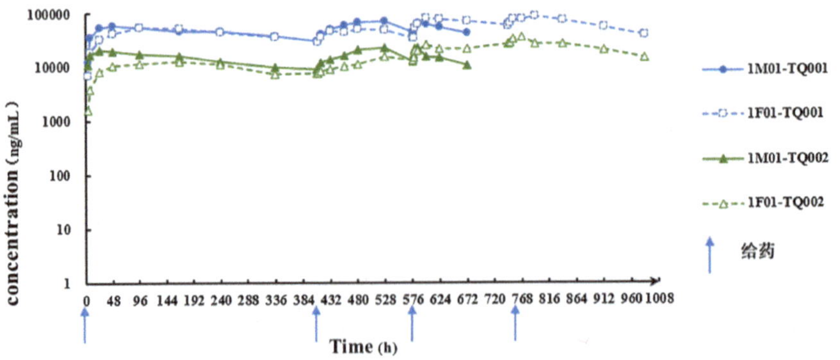

Fig. 6.42 Individual serum drug concentration–time curves of cynomolgus monkeys injected subcutaneously with repeated administration of TQ001 and TQ002

Table 6.35 Mean pharmacokinetic parameters after cynomolgus monkeys were given TQ001 and TQ002 via subcutaneous injection

Pharmacokinetic parameters	TQ001 (5 mg/kg)		TQ002 (3 mg/kg)	
	Female pregnant animals	Male animals	Female pregnant animals	Male animals
$T_{1/2}$ (h)	251.84 ± 50.99	373.56 ± 121.14	168.83 ± 7.19	208.66 ± 95.08
T_{max} (h)	96–168	48	48–168	24–48
C_{max} (ng/mL)	42541 ± 13086	60158 ± 1460	13454 ± 1730	23907 ± 4089
AUC_{0-t} (h*ng/mL)	15717624 ± 689176	20764796 ± 5103548	4874580 ± 1202806	6570217 ± 1316733
$AUC_{0-\infty}$ (h*ng/mL)	21540625 ± 8295260	31909615 ± 11245418	5723451 ± 69072	7864934 ± 667504
V_d (mL/kg)	87.9 ± 13.87	85.68 ± 11.97	127.64 ± 3.9	116.16 ± 57.7
Cl (mL/h/kg)	0.253 ± 0.081	0.169 ± 0.055	0.524 ± 0.006	0.383 ± 0.032
$MRT_{0-1176h}$ (h)	260.84 ± 94.06	263.43 ± 90.58	258.19 ± 82.97	209.29 ± 63.8
$MRT_{0-\infty}$ (h)	394.82 ± 106.99	532.74 ± 186.65	328.91 ± 46	305.72 ± 85.46

is shown in Table 6.41. The 2F01 and 3F01 animals produced antidrug antibodies against TQ001, and the 2M01, 1F01, 2F01, and 3F01 animals produced antidrug antibodies against TQ002, and the immunogenicity of TQ002 was slightly stronger than that of TQ001.

(9) Production of antidrug antibodies against TQ001 and TQ002 in each tissue: For each tissue homogenate, antidrug antibodies against TQ001 and TQ002 were detected. The detection results of male animals showed that no antidrug antibodies against TQ001 and TQ002 were detected in the testis, epididymis, seminal vesicle and adrenal gland of 1M01. When the mother produced antidrug antibodies against TQ001 or antidrug antibodies against TQ002, antidrug antibodies could be detected in both placenta and fetal serum, and the antidrug antibody titer in fetal serum was stronger than that of the mother, but it was not clear whether the antidrug antibodies in fetal serum were all from the mother. The detailed results are shown in Table 6.42.

10. Discussion After subcutaneous administration of 5 mg/kg TQ001 and 3 mg/kg TQ002 for the first time in all animals, there were no statistically significant differences in major pharmacokinetic parameters $T_{1/2}$, C_{max}, AUC_{0-t}, $AUC_{0-\infty}$, Vd, Cl, MRT_{0-t} and $MRT_{0-\infty}$ in pregnant animals and male animals (P>0.05), the ratio was greater than 0.5 and less than 2, no statistical difference was observed, but the T_{max} of female animals during pregnancy was greater than that of male animals, and the drug exposure was less than that of male animals. This trend was not observed in nonpregnant females or males. This phenomenon may be related to increased blood volume in pregnant animals.

After 1M01 was simultaneously administered 5 mg/kg TQ001 and 3 mg/kg TQ002 on D_1, D_{18}, and D_{25}, respectively, the animal was found died on D_{30}. After sampling testis, epididymis, seminal gland, adrenal gland, and serum, the concentration of the drug in the homogenate of male reproductive organs was detected. The results showed that a small amount of the drug was distributed to the male reproductive organs.

Table 6.36 Individual pharmacokinetic parameters of cynomolgus monkeys after subcutaneous injection of TQ001 (5 mg/kg)

Animal name	$T_{1/2}$(h)	T_{max}(h)	C_{max}(ng/mL)	AUC_{0-t}(h*ng/mL)	$AUC_{0-\infty}$(h*ng/mL)	$AUC_{\_\%Extrap}$(%)	V_d(mL/kg)	Cl(mL/h/kg)	MRT_{0-840h}(h)	$MRT_{0-\infty}$(h)
1F01	309.71	96	55,947	15,074,567	31,066,285	51.48	71.91	0.161	168.14	484.55
2F01	213.53	168	41,876	15,633,170	15,907,339	1.72	96.83	0.314	258.18	276.41
3F01	232.29	96	29,801	16,445,136	17,648,252	6.82	94.95	0.283	356.20	423.48
1M01	513.42	48	58,805	15,924,153	44,309,446	64.06	83.58	0.113	160.22	747.33
2M01	301.61	48	61,706	26,095,845	29,047,750	10.16	74.90	0.172	329.68	442.83
3M01	305.66	48	59,962	20,274,392	22,371,651	9.37	98.56	0.223	300.40	408.07
Female mean	251.84	96–168	42,541	15,717,624	21,540,625	20.01	87.90	0.253	260.84	394.82
SD	50.99	–	13,086	6,89,176	8,295,260	27.37	13.87	0.081	94.06	106.99
%CV	20.2	–	30.8	4.4	38.5	136.8	15.8	32.1	36.1	27.1
n	3	3	3	3	3	3	3	3	3	3
Male mean	373.56	48	60,158	20,764,796	31,909,615	27.87	85.68	0.169	263.43	532.74
SD	121.14	–	1460	5,103,548	11,245,418	31.35	11.97	0.055	90.58	186.65
%CV	32.4	–	2.4	24.6	35.2	112.5	14.0	32.7	34.4	35.0
n	3	3	3	3	3	3	3	3	3	3
Female–male ratio	0.7	/	0.7	0.8	0.7	/	1.0	1.5	1.0	0.7

Note: –, no relevant statistical data. Among them, the parameter T_{max} was a range value. The AUC_{0-t} of 1F01 and 1M01 represented 0–336 h, while that of the remaining animals represented 0–1008 h

Table 6.37 Individual pharmacokinetic parameters of cynomolgus monkeys after subcutaneous injection of TQ002 (3 mg/kg)

Animal name	$T_{1/2}$(h)	T_{max}(h)	C_{max}(ng/mL)	AUC_{0-t}(h*ng/mL)	$AUC_{0-\infty}$(h*ng/mL)	$AUC_{\_\%Extrap}$(%)	V_d(mL/kg)	Cl(mL/h/kg)	$MRT_{0-840\,h}$(h)	$MRT_{0-\infty}$(h)
1F01		168	12,654	3,485,754					167.57	
2F01	163.74	96	15,440	5,558,385	5,674,610	2.05	124.89	0.529	276.56	296.38
3F01	173.91	48	12,269	5,579,603	5,772,292	3.34	130.40	0.520	330.44	361.43
1M01	235.41	24	21,398	5,184,765	8,553,214	39.38	119.12	0.351	147.68	355.60
2M01	103.07	48	28,625	7,805,324	7,821,235	0.20	57.04	0.384	205.10	207.03
3M01	287.49	48	21,697	6,720,563	7,220,353	6.92	172.33	0.415	275.07	354.52
Female mean	168.83	48–168	13,454	4,874,580	5,723,451	2.69	127.64	0.524	258.19	328.91
SD	7.19	–	1730	1,202,806	69,072	0.91	3.90	0.006	82.97	46.00
%CV	4.3	–	12.9	24.7	1.2	33.9	3.1	1.2	32.1	14.0
n	2	3	3	3	2	2	2	2	3	2
Male mean	208.66	24–48	23,907	6,570,217	7,864,934	15.50	116.16	0.383	209.29	305.72
SD	95.08	–	4089	1,316,733	6,67,504	20.95	57.70	0.032	63.80	85.46
%CV	45.6	–	17.1	20.0	8.5	135.1	49.7	8.4	30.5	28.0
n	3	3	3	3	3	3	3	3	3	3
Female–male ratio	0.8	–	0.6	0.7	0.7	–	1.1	1.4	1.2	1.1

Note: –, no relevant statistical data. Among them, the parameter T_{max} was a range value. The AUC_{0-t} of 1F01 and 1M01 represented 0–336 h, while that of the remaining animals represented 0–1008 h

Table 6.38 Drug concentrations in the reproductive organs and serum of male cynomolgus monkeys after subcutaneous injection of TQ001 and TQ002

Tissue type	TQ001 5 mg/kg		TQ002 3 mg/kg	
	Concentration (ng/mL)	Ratio to serum %	Concentration (ng/mL)	Ratio to serum %
Testis	500	1.19	228	1.77
Epididymis	796	1.89	291	2.26
Seminal vesicle gland	467	1.11	178	1.38
Adrenal gland	347	0.82	196	1.52
Serum	42088	–	12861	–

Note: –, no such item

Table 6.39 Drug concentrations in the reproductive system and serum of female cynomolgus monkeys after subcutaneous injection of TQ001 and TQ002

Tissue type	TQ001 5 mg/kg			TQ002 3 mg/kg		
	1F01	2F01	3F01	1F01	2F01	3F01
Maternal serum	40,151	979	3037	15,043	582	511
Placenta	1110	BLQ	BLQ	632	BLQ	BLQ
Umbilical cord	BLQ	BLQ	–	36	BLQ	–
Amniotic fluid	3084	–	–	1238	–	–
Fetal serum	9083	BLQ	1855	1913	BLQ	38
Amniotic fluid/mother	7.68%	–	–	8.23%	–	–
Fetus/mother	22.62%	–	61.08%	12.72%	–	7.44%

Note: –, no such item. Among them, the fetuses of 1F01 and 3F01 died after birth. The serum of both the mother and the fetuses was collected at the time of parturition. For 2F01, the blood of the fetus was collected on the fifth day after birth, and the blood of its mother was also collected on the fifth day after parturition

The placenta, umbilical cord, amniotic fluid, and fetal serum were collected after delivery of 1F01 on D_{42}. The placenta and umbilical cord of the 2F01 were collected after delivery on D_{35}, and maternal and fetal serum were collected on day 5 after delivery. After the birth of 3F01 on D_{45}, the placenta and fetal serum were collected. The results showed that drugs could cross the placental barrier into the placenta, amniotic fluid, and the fetus, but were less distributed in the umbilical cord tissue.

To observe the blood–milk barrier, 2F01 was administered 0.5 mg/kg TQ002 on D_{50} (day 15 after delivery), and 3F01 was administered 3 mg/kg TQ002 on D_{50} (day 5 after delivery). The sampling points of milk and maternal serum were designed as follows: Before the second dose (0 h), 1 h, 6 h, 24 h (D_2), 48 h (D_3), 72 h (D_4), 120 h (D_6), 168 h (D_8), 240 h (D_{11}), 336 h (D_{15}), and 408 h (D_{18}) after the second dose. Drug concentrations in the serum and milk of TQ001 and TQ002 female monkeys were

Table 6.40 Drug concentrations in the serum and milk of cynomolgus monkeys dosed TQ001 and TQ002 via subcutaneous injection after parturition

Time (h)	TQ001				TQ002			
	Milk		Serum		Milk		Serum	
	2F01	3F01	2F01	3F01	2F01	3F01	2F01	3F01
0	BLQ	BLQ	439	2422	BLQ	BLQ	288	164
1	BLQ	BLQ	402	2251	34	BLQ	898	325
6	–	BLQ	410	1966	BLQ	BLQ	1643	3184
24	BLQ	BLQ	329	1758	BLQ	BLQ	2023	15,312
48	BLQ	BLQ	316	1613	32	31	2155	13,970
72	BLQ	BLQ	296	1593	BLQ	30	2091	18,076
120	BLQ	BLQ	243	1645	BLQ	72	2003	20,674
168	BLQ	BLQ	210	1566	BLQ	124	1859	18,945
240	BLQ	BLQ	BLQ	1044	BLQ	221	1139	14,352
336	BLQ	BLQ	BLQ	BLQ	BLQ	66	389	218
408	BLQ	BLQ	BLQ	BLQ	BLQ	BLQ	98	40

Note: –, Samples were not collected. BLQ indicated that the detected drug concentration was below LLOW. 2F01 was given TQ002 at a dose of 0.5 mg/kg subcutaneously on the 15th day after parturition. 3F01 was given TQ002 at a dose of 3 mg/kg subcutaneously on the 5th day after parturition. The drug concentration of TQ001 in the serum was the remaining drug after the first administration. 0 h was the moment when the TQ002 test article was administered on D_{50}

measured, and results showed that only a small amount of drugs could cross the blood–milk barrier into mature milk.

The results of serum antidrug antibodies against TQ001 and TQ002 showed that 2F01 and 3F01 produced antidrug antibodies against TQ001, and 2M01, 1F01, 2F01, and 3F01 produced antidrug antibodies against TQ002, and the immunogenicity of TQ002 was slightly stronger than that of TQ001.

For each tissue homogenate, antidrug antibodies against TQ001 and TQ002 were detected. The detection results of male animals showed that no antidrug antibodies against TQ001 and TQ002 were detected in the testis, epididymis, seminal vesicle, and adrenal gland of 1M01. When the mother produced antidrug antibodies against TQ001 or antidrug antibodies against TQ002, antidrug antibodies could be detected in both placenta and fetal serum, and the antidrug antibody titer in fetal serum was stronger than that of the mother, but it was not clear whether the antidrug antibodies in fetal serum were all from the mother.

11. Conclusion: Under the conditions of this experiment, it could be seen that the increase of blood volume in pregnant animals may lead to a delay in peak time and a decrease in peak concentration of antibody drugs. Antibody drugs could distribute across the placental barrier to the placenta, amniotic fluid, and the fetus. Very small amounts of antibody drugs could enter mature milk through the blood–milk barrier. A small amount of the antibody–drug could distribute to the male reproductive organs. antidrug antibody fluid produced by animals could be transferred to the placenta and amniotic fluid through the placental barrier. The titer of drug-resistant antibodies

Table 6.41 Antidrug antibodies in the serum of cynomolgus monkeys after subcutaneous injection of TQ001 and TQ002

Time	TQ001						TQ002					
	1M01	2M01	3M01	1F01	2F01	3F01	1M01	2M01	3M01	1F01	2F01	3F01
D_1	1	–	–	–	<1	–	–	–	–	–	–	
D_{15}	–	–	–	–	58	<1	–	6	–	51	123	–
D_{22}	–	–	–	–	187	–	–	14	–	27	209	4
D_{25}	–	NA	NA	–	NA	NA	–	NA	NA	14	NA	NA
D_{29}	NA	–	–	NA	50	–	NA	27	–	NA	60	11
D_{39}	NA			–	NA	NA	NA			6	NA	NA
Parturition				–	21	11				22	32	231

Note: – indicated screened as negative. The numbers represented the results of titer detection after being screened as positive. NA indicated no such item. The parturition time of 1F01 was D_{42}, that of 2F01 was D_{35}, and that of 3F01 was D_{45}

Table 6.42 Antidrug antibodies in each tissue at the time of parturition after cynomolgus monkeys were dosed with TQ001 and TQ002 via subcutaneous injection

Tissue types	TQ001			TQ002		
	1F01	2F01	3F01	1F01	2F01	3F01
Maternal body	–	21	11	13	15	231
Placenta	–	19	12	8	12	9
Umbilical cord	NA	–	NA	–	–	NA
Amniotic fluid	–	NA	NA	2	NA	NA
Fetus	–	245	8	45	637	589
Milk	NA	–	2	NA	–	–

Note: – indicated screened as negative. The numbers represented the results of titer detection after being screened as positive. NA meant no such item. The milk of 2F01 was the milk on the 15th day after parturition, and the milk of 3F01 represented the milk on the 5th day after parturition

in the fetus was higher than that of the mother, but it was not possible to determine whether the antidrug antibodies in the fetal serum were produced by the mother or the immune system.

Ethical approval

All animal experiments conducted in this study complied with the Guide for the Care and Use of Laboratory Animals (2011) published by the US National Academy Press and the Regulations for the Administration of Laboratory Animals (revised in 2017) issued by the National Science and Technology Commission of China. The management, use, and related procedures involving animals were reviewed and approved by the Institutional Animal Care and Use Committee (IACUC).

References

1. IC, H.S5 (R3): Guidance on Detection of Reproductive and Developmental Toxicity for Human Pharmaceuticals [EB/OL]. (20200218). https://www.cde.org.cn/ichWeb/guideIch/downloadAtt/1/ad236edc7b83a68721fb4aeacd93a61e.
2. Sun L et al. (2018) Pharmacokinetics of recombinant humanized anti-human interleukin 6 receptor monoclonal antibody BAT-1806 injection after single administration. Chin J Pharm Anal 38(10):1775–1780
3. IC, H.M3 (R2) Guidance on nonclinical safety studies for the conduct of human clinical trials and for pharmaceuticals [EB/OL]. (20090611). https://www.cde.org.cn/ichWeb/guideIch/downloadAtt/2/2c8ffc7b2f2ade324bf083f3372b5cc0.
4. Lacy S (1998) Effect of oral probenecid coadministration on the chronic toxicity and pharmacokinetics of intravenous cidofovir in cynomolgus monkeys. Toxicol Sci 44(2):97–106
5. Wei M, Zhao M (2008) Pharmacokinetics research and evaluation on new drugs. Peking University Medical Press, Beijing

6. Meibohm (2010) Pharmacokinetics and Pharmacodynamics of Biotech Drugs: Principles and Case Studies in Drug Development. People's Military Medical Press, Beijing
7. Iwasaki K, Uno Y, Utoh M et al (2019) Importance of cynomolgus monkeys in development of monoclonal antibody drugs. Drug Metab Pharmacokinet 34(1):55–63
8. Moffat GJ, Davies R, Kwon G et al (2014) Investigation of maternal and fetal exposure to an IgG2 monoclonal antibody following biweekly intravaginal administration to cynomolgus monkeys throughout pregnancy. Reprod Toxicol 8:132–137
9. Moffat GJ, Retter MW, Kwon G et al (2014) Placental transfer of a fully human IgG2 monoclonal antibody in the cynomolgus monkey, rat, and rabbit: a comparative assessment from during organogenesis to late gestation. Birth Defects Res B Dev Reprod Toxicol 101(2):178–188
10. IC, H. S6 (R1): Preclinical Safety Evaluation of Biotechnology-Derived Pharmaceuticals [EB/OL]. (20110612). https://www.cde.org.cn/ichWeb/guideIch/downloadAtt/2/6830b4148ba442d75378ae7c0e160777.
11. Ovacik M, Lin K (2018) Tutorial on monoclonal antibody pharmacokinetics and its considerations in early development. Clin Transl. Sci 11(6):540–552
12. Kiskova T, Mytsko Y, Schepelmann M et al (2019) Expression of the neonatal Fc-receptor in placental-fetal endothelium and in cells of the placental immune system. Placenta 78:36–43
13. Liu C, Cai Y, Fan H (2014) Thinking on pharmacokinetic studies of therapeutic antibody drugs. Chin Pharm J 49(04):257–264
14. Zhou J, Hhuang Y, Zheng M (2020) Advances in biologics for generalized pustular psoriasis. Dermatol Bull 37(05):472–476
15. Fujimoto K, Terao K, Cho F et al. (1983) The placental transfer of IgG in the cynomolgus monkey. Jpn J Med Sci Biol 36(3):171–176
16. Gong X, Shao X, Zhang M, Wang H et al (2018) Research progress on hypersensitivity reactions induced by monoclonal antibody products. Chin J New Drugs 28(21):507–520
17. Patyna S, Arrigoni C, Terron A et al (2008) Nonclinical safety evaluation of sunitinib: a potent inhibitor of VEGF, PDGF, KIT, FLT3, and RET receptors. Toxicol Pathol 36(7):905–916
18. Wei M Li K (2014) Bioanalysis performed according to regulations and guidelines. Chin J Pharm Anal 34(1):12

Common Techniques and Methods for Reproductive and Developmental Toxicology Studies in Cynomolgus Monkeys

7

Mao Shanshan, Pang Cong and Gong Xiashi

Abstract

This chapter systematically describes common techniques and methods used in reproductive and developmental toxicology studies of cynomolgus monkeys. It covers key definitions and parameters, including sexual maturity, extragestational weight gain, teratogen-sensitive period, maternal toxicity, embryotoxicity, placental toxicity, gestation diagnosis, ovarian cycle, menstrual cycle, implantation index, preimplantation loss, postimplantation loss, average gestation length, birth survival rate, and survival index. The chapter then details practical procedures for mating, pregnancy diagnosis, and estrous cycle examination, such as natural mating, artificial insemination, ultrasound examination, palpation, progesterone and monkey chorionic gonadotropin measurement, vaginal smear dynamics, and sexual skin observation. It also introduces parental animal observation and terminal procedures, fetal appearance, internal organ and skeletal examination, amniotic fluid collection, sperm collection via rectal probe electrostimulation, penile electrostimulation, penile vibratory stimulation, and natural collection, as well as laparoscopic reproductive interventions for female nonhuman primates. Ethical and animal welfare considerations are emphasized throughout.

Keywords

Cynomolgus monkey · Reproductive and developmental toxicology · Experimental techniques · Pregnancy diagnosis · Vaginal smear · Sperm collection · Laparoscopy

M. Shanshan (✉) · P. Cong · G. Xiashi
Hubei Topgene Biotechnology Co., Ltd., Wuhan, China
e-mail: maoshanshan@topgenebio.com

L. Zhou and Z. Sun (eds.), *Reproductive and Developmental Toxicology on Macaca Fascicularis*, https://doi.org/10.1007/978-981-92-3834-7_7

7.1 Main Terms and Concepts

1. **Sexual maturity** In female Cynomolgus Monkeys, this is indicated by the presence of regular menstrual cycles and well-developed mammary glands. In males, it is indicated by well-developed genitalia or the presence of sperm in semen.
2. **Extragestational weight gain** The average body weight of the mother monkey at necropsy and the amount of weight gained during pregnancy, or the total maternal weight gain. Extragestational weight gain in female monkeys = ((GD100 − GD20 − uterine and fetal weight) × 100%).
3. **Teratogen-sensitive period** The period of organogenesis, extending from implantation to the closure of the hard palate. During this period, the embryo is most sensitive to exogenous substances and is prone to malformations.
4. **Teratogen** Substances capable of inducing structural or functional abnormalities in a developing embryo or fetus, or significantly increasing the incidence of birth defects after exposure to either parent before conception, to the female during pregnancy, or directly to the developing organism. The term is sometimes used more broadly to include any substance causing embryonic developmental abnormalities; it is therefore also known as a developmental toxicant. Teratogens can be environmental (drugs, viruses, radiation) or genetic (mutant genes, chromosomal abnormalities). Teratogenicity refers to the inherent capacity of a teratogen to induce embryonic malformations, whereas teratogenesis refers to the processes and mechanisms by which these malformations arise during embryonic development.
5. **Maternal toxicity** The organ and functional damage in the mother resulting from drug exposure. Clinical manifestations may include, but are not limited to, decreased weight gain, organ dysfunction, and mortality.
6. **Embryotoxicity** The selective toxic effects of a drug on the embryo, resulting in potential embryo death, developmental retardation, malformations, and functional impairment. Substances that cause embryotoxicity are called embryotoxins.
7. **Placental toxicity** The toxic effects of a drug on the placenta are mainly manifested as placental injury, altered placental blood flow, reduced placental transport of nutrients, and abnormal placental function (such as endocrine and metabolic functions).
8. **Gestation diagnosis** Several methods can be applied to determine pregnancy in Cynomolgus Monkeys. ① Chorionic Gonadotropin (CG) Measurement: Pregnancy can be diagnosed by measuring the presence of chorionic gonadotropin (CG) in excreta throughout pregnancy. Peak concentrations are detectable around weeks 8–9 of pregnancy. During early pregnancy, significantly elevated levels of relaxin, produced by the uterus and placenta, along with CG, serve as markers in the first trimester. Serum relaxin concentrations reach approximately 1 ng/mL during this period, and may increase to 15 ng/mL in mid-trimester of pregnancy, coinciding with a decrease in progesterone levels. In the third trimester, relaxin decreases

while progesterone increases. ② Ultrasonography: Around gestational day (GD) 20, Ultrasound Examination can be applied to observe the gestational sac. The image shows a bright, oval area within the uterus. A hypoechoic area (the embryo) is visible between the uterine wall and the fully developed gestational sac, confirming pregnancy. Fetal heart rate is detectable around GD50.

9. **Ovarian cycle** The periodic changes in the morphology and function of the ovaries from puberty to menopause.
10. **Sexual skin** Typically located at the base of the tail, the skin of the perineal region and the posterior legs becomes visibly swollen as the animal reaches puberty. After the swelling goes down, the affected skin turns red. In adult animals, the color of this skin changes with hormonal fluctuations throughout their menstrual cycle, becoming palest during menstruation. In some animal species, this skin area swells slightly as ovulation nears.
11. **Menstrual cycle** The duration between the start of two consecutive menstrual periods in Cynomolgus Monkeys, typically measured in days and inclusive of the bleeding period.
12. **Implantation index** The ratio of the number of implantation sites to that of corpora lutea, expressed as a percentage. Implantation Index = (Number of Implantation Sites/Number of Corpora Lutea) × 100%.
13. **Preimplantation loss** The ratio of number of fertilized eggs that fail to implant to the total number of fertilized eggs, expressed as a percentage. Interruptions in early development can significantly reduce the fertilization rate and increase the mortality rate of preimplantation embryos. The preimplantation loss can be calculated using the following formula: the difference between the number of corpora lutea and the number of implantations, divided by the number of corpora lutea, resulting in a ratio. Preimplantation loss = [(Number of Corpora Lutea − Number of Implantation Sites)/Number of Implantation Sites] × 100%.
14. **Post-implantation loss** The percentage of the number of embryos that did not survive to the total number of implants. In studies of complete reproductive function, the post-implantation loss rate is determined after fetal delivery. Specifically, the uterus and implantation sites are examined during the necropsy of the dam after the fetuses are weaned. The post-implantation loss rate is calculated as the number of implantations minus the number of surviving fetuses after full-term delivery, divided by the number of implantations. Post-implantation loss = [(Number of implantation sites − Number of live fetuses)/Number of implantation sites] × 100%.
15. **Average gestation length** The duration from the day of conception (GD0, defined as the day of successful mating) to the day of parturition. If all offspring are delivered between the last observation on the day of parturition and the first observation on the following day, then 0.5 days should be subtracted from the interval (GD0 to the day of parturition observed).
16. **Birth survival rate** The percentage of offspring that survive at birth out of the total number of offspring.

17. **Survival index** It also known as the survival ability index, which refers to a time-specific measure that quantifies the percentage of offspring surviving to a designated point in time after birth.
18. **Highest nonseverely toxic dose (HNSTD)** The maximum dose of an anti-tumor drug that does not cause life-threatening or irreversible toxicities in nonrodents. The HNSTD of a substance is the specific concentration at which, when exceeded, the substance has the potential to cause irreversible or intolerable toxicities in nontarget organisms.
19. **Severely toxic dose in 10% (STD10)** For rodents, the STD10 is defined as the dose of an anti-tumor drug that induces severe toxic reactions in 10% of the treated animals.

7.2 Common Experimental Techniques and Operating Methods

7.2.1 Mating, Diagnosis of Pregnancy, and Estrous Cycle Examination in Cynomolgus Monkeys

The reproductive physiology and embryogenesis of Cynomolgus Monkeys are very similar to those of humans, and their mating and pregnancy are not seasonally limited, making them an ideal model for studying the developmental toxicity of drugs. Cynomolgus Monkeys must reach sexual maturity (preferably physical maturity) before mating. It is recommended that male animals should be ≥5 years old and female animals should be at least 3.5 years old or 4 years old. In the toxicity studies of embryonic and fetal development (EFD) and pre- and postnatal development (PPND), male monkeys were used only as breeding animals to mate with females. Teratogenicity refers to in [1–5].

1. Natural mating The sexual maturity of female and male animals is confirmed through biological endpoints, such as a regular menstrual cycle in females, the development of sex organs in males, or the presence of sperm in semen. The regular menstrual cycle of female monkeys is beneficial for selecting the appropriate mating time and maximizing the conception rate. Male and female animals were placed in mating cages in ratios of 1:1 (one female, one male), 2:1 (two females, one male), and even 6:1 (six females, one male), and their mating behavior and status were confirmed through video recording [6].

Given the low mating and conception rates, and spontaneous abortion rates of 10%–15% around GD100 in Cynomolgus Monkeys, the ICH S5 (R3) guidelines for Detection of Reproductive and Developmental Toxicity for Human Pharmaceuticals in 2020 recommend a minimum of 16 pregnant females for EFD toxicity studies. This ensures sufficient offspring for evaluating potential adverse effects on morphological development. Enhanced PPND toxicity studies typically employ approximately 16 pregnant females. This group size is designed to yield a sufficient number of offspring to comprehensively assess potential adverse effects on pregnancy outcomes, malformations, and postnatal development, allowing for targeted investigations (e.g., the immune system) where necessary. Most pregnant animals in enhanced PPND toxicity tests are obtained within a few months. A larger number of female monkeys need to be bred to obtain the necessary number of pregnant monkeys for the study [7–10].

2. Artificial insemination Artificial insemination (AI) in nonhuman primates (NHPs) is a technique whereby sperm from a male is artificially introduced into the female reproductive tract to facilitate fertilization and subsequent pregnancy.

AI is a two-step process. First, semen is collected from the male using manual or electrical stimulation. Subsequently, the collected semen is introduced into the female reproductive tract using specialized equipment or tools (e.g., a syringe). Typically, the syringe tip is placed into the female's vagina with the tip pointing upward. The semen is then injected, traveling towards the cervix, completing the AI procedure.

Before injection, the collected semen should be stored at an appropriate temperature, typically around 37°C. Temperatures that are too high or too low will affect sperm viability and quality. Furthermore, freezing the collected sperm should be avoided [11].

3. Gestation diagnosis

(1) Ultrasound examination: Cynomolgus Monkeys cohabitate for mating from menstrual cycle days 10–12. Confirmation of mating is achieved through behavioral observation. On the 18–20 days of mating, ultrasound examination can be applied to observe the gestational sac. The image showed an oval, bright area within the uterus. An anechoic area (the embryo) was visible in the uterus, confirming pregnancy. The ultrasound examination method has high accuracy and is the gold standard for early pregnancy diagnosis in Cynomolgus Monkeys [12].

An ultrasound examination was conducted to observe the development of the gestational sac in the uterus of female Cynomolgus Monkeys. Starting from GD14-GD15, the gestational sac was observed at GD16-GD18, while the embryo, yolk sac, and fetal heart rate were observed at GD21-GD25, confirming pregnancy. After the embryo was found, growth could be evaluated, or gestational age could be predicted. Various embryonic growth parameters help assess fetal growth. At GD70-GD75, fetal sex can be accurately determined. Observation of the embryo/fetus's heart rate and gross body movements helps determine fetal viability and condition. The detailed operation process is shown in Fig. 7.1.

(2) Palpation: Palpation is a technique for assessing the genital status of animals through abdominal or rectal palpation. This method offers convenience and cost-effectiveness, making it suitable for large-scale pregnancy diagnosis in animal production. Experienced personnel are essential in monkey breeding facilities. Rectal palpation is the standard method for diagnosing pregnancy in cattle and sheep. Rectal palpation of the uterus and ovaries is a common method for diagnosing pregnancy in NHPs such as macaques and baboons.

Abdominal palpation: Transabdominal palpation is used for pregnancy diagnosis in macaques. The operator performed a physical examination, restraining the female macaque in a vertical position with legs fully extended towards the tail. The operator wore thin gloves to maximize tactile sensitivity. One hand supported the animal's pubic

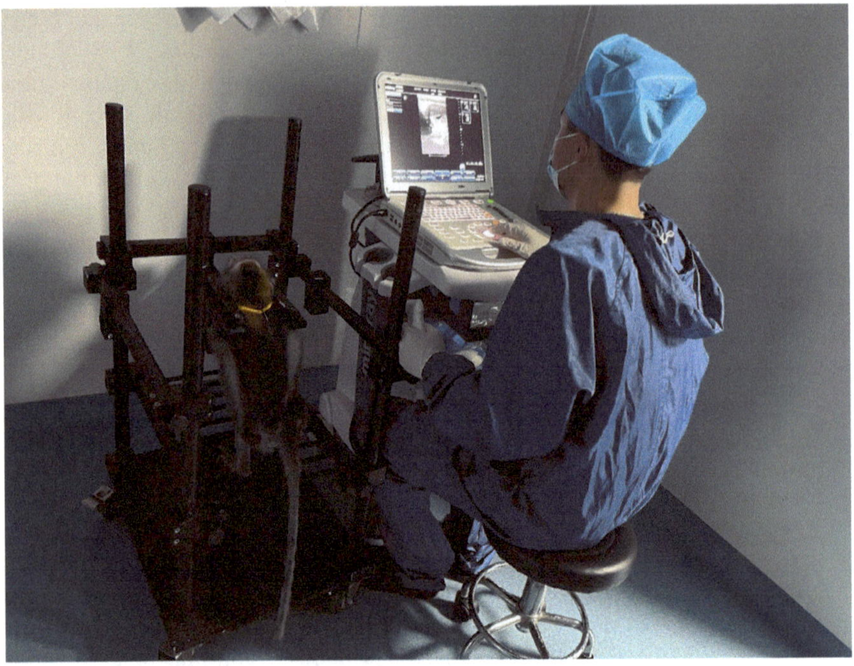

Fig. 7.1 Ultrasound examination of female Cynomolgus Monkeys

region at the sacroiliac joint, while the thumb and index finger of the other hand palpated the uterus and ovaries transabdominal. The thumb and index finger were placed around the uterus to measure its size. Two fingers were applied as "calipers" to measure uterine size. If possible, two operators performed measurements independently. The fingers were slightly closed as they were withdrawn. Therefore, in practice, the measurable size is between 1 and 2 mm.

The uterus of an animal that has not given birth is firm and rod-shaped, measuring 1–5 cm in length and 4–5 mm in width. The ovaries are initially impalpable; however, in sexually mature animals, firm, ovoid structures, measuring 3–4mm in diameter, become palpable cranial to the uterus. The uterus of a female animal experiencing her first pregnancy is located close to the rectum on the back side. In contrast, during pregnancies with multiple fetuses, the uterus is more easily palpated above the top of the pubic symphysis in the lower abdomen. Pregnancy is suspected 15–20 days after mating and confirmed by 25–30 days, based on uterine and ovarian changes. The uterus transforms from a rod-shaped to a firm sphere, slightly increasing in size (about one or two ovarian volumes).

(3) Progesterone level: Within the Cynomolgus Monkeys model for evaluating EFD toxicity, drug administration to pregnant monkeys is typically initiated at GD20-GD50

(the period of organogenesis). Terminal anatomy and fetal examination are performed at GD100. Analysis of serum hormone concentrations provides a crucial metric for assessing maternal toxicity.

The progesterone detection can be used as an auxiliary method for early pregnancy diagnosis. The hormonal pattern for maintaining menstrual cycles in Cynomolgus Monkeys is similar to that in humans. GD0 (the second day of mating between male and female animals in the same cage) is the 13th day of menstruation in female monkeys, and the corpus luteum has formed but is not yet mature, with lower progesterone levels. At GD20, the corpus luteum of nonpregnant female monkeys atrophied, and progesterone levels returned to low levels before ovulation. The corpus luteum of pregnant female monkeys continues to secrete progesterone, and the progesterone level increases. Therefore, comparing progesterone levels at GD0 and GD20 can help diagnose pregnancy in female monkeys. Progesterone levels vary significantly between animals, possibly due to menstrual cycle length or other hormone influences. Therefore, it is necessary to consider an individual's baseline hormone levels for a comprehensive assessment, thereby improving diagnostic accuracy [13].

The secretion of estradiol and progesterone during pregnancy in Cynomolgus Monkeys is also similar to that in humans. The corpus luteum produces estrogen and progesterone in early pregnancy, essential for the maintenance of pregnancy. In late pregnancy, this function is taken over by the placenta. In addition, estrogen increases the number and volume of pituitary prolactin cells, with prolactin levels rising around GD48.

To help improve the accuracy of early pregnancy diagnosis and hormone testing in EFD toxicity studies on Cynomolgus Monkeys, researchers measured progesterone levels in both pregnant and nonpregnant monkeys at the beginning of the study (GD0) and 20 days later (GD20). Changes in the levels of progesterone, estradiol, and prolactin in the blood of pregnant monkeys were also detected throughout their pregnancies (GD0 to GD100). This data will support the conduct of EFD toxicity tests in Cynomolgus Monkeys.

(4) Monkey chorionic gonadotropin: It is reported that monkey chorionic gonadotropin (mCG) can also serve as an auxiliary method for early pregnancy diagnosis in Cynomolgus Monkeys. MCG increases rapidly from around GD18, peaks around GD22 and then decreases rapidly until it is almost undetectable around GD32. Human chorionic gonadotropin (hCG) early pregnancy test strips were applied to measure the urine of pregnant female monkeys at GD20; the reaction results were all negative. The causes for negative results may include: ① The different structures of subunits of hCG and mCG result in the inability to detect mCG using hCG detection methods; ② The concentration of mCG in the urine of pregnant Cynomolgus Monkeys is below the lower limit of the minimum detectable value [14].

mCG is the first clear embryonic signal of early pregnancy in primates. Chorionic gonadotropin (CG) is similar in structure and function to pituitary luteinizing hormone (LH), which is regulated by gonadotropin-releasing hormone (GnRH).

mCG in the placenta, blood, and urine can be measured by radioimmunoassay and bioassay. Throughout gestation, mCG is readily detectable in monkey placenta, blood, and urine during a brief period in early pregnancy. However, mCG is undetectable in placental extracts, serum, or 40-fold concentrated urine from GD40 to full-term pregnancy, indicating a marked absence of mCG after GD40. Macaques need to undergo CG testing before they can be used as a model in pregnancy research. Unlike humans and some higher primates, research on fetal, placental, and maternal endocrine function of macaques can be conducted in the absence of CG.

4. Menstrual cycle The menstrual cycle of NHPs is generally 28 days, with approximately 77% ranging from 23 to 33 days. It should be noted that the menstrual cycle and fertility of captive macaques are affected by seasonal variation. The animals used in this research have menstrual cycles that are known to be affected by the seasons in their natural environment. However, these animals are housed in a temperature-controlled environment, eliminating seasonal effects on menstrual cycles. The gonadal function of the species has been shown to be unaffected by light-dark changes.

Rhesus macaques in semi-natural environments exhibit distinct seasonal mating cycles, with conception limited to autumn and winter. Although changes in the menstrual cycle are observed throughout the year, ovulation is only observed in females in autumn and winter. Irregular menstruation in spring and summer is also related to anovulatory cycles. These female animals ovulate two to six times during the breeding season, which is positively correlated with body weight, average progesterone levels during the luteal phase of the normal cycle, and dominance hierarchy. Within the seasonally limited ovulatory period, female animals exhibit predictable specific physical and behavioral characteristics within a certain range of ovum quality and quantity [15].

In most animals, the resumption of menstrual cycles causes embryo death. Animals that have multiple offspring at a time are less able to cope with the physiological disruptions caused by stress. In some NHPs, the secretion of adrenal corticosteroids may reduce estrogen-induced preovulatory surge in LH. Disruption of the hypothalamic-pituitary-gonadal axis can delay ovulation, thereby affecting the timing of fertilization and causing embryo-endometrial developmental asynchrony, reducing the survival rate of the embryo.

The ovarian cycle of the Cynomolgus Monkeys is a physiological event that promotes follicle maturation, followed by luteal phase formation of the corpus luteum, subsequent corpus luteum regression, and finally the menstrual phase. The follicular phase duration is 12–14 days, the interovulatory interval is approximately 3 days, and the luteal phase duration is 14–16 days. Estradiol is the main ovarian hormone during the follicular phase. While estradiol gradually increases, LH and FSH levels typically remain low or even decrease, and progesterone levels also remain low. The midcycle peak of the ovarian cycle begins with a sharp rise in estradiol levels, followed by rapid increases in LH and FSH, with little change in progesterone. A study by Weinbauer et al. found that in monkeys, the estradiol reaches its peak on day 12 of the menstrual cycle. This is followed by peaks in LH (on day 12.5) and FSH (on day 13). The levels of inhibin B are higher during the follicular phase, while inhibin A levels are higher in the luteal phase. Progesterone levels reach their peak on the 22nd day of the ovarian cycle (luteal phase), while gonadotropin levels return to levels similar to the follicular phase.

Inhibins are important biomarkers of ovarian function in monkeys and humans. In female fertility testing, studies need to be scheduled according to the menstrual cycle, especially when assessing reproductive hormone levels. Administering medication on day 1 of the menstrual cycle provides more comprehensive data and allows for better interpretation. Blood samples are collected at various stages of the menstrual cycle. Following Chellman et al.'s recommendation, samples are taken every 2 days during the follicular phase (to capture estrogen and LH peaks) and every 3 days during the luteal phase. A 6-week sampling period covers longer cycles.

5. Dynamic observation of vaginal smears of Cynomolgus Monkeys In the practice of artificial breeding of Cynomolgus Monkeys, it has been observed that, similar to other NHPs, they exhibit periodic changes in sexual skin. However, the skin changes in some Cynomolgus Monkeys are not very pronounced. Therefore, it is not possible to accurately determine their estrous cycle based solely on changes in the sexual skin. Accurate determination of estrus and ovulation timing is crucial for timely mating and AI in reproductive biotechnology and embryo engineering research on Cynomolgus Monkeys.

(1) Observation of sexual skin signs: Daily monitoring and recording of color and swelling changes in the tail base, calluses, perineum, thighs, back, and face (areas exhibiting obvious sexual skin changes) throughout the Cynomolgus Monkeys's estrous cycle, and recording of vaginal discharge and menstruation.

(2) Vaginal smears: A sterile cotton swab is used to collect a vaginal sample from the Cynomolgus Monkeys. The sample is spread evenly onto two slides, air-dried, and stained with Wright-Giemsa solution (for 1 min), followed by a buffered solution (with dilution ratio of 1:1 or 1:2, for 5–10 min). Slides are finally rinsed and air-dried. One of the well-stained slides is selected and observed under a 400× biological microscope. The number of cells (leukocytes, keratinocytes, intermediate basal cells) and cell debris is counted. Five fields of view are randomly selected per slide for cell counts and photographs, with a total of 200 cells counted.

Vaginal smears are performed every other day for each female monkey. If estrus signs are observed, vaginal smears are performed daily. The experiment lasts for one menstrual cycle, from the end of menstruation (vaginal bleeding) to the end of the next menstruation. Each menstrual cycle is divided into seven phases based on the research on the menstrual cycles of macaques and baboons by Zeng Zhongxing et al.: menstruation, post-menstruation, pre-ovulation, ovulation, post-ovulation, luteal phase, and pre-menstruation. Based on the daily observations and records of sexual skin changes, data from female monkeys whose menstrual cycles clearly show the above-mentioned phases are selected for statistical analysis.

(3) Characteristics of sexual skin changes: The main indicators are the changes in the intensity of the color and the degree of swelling. Observations and statistical analysis indicate that the normal skin color of female Cynomolgus Monkeys is dull gray. Their sexual skin color can be broadly categorized as pale pink, light red, red, and dark red or purplish-red. In female Cynomolgus Monkeys, sexual skin swelling commonly occurs in the tail base, perineum, and calluses, exhibiting bright red or purplish-red coloration. Color intensity, swelling, and regression fluctuate cyclically with the menstrual cycle. From menstruation to the proestrus phase, the sexual skin at the tail base and perineum gradually reddens, then swells, wrinkles, and develops into elastic, red skin. The most pronounced swelling and vivid coloration of the sexual skin occur at the peak of estrus. Four- to five-years-old females show pronounced swelling on the thighs and back, with prominent wrinkling. However, in females over 6 years old, the thighs only redden, with minimal swelling. Sexual skin swelling and redness decrease in mid to late estrus, returning to a resting state by the luteal phase. Changes in the sexual skin of female Cynomolgus Monkeys in different phases: the tail base and perineum region change from light red during menstruation to slightly swollen and light red in the post-menstruation phase, swollen and red with wrinkles in the pre-ovulation phase, extensively swollen, dark red or purplish-red with numerous wrinkles during ovulation, less swollen and light red with fewer wrinkles in the post-ovulation phase, dark gray with few wrinkles in the luteal phase, and light red with no wrinkles in the pre-menstruation phase. During the seven phases described above, the facial skin color changes as follows: pale red, light red, red, dark red, dull gray, dull gray, and pale red.

Based on observations and records of sexual skin changes and menstrual bleeding, among 30 female monkeys, 13 (approximately 43.33%) showed clearly distinguishable seven phases of sexual skin changes within one sexual cycle. Another 12 (approximately 40%) showed consistently bright red or purplish-red color at the tail base and calluses. The remaining five (approximately 16.67%) showed no significant changes in sexual skin. Therefore, observation of sexual skin can help determine the ovulation period in some Cynomolgus Monkeys, but it cannot be used as an accurate method for determining the exact day of estrus and ovulation.

(4) Cell morphology of vaginal smears from Cynomolgus Monkeys: The following cell components are mainly observed in vaginal smears from Cynomolgus Monkeys.

Leukocytes: Predominantly polymorphonuclear leukocytes. The cytoplasm is lightly stained, and the nuclei are pink, often appearing kidney-shaped or multilobed (four or more lobes). Keratinocytes: These are large, polygonal cells with irregular borders. Nuclei are small and centrally located, with chromatin condensation. The cytoplasm is abundant; some cells have thin, transparent cytoplasm and easily curl at the edges.

Keratinized epithelial cells: The degree of keratinization varies, resulting in different staining results. In cells that have just begun keratinization, the nuclear membrane is blurred, and the staining around the nucleus is deeper than at the cytoplasmic periphery. In fully keratinized cells, the nucleus disappears, and the entire cytoplasm shows a uniform pale red color.

Intermediate basal cells: These cells are typically round, oval, or irregularly shaped with abundant, lightly stained cytoplasm. Their nuclei are relatively small, deep purplish-red, centrally located, and show a defined nuclear boundary. Cell fragments are randomly distributed, anucleated cytoplasmic fragments and debris of varying sizes, typically staining pink. They may arise from the breakdown of epithelial cells in the late menstrual phase. Smears taken during the pre-ovulation and ovulation phases show streaks resulting from dried mucus.

(5) Changes in cellular components during different estrous cycles: Subjects were selected with menstrual cycles of approximately 30–34 days in length, based on observations of sexual skin changes and menstrual bleeding in the Cynomolgus Monkeys.

Menstruation: During this phase, numerous red blood cells are present. Keratinized epithelial cells are stained bright pink, exhibiting visible protoplasm, and a few basal keratinocytes are also observed. White blood cells are abundant, accounting for about 48% of the total number of various cellular components; intermediate-layer basal cells account for 7%; keratinized epithelial cells account for approximately 37%; there is a significant amount of cellular debris (7%) and minimal mucus. Menstrual bleeding typically lasts 3–5 days.

Post-menstruation: During this phase, red blood cells are absent, while keratinized epithelial cells increase, comprising approximately 58% of the total number of various cellular components. There is a slight decrease in mucus and white blood cells, and basal keratinocytes also diminish.

Pre-ovulation: Keratinized epithelial cells account for 76%, with a dramatic increase in mucus.

Ovulation: Keratinized epithelial cells constitute 96% of the cellular components. Intermediate basal cells and white blood cells are reduced or absent, as are cellular fragments. Mucus is significantly increased.

Post-ovulation: There is an increase in white blood cells, with cells exhibiting a tendency toward clustering. Intermediate basal cells are absent, and mucus is virtually nonexistent.

Luteal phase: There's been a sharp decrease in keratinized epithelial cells, only representing 27% of the total. White blood cells have increased, making up approximately 41%.

Pre-menstruation: Keratinized epithelial cells are slightly increased, reaching approximately 37%.

Of the three cell types, keratinized epithelial cells are most prevalent, reaching a maximum of 96% during ovulation. This cell type also exhibits the widest range of variation (1%–96%). White blood cells show a variation of 2%–48%, while intermediate basal cells range from only 1%–14%. White blood cells, intermediate basal cells, and cell debris decrease progressively from menstruation to ovulation, reaching their lowest levels, then increase progressively from ovulation to menstruation. Keratinized epithelial cells follow the opposite pattern. During ovulation in Cynomolgus Monkeys, vaginal intermediate basal cells and white blood cells decrease significantly. Conversely, the proportion of keratinocytes increases, averaging 96% and reaching up to 99%. In

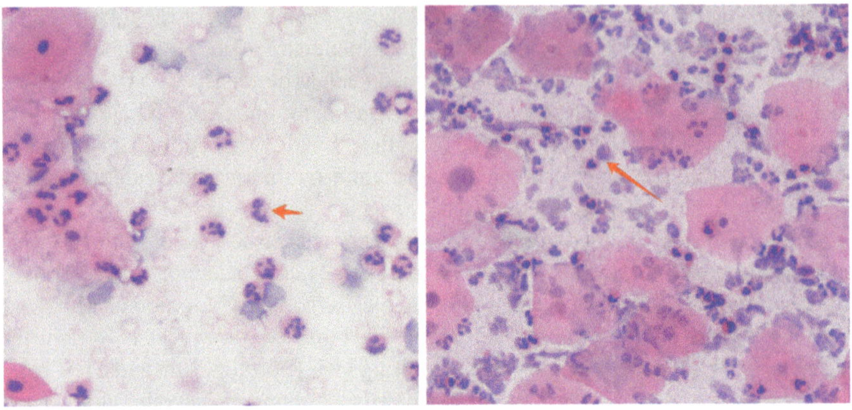

Fig. 7.2 White blood cells (arrow) (HE Staining, ×200)

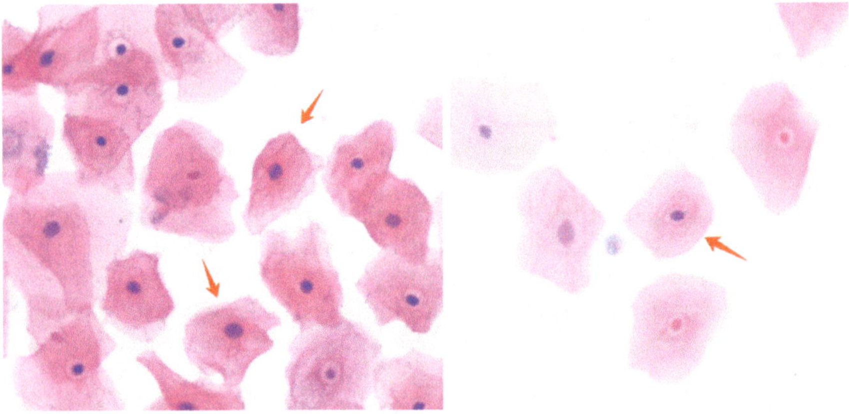

Fig. 7.3 Keratinized epithelial cells (arrow) (HE Staining, ×200)

most female monkeys, when keratinized cells reach their peak, the sexual skin exhibits the most vibrant color and the highest degree of swelling with the largest area, which are signs of estrus. They also show a preference for proximity to male monkeys, often exhibiting restlessness and low calls when a male is present, and are willing to mate. This indicates that changes in sexual skin and the number of vaginal keratinized epithelial cells are consistent with changes in the sexual cycle. Furthermore, it should be noted that an increase in keratinized epithelial cells to 76%, accompanied by a sharp rise in mucus, signifies the pre-ovulation phase and the imminent onset of ovulation.

Cynomolgus Monkeys vaginal smears show >96% keratinized epithelial cells during ovulation, significantly more than in other cycle phases; white blood cells and intermediate basal cells are inversely related. The data demonstrate that monitoring

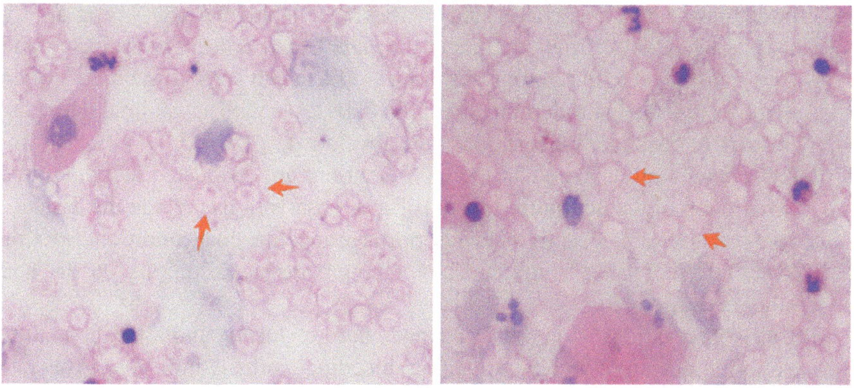

Fig. 7.4 Red blood cells (arrow) (HE Staining, ×200)

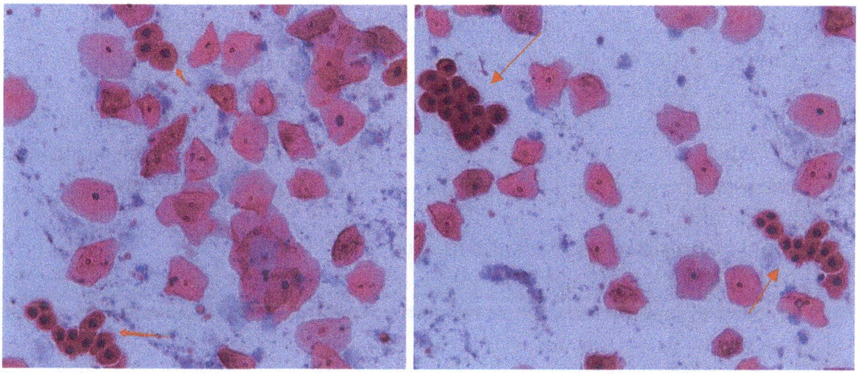

Fig. 7.5 Stratum basale cells (arrow) (HE Staining, ×200)

vaginal keratinized epithelial cell counts is a highly effective method for determining the timing of ovulation in Cynomolgus Monkeys. This approach, combined with observations of sexual skin changes, provides a robust and reliable means of assessing estrus and ovulation in Cynomolgus Monkeys. Figures 7.2–7.5 show vaginal smears from a female Cynomolgus Monkeys at different phases.

7.2.2 Parental Animal Observation and Terminal Procedures

1. Parental animal observation

(1) Microbiological quality control in NHPs involves a comprehensive approach that includes appropriate pre-acquisition evaluations of source colonies and individual animals, rigorous quarantine procedures, a robust infectious disease prevention and health program, eradication and control measures for specific

infectious agents, and a dedicated occupational health and safety program for animal keepers. Animals that meet the established criteria are selected and then transferred to quarantine authorities. The health screening process often involves repeated intradermal tuberculin (TB) tests, with any animals showing positive or questionable reactions being excluded.

(2) After parent animals are admitted, observations are conducted daily until the completion of the quarantine period. These observations include the animals' physical appearance, activity levels, posture, appetite, coat condition, reaction to stimuli, secretions from glands, breathing patterns, excretions, deaths, and other relevant factors.

(3) Daily observations should also be made before, during, and after the mating period, focusing on behavior, vaginal bleeding, and any mortality. After the drug administration period for the test animals, the animals are observed for any abnormal symptoms until necropsy. The time of onset and duration of any abnormal symptoms are also observed.

(4) In PPND toxicity studies, animals are observed daily prior to parturition, with particular attention to behavior and activities, vaginal bleeding, and mortality. During parturition, the occurrence of any complications, such as dystocia or abortion, is meticulously recorded. Postnatal observations focus on maternal behavior, including lactation and pup rearing. Necropsy is conducted following weaning. Any abnormal signs observed before, during, and after parturition (until necropsy) should be recorded, including the onset and duration of the abnormality.

2. Terminal examination of parental animals

(1) Following anesthesia and blood collection, the parent animals are euthanized via inguinal exsanguination. The animals are placed on the autopsy table with their abdomens facing upward, and the abdomen is disinfected with 75% ethanol. Using a scalpel, an incision is made through the skin from the chin along the abdominal midline, opening the thoracic and abdominal cavities to expose the internal organs. The internal organs of the parent animals are inspected for any abnormalities. If necessary, professional pathologists and veterinarians should be consulted for verification.

(2) The abdominal wall skin is lifted with forceps, and an incision is made with a scalpel along the ventral midline, extending to the pubis.

(3) The abdominal organs and peritoneal surface are examined for any abnormalities; macroscopic abnormalities are recorded and inspected. Any abnormal fluid or discoloration within the abdominal cavity is sampled for cytology and bacterial culture, and the volume and appearance of the fluid are recorded.

(4) Through an incision in the diaphragm and by cutting through the ribs or costochondral junctions, the thoracic cavity can be exposed.

(5) The thoracic organs and pleural surfaces are examined for any abnormalities, and the findings are recorded. Excessive fluid or discoloration within the thoracic cavity is sampled for cytology and bacterial culture, and the volume and appearance of the fluid are recorded.

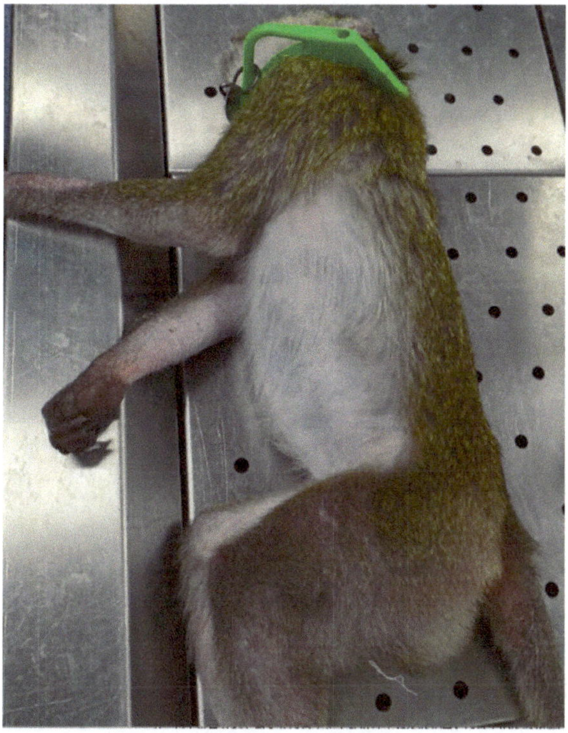

Fig. 7.6 GD_{100} pregnant cynomolgus monkey, lateral view

(6) To examine the brain, a midline incision is made over the cranium. The skin and muscles covering the cranium are incised transversely. Using a bone-cutting saw, the cranium is incised along the mandibular, lateral, and occipital aspects.
(7) Finally, the reproductive organs are examined. In male monkeys, the testes, epididymis, seminal vesicles, and prostate gland are mainly inspected. In female monkeys, the uterus, ovaries, and vagina are examined for any pathological changes.
(8) At each step of the dissection, tissues designated for collection in the study protocol are identified. Small organs (such as the thyroid gland, adrenal glands, and lymph nodes) are placed in labeled tissue cassettes for ease of identification during processing.
(9) Following completion of the necropsy, the carcass is placed in a plastic bag, and all instruments and surgical tools are thoroughly cleaned. The plastic bag containing the carcass is placed in a refrigerator until disposal can be arranged with a compliant waste disposal facility.

3. Post-cesarean evaluation [16]

(1) Examination time: EFD toxicity studies are conducted at GD100, while PPND toxicity studies are conducted at the end of the lactation period (approximately

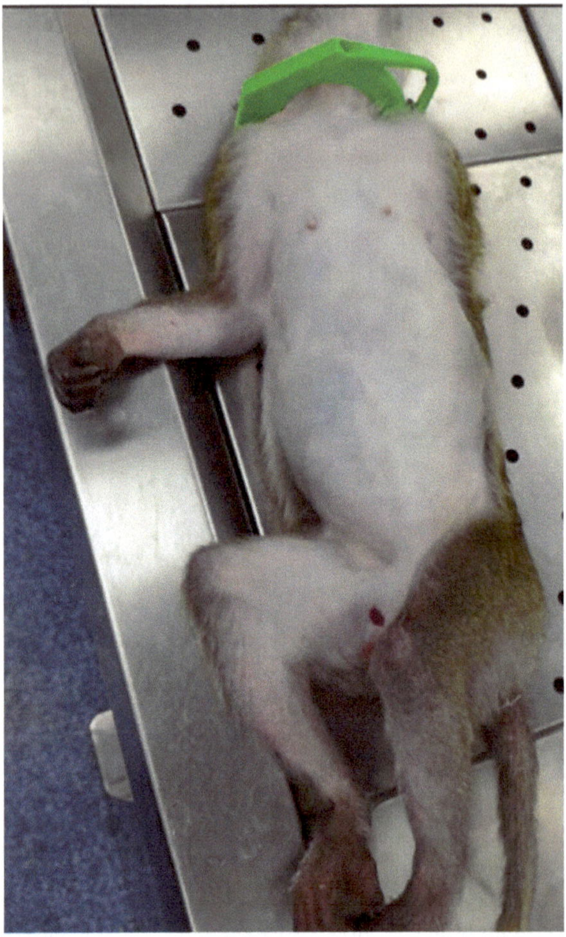

Fig. 7.7 GD_{100} pregnant cynomolgus monkey, frontal view

6 months). Terminal necropsy of dams is performed when necessary (Figs. 7.6–7.12).

(2) Cesarean section is generally performed at GD100. The assessment includes evaluation of the amniotic fluid (volume and clarity), placenta (weight, number of placental lobes, and placental diameter), fetal appearance and weight, umbilical cord insertion site, and umbilical cord length.

(3) Prior to dissection, the dam's abdomen is moistened with 75% ethanol to prevent hair loss from interfering with the uterine excision during the procedure.

(4) After opening the dam's abdominal cavity along the midline, the uterus is exposed. Tissues with macroscopic abnormalities are preserved; corresponding tissues from control animals are also preserved. All abnormal tissues are

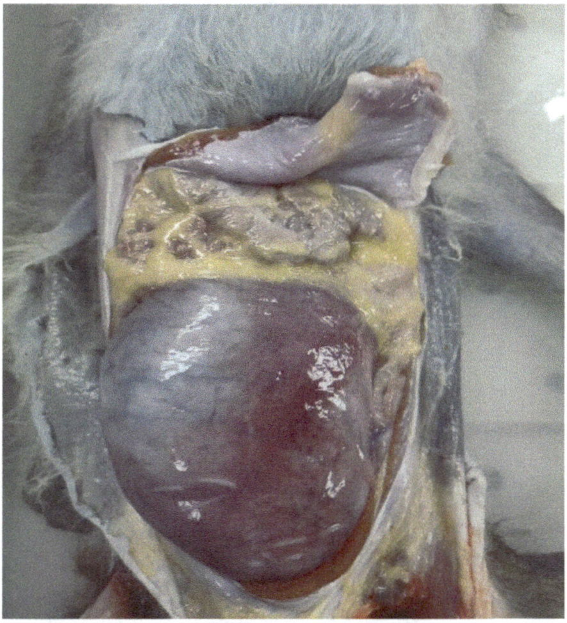

Fig. 7.8 Cynomolgus monkey on GD_{100}, gravid uterus with visible embryo (arrow)

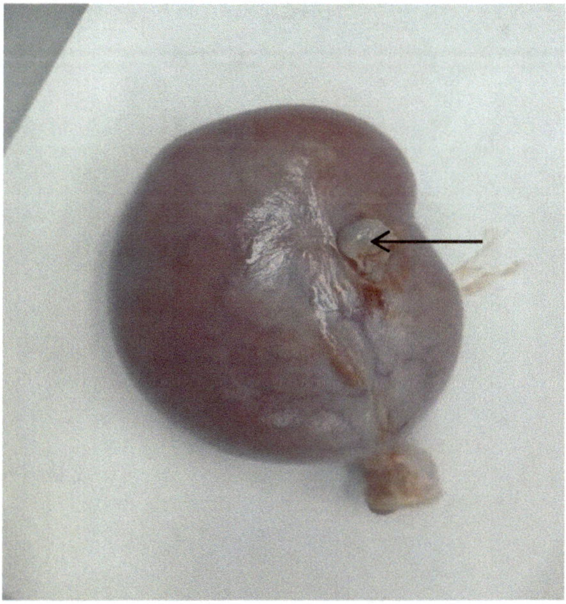

Fig. 7.9 Cynomolgus monkey on GD_{100}, gravid uterus with visible ovary (arrow)

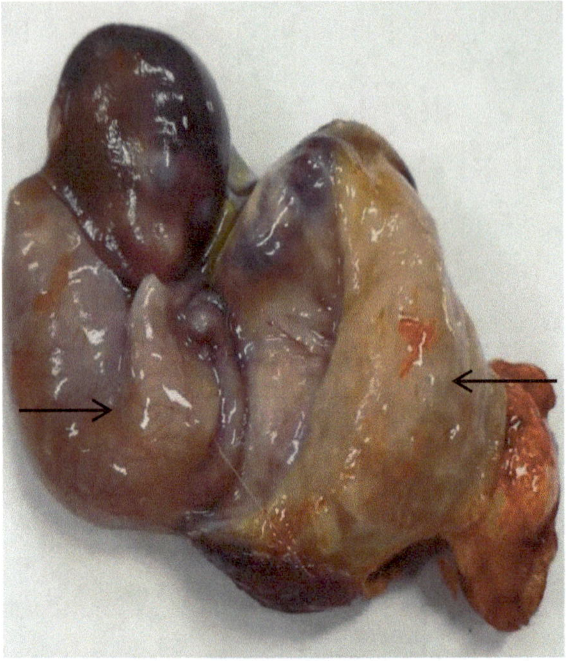

Fig. 7.10 Cynomolgus monkey on GD_{100}, gravid uterus with visible embryo (arrow)

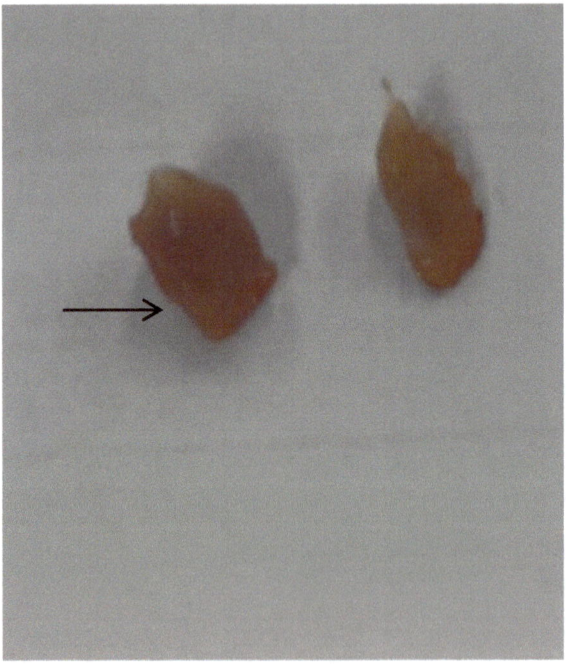

Fig. 7.11 Ovary of a cynomolgus monkey on GD_{100} (arrow)

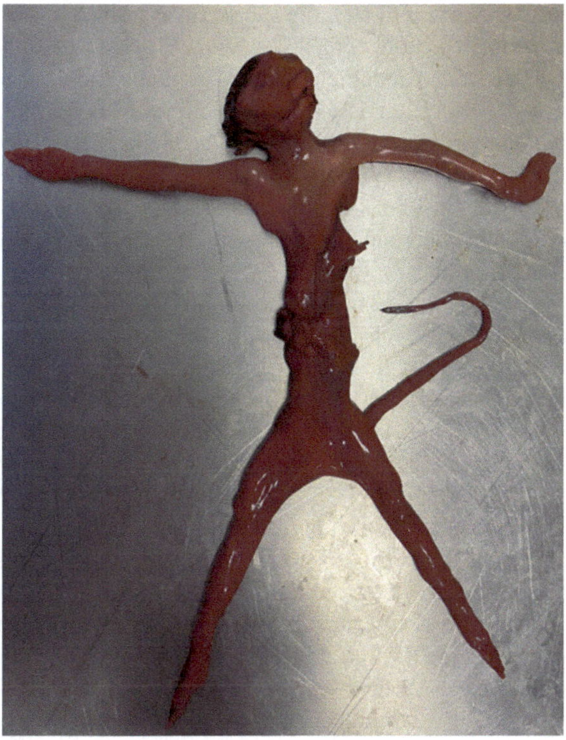

Fig. 7.12 Aborted embryo of a Cynomolgus Monkey on GD_{134}

collected and placed in 10% neutral buffered formalin for further histopathological examination.

(5) The weight of the uterus and fetus is recorded.

(6) An incision is made at the cervix to expose the implant. The uterus and fetuses are examined. The fetal membranes are gently torn, the umbilical cord is severed, and the fetuses are removed. Amniotic fluid adhering to the fetuses is removed, and fetal weight, appearance, crown-rump length, and tail length are recorded.

(7) To assess amniotic fluid volume and color, care is taken to avoid damaging the fetal membranes after making an incision in the uterus. Amniotic fluid is then aspirated using a syringe, and the volume is recorded. The color of the amniotic fluid is recorded before aspiration.

7.2.3 Examination of Fetal Appearance, Internal Organs, and Bones

1. Examination of fetal appearance

(1) Observation parameters: Shape, size, number, and color are observed. Eyes and ears, as well as limbs, are compared bilaterally (left and right sides).

(2) Examination sequence: Firstly, the subject is examined in a supine position, from head to tail, in the following order: forehead, ears, face, mouth, tongue and palate, neck, chest and abdomen, external genitalia and anus, tail, and limbs. Subsequently, the subject is examined in a prone position, from head to tail, in the following order: crown of the head, nape, hindquarters, and spine.

(3) Appearance inspection: This includes assessing the animal's physical condition (fetal monkey weight, head circumference, and length of long bones), skin, eyes, ears, nose, mouth, anus, and the openings of the urogenital system.

(4) Observation procedures

1) Observation of head: Examine the skull for completeness, and note any protrusions or depressions; Observe the size, shape, and position of the eyes, ears, nose, mouth, and lips for any abnormalities.

2) Trunk examination: Check for body symmetry; note any hematomas, gastroschisis, umbilical hernias, spinal deformities, or other abnormalities.

3) Limb examination: Examine the limbs for symmetry; note the number, shape, and length of digits.

4) Tail examination: check the tail for length and shape.

5) External genitalia and anus examination: examine the external genitalia for shape, size, position, and openings.

6) Record of examination results: record any observed abnormalities and take photographs during the visual inspection.

(5) Fetal sex determination: fetal sex is determined by direct examination of the external genitalia. The urethral opening is first inspected. Female animals have a relatively larger clitoris, with a groove-like formation on the ventral side leading to the urethral orifice. In male animals, the urethral orifice is located at the tip of the penis.

2. Internal organ examination of the fetus [17–19]

After visual inspection, the fetus is removed from the uterus. The fresh internal organs of the fetal monkey (excluding the heart, which is fixed first) are then examined.

(1) Lungs: Check for situs inversus (reversed position), hypoplasia, and supernumerary lobes. (Note: The left lung typically has two to three lobes, and the right lung three to four lobes).

(2) Heart: Check for position, septal defects, and single ventricle.

(3) Liver: Check for heterotopia, hypoplasia, and supernumerary lobes. (Note: The liver typically has six lobes).

(4) Gastrointestinal Tract: Check for intestinal hernias.

(5) Kidneys: Check for horseshoe kidney, hydronephrosis, renal agenesis, asymmetry, and heterotopia.

(6) Ureters: Check for hydroureter and bladder agenesis.

(7) Reproductive Organs: Check for uterine agenesis, cryptorchidism, and hypoplasia.

(8) Brain: Without disrupting the cranial bones, the brain tissue can be retrieved through the fontanelles (anterior and posterior) for examination after fixation.

3. Skeletal examination [20]

Fetal monkey skeletons are prepared for examination by double staining with Alcian blue and Alizarin red. If a cesarean section is performed in the third trimester of pregnancy, skeletal development can be assessed using X-ray imaging. If any skeletal abnormalities are observed, they should be photographed and the abnormalities documented.

(1) Skull: The skull is comprised of the supraoccipital bone, exoccipital bone, interparietal bone, parietal bone, frontal bone, nasal bone, incisive bone, maxilla, zygomatic bone, temporal bone, and mandible. The size, shape, and degree of ossification of the bones should be examined. Any abnormalities, such as incomplete or absent ossification or malformations, should be noted and recorded.

(2) Intrauterine ultrasound examination measurements of the fetus, such as body length, the length of long bones, abdominal circumference, head circumference, biparietal diameter, and occipitofrontal diameter should be taken.

(3) Sternal segments: Under normal circumstances, there are six sternal segments. The sternal segments are examined for fusion, increase or decrease in number, disorganization (indicated by segments being misaligned by at least 1/3 of their length or all 6 segments being misaligned), and incomplete ossification.

(4) Spine: The monkey's spine consists of approximately 41 vertebrae, including seven cervical vertebrae, 12–13 thoracic vertebrae, seven lumbar vertebrae, one to three sacral vertebrae, and 13–15 coccygeal vertebrae.

(5) Ribs: Ribs are normally 12 pairs, corresponding to the number of thoracic vertebrae. The presence of rib abnormalities such as fewer ribs, short ribs, bifurcated ribs, wavy ribs, or fused ribs is assessed.

(6) Carpal Bones: There are nine carpal bones.

(7) Limb bones: The limb bones of fetal monkeys include the shoulder girdle, forelimb bones (humerus, radius, ulna, metacarpals), hindlimb bones (femur, tibia, fibula, metatarsals), and pelvic bones (ilium, ischium, pubis). Any absence, presence of extra bones, degree of ossification, and abnormalities in shape and size are examined.

7.2.4 Assessment of Infant Monkey Development, Reflexes, Learning Abilities, Memory Function, and Neurobehavioral Activities [21]

1. Infant monkey development assessment includes: ① Physical development assessment: Physical examinations of the infant monkeys begin at birth (PND_0) and include measurements of body weight, tibia length, head circumference, tail length, crown-rump length, and anogenital distance; ② Grip strength assessment: The infant monkey's grip strength is assessed by measuring the duration it maintains its grip on a rope. A grip lasting 30 s or longer is considered satisfactory.

The reproductive physiology and endocrinology of macaques are similar to those of humans. Macaques have regular menstrual cycles, similar to humans (28 days). The time required for spermatogenesis is 40–46 days in macaques, while it is 64–74 days in humans. Humans and macaques exhibit similar organ development patterns between GD_{20} and GD_{50}. Following embryonic organogenesis, macaques undergo a period of accelerated development relative to humans. Consequently, the development of macaques at birth is the same as that of humans, or even exceeds that of humans. Thus, developmental studies conducted on newborn macaques (which are necessary for the development of certain rodent species) encompass all stages of human embryonic and fetal development [22].

The timing of embryonic development in Cynomolgus Monkeys is very similar to that of other macaques and baboons, with limb buds forming between GD_{25} and GD_{27}. Limb buds also develop within the same gestational time period in rhesus macaques, bonnet macaques, and baboons. Relevant studies indicate that thalidomide administration to pregnant NHPs can induce limb malformations if given before or during the period of limb bud formation. The period of sensitivity for limb development in rhesus macaque embryos spans from GD_{25} to GD_{30}, for baboons from GD_{25} to GD_{29}, and for bonnet macaques from GD_{25} to GD_{28}, which is consistent with the pattern observed in Cynomolgus Monkeys. The incidence of limb deficiencies in the embryos of stump-tailed macaques and Japanese monkeys occurs, respectively, during GD_{25}-GD_{27} and GD_{24}-GD_{26}. By increasing the dosage, the sensitive period for both the rhesus macaque and the baboon can be extended. If the drug is administered at GD_{24} or earlier, the rhesus macaque, the Cynomolgus Monkey, and the baboon can all give birth to normal offspring.

Abnormal fetal development in the Cynomolgus Monkeys can lead to fetal death, and structural and functional disorders from various causes can also result in lifelong disabilities. Although the study of human fetal biology has emerged, there are very few instances where a normal human fetus is available for analysis. Therefore, various experimental animals are applied as models for the study of normal fetal biology. The growth process and placental morphology of many animal fetuses differ significantly from those of higher primates, and the data generated may not be directly applicable to human embryos.

The development of macaques is relatively close to that of humans, and the embryonic organogenesis of Cynomolgus Monkeys has research significance. Comparative analysis of data from healthy adult Cynomolgus Monkeys at GD_{50}, GD_{75}, GD_{100}, GD_{125}, GD_{150}, and GD_{175} revealed variations in the biochemical maturation rate and relative water content of different organs. As fetal and postnatal development progresses, the liver consistently shows the lowest values at each stage. The relative water content of the lungs does not change, and the relative water content of the fetus does not change before structural maturation and extrauterine respiration. The numerical values for fetal muscle decrease as gestation progresses, while the relative nitrogen and protein content in the lungs increase in the third trimester of pregnancy.

The lung is the sole organ where relative size does not appreciably increase between birth and adulthood. The relative protein content of muscle grows at the highest rate in the fetal period, with liver values decreasing specifically between days 75 and 100. The relative lipid content in fetuses significantly influences their growth and development. Additionally, as the pregnancy progresses to full term, the relative lipid content in various fetal organs also shows specific patterns of change. The liver exhibits a higher relative fat content compared to other organs, with minimal change during the fetal period. A substantial increase in fat content is observed in the liver of infant monkeys from birth to adulthood.

The relative lipid content of the brain is higher than that of any other organ. By the end of the fetal period, the relative lipid content in the brain exceeds that in all other organs. During the third trimester of pregnancy, the content significantly increases and continues to rise after birth. The relative glycogen content of the kidneys and brain is low across all age groups studied. The glycogen content in the lungs is relatively high in the early trimester of pregnancy and decreases as the structure matures. The values for fetal muscle gradually increase, peaking at GD150, then decline towards levels observed in adult tissue.

2. Memory function and neurobehavioral activities Behavioral and neurofunctional assessments can be performed on infant monkeys 3 months after birth [23]. The specific operation process and scoring standards are provided in Table 7.1.

Recent studies demonstrate that hypothalamic neurohormones play a regulatory role in the higher neural activities of NHPs, and have a compensatory effect on advanced neurological disorders of aged animals. The neurohormonal effects in aged animals are particularly evident in genetic behavioral patterns and simple neural activities. These effects last longer in older animals and, while being similar to those in younger animals, are more pronounced. The impact of neurohormones on memory is complex and varied. Specifically, antidiuretic hormone (ADH), thyrotropin-releasing factor (TRF), and adrenocorticotropic hormone (ACTH) show different compensatory effects depending on the type of memory involved. Furthermore, older monkeys have homeostatic systems that operate differently from those in younger monkeys.

Studies show that neurohormonal compensation for advanced neurological disorders in elderly monkeys differs from that in young animals, mainly due to thyrotropin. The duration of ADH's compensatory effect is significantly reduced in aged monkeys. Administration of even extremely low doses of ADH results in pronounced sedation. Furthermore, in aged monkeys, ADH modulates neuronal metabolic processes, thereby facilitating the restoration of neuronal activity, the establishment of novel inter-brain connectivities, and a consequent enhancement of overall brain function. Consistent with this conclusion, Jolles' data shows that ADH directly impacts the central nervous system, stimulating motor activity, memory, learning, and emotional-motivational domains. Acting on subcortical centres enables comprehensive control and initiation of these processes. The anxiolytic and anti-stress effects of ADH likely result from the increased levels of γ-aminobutyric acid (GABA) and serotonin in neurons. Substantial experimental evidence suggests that ADH functions as a neuromodulator in the brain, modulating the activity of distinct neurotransmitter systems by upregulating or downregulating their levels. Notably, it has been shown to stimulate the impulse activity of catecholaminergic neurons. Importantly, reduced bioactive vasopressin levels in animals are associated with lower catecholamine levels, while elevated vasopressin leads to increased catecholamines, highlighting the antidiuretic hormone's regulatory influence.

Trace conditioning involves a reflex response where the conditioned stimulus appears first, disappears for a period, and is followed by the unconditioned stimulus.

Table 7.1 Operation methods and scoring criteria for behavioral and neurological function evaluation

Category	Item	Standard score	Operation method and scoring criteria
Locomotion ability	Visual orient	1	Eyes orient toward the objects in four positions of infant's periphery (0 = not facing; 1 = brief direct gaze; 2 = long-term direct gaze)
	Visual follow	1	Eyes follow a moving object in both horizontal and vertical directions (0 = contact but no following; 1 = starts to follow then stops; 2 = complete follow).
	Duration of looking	1	Length of looks on visual orientation and follow (0 = no looking; 1 = brief looks; 2 = 1- to 2-s looks)
	Attention	1	Rating of attention on visual orienting items (0 = no attention; 1 = slight attention (25% of time); 2 = definite attention (75% of time).
	Reaching and grasping	2	Attempts to grasp toy from orientation items (0=no attempts to grasp; 1 = swat, no finger flexion; 2 = intentional grasp with finger flexion)
Status assessment	Irritability	1	Amount of distress during examination (0 = extreme, constant distress; 1 = slight, distress few times; 2 = none, no distress)
	Vocalizations	3–5 times	Number of "whoo" vocalizations during a 1-min period in which the infant is placed alone in an enclosed Plexiglas area, approximately
	Struggling during. test	2	Amount of squirming during examination (0 = little, 25% of time; 1 = moderate, when appropriate; 2 = difficult, continuous squirming)
	Soothability	2	Ease of consoling infant during examination (0 = cannot console, nothing works; 1 = consoles with difficulty, pick up, rock and pat gently; 2 = easy to console, pick up only)
	Necessity of soothing	1	Necessity and frequency of soothing infant during examination (0 = less than average, intervention seldom necessary; 1 = moderate, intervention often necessary; 2 = harder than average, continuous intervention necessary)
	Predominant state	0	State of infant during examination (0 = alert, awake, and aware; 1 = alert but somewhat agitated; 2 = extreme agitation, body jerks and screams)

Table 7.1 (Continued)

Category	Item	Standard score	Operation method and scoring criteria
Activity	Response intensity	0	Quality of vocal reactions during 1-min vocalizations test (0 = low, "laid back"; 1 = moderate; 2 = high distress, intense in expression)
	Motor activity	1	Observation of motor activity during 1-min vocalizations test (0 = slight, 25% of time moving; 1 = normal, 50% of time moving; 2 = excessive, in continuous movement)
	Coordination	2	Quality of movement rated during 1-min vocalizations test (0 = poor, clumsy; 1 = adequate; 2 = excellent, agile)
	Spontaneous crawl	2	Quality of crawl locomotion (0 = absent, no crawl; 1 = weak try, uncoordinated; 2 = coordinated crawl)
	Passive resistance	2	Degree of resistance to passive flexion and extension of limbs (0 = barely discernible resistance; 1 = moderate resistance; 2 = strong resistance)
	Balance	2	Infant is held in the sitting position and support is withdrawn (0 = infant falls; 1 = places arms out but falls; 2 = uses arms for support, no fall)

(Adapted from Laughlin et al. [24]

In elderly monkeys, conditioned memory is significantly compromised, making it difficult for them to form trace conditioning. This can only be achieved with very short delay intervals. Long-delay trace conditioning (with delays up to 30 s) is often accompanied by a weakening of higher nervous activity, manifesting as stereotypy, tension responses, and pathological EEG changes. Analysis of brain morphology and cytoarchitecture has demonstrated that in aged monkeys, the cerebral cortex exhibits changes, including a reduction in capillary luminal diameter in the frontal and temporal cortices and impaired metabolite transport. Impaired excitability in hippocampal neurons correlates with cognitive impairment. Although efforts have focused on evaluating the distinct contributions of different brain structures to various memory parameters, the experimental data largely originate from studies on lower mammals, specifically rats and rabbits, which lack the differentiated association cortices found in higher mammals. According to data provided by some scholars, memory processes and disorders (amnesia and dementia) in primates are similar to those in humans. These data also suggest that trace conditioning in aged monkeys and lower animals is comparable. It has been noted that achieving trace conditioning in hedgehogs and rabbits is particularly challenging. Specifically, the short inter-stimulus interval can reach 15 s for hedgehogs and 25 s for rabbits.

7.2.5 Amniotic Fluid Collection [25]

Amniotic fluid is the liquid within the amniotic sac, secreted mainly by the amniotic membrane. Once blood vessels form on the amniotic sac wall, some fluid is derived from vascular permeation. As fetal swallowing and urination develop, the amniotic fluid enters a dynamic circulation. During late pregnancy, fetal vernix, shed epithelial cells, and meconium also enter the amniotic fluid. The fetus is enveloped by and develops within this fluid, which cushions against external impacts and acts as a lubricant for the birth canal during parturition. In a full-term fetus, the approximate volume of amniotic fluid is 1000 mL. The volume of amniotic fluid can be diagnosed during late pregnancy through ultrasound. Amniocentesis is the most common prenatal diagnostic technique, involving the use of a needle to aspirate amniotic fluid from the uterine cavity. Under continuous ultrasound guidance, a needle is transabdominally inserted into the uterine cavity to aspirate amniotic fluid, obtaining a sample containing exfoliated cells, exudates, urine, or secretions of the fetus. Amniotic fluid contains amniotic epithelial cells and fetal epithelial cells. It can be detected directly or cultured in various media for chromosomal, biochemical, molecular, and microbiological studies.

In clinical practice, amniocentesis for genetic testing is typically performed between 16 and 20 weeks of gestation. Diagnostic amniocentesis is commonly used for prenatal diagnosis of chromosomal abnormalities, single-gene disorders, fetal infections, and chorioamnionitis. Before undergoing amniocentesis, both preoperative design and ultrasound screening are essential. The procedure is conducted entirely under real-time ultrasound guidance, adhering to appropriate sterile techniques, and involves continuous observation of the needle's position throughout. Following the surgery, an immediate ultrasound is conducted to assess the fetus's viability.

Comprehensive clinical data recording and necessary checks are indispensable preconditions. Pre-operative ultrasound assessment includes a comprehensive intrauterine fetal scan. This assessment is accomplished through continuous scanning of the uterine cavity and obtaining transverse views of the pregnant monkey's abdomen to evaluate several critical factors: placental location, fetal position, chorionicity in multiple pregnancies, fetal movements, gestational age and viability, amniotic fluid volume, cervical length, and to rule out chorioamniotic separation.

The following precautions are critical when performing amniocentesis collection of amniotic fluid: ① Ensure that the needle maintains a perpendicular orientation with respect to the abdominal surface of the pregnant monkey; ② Select the appropriate needle length, taking into consideration the body size of the pregnant monkey; ③ Select the largest vertical amniotic fluid pocket visualized on a transverse abdominal ultrasound, avoiding oblique or lateral approaches; ④ Magnify the ultrasound image to ensure complete visualization of the maternal skin and amniotic fluid pocket. Documentation of placentocentesis should only be performed if there is a risk of surgical failure. This technique should only be used for malpresentations. ⑤ To prevent sample misidentification in multiple pregnancies, separate amniocenteses should be performed using two distinct needles for each fetus. This aims to extract amniotic fluid and perform angiography. ⑥ Aseptic preparation of the abdomen and transducer is essential for real-time visualization of needle placement.

In ultrasound-guided amniocentesis, a free-hand technique is employed, wherein a trained professional performing the procedure uses one hand to maneuver the ultrasound transducer and the other hand to guide the needle. The entire procedure is conducted under continuous ultrasound guidance, with real-time visualization of the needle throughout the process. Needle insertion has four stages: abdominal skin puncture, uterine puncture, entry into the amniotic cavity, and advancement of the needle. The needle is inserted at a 45° angle to the midline of the pregnant monkey, and at 90° contralateral to the transducer. Careful observation of the full transducer pathway is necessary to avoid injury to adjacent intestinal loops. The uterine puncture may induce discomfort or localized uterine contractions, potentially causing distress or startling the subject. If uterine muscle contractions cause distress, it may be necessary to readjust the needle's direction. Adjustment is required.

During amniocentesis, a needle is advanced into the amniotic cavity via a controlled puncture. This technique is necessary to avoid rupture of the amniotic membrane and ensure successful aspiration of amniotic fluid. There is a possibility of unsuccessful aspiration of the amniotic membrane or amniotic fluid. If amniotic membrane tenting occurs, needle puncture or rotation may aid in successful amniotic fluid aspiration. Optimal needle advancement into the amniotic cavity should be performed under full visualization. After proper placement within the cavity, the needle is withdrawn, and the necessary volume of amniotic fluid is aspirated, with the initial 2 mL discarded. Amniotic fluid should be collected into two to three sterile tubes. If the initial aspirate contains blood, the first 2–3 mm of amniotic fluid should be discarded.

The needle may remain within the amniotic cavity for approximately 1 min. If the aspiration is unsuccessful after 1 min, the needle should be withdrawn. A new puncture site and a new needle should be employed to avoid contamination. A new puncture site must be chosen, and the needle should be changed to avoid contamination. No more than two attempts are recommended. If a satisfactory sample is not obtained, the procedure should be repeated 1 week later.

During cesarean delivery, amniotic fluid can be aspirated by inserting a sterile syringe into the amniotic cavity. Appropriate care should be taken throughout the procedure to prevent contamination.

7.2.6 Sperm Collection

Spermatogenesis is a complex process, especially when considering the development of germ cells. During this process, spermatogenic cells, with the support of Sertoli cells, undergo mitotic and meiotic divisions and differentiation to generate elongated spermatozoa. The duration of spermatogenesis in monkeys is 40–46 days, and the transit time of spermatozoa through the epididymis is 5–10 days. The male reproductive system is classified into six developmental stages, ranging from "immature" to "mature" (refer to Chap. 8). At stage 6, the epididymis of the male animal exhibits a large quantity of mature spermatozoa [26].

In biomedical research, the most common methods for sperm collection are electroejaculation and vibratory stimulation. Electroejaculation is the process of using an electric current to produce an ejaculation. The most frequently used electroejaculation procedural approaches are rectal probe electrostimulation and penile electrostimulation.

The sperm samples collected through rectal probe electroejaculation typically exhibit low sperm concentrations, which renders them less appropriate for quantitative assessments of semen samples. Nevertheless, these samples are highly valuable for qualitative analyses, such as determining the presence of sperm in ejaculates to confirm sexual maturity and evaluate the sperm morphology. Penile electrostimulation is most frequently used for the collection of sperm for quantitative analysis due to higher semen volumes and is the recommended semen collection method for in vitro fertilization (IVF) or intracytoplasmic sperm injection. Most semen parameters yield low statistical power for evaluating reproductive function; only sperm motility and, to a lesser extent, sperm morphology have higher statistical power (between 70% and 90%), thereby rendering them more useful in the evaluation of reproductive function.

1. Rectal probe electrostimulation (RPE) The RPE procedure is the historical method for semen collection in NHPs. The mechanism of ejaculation is by direct stimulation of peripheral neuromuscular junctions, resulting in the contraction and relaxation of pelvic organs. This stimulation results in the release of the contents of those organs [27].

The procedure requires sedation to light anesthesia but does not require training of the animal. However, operator skill and training are integral to the success of the procedure. Once lightly anesthetized, the animal is placed in lateral recumbency. Alternatively, a sling can be used to suspend the animal in ventral recumbency, which provides good access to the penis and improves the positioning for semen collection. The size of the probe is species dependent. It should fit easily into the rectum, and the probe electrode footprint should be oriented directly over the prostate. Prior to use, the electrodes are lightly sanded, rinsed, and sanitized. The penis is gently exteriorized from the prepuce and cleaned to remove particulate matter if necessary (e.g., sterile saline). The penis is held with powder-free gloves during the collection procedure. The prostate is gently palpated to determine depth and to facilitate placement of the probe electrodes directly over the prostate. A thin layer of sterile water-soluble lubricating gel is applied to the probe prior to insertion. To ensure contact of the electrodes with the prostate, the tip of the probe is gently pressed downward by lifting the other end of the probe. The probe is activated by slowly increasing the voltage until the animal responds with leg extension, with or without clasping. The voltage setting to which the animal responds becomes the animal's voltage set point (the lowest voltage that elicits a response). Each stimulus is comprised of a slowly increasing response voltage that remains steady for a brief period (up to about 5 s) before decreasing. As the stimulus is applied, the penis is observed for extension, rigidity, engorgement, and pre-ejaculate. Multiple repetitions comprise a set of stimuli. On average, three sets of stimulations will produce an ejaculation. During the entire course of stimulation, the tip of the penis is held over a pre-warmed glass beaker for reproductive purposes or other collection receptacle (e.g., 15 mL conical tube).

Animal welfare considerations: This procedure is more invasive than other techniques, and it is important to check the animal and the probe regularly to ensure that no blood is present. The rectum is gently manually palpated to check for evidence of blood and to determine if there is an increase in internal temperature in the tissue overlying the prostate. If blood is present or there is a subjectively increased temperature above the prostate, the procedure is immediately stopped, and the animal is allowed to recover. Post-procedure care is up to the veterinary judgment. The procedure should be limited to no more than twice-weekly collection.

2. Penile electrostimulation procedure (PEP) The PEP operates by stimulating afferent nerve endings in the penis, thereby triggering the sympathetic efferent pathways that mediate penile erection and the process of ejaculation.

Male Cynomolgus Monkeys, with an age of 5 years or greater, are chosen for semen collection via a modified penile electroejaculation technique. During semen collection, monkeys are restrained in a chair, with manual assistance from personnel if necessary, to minimize stress on the animals. Traditional restraint methods for this procedure involve placing the animal in an open restraint chair and using the pole-and-collar technique for conscious sample collection. However, recent studies demonstrate that training the animal to enter directly from its home cage into a closed box chair is a viable alternative to open chair restraint, potentially representing a significant refinement for animal welfare, semen quality (increased sample volume and sperm concentration), and training time, so it may be a preferred method of restraint. Additional guidelines for NHP restraint are available for reference.

To begin, the penis is gently extricated, gel defibrillator pads with lubricating gel are wrapped around the penis, and electrodes are attached to the gel pads and then connected to the electroejaculation stimulator device. A stimulating current is administered, with the first pulsation given at a low voltage (appropriate for the species and size of the animal) for approximately 10–15 , followed by slow incremental increases up to a predetermined maximum. Generally, no more than three trials are attempted at one session (depending on the specific procedure and the animal response). Species-specific voltages vary widely based on a number of variables and are described in the literature. For example, in Cynomolgus Monkeys, a trial may start at 10–30 volts, with a duration of 1–3 ms. The voltage can be increased in 5–10 V increments, as needed, reaching a maximum of 50 V or more. At each stimulation, the animal is carefully observed for physiologic response and ejaculation. If ejaculation is not observed, the animal should rest for at least 1 min. The animal is stimulated until an ejaculate is obtained or the last trial attempt has been reached. In the event that ejaculation is not observed within 10 min, the animal is returned to its cage. A collection tube is placed at the tip of the penis to collect the ejaculated semen sample, which is then processed for evaluation. Semen collection can be performed multiple times in a row over days/weeks without ill effects. Sperm numbers are maintained through several electroejaculations, but will eventually decrease with multiple collections. In consideration of both animal welfare and sperm production rates, the procedure is usually not attempted more frequently than weekly (e.g., during a 2-week pre-study period for baseline determinations) and monthly/quarterly (e.g., during the dosing phase of a study). If sampling is conducted over longer durations for quantitative assessment, sampling at more frequent intervals (e.g., every other week) may be appropriate. The initial semen collection has an 80% success rate, increasing to 100% success rate for the second collection within a 2-day timeframe. The frequency of collection may increase depending on the study requirements. Animals collected for gamete preservation, IVF/ICSI, or genetic preservation should be given approximately 48 h of rest between samplings. Once animals are trained and experienced with the procedure, they should be observed carefully for possible spontaneous ejaculation prior to electrostimulation being applied.

Most reports of direct penile electrostimulation indicate higher numbers of sperm per ejaculate compared to the rectal probe method and higher sperm quality based on the ability of sperm to fertilize oocytes in vitro. The direct penile method has been proven to achieve better stimulation of the entire reproductive tract and has fewer problems with urine contamination and semen sample dilution due to the lack of anesthesia. Also, the potential for retrograde ejaculation into the bladder, which has been associated with the rectal probe method, is minimized with penile electrostimulation. This noninvasive technique requires that the animal be trained and the experimental environment be controlled (e.g., a quiet room and staff familiar with the animals). It may also take longer to obtain a sample with this method than with the rectal probe electroejaculation technique, but generally no longer than several minutes. A potential drawback of penile electrostimulation is that some animals do not respond to penile stimulation and will not provide a semen sample. Additionally, because this method involves working with conscious, chair-restrained animals, animal health status, such as endogenous and exogenous viral status, and the occupational risk therein, should be taken into consideration.

Semen samples are collected and sealed in test tubes or collection tubes, then equilibrated at 4°C for 30 min. Subsequently, samples are cryopreserved by freezing for 10 min and stored in liquid nitrogen. Following a storage period of 2–180 days in liquid nitrogen, the cryovials were rapidly thawed in a 37°C water bath. Cryopreserved spermatozoa are utilized for artificial insemination to propagate Cynomolgus Monkeys [28, 29].

Animal welfare considerations: Penile electrostimulation is a noninvasive procedure. Use of defibrillator pads and gel for application of stimulating current to the penis increases the animal's comfort during the procedure and eliminates issues associated with older methods, such as metal foil electrodes, which can lead to dermal trauma. Animals are not anesthetized for the procedure, but rather acclimated and trained for restraint. The stimulating current is administered in a conservative and carefully controlled manner. Even for animals that have undergone the procedure, no more than three attempts to collect an ejaculate should be made in a single session on any given day. The animal is rewarded for its participation regardless of the outcome of the procedure.

3. Penile vibratory stimulation (PVS) Vibratory stimulation is a procedure involving the natural reflex sequence resulting in a normal emission and ejaculation response, yielding a natural ejaculation. This technique uses a modified human vibratory device equipped with a collection vessel. The glass collecting tube has an internal diameter appropriate to achieve good contact with the penis and the required level of stimulation.

It is commonly used with the animal awake and chair-restrained, with novel rewards provided to encourage participation, while working in a darkened room to reduce the animal's excitement. For the collection of sperm, the penis is gently extruded from the preputial sheath, and the vibrating glass tube is turned over the tip of the penis and held against the preputial orifice. Vibratory parameters used depend on the response of the animal to stimulation, which is increased gradually with allowance for rest periods. If ejaculation is not achieved within 15–20 min, stimulation is discontinued.

Animal welfare considerations: PVS may not be the preferred method for semen collection in macaques, such as Cynomolgus Monkeys.

Animal selection: Careful consideration must be given to the physiological status of the animal when collecting semen, irrespective of the method utilized. The most reliable indicator of sexual maturity in NHPs is the confirmation of spermatogenesis, evidenced by the presence of spermatozoa in the ejaculate. Seasonal variations should be taken into account when scheduling semen collection in some NHP species. Before undertaking this confirmation, animal selection can be enhanced through the application of standard criteria such as age, body weight, and testicular volume. Testosterone levels are not a dependable metric due to considerable pulsatile/diurnal variation and variability among individual animals. These parameters are not individually predictive of sexual maturity, and the definitive standards for maturity are subject to variation based on animal species and, in some cases, even geographical provenance. Studies have shown that the onset of sexual maturity, marked by the presence of sperm in the ejaculate, occurs at 3–4 years of age in Cynomolgus Monkeys from Mauritius, while the same species from the Asian mainland exhibits delayed maturity, requiring more than 4 years. In the published literature on Cynomolgus Monkeys and Rhesus Macaques, evidence suggests that sexual maturation is improbable in animals under 4 years old and with a body weight below 4 kg.

Before the procedure, a comprehensive physical examination of the animal is necessary, with particular attention to the rectum to check for any irregularities, including scars, stenosis, or hemorrhoids. Additionally, animals that exhibit characteristics likely to cause stress or adversely affect procedural success, including signs of tension or anxiety, are unsuitable and should be excluded. Similarly, animals unable to tolerate chair restraint or electrode placement are also inappropriate for inclusion in the study.

Collection methods should be selected based on the animal's size. In particular, smaller animals, such as New World nonhuman primates (squirrel monkeys and marmosets), are more amenable to PVS than the other two methods discussed. There is currently no evidence to support the successful application of this technique in macaques.

4. Natural collection The female monkey's external genitalia are cleaned with a 2% benzalkonium chloride solution. Vaginal mucus is then aspirated with a syringe and wiped with a sterile swab before the female is introduced to a cage with male monkeys for mating.

Semen collection: Semen is collected 15 min after or upon confirmation of ejaculation. The female animal is separated from the male, and the animal is secured with its tail positioned upward. A pipette is carefully inserted into the vagina, and the ejaculated semen is then slowly collected using the pipette.

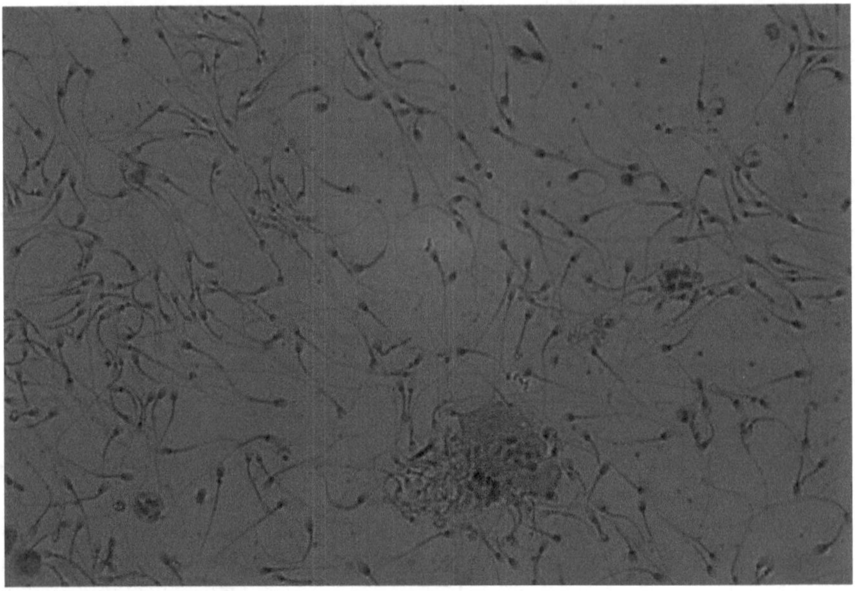

Fig. 7.13 Cynomolgus Monkey sperm (Giemsa staining, ×400)

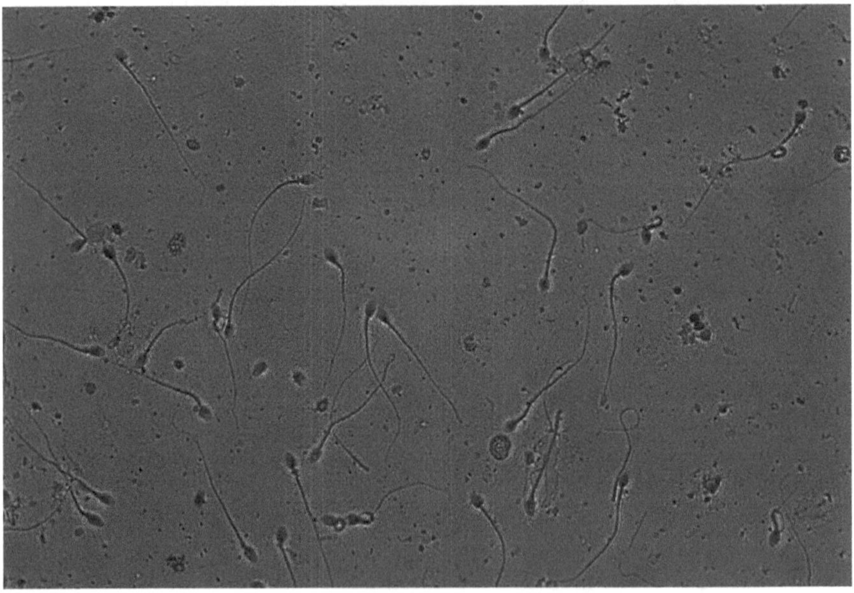

Fig. 7.14 Cynomolgus Monkey sperm (Giemsa staining, ×400)

Cryopreservation of semen: Following collection, semen is transferred to a small tube and incubated in a 37°C water bath for approximately 10 min. Subsequently, the semen is diluted at a ratio of 1:5 and incubated at 37°C for an additional 10 min. Finally, approximately 0.1 mL of the diluted semen is directly dripped into wells formed on the surface of a dry ice block within a freezing container. This technique is known as "vitrification." Alternatively, the diluted semen is placed into a small vial, and the vial is then positioned in a beaker containing approximately 50 mL of 37°C warm water, where it is gradually cooled to 4°C in a cryogenic freezer.

The semen is allowed to acclimate to the lower temperature over a period of 30 min or more. Furthermore, this 30-min duration may aid in achieving a glycerol equilibration, which plays a crucial role in protecting sperm from damage during freezing. The glycerol concentration in the extender used by Rousse et al. is approximately 14%.

This collection and preservation technique is capable of ensuring a sufficient quantity of high-quality semen in a fluid state. Semen collection from the vagina of a female macaque after mating is relatively simple. Macaques form a semen coagulum immediately during or after ejaculation, making it easy to obtain liquid semen containing a small amount of coagulum (Fig. 7.13). Compared with electroejaculation, naturally collected semen typically consists of both liquid and coagulum and exhibits higher sperm viability (Fig. 7.14).

7.2.7 Laparoscopic Reproductive Interventions for Female NHPs

In reproductive medical research, the use of laparoscopic surgical techniques in reproductive procedures of female NHPs is becoming increasingly common. Laparoscopic methods are generally considered minor surgeries, thereby reducing the number of major surgical procedures that animals experience throughout their lives. Minimally invasive laparoscopic approaches are recommended to replace open surgical techniques whenever feasible, in order to minimize pain and distress while reducing postoperative recovery time. The substitution of laparoscopic examination for laparotomy contributes to the refinement of the 3Rs (Replacement, Reduction and Refinement). The implementation of laparoscopic techniques necessitates approval by the Institutional Animal Care and Use Committee (IACUC), demonstrable laparoscopic proficiency by the veterinary surgeon, access to appropriate equipment, and the cultivation of a robust collaborative relationship between veterinary and research personnel.

Laparoscopic examination is a surgical procedure performed within the abdominal cavity using a camera or laparoscope through small incisions (typically 3–10 mm). It has been employed for various reproductive techniques in both human and NHP medicine. Common laparoscopic reproductive procedures in NHPs encompass follicular aspiration for the purpose of oocyte collection, ovariectomy, endometrial biopsy, diagnostic laparoscopy, and embryo transfer. Furthermore, the application of laparoscopy extends to specialized reproductive evaluations, the induction of disease models, and therapeutic interventions in NHPs [30].

In comparison to open abdominal surgery, laparoscopic procedures utilize smaller incisions, thereby generally resulting in less tissue inflammation, alleviated post-operative incisional pain, decreased blood loss, and a lower risk of post-operative infection. Moreover, the likelihood of post-operative adhesion formation is diminished. Similar to human patients, these combined benefits result in reduced overall veterinary care time, potentially lessen the need for prolonged post-operative analgesia, and for NHPs, facilitate a faster return to be housed in social groups.

Animal selection: Female NHPs selected for laparoscopic procedures should generally be sexually mature. Detailed consideration is warranted regarding any active reproductive history or prior surgical procedures related to reproductive manipulation. If recent blood tests have not been performed, animals scheduled for laparoscopic examination should undergo routine screening. This screening should comprise a comprehensive medical history review, along with a complete blood cell count and biochemical analysis as part of the physical examination. The review of past medical history should encompass a detailed assessment of prior parturitions and reproductive manipulation procedures. Special consideration must be given to any complications or sequelae. Abnormalities observed during previous surgical procedures involving reproductive manipulation, such as aberrant anatomy, adhesions, or cysts, could serve as exclusion criteria for the animal's participation in studies, including laparoscopic procedures. Depending on the research purposes, a documented history of normal menstrual cycles may be significant. The physical examination should involve bimanual (rectal and abdominal) palpation to assess the reproductive function of uterine structures, which typically move freely and unrestricted in the caudal abdomen. When selecting animal models for studies that include laparoscopic reproductive surgery, it is critical to assess the potential for physiological damage, such as reproductive impairment. The impact of such harm on the animals' long-term usability in future research and breeding initiatives must be carefully evaluated.

Surgical considerations: The specific laparoscopic techniques, equipment, and preoperative evaluations employed will be tailored to the objectives and procedural details of each individual study. This surgical procedure can be adapted for specific species or animals that have undergone previous procedures. In species prone to abdominal adhesions, such as apes, preoperative ultrasound is important for selecting either a paramedian or a supraumbilical midline approach to avoid existing tissue adhesions. Prior reproductive or cesarean surgeries in animals can often lead to the formation of abdominal midline adhesions. Consequently, paramedian placement of laparoscopic ports is critical during surgery in these cases to facilitate adequate visualization of the surgical field.

Surgical complications in both humans and animals can be associated with laparoscopic procedures. These complications may arise from the processes of entering the abdomen, creating pneumoperitoneum, as well as positioning and/or visualization and manipulation within the surgical field. Inappropriately large port site incisions can result in the loss of pneumoperitoneum and subsequently impair the ability to maintain proper visualization of the reproductive organs. The incision should be kept to a minimum size to allow for the placement of ports while avoiding trauma to adjacent tissues, thereby minimizing carbonic oxide leakage. The use of trocars can lead to a variety of mechanical injuries, such as damage to major blood vessels or the gastrointestinal system, abdominal wall hematomas, bladder perforations, hernias, and/or ureteral injuries. The potential for injury to abdominal structures exists during laparoscopic manipulation of the abdominal cavity, particularly when tissue handling is not meticulous or if poor visualization makes it challenging to accurately identify structures. Pneumoperitoneum, achieved through the insufflation of carbon dioxide into the abdominal cavity to enhance visualization and manipulation of intra-abdominal structures, is associated with intraoperative complications such as respiratory acidosis, deep vein thrombosis, subcutaneous emphysema, gas embolism, decreased dynamic lung compliance, and increased peak and plateau inspiratory pressures. Clinically, shoulder pain is also observed following laparoscopic surgery, attributed to diaphragmatic irritation and/or phrenic nerve stretching. Animals positioned in the Trendelenburg position (defined as a supine position with a 15°–30° head-down tilt, with the feet elevated above the head; a standard position for female laparoscopy procedures) may experience increased mechanical impedance to lung inflation compared to animals with abdominal insufflation of carbon dioxide; therefore, mechanical ventilation is recommended.

Postoperative precautions: Postoperative monitoring should be continuously conducted until the patient can consistently maintain an upright posture. Furthermore, daily postoperative monitoring, including assessment of basic NHP physiological and behavioral parameters, should be performed for 3–7 days post-surgery. Postoperative analgesia following routine laparoscopic procedures should be administered for a minimum of 48–72 h and may be achieved through the use of opioids, nonsteroidal anti-inflammatory drugs (NSAIDs), or a combination as determined by veterinary assessment.

Short-term complications associated with laparoscopic examinations are generally related to surgical incisions. However, postoperative abdominal discomfort, particularly increased abdominal pressure or bleeding during inflation, should be closely monitored. Postoperative surveillance should focus on erythema, inflammation, and discharge at the incision site, which may indicate a surgical site infection. The potential for fascial dehiscence and herniation of abdominal contents through the incision site also exists. Because of the small incision size, the omentum is typically the most common abdominal tissue involved in laparoscopic incisional hernias. While edema at the incision site may be misconstrued as a hernia, it usually resolves without intervention.

Long-term complications associated with laparoscopic procedures are primarily impaired fertility, endometriosis, and adhesion formation. Trauma or injury to the ovaries, fallopian tubes, uterus, or related vasculature during laparoscopic surgery can compromise fertility. The formation of adhesions is a frequent consequence of laparoscopic reproductive surgeries in NHPs. Adhesions are often mild, involving minor omental attachments to the ovaries, uterus, or laparoscopic port sites. However, more extensive adhesions can occur, leading to distortions of normal reproductive anatomy. The presence of adhesions can be evaluated using bimanual palpation and reproductive ultrasound during follow-up physical examinations. Adhering strictly to hemostasis at the incision/trocar sites and performing thorough abdominal lavage after laparoscopic procedures to eliminate blood and foreign material may help to minimize the risk of adhesions. Under the guidance of hysteroscopy (e.g., endometrial biopsy), abdominal flushing may reduce the risk of endometriosis. Overall, when performed properly in healthy animals, the risk of postoperative complications is very low.

Ethical Approval

This chapter is a review of previously published accounts; as such, no animal or human studies were performed.

References

1. Zeng Z, Chen Y, Bai S (1982) Regarding the sexual cycle of *Macaca mulatta*. Chin J Wildlife 000(002):3035
2. Aslam H, Rosiepen G, Krishnamurthy H, et al. (1999) The cycle duration of the seminiferous epithelium remains unaltered during GnRH antagonist-induced testicular involution in rats and monkeys. J Endocrinol 161:281–288
3. Bhehre HM, Nashan D, Nieschlag E (1989) Objective measurement of testicular volume by ultrasonography: evaluation of the technique and comparison with orchidometer estimates. Int J Androl 12:395–403
4. Chellman GJ, Bussiere JL, Makori N et al (2009) Developmental and reproductive toxicology studies in nonhuman primates. Birth Defects Res B Dev Reprod Toxicol 83:446.
5. Smedley JV, Bailey SA, Perry RW, et al. (2002) Methods for predicting sexual maturity in male cynomolgus macaques on the basis of age, body weight, and histologic evaluation of the testes. Contemp Top Lab Anim Sci 41:18–20
6. Boot R, Leussink AB, Vlug RF (1985) Influence of housing conditions on pregnancy outcome in cynomolgus monkeys (Cynomolgus Monkeys). Lab Anim 19(1):42
7. Buse E, Habermann G, Osterburg I, et al. (2003) Reproductive/developmental toxicity and immune toxicity assessment in the nonhuman primate model. Toxicology 185(3):221–227
8. Henck JW, Hilbish KG, Serabian MA, et al. (1996) Reproductive toxicity testing of therapeutic biotechnology agents. Teratology 53(2):185–195
9. Meyer JK, Fitzsimmons D, Hastings TF, et al. (2006) Methods for the prediction of breeding success in male cynomolgus monkeys (Cynomolgus Monkeys) used for reproductive toxicology studies. J Am Assoc Lab Anim Sci 45:31–36
10. Weinbauer GF, Frings W, Fuchs A et al (2007) Reproductive/developmental toxicity assessment of biopharmaceuticals in nonhuman primates. John Wiley & Sons, Inc.
11. Amann RP, Johnson L, Thompson JrDL, et al. (1976) Daily spermatozoal production, epididymal spermatozoal reserves and transit time of spermatozoa through the epididymis of the rhesus monkey. Biol Reprod 15:586–592
12. Cruz-Lemini M, Parra-Saavedra M, Borobio V, et al. (2014) How to perform an amniocentesis. Ultrasound Obstet Gynecol 44:727–731
13. Hearn JP, Hodges JK, Gems S (1988) Early secretion of chorionic gonadotrophin by marmoset embryos in vivo and in vitro. J Endocrinol 119:249–255
14. Roland KM (1991) Chorionic gonadotrophin corpus luteum function and embryo implantation in the rhesus monkey: in the use of non-human primates in research on human reproduction. WHO Symposiums, Sukhumi. pp 214–217
15. Fraser HM, Lunn SF (1999) Nonhuman primates and female reproductive medicine. In: Weinbauer GF, Korte R (eds.) Reproduction in nonhuman primates: a model system for human reproductive physiology and toxicology. Münster: Waxmann. pp 27–59
16. Holsapple MP, West LJ, Landreth KS (2003) Species comparison of anatomical and functional immune system development. Birth Defects Res B 68:321–334

17. Makori N, Rodriguez CG, Cukierski MA, et al. (1996) Development of the brain in staged embryos of the long-tailed monkey (Cynomolgus Monkeys). Primates 37:351–361
18. Zoetis T, Hurtt ME (2003) Species comparison of anatomical and functional renal development. Birth Defects Res B 68:111–120
19. Zoetis T, Hurtt ME (2003) Species comparison of lung development. Birth Defects Res B 68:121–124
20. Zoetis T, Tassinari MS, Bagi C, et al. (2003) Species comparison of postnatal bone growth and development. Birth Defects Res B 68:86–110
21. Testard C, Tremblay S, Platt M (2021) From the field to the lab and back: neuroethology of primate social behavior. Curr Opin Neurobiol 68:76–83
22. Wood SL, Beyer BK, Cappon GD (2003) Species comparison of postnatal CNS development: functional measures. Birth Defects Res B 68:391–407
23. Ausderau KK, Dammann C, Mcmanus K, et al. (2017) Cross species comparison of behavioral neurodevelopmental milestones in the common marmoset monkey and human child. Dev Psychobiol 59(4):807–821
24. Laughlin NK, Lasky RE, Giles NL et al (1999) Lead effects on neurobehavioral development in the neonatal rhesus monkey (*Macaca mulatta*). Neurotoxicol Teratol 21(6): 627–638
25. Dimri N, Baijal A (2016) Amniocentesis. Fetal Med 3:131–135
26. Ehmcke J, Wistuba J, Schlatt AS (2006) Spermatogonial stem cells: questions, models and perspectives. Hum Reprod Update 12(3):275–282
27. Gould KG, Mann DR (1988) Comparison of electrostimulation methods for semen recovery in rhesus monkey (*Macaca mulatta*). J Med Primatol 17:95–103
28. Roussel JD, Austin CR (1967) Preservation of primate spermatozoa by freezing. J Reprod Fertil 13:333–335
29. Sankai T, Terao K, Yanagimachi R, et al. (1994) Cryopreservation of spermatozoa from cynomolgus monkeys (Cynomolgus Monkeys). J Reprod Fertil 101:273–278
30. Walthall K, Cappon GD, Hurtt ME, et al. (2005) Postnatal development of the gastrointestinal system: a species comparison. Birth Defects Res B 74:132–156

A Case Study of Reproductive and Developmental Toxicology in Cynomolgus Monkeys

8

Fang Pan, Mao Shanshan, Zhou Li and Sun Zuyue

Abstract

This chapter mainly presents fertility evaluation with toxicokinetics in cynomolgus monkeys (Phase I), repeated-dose administration with fertility evaluation, embryo-fetal developmental toxicity with toxicokinetics (Phase I), and enhanced perinatal toxicity with toxicokinetics. These studies were conducted mainly in accordance with ICH S5(R3) "Detection of Reproductive and Developmental Toxicity for Human Pharmaceuticals" (February 2020). In particular, the research cases in this chapter are all from the accumulated work of the chief editor's laboratory in recent years and are original materials; their authenticity is beyond doubt. Their scientific and normative quality is basically consistent with the most advanced and cutting-edge scientific and technological level and relevant regulations and guidelines. However, due to the complexity of such studies, some considerations may inevitably be insufficient. In the report content of this chapter, while establishing a nonclinical evaluation research system for cynomolgus monkey reproduction and development, we also summarize shortcomings and reflect on them, and believe that these experiences have certain reference value. For confidentiality, the names of test articles were specially concealed and replaced with "AAA", "BBB", "CCC", etc. Other information inconvenient to

F. Pan (✉) · M. Shanshan · Z. Li
Hubei Topgene Biotechnology Co., Ltd., Wuhan, China
e-mail: fangpan@topgenebio.com

S. Zuyue
The GBA National Institute for Nanotechnology Innovation, Guangdong Canosafe Pharmtech Co., Ltd, Guangdong, China

L. Zhou and Z. Sun (eds.), *Reproductive and Developmental Toxicology on Macaca Fascicularis*, https://doi.org/10.1007/978-981-92-3834-7_8

disclose, such as company names, drug names, and institutional codes, has been uniformly replaced with "XXX".

Keywords

Cynomolgus monkey · Reproductive and developmental toxicology · Case study · Positive drug validation · Fertility evaluation · Toxicokinetics · Embryo-fetal developmental toxicity · Enhanced perinatal developmental toxicity · Cyclophosphamide · Testosterone undecanoate · Thalidomide

This chapter mainly presents the studies of fertility evaluation with toxicokinetics in cynomolgus monkeys (stage I), repeated administration with fertility evaluation, fetal developmental toxicity with toxicokinetics (stage II), and enhanced perinatal toxicity with toxicokinetics. These studies were conducted in compliance with ICH S5 (R3) Detection of Reproductive and Developmental Toxicity for Human Pharmaceuticals (February 2020).

The format of the content of each case study follows the principle of "summarizing the main contents of the report" in the *Good Laboratory Practice for Nonclinical Laboratory Studies* issued by the National Medical Products Administration (CFDA) on August 2, 2017.

In particular, the research cases in this chapter are all from the accumulated work of the chief editor's laboratory in recent years, which belong to the original materials, its authenticity is beyond doubt, and their scientific and normative aspects are basically in line with the most advanced and cutting-edge scientific and technological level and relevant regulations and guidelines. However, due to the complexity of such experiments, there will inevitably be some ill-considered points. In the report content of this chapter, while establishing the nonclinical evaluation research system of reproduction and development of cynomolgus monkeys, we are also summarizing and reflecting on the shortcomings, and believe that these experiences have certain reference value.

In order to keep confidentiality, the identity of the test article was specially hidden, replaced with "AAA," "BBB," "CCC," etc., and other inconvenient information, such as company name, drug name, and institutional code, will be uniformly replaced by "XXX."

8.1 Study on Fertility Evaluation and Toxokinetics of Cynomolgus Monkeys (Phase I)

8.1.1 Study Purpose

According to ICH S5 (R3), a fertility and early embryonic development toxicity study in cynomolgus monkeys was designed to evaluate the side effects of administration in male and/or female animals before mating and continued after mating and implantation. The purpose of the study was to evaluate the maturation of gametes, mating behavior, fertility, preimplantation development, and implantation of embryos. For female animals, including the effects on the estrous cycle, fallopian tube transport; In male animals, this includes the detection of functional effects (e.g., epididymal sperm maturation) that cannot be obtained by histological examination of male reproductive organs.

This study is a systematic validation study of positive drugs that cause damage to the male and female reproductive systems. Therefore, positive drugs [1, 2] known to have reproductive toxicity were selected: cyclophosphamide and testosterone undecanoate. Due to the rapid and sensitive effects of positive drug toxicity, the administration was performed in a specific time period.

Cyclophosphamide and testosterone undecanoate were used as positive drugs, and the effects of cyclophosphamide and testosterone undecanoate on gamete formation, mating behavior, fertility, growth, and development of embryos before and after implantation were observed for more than 60 days after continuous administration for 7 days. At the same time, the blood drug concentration and drug concentration in testicular tissue (through the blood–testis barrier) of animals at different time points were measured to describe the relationship between the dose, time of administration and the results of fertility evaluation test after the above two drugs were administrated in cynomolgus monkeys, and to evaluate the toxicity or interference effect on animal fertility, so as to provide reference information for clinical drug risk assessment.

8.1.2 Test Article 1

(1) Identity: Cyclophosphamide.
(2) Abbreviation: CP (cyclophosphamide).
(3) Test Article No.: H1927.
(4) Batch Number: 602200401 and 220201CD.
(5) Component: C7H17Cl2N2O3P.
(6) Content: 99.5% and 99.8%, corresponding to the batch number above.
(7) Supplier: xxx technology company and xxx pharmaceutical company, corresponding to the above batch number.
(8) Expiration date: Three years after opening.
(9) Storage condition: Ambient temperature.
(10) Preparation method: Prepared with 0.9% sodium chloride injection.
(11) Sample retention: The archives room is responsible for the retention of samples, which are stored in the sample retention room of the institution.
(12) After the end of this study, the remaining test articles were used for a follow-up study.

8.1.3 Test Article 2

(1) Identity: Testosterone undecanoate.
(2) Abbreviation: TU (testosterone undecanoate).
(3) Test Article No.: H1927.
(4) Batch Number: HH20210816.

(5) Component: C30H48O3.
(6) Content: 99.4%.
(7) Supplier: XXX pharmaceutical company.
(8) Expiration date: 3 years after opening.
(9) Storage condition: Ambient temperature.
(10) Preparation method: Prepared with olive oil.
(11) Sample retention: The archives room is responsible for the retention of samples, which are stored in the sample retention room of the institution.
(12) Disposal of remaining test article: After the end of the study, the remaining test articles were used for a follow-up study.

8.1.4 Vehicle 1

(1) Identity: Sodium chloride injection
(2) Batch Number: 220103522 and 220411D03.
(3) Specification: 100Ml: 0.9 g.
(4) Component: The main component of this product is sodium chloride, and the auxiliary material is water for injection.
(5) Supplier: xxx Pharmaceutical Company, corresponding to the above batch number.
(6) Concentration in use: 0.9%.
(7) Expiration date: July 02, xxxx, and April 10, xxxx, corresponding to the above batch numbers one by one.
(8) Storage condition: Sealed storage.
(9) Preparation method: Direct use without preparation.

8.1.5 Vehicle 2

(1) Identity: XXX Extra virgin olive oil.
(2) Batch Number: 20210318.
(3) Specification: 1 L
(4) Supplier: xxx Company.
(5) Expiration date: 24 months.
(6) Storage condition: Store in a cool and dry place, away from light.
(7) Preparation method: Direct use without preparation.

8.1.6 Other Main Reagents

(1) Identity: Zoletil 50 (Teletamine hydrochloride, zolazepam hydrochloride for injection).
(2) Batch Number: 8KM7 and 8V8K.

(3) Dispensing/Component: 125 mg Tiletamine + 125 mg Zolazepam + Excipient (Q.S. 1 bottle).
(4) Concentration in use: 50 mg/mL.
(5) Expiration date: October ×××× and March ××××, corresponding to the above batch numbers.
(6) Storage condition: Room temperature, airtight, shading.
(7) Preparation method: Dissolve the powder in the solid bottle with sterile water for injection in the package (batch number ××× and ××× ×) before use, i.e., the concentration is 50 mg/mL.
(8) Preparation date: on November 2nd, January 05, January 06, ××××, February 23, ×××× and February 27th, ××××.
(9) Supplier: ××× limited company.
(10) Disposal of remaining narcotics: The remaining narcotics were returned to the narcotics room for unified treatment after registration.

8.1.7 Test System

(1) Species, strain, and grade: Cynomolgus monkey, conventional.
(2) Sex and quantity: 30 spare animals (half male and half female) were applied, and 30 animals (half male and half female) were used in the testing.
(3) Age range: 3.6–5.7 years old; Healthy, sexually mature cynomolgus monkeys.
(4) Body weight range: At the time of receiving, the female weighed 2.42–3.48 kg. Male monkeys weighed 3.42–5.98 kg.
(5) Animal source: Spare animals of the institution were used to carry out the study; spare animals were purchased from ××× company.
(6) Laboratory animal production permission number: SCXK(X)20180043, issued by the xxx Science and Technology Department. SCXK(Gui)20180006, issued by xxx Science and Technology Department.
(7) Laboratory animal use certificate numbers: 44818300000306, 44818300000310, 0005078, 0005079, 0005080, 0005086, 0005088, 0005095, 0005098, and 0005113.
(8) Laboratory animal use permission number: SYXK(X)20210090, issued by the xxx Science and Technology Department.
(9) Rationale for Study System: Cynomolgus monkey is one of the recognized standard animals in toxicological reproductive toxicity studies. ICH S5(R3) "Detection of Reproductive and Developmental Toxicity for Human Pharmaceuticals" recommends the use of this animal, and the sponsor agrees to use this animal, so the cynomolgus monkey is used in this test.
(10) Animal identification: Animals are numbered in accordance with the laboratory animal numbering and grouping procedures of the institution, and the collar and cage card (each animal has its own unique collar number, and the grouped animal number corresponds to the collar number one by one) are used as animal identification marks.

(11) Animal reception date: Laboratory animals arrived at the institution in 10 batches (August 12th xxx, September 30 xxx, October 29, xxx, December 23 xxx, February 26 xxx, April 12, xxx, June 7 xxx, August 9, xxx, August 18 xxx, and September 22 xxx). After entering the facility, laboratory animals were quarantined according to the relevant SOP requirements of the institution and transferred to the reserve animal library of the institution after passing the quarantine. The laboratory animals were transferred to this study three times on June 08, ×××, October 24, ×××, and November 09, ×××.

(12) Feed and Drinking Water

1) Feed: The maintenance feed of monkeys was manufactured by xxx, Ltd., batch No. 22088221, 22118211, 22048211, etc. Feed nutritional components, microorganism parameters, and chemical contaminants were tested by a supplier entrusted with a qualified unit, and the reports were submitted to the facility. The test parameters met GB 14924.32010 and GB 14924.22001. Microorganism parameters and chemical contaminants were tested by a facility entrusted with a qualified unit every year, and the test parameters met GB 14924.22001. Feed colony population was tested quarterly by the facility, and the test parameters met GB 4789.22016. The above test results of the feed used met the requirements.

2) Drinking water: Drinking water for laboratory animals was purified by the facility. Microorganisms, chemical contaminants, and toxic substances in animal drinking water were tested by a facility entrusted with a qualified unit every year, and the testing parameters met GB 57492006. Total bacterial colonies were tested once a quarter by the facility, and the test parameters met GB 57492006. The above test results of the drinking water used met the requirements.

(13) Animal husbandry and environment: Animals were housed in the conventional laboratory. The feeding cages were stainless steel monkey cages, the size was 900 mm × 1000 mm × 2080 mm, and the animals were housed one to two animals per cage during the adaptive training period and were housed individually after grouping with free access to drinking water and feed. The temperature was set at room temperature (19.6°C–25.5°C), relative humidity was set at 15.5%–100%, ventilation rate ≥8 times/h, working illuminance ≥200 Lux, animal illuminance 100 Lux–200 Lux, with automatic illumination, on a 12-h alternative cycle of light and darkness.

(14) Animal welfare: All animal welfare involved in this study was in compliance with the Animals Welfare Guidelines of xxx company. The management and use of animals during the study were in line with the Guide for the Care and Use of Laboratory Animals (2011) published by the National Academy Press (NAP) and the Laboratory Animal Management Regulations revised in 2017 by the State Scientific and Technological Commission. The management, use, and relevant procedures of the animals involved in this study were reviewed and approved by the Institutional Animal Care and Use Committee (IACUC) of xxx company. Approval No.: IACUC (Approved)xxx-161.

(15) Veterinary treatment: None of the animals required veterinary treatment/care, or other related conditions during the study.

8.1.8 Group Assignment and Dosage Design

(1) Grouping: Animals were randomly divided into vehicle control group (saline), cyclophosphamide subcutaneous group, and testosterone undecanoate subcutaneous group, a total of three groups, ten in each group, half male and half female.
(2) Dosage setting basis: According to the literature.
(3) Dose multiples: None.
(4) Dosage: See Table 8.1.

8.1.9 Administration Method

(1) Administration route: cyclophosphamide subcutaneous injection (sc); testosterone undecanoate subcutaneous injection
(2) Administration volume: 1 mL/kg
(3) Administration time: 08:53–15:59
(4) Administration frequency and duration
   1) Male cynomolgus monkeys: The male cynomolgus monkeys were administered cyclophosphamide or testosterone undecanoate once a day and observed for more than 60 days after continuous administration for 7 days (considering the duration of spermatogenesis and the time of sperm transport through the epididymis of cynomolgus monkeys, the administration period should not be less than 60 days to evaluate the effect on germ cell production, that is, the spermatogenesis time of male cynomolgus monkeys is 40–46 days. The transit time of sperm through the epididymis is 5–10 days).
   2) The female cynomolgus monkeys were administered cyclophosphamide or testosterone undecanoate once a day in each group on the 2nd day after the start of menstruation, and more than two menstrual cycles were observed after continuous administration for 7 days.

Table 8.1 Group information and dose design

Group	Dosage (mg/kg)	Animal Number	
		♂	♀
Vehicle control group (saline)	–	1M01–1M05	1F01–1F05
Cyclophosphamide (sc)	15	2M01–2M05	2F01–2F05
Testosterone undecanoate (sc)	20	3M01–3M05	3F01–3F05

Table. 8.2 Test article preparation

Group	Dosage (mg/kg)	Test article volume (mg)	Solution volume (mL)	Target conc. (mg/mL)
Vehicle control group (Saline)	–	–	–	–
Cyclophosphamide (sc)	15	750	50	15
Testosterone undecanoate (sc)	20	1000	50	20

Note: The total dosage of each dose group changes with the number and weight of animals administered. This table shows the preparation method for the first dose

(5) Description of the administration route of the test article: The same as the clinical proposed route, cyclophosphamide subcutaneous injection, and testosterone undecanoate subcutaneous injection.
(6) Preparation method of the test article and control article: Before clinical use, according to the preparation requirements of the test article, the test article was prepared with saline (cyclophosphamide) and olive oil (testosterone undecanoate) into different concentrations. The formulation was prepared once before administration, and the specific preparation method was shown in Table 8.2. The remaining test article formulations were returned by the experimenter to the test article preparation room for operation according to SOP.
(7) Administration method of the test article and control article: The operation was performed according to the monkey administration method in SOP.

8.1.10 Test Method

(1) Animal quarantine: Upon reception, the animals were quarantined according to the requirements of laboratory animal quarantine in SOP and quarantined for 14 days after receiving.
(2) Adaptive feeding: During the quarantine period, adaptive feeding observation was carried out at the same time, and the adaptive feeding time was determined according to the weight increase. The general condition of the animals was observed once a day.
(3) Administration in male monkeys: The dosage volume was adjusted according to the change in body weight. Cyclophosphamide, testosterone undecanoate, and vehicle control groups were observed for 60 days after 7 days of administration.
(4) Sperm collection: Semen was collected manually with the help of an electric stimulator, and the cynomolgus monkey was first kept on the monkey chair. The experimenter (semen collector) held the prepared cup for collecting semen between the fingertips of the middle finger and ring finger of the right hand (the cup mouth is outward), and inserted the electrode rod in the right hand into the anus of the cynomolgus monkey at a depth of 15–20 cm. The switch of the semen collector was electrically stimulated by another person. At the same time, the collecting person held the electrode in his right

hand in a circular motion around the rectal wall. Repeat electric stimulation three to five times, each time for 1 s, 1 s off, and according to the animal's reaction, constantly increase the voltage to spermatogenesis. When the animal had sperm discharge, the collecting person's right hand quickly reversed and immediately moved the mouth of the cup to the lower part of the penile mouth to collect semen.

(5) Blood collection in male monkeys: Collect blood twice pre-dose (7-day interval) and collect about 2 mL blood from male monkeys post-dose every 2 weeks. Separate serum, and determine the hormone levels of DHT, estradiol (E_2), and testosterone (T) in male monkeys by the ELISA method. Absorbance (OD) was determined by a microplate reader at 450 nm wavelength according to the test instructions of the kit, and the hormone levels to be measured in the samples were calculated using a standard curve.

(6) Testicular volume detection of male monkeys: The size of the testis was measured with an ultrasound instrument. The cynomolgus monkey was first kept on the monkey chair. The experimenter separated the hind legs of the animal and exposed the scrotum of the animal. After adjusting the ultrasound instrument, the experimenter applied the coupling agent on the skin surface of the scrotum first, and then moved the probe back and forth on the skin surface of the scrotum until the complete testicle image appeared on the screen. Then the images of the left and right testis were collected and saved, and the volume size of the left and right testis was calculated using the tools included in the ultrasound instrument (Fig. 8.1).

(7) Monitoring of menstrual cycle in female monkeys: Insert a cotton swab into the vagina, check whether the swab contains blood, to determine whether there is menstruation, and record.

(8) Blood collection in female monkeys: Blood was collected twice (7-day interval) pre-dose, and about 2 mL blood was collected every 2 weeks from administration to necropsy of female monkeys. The hormone levels of luteinizing hormone (LH), follicle-stimulating hormone (FSH), testosterone, E_2, and progesterone (P) in female monkeys were measured by the ELISA method. Absorbance (OD value) was measured at 450 nm wavelength by a microplate reader, and the hormone level was calculated by a standard curve.

(9) TK: Blood drug concentration and testicular tissue drug concentration were detected to determine whether the test article had penetrated the blood-testis barrier.

1) According to the TK detection methods provided in the literature and the detection methods established in the preliminary test in the laboratory, the TK detection method for monkeys was proposed to use tolbutamide as the internal standard, and the methodology was validated.

2) Blood sample treatment: No less than 1 mL blood was collected from the veins of the limbs, whole blood was collected into the collection vessels containing heparin sodium, thoroughly mixed, left for 0.5–1 h, at 2°C–8°C, $1800 \times g$, centrifuged for 10 min, and the upper plasma was absorbed, divided, and placed in an ultra-low temperature refrigerator at −80°C.

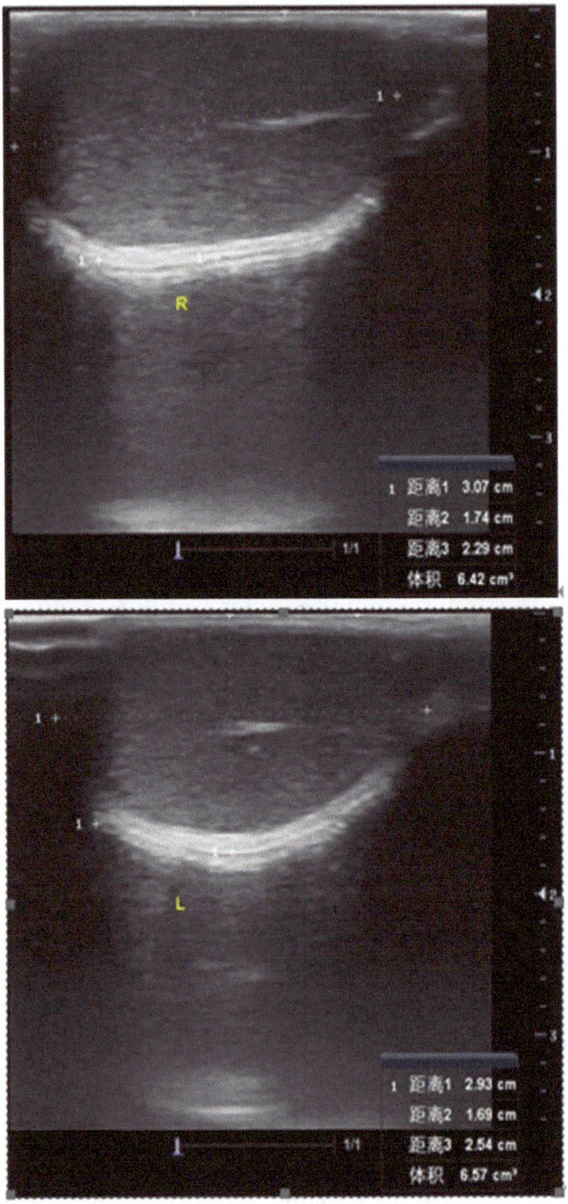

Fig. 8.1 Testicular image measured by ultrasound. The image above is of the left testicle. The image below shows the testicle on the right

3) Collection time: ① Male monkeys: Blood was collected pre-dose and 10 min, 30 min, 45 min, 1 h, 2 h, 4 h, 6 h and 24 h post-dose during the first dose (D_1) and the last dose. ② Female monkeys: Blood was collected pre-dose and

10 min, 30 min, 45 min, 1 h, 2 h, 4 h, 6 h, and 24 h post-dose during the first dose (D_1) and the last dose.

4) Sample collection: ① When collecting sperm, prepare TK samples for back up; weigh semen (first weigh EP tube), add quantitative incubation solution (weigh 0.05 g bovine serum albumin BSA, add 10 mL cream sugar DMEM and mix well to obtain the incubation solution) and dilute (dilution ratio is 1:9 or 1:99), divide the solution in EP tubes and place the tubes at −80°C for testing. ②Male monkey tissue: Considering the need of sample collection, five male monkeys in each group could be administrated again before necropsy. When the peak blood concentration time point was reached, testicle and epididymis tissues of male monkeys (at least four valid data points) were collected and homogenized, the homogenate was centrifuged at 3000 rmp/min for 10 min, divided into the solution in EP tubes, and placed at −80°C for testing.

(10) Euthanasia: After the last administration, the male monkeys were euthanized by acute blood loss after anesthesia with Zoletil 50 (0.1 mL/kg), and the abdomen was opened to expose the testicles, epididymis, and internal organs on both sides. After 7 days of continuous administration and two menstrual cycles of observation, female monkeys were anesthetized by Zoletil 50 (0.1 mL/kg) and euthanized by acute blood loss, and the abdomen was opened to expose the ovaries, uterus, and internal organs. A gross necropsy of male and female monkeys was performed.

8.1.11 Observation Indicator

(1) General condition observation: Observe the general condition of the animal once a day, record the appearance, behavior, or abnormal signs of the animal; Found dead or moribund animals should be necropsied in time.
(2) Body weight: Be measured every 2 weeks.
(3) Food consumption: The animal diet was recorded every day, and the feed residual of less than one-third was normal, the feed residual of one-third to two-third was borderline, and the feed residual more than two-third was poor.
(4) Body temperature: Body temperature was measured every 2 days.
(5) Sperm test: Sperm were collected twice pre-dose and collected every 2 weeks from the beginning of administration until necropsy. Sperm were removed and incubated in DMEM culture solution, and sperm number, density, and motility were detected by TOX IVOS II sperm analyzer.
(6) Testicular volume detection: The testicular volume was measured by an ultrasonic instrument, and was detected once pre-dose and once every 2 weeks post-dose.
(7) Menstrual cycle monitoring of female monkeys: The menstrual cycle of female cynomolgus monkeys was examined 2 months before and 2 months after administration to determine the length and change of the cycle.

(8) Final examination of female and male monkeys: ① The ovaries, uterus, testis, epididymis, prostate gland, seminal vesicle, levator ani, and sphincter were taken and weighed, and the organ coefficients were calculated. ② The ovaries, uterus, one side testicle, one side epididymis, prostate gland, seminal vesicle gland, levator anal muscle, and sphincter and organs with abnormal visual observation were preserved and fixed with 10% formalin, and histopathological examination was performed.
(9) Hormone detection: DHT, E_2, and testosterone in male monkeys; Levels of LH, FSH, E2, testosterone, and progesterone in female monkeys.
(10) TK: ① The blood concentration of each sampling point of female and male monkeys; ② The concentration of drugs in semen, testis, and epididymis tissues, and the passage of drugs through the blood-testis barrier were detected.

8.1.12 Statistical Analysis of Data

Test measurement data were expressed as $X \pm \text{SD}$.

8.1.13 Results and Conclusion

(1) General condition observation: ① Death of animals: On D9, 2M04 animals in the cyclophosphamide group were found to have died spontaneously. Before death, the animals were observed to have decreased activity, decreased food consumption, low body temperature, listlessness, prone lying, slow breathing, pale mucous membranes, and blood in vomit and feces. Gross necropsy and histopathological examination showed no obvious abnormality; no obvious cause of death was found. ② Observation of symptoms: During the study, no abnormalities were observed in appearance, behavior, posture, diet, hair, irritation response, glandular secretions, excrement, and respiratory status of animals in the other groups, except for the loose stool/water stool of the 3F01 animal in the testosterone undecanoate group during D_{56}–D_{59}.
The spontaneous death of 2M04 in the cyclophosphamide group was considered to be related to the toxic effects of cyclophosphamide in combination with the symptoms observed before death and the characteristics of cyclophosphamide itself (nausea, vomiting, and gastrointestinal irritation). 3F01 in the testosterone undecanoate group developed loose/watery stools during D_{56}–D_{59}, and the duration was relatively short, which was considered not related to the administration of testosterone undecanoate, and was considered to be individual animal differences.
(2) Body weight and weight gain: Summary data are presented in Tables 8.3 and 8.4. There was no significant trend change in body weight and weight gain of male and femdale animals in each dose group before and after administration. It was considered that subcutaneous injection of cyclophosphamide or testosterone undecanoate had no significant effect on body weight and weight gain of cynomolgus monkeys.

Table. 8.3 Summary of body weight and weight gain (male, kg, $\overline{X}\pm SD$)

Time (day)	Animal number (number/group)	Vehicle control group	Cyclophosphamide group[1]	Testosterone undecanoate group
D_{-9}	5	3.91±0.48	4.39±0.94	3.96±0.82
D_{-1}	5	3.95±0.49	4.35±0.94	3.96±0.86
D_{15}	5	3.92±0.43	3.95±0.32	4.02±0.71
D_{29}	5	3.90±0.47	3.85±0.23	3.94±0.68
D_{43}	5	3.80±0.39	3.85±0.26	3.98±0.75
D_{57}	5	3.62±0.21	3.90±0.25	4.03±0.84
D_{-9}–D_{-1}	5	0.04±0.07	−0.04±0.11	0.01±0.07
D_{-1}–D_{15}	5	−0.03±0.16	−0.02±0.18	0.06±0.17
D_{15}–D_{29}	5	−0.02±0.08	−0.10±0.12	−0.08±0.07
D_{29}–D_{43}	5	−0.10±0.11	−0.01±0.07	0.03±0.11
D_{43}–D_{57}	5	−0.18±0.43	0.05±0.04	0.06±0.08

[1]2M04 in cyclophosphamide group was found died on D_9, During D_{15}– D_{57}, animal number was four and during D_{-1}–D_{15} and D_{43}–D_{57} animal number was four

Table. 8.4 Summary of body weight and weight gain (female, kg, $\overline{X}\pm SD$)

Time (day)	Animal number (number/group)	Vehicle control group	Cyclophosphamide group	Testosterone undecanoate group
D_{-9}	5	3.07±0.41	2.64±0.11	2.60±0.10
D_{-1}	5	3.00±0.31	2.68±0.16	2.56±0.08
D_{15}	5	2.88±0.20	2.64±0.20	2.60±0.07
D_{29}	5	2.94±0.19	2.74±0.21	2.63±0.09
D_{43}	5	2.96±0.13	2.76±0.20	2.60±0.11
D_{57}	5	2.99±0.17	2.76±0.19	2.64±0.11
D_{-9}–D_{-1}	5	−0.07±0.15	0.04±0.08	0.05±0.08
D_{-1}–D_{15}	5	−0.12±0.17	−0.04±0.08	0.05±0.02
D_{15}–D_{29}	5	0.06±0.07	0.10±0.09	0.02±0.03
D_{29}–D_{43}	5	0.02±0.11	0.03±0.02	−0.02±0.05
D_{43}–D_{57}	5	0.03±0.09	0.00±0.03	0.04±0.06

(3) Food consumption: During the study, the feed surplus of male and female animals in each dose group was between one-third and two-third or less than one-third, and there was no significant reduction in food consumption. It was considered that subcutaneous injection of cyclophosphamide or testosterone undecanoate had no significant effect on the food consumption of cynomolgus monkeys.
(4) Body temperature: The summary data are shown in Tables 8.5 and 8.6. There was no significant trend change in the body temperature of male and female animals in each dose group compared with the vehicle control group before and after administration. It was considered that subcutaneous injection of

Table. 8.5 Summary of body temperature (male, °C, $\overline{X}\pm$SD)

Time (day)	Animal number (number/group)	Vehicle control group	Cyclophosphamide group[1]	Testosterone undecanoate group
D_{-1}	5	36.4±0.3	36.2±0.2	36.2±0.2
D_3	5	36.4±0.3	36.7±0.3	36.5±0.3
D_6	5	36.3±0.3	36.3±0.1	36.4±0.3
D_9	5	36.6±0.2	35.8±1.6	36.6±0.2
D_{12}	5	35.9±0.2	36.0±0.2	36.1±0.2
D_{15}	5	36.6±0.4	36.5±0.2	36.7±0.2
D_{18}	5	36.6±0.4	36.7±0.3	36.5±0.3
D_{21}	5	36.3±0.2	36.1±0.1	36.3±0.3
D_{24}	5	36.3±0.2	36.6±0.3	36.3±0.3
D_{27}	5	36.4±0.4	36.3±0.5	36.5±0.2
D_{30}	5	36.6±0.3	36.4±0.1	36.6±0.3
D_{33}	5	36.7±0.1	36.6±0.2	36.4±0.1
D_{36}	5	36.6±0.2	36.7±0.1	36.4±0.3
D_{39}	5	35.7±0.4	35.9±0.5	35.8±0.6
D_{42}	5	36.5±0.2	36.7±0.2	36.5±0.2
D_{45}	5	36.5±0.2	36.4±0.1	36.5±0.2
D_{48}	5	36.5±0.2	36.6±0.2	36.6±0.2
D_{51}	5	36.4±0.3	36.5±0.2	36.3±0.1
D_{54}	5	36.4±0.1	36.5±0.2	36.4±0.1
D_{57}	5	36.3±0.2	36.3±0.4	36.4±0.3
D_{60}	5	35.9±0.4	35.9±0.2	35.9±0.5

[1]2M04 in the cyclophosphamide group was found to have died on D_9, D_{12}–D_{60}. Animal number was four

cyclophosphamide or testosterone undecanoate had no significant effect on the body temperature of cynomolgus monkeys.

(5) Analysis of male monkey semen: Summary data are shown in Tables 8.7–8.9. Self-control comparisons before and after administration and comparisons with the vehicle control group suggest that the semen weight, sperm density, motile sperm density, forward motile sperm density, sperm motility percentage, rapid motility percentage, and sperm motility distribution of the cyclophosphamide group showed a significant decrease trend after the administration on D_{43}, and all indexes exhibited a recovery trend after administration on D_{57}. The indices of sperm analysis in the testosterone undecanoate group did not significantly decrease or increase during the whole administration period, which was consistent with the trend in the vehicle control group.

Cyclophosphamide has the side effect of reducing the quality of male sperm in clinical practice. Comprehensive analysis suggests that the changes in various sperm analysis indexes of male animals in the cyclophosphamide group may be related to the toxic effect of cyclophosphamide, as well as the sexual maturity and number of

Table. 8.6 Summary of body temperature (female, °C, $\overline{X}\pm$SD)

Time (day)	Animal number (number/group)	Vehicle control group	Cyclophosphamide group	Testosterone undecanoate group
D_{-1}	5	36.4±0.3	36.2±0.1	36.5±0.2
D_3	5	36.5±0.3	36.2±0.7	36.2±0.2
D_6	5	36.5±0.3	36.5±0.4	36.5±0.2
D_9	5	36.4±0.4	36.6±0.3	36.6±0.3
D_{12}	5	36.2±0.4	36.6±0.3	36.3±0.3
D_{15}	5	36.2±0.5	36.4±0.2	36.6±0.2
D_{18}	5	36.3±0.2	36.2±0.2	36.4±0.3
D_{21}	5	36.5±0.1	36.6±0.2	36.2±0.2
D_{24}	5	36.3±0.2	36.3±0.3	36.5±0.3
D_{27}	5	36.4±0.4	36.4±0.1	36.4±0.2
D_{30}	5	36.5±0.3	36.4±0.2	36.5±0.1
D_{33}	5	36.2±0.2	36.4±0.1	36.4±0.4
D_{36}	5	36.6±0.2	36.4±0.3	35.7±0.8
D_{39}	5	36.3±0.2	35.7±0.3	36.3±0.3
D_{42}	5	36.3±0.2	36.4±0.3	35.5±1.0
D_{45}	5	36.5±0.1	36.1±0.5	36.3±0.3
D_{48}	5	36.4±0.2	36.3±0.1	36.4±0.3
D_{51}	5	36.6±0.3	36.6±0.2	36.6±0.3
D_{54}	5	36.3±0.2	36.5±0.1	36.5±0.3
D_{57}	5	36.0±0.6	36.5±0.2	36.3±0.5
D_{60}	5	36.2±0.3	36.4±0.1	36.4±0.4

animals. Therefore, sexually mature animals should be selected for the reproductive toxicity test of nonhuman primates, and the sample size may be larger. Try to eliminate the judgment of the test results due to the problems of the test system.

(6) Testicular volume of male monkeys: Summary data are shown in Table 8.10. There was no significant trend change in testicular volume of male animals in each dose group before and after administration. It was considered that subcutaneous injection of cyclophosphamide or testosterone undecanoate had no effect on the testicular volume of cynomolgus monkeys.
(7) Menstrual cycle monitoring of female monkeys: Data are summarized in Table 8.11. Compared with the vehicle control group, the number of menstrual cycles and the total duration of menstruation in the cyclophosphamide group and the testosterone undecanoate group exhibited a significant decreasing trend. Cyclophosphamide or testosterone undecanoate have clinical side effects that affect women's menstrual disorders. Comprehensive analysis suggests that the changes in the menstrual cycle indicators of female animals in the cyclophosphamide and testosterone undecanoate groups may be related to the administration of cyclophosphamide or testosterone undecanoate groups, and may also be related

Table. 8.7 Summary of vitality indicator of male monkey semen ($\overline{X}$ ±SD) (vehicle control group)

Item	D_{-8}	D_{-1}	D_{15}	D_{29}	D_{43}	D_{57}
Animal number (*n*)	5	5	5	5	5	5
Weight of semen (g)	0.06 ± 0.04	0.02 ± 0.02	0.07 ± 0.04	0.05 ± 0.03	0.07 ± 0.08	0.03 ± 0.01
Sperm density (mol/mL)	313.8 ± 333.7	139.3 ± 162.2	118.6 ± 175.3	325.9 ± 316.6	155.4 ± 193.8	246.3 ± 241.8
Motile sperm density (mol/mL)	270.4 ± 323.8	81.6 ± 82.4	74.6 ± 136.7	277.6 ± 276.8	106.2 ± 148.6	193.5 ± 228.3
Forward motile sperm density (mol/mL)	142.5 ± 188.5	39.1 ± 42.1	53.0 ± 105.4	143.5 ± 173.1	64.0 ± 117.6	49.6 ± 60.8
Percentage of motile sperm (%)	73 ± 17	65 ± 28	49 ± 22	78 ± 16	47 ± 29	60 ± 37
Percentage of rapid activity (%)	50 ± 30	36 ± 34	29 ± 26	51 ± 25	27 ± 30	18 ± 16
Activity-Release						
Rapid (mol/mL)	204.3 ± 276.1	51.1 ± 52.8	64.2 ± 127.2	196.3 ± 247.4	86.1 ± 149.3	73.7 ± 87.4
Medium (mol/mL)	39.6 ± 49.0	23.7 ± 37.6	6.9 ± 11.4	47.8 ± 46.6	8.6 ± 6.7	76.7 ± 97.8
Slow (mol/mL)	51.4 ± 46.9	29.6 ± 47.4	12.6 ± 18.5	56.9 ± 50.8	19.8 ± 15.8	66.7 ± 56.7
Static (mol/mL)	18.5 ± 17.4	34.9 ± 43.7	34.9 ± 31.0	24.9 ± 29.6	41.0 ± 32.0	29.2 ± 39.5
Average path velocity (μm/s)	125.9 ± 61.7	91.8 ± 55.5	94.6 ± 49.0	108.8 ± 43.0	66.9 ± 62.0	44.3 ± 33.6
Linear velocity of motion (μ m/s)	114.8 ± 59.5	80.5 ± 50.9	84.3 ± 47.8	96.6 ± 41.3	56.4 ± 52.8	37.7 ± 29.6
Rate of curvilinear motion (μ m/s)	172.7 ± 70.2	135.3 ± 75.1	156.4 ± 53.4	167.0 ± 53.9	113.3 ± 103.8	70.1 ± 49.3
Amplitude of lateral head displacement (μm)	6.4 ± 0.8	4.7 ± 2.8	7.2 ± 3.5	6.1 ± 0.8	4.3 ± 4.0	4.4 ± 2.6
Beat cross frequency (Hz)	34.6 ± 3.4	30.9 ± 6.1	34.5 ± 7.2	34.8 ± 3.6	21.3 ± 15.9	23.7 ± 13.7
Forward (%)	86 ± 5	84 ± 6	85 ± 7	84 ± 5	67 ± 38	65 ± 37
Linearity (%)	59 ± 10	55 ± 7	50 ± 16	54 ± 9	41 ± 24	40 ± 24
Elongation (%)	59 ± 7	63 ± 5	57 ± 9	60 ± 4	51 ± 30	45 ± 25
Area (μmsq)	4 ± 1	4 ± 0	4 ± 0	4 ± 0	3 ± 2	4 ± 2

Table. 8.8 Summary of vitality indicator of male monkey semen ($\overline{X}$±SD) (cyclophosphamide group)

Item	D_{-8}	D_{-1}	D_{15}	D_{29}	D_{43}	D_{57}
Animal number (*n*)	4	4	4	4	3	4
Weight of semen (g)	0.14±0.10	0.10±0.12	0.12±0.07	0.05±0.04	0.04±0.01	0.05±0.02
Sperm density (mol/mL)	394.3±497.8	243.3±262.6	247.8±373.5	231.8±393.3	10.9±17.4	55.5±64.1
Motile sperm density (mol/mL)	295.5±495.8	234.3±260.8	225.1±380.4	222.0±389.6	8.0±13.9	31.3±40.7
Forward motile sperm density (mol/mL)	191.9±342.9	80.7±99.7	90.5±179.5	64.6±117.8	0.6±1.0	1.1±0.7
Percentage of motile sperm (%)	52±32	69±47	53±41	58±44	26±45	55±31
Percentage of rapid activity (%)	40±29	43±45	20±35	22±26	5±9	21±23
Activity release						
Rapid (mol/mL)	231.7±404.4	100.8±118.0	146.8±286.6	112.2±201.3	1.7±2.9	1.7±1.3
Medium (mol/mL)	38.7±43.9	95.4±183.9	31.6±44.7	72.9±132.7	0.9±1.6	20.1±23.3
Slow (mol/mL)	45.4±44.4	38.2±67.3	52.0±52.4	37.0±56.1	5.5±9.5	31.3±41.3
Static (mol/mL)	78.5±73.9	9.0±8.3	17.4±15.5	9.8±6.6	2.9±3.5	2.4±3.0
Average path velocity (μm/s)	116.3±44.3	110.3±116.1	48.6±64.7	49.4±58.1	27.0±46.8	72.3±60.9
Linear velocity of motion (μm/s)	101.4±41.5	101.6±107.0	40.4±56.2	39.3±45.6	19.3±33.4	65.9±57.1
Rate of curvilinear motion (μm/s)	181.6±73.2	132.8±130.6	77.4±83.2	83.6±101.9	49.3±85.4	128.6±105.7
Amplitude of lateral head displacement (μm)	8.5±2.8	4.3±2.8	2.8±3.3	4.0±5.0	2.5±4.3	8.6±5.6
Beat cross frequency (Hz)	31.8±6.3	23.3±15.8	25.9±17.6	16.8±19.4	8.4±14.5	37.6±6.1
Forward (%)	82±6	67±45	61±40	39±45	25±44	91±6
Linearity (%)	53±4	52±36	34±25	23±27	16±28	52±11
Elongation (%)	62±9	47±31	40±29	29±34	18±31	70±10
Area (μmsq)	4±0	3±2	3±2	2±3	1±2	5±1

to the sexual maturity and number of animals. Therefore, when conducting reproductive toxicity tests in nonhuman primates, it is recommended to select sexually mature animals, observe the menstrual cycle of female animals before administration, select female animals with regular menstruation for the test, and the sample size may be larger, so as to eliminate the judgment of the test results caused by the problems of the test system.

(8) Organ weight and coefficient of male and female animals: Summary data are shown in Tables 8.12 and 8.13. Compared with the vehicle control group, there

Table. 8.9 Summary of vitality indicator of male monkey semen ($\overline{X}$±SD) (testosterone undecanoate group)

Item	D_{-8}	D_{-1}	D_{15}	D_{29}	D_{43}	D_{57}
Animal number (*n*)	5	5	5	4	5	5
Weight of semen (g)	0.03±0.02	0.07±0.12	0.12±0.09	0.09±0.07	0.02±0.01	0.10±0.10
Sperm density (mol/mL)	440.1±772.4	266.0±360.5	52.2±32.1	539.0±588.4	303.9±250.2	304.1±368.2
Motile sperm density (mol/mL)	339.3±640.8	259.3±358.3	36.0±22.7	356.8±367.9	279.3±254.4	286.9±354.4
Forward motile sperm density (mol/mL)	238.5±456.0	185.3±261.2	23.0±18.8	73.3±64.5	181.1±197.1	121.7±162.8
Percentage of motile sperm (%)	54±32	83±36	68±24	57±32	67±43	72±41
Percentage of rapid activity (%)	30±28	35±43	44±35	25±14	47±36	35±34
Activity Release						
Rapid (mol/mL)	280.4±544.1	211.0±291.1	26.6±20.2	132.7±116.2	215.5±235.6	169.9±232.0
Medium (mol/mL)	53.1±100.4	31.8±55.0	5.8±7.4	79.6±74.1	33.9±29.1	52.9±82.6
Slow (mol/mL)	51.4±88.9	16.6±19.6	7.2±7.0	145.0±191.2	38.7±28.0	64.5±78.1
Static (mol/mL)	55.3±64.6	6.6±6.5	12.6±13.9	181.7±248.9	15.8±9.9	16.7±15.6
Average path velocity (μm/s)	95.9±80.9	90.6±82.0	107.4±85.5	75.9±27.4	106.3±76.4	83.8±75.5
Linear velocity of motion (μm/s)	88.2±77.4	84.4±76.4	99.0±80.7	62.6±27.1	97.7±70.6	75.2±67.7
Rate of curvilinear motion (μm/s)	124.8±96.3	127.5±109.1	152.0±108.0	124.2±44.1	142.8±99.5	114.8±94.8
Amplitude of lateral head displacement (μm)	4.3±2.5	4.0±3.6	5.0±2.8	5.3±0.5	4.7±2.8	3.3±3.2
Beat cross frequency (Hz)	28.8±16.4	28.1±17.3	30.0±16.8	30.1±4.8	18.6±11.9	29.4±17.2
Forward (%)	70±39	72±41	70±39	78±8	70±39	67±38
Linearity (%)	50±30	50±29	48±29	49±7	51±30	44±27
Elongation (%)	46±27	55±33	48±28	55±12	55±31	48±27
Area (μmsq)	3±2	3±2	3±2	4±0	3±2	4±2

was no significant trend change in the reproductive organ weight and the coefficient of male and female animals in each dose group. It was considered that subcutaneous injection of cyclophosphamide or testosterone undecanoate had no significant effect on the reproductive organ weight and coefficient of cynomolgus monkeys.

Table. 8.10 Summary of testicular volume data of male monkeys (cm^3, $\overline{X}$±SD)

Time (day)	Animal number (number/group)	Vehicle control group	Cyclophosphamide group[1]	Testosterone undecanoate group
D_{-1}	5	6.90±2.52	4.99±1.74	6.61±5.19
D_{15}	5	3.95±1.44	3.49±0.65	6.09±6.34
D_{29}	5	4.08±1.20	3.14±0.62	5.63±3.75
D_{43}	5	4.39±1.70	3.24±0.84	6.00±4.80
D_{57}	5	4.73±1.26	4.05±1.30	5.48±3.76

[1]2M04 in the cyclophosphamide group died on D_9, during D_{-1}–D_{57}, animal number was four; testicular volume was the average volume of the left and right testis of the animal

Table. 8.11 Summary of menstrual cycle data of female monkeys ($\overline{X}$±SD)

Test indicator	Animal number (number/group)	Vehicle control group	Cyclophosphamide group[a]	Testosterone undecanoate group
Number of menstrual cycles (number)	5	2.4±1.5	1.6±0.6	1.6±0.6
Total number of days the menstrual period lasts (day)	5	12.8±10.2	10.4±4.7	9.0±5.3

Table. 8.12 Summary of organ weight and coefficient (male, n = 5, $\overline{X}$±SD)

Test indicator		Vehicle control group	Cyclophosphamide group[1]	Testosterone undecanoate group
Testis	Weight (g)	15.40±5.63	13.19±2.38	18.24±13.18
	Organ-to-body weight ratio (%)	0.004±0.001	0.003±0.001	0.004±0.002
Epididymis	Weight (g)	2.81±0.72	2.34±0.58	3.07±1.81
	Organ-to-body weight ratio (%)	0.001±0.000	0.001±0.000	0.001±0.000
Prostate	Weight (g)	1.62±0.60	1.78±0.48	1.77±1.12
	Organ-to-body weight ratio (%)	0.000±0.000	0.000±0.000	0.000±0.000
Seminal vesicle	Weight (g)	5.52±2.57	4.39±1.00	5.17±2.76
	Organ-to-body weight ratio (%)	0.001±0.001	0.001±0.000	0.001±0.000
Sphincter	Weight (g)	0.70±0.20	0.86±0.21	0.95±0.13
	Organ-to-body weight ratio (%)	0.000±0.000	0.000±0.000	0.000±0.000
Levator ani	Weight (g)	2.23±0.53	2.88±0.85	2.56±1.04
	Organ-to-body weight ratio (%)	0.001±0.000	0.001±0.000	0.001±0.000

[1]2M04 in cyclophosphamide group was found died on D_9, and animal number was four

Table. 8.13 Summary of organ weight and coefficient (female, n = 5, $\overline{X}$ ±SD)

Test indicator		Vehicle control group	Cyclophosphamide group	Testosterone undecanoate group
Ovary	Weight (g)	0.29±0.07	0.19±0.05	0.19±0.09
	Organ-to-body weight ratio (%)	0.000±0.000	0.000±0.000	0.000±0.000
Uterus	Weight (g)	5.53±1.56	5.23±1.74	4.42±1.48
	Organ-to-body weight ratio (%)	0.002±0.000	0.002±0.001	0.002±0.001

Table. 8.14 Summary of hormone indicators (male, $\overline{X}$ ±SD)

Test indicator	Test stage	Animal number (number/group)	Vehicle control group	Cyclophosphamide group[1]	Testosterone undecanoate group
E_2 (pg/mL)	First time pre-dose	5	172.261±49.597	249.224±123.131	266.613±73.150
	$D-_1$	5	195.202±36.253	284.638±136.471	219.985±102.950
	D_{15}	5	192.428±46.293	239.412±97.624	223.310±81.435
	D_{29}	5	221.984±50.313	305.739±173.707	227.898±87.052
	D_{43}	5	216.826±60.889	254.644±114.353	299.842±121.151
	D_{57}	5	216.157±67.325	193.896±25.211	310.955±145.066
T (ng/mL)	First time pre-dose	5	1.125±0.331	1.357±0.552	0.983±0.571
	$D-_1$	5	0.971±0.749	0.953±0.473	0.947±0.333
	D_{15}	5	0.929±0.467	0.855±0.358	1.154±0.723
	D_{29}	5	1.130±0.869	0.900±0.723	0.827±0.353
	D_{43}	5	0.796±0.262	0.795±0.220	0.848±0.470
	D_{57}	5	0.740±0.283	0.822±0.434	0.632±0.315
DHT (pg/mL)	First time pre-dose	5	222.988±105.358	231.492±130.404	193.059±167.635
	$D-_1$	5	168.970±59.451	157.420±35.643	172.178±77.900
	D_{15}	5	159.634±35.205	142.854±44.706	173.070±135.718
	D_{29}	5	118.223±38.855	123.818±38.753	149.726±73.077
	D_{43}	5	147.123±45.294	139.445±42.459	97.924±30.498
	D_{57}	5	94.182±26.121	75.828±26.855	79.238±45.067

[1]2M04 in cyclophosphamide group was found died on D_9, during D_{15}–D_{57}, animal number was four

(9) Hormone indicators:

Summary data are shown in Tables 8.14 and 8.15. Self-control comparisons before and after administration and comparisons with the vehicle control group suggested there was no obvious trend change in the indexes of male and female animal hormones in each dose group, and the changes were of the same order of magnitude. Due to the lower frequency and long interval of blood collection (blood collection once every 2

Table. 8.15 Summary of hormone indicators (female, $\overline{X}$±SD)

Test indicator	Test stage	Animal number (number/group)	Vehicle control group	Cyclophosphamide group	Testosterone undecanoate group
E_2 (pg/mL)	First time pre-dose	5	266.673±78.413	464.055±321.791	440.970±195.278
	D_{-1}	5	267.842±116.599	558.628±393.941	351.438±202.065
	D_{15}	5	270.076±121.492	376.837±206.598	339.752±180.977
	D_{29}	5	306.591±137.228	629.315±513.598	386.774±203.776
	D_{43}	5	287.707±118.065	630.745±415.297	371.504±205.348
	D_{57}	5	259.263±102.509	678.589±479.531	361.226±176.495
T (ng/mL)	First time pre-dose	5	0.948±0.501	1.295±0.583	1.170±0.375
	D_{-1}	5	0.840±0.214	0.805±0.194	0.976±0.160
	D_{15}	5	0.863±0.321	1.477±1.085	1.039±0.249
	D_{29}	5	1.074±0.292	1.113±0.174	1.454±0.759
	D_{43}	5	0.876±0.458	1.636±0.544	0.856±0.093
	D_{57}	5	1.274±0.404	0.682±0.114	0.861±0.036
FSH (mIU/mL)	First time pre-dose	5	362.424±287.611	324.737±186.286	473.847±253.680
	D_{-1}	5	381.219±184.241	400.147±166.998	474.346±231.058
	D_{15}	5	449.587±202.306	378.294±143.012	511.620±262.262
	D_{29}	5	347.909±258.907	321.566±176.183	406.716±220.511
	D_{43}	5	324.791±246.944	251.873±157.270	400.419±224.103
	D_{57}	5	307.902±223.675	362.076±207.855	443.164±240.438
P (pg/mL)	First time pre-dose	5	1426.529±511.216	4209.169±2330.863	3972.163±2610.302
	D_{-1}	5	1154.553±473.832	5885.031±4725.422	2957.982±2126.566
	D_{15}	5	2116.475±2347.238	4812.777±2940.052	2752.287±2671.395
	D_{29}	5	922.829±408.396	6910.558±4412.893	2924.631±2887.070
	D_{43}	5	1532.930±1389.028	6802.842±6903.580	2284.695±1635.271
	D_{57}	5	831.390±357.054	6929.862±4757.037	2653.449±2019.053
LH (mIU/mL)	First time pre-dose	5	32.964±2.962	32.103±6.536	35.923±7.517
	D_{-1}	5	32.945±3.892	34.139±6.649	30.972±7.969
	D_{15}	5	39.156±12.003	34.815±7.100	33.528±6.013
	D_{29}	5	34.302±9.088	31.653±10.848	28.422±9.839
	D_{43}	5	23.471±5.160	26.270±5.662	26.182±5.430
	D_{57}	5	24.081±3.444	38.507±17.348	26.212±4.430

weeks) in this test, it is not possible to monitor the changes in hormone indexes well, and it is not possible to judge whether the administration of cyclophosphamide or testosterone undecanoate has an effect on the hormone indexes of male and female animals. Therefore, it is recommended to pay attention to the frequency and interval of blood collection when conducting reproductive toxicity tests in nonhuman primates. It is best to take blood samples of female animals every 2 days during the follicular phase (to ensure capturing estrogen and LH peaks) and every 3 days during the luteal phase; male animals shall undergo blood collection every 3 days.

(10) Toxicokinetics: See "Appendix I Report on Toxicity Analysis."
   1) The blood concentration of each sampling point of female and male monkeys: ① After the administration on D_1, the peak time of blood concentration of cynomolgus monkeys in subcutaneous cyclophosphamide group was 0.17–0.5 h; The C_{max} was (7641.29 ± 1351) ng/mL, AUC_{0t} was (10329 ± 1895) h ng/mL. ②After D_7 administration, the peak time of blood concentration of cynomolgus monkeys in subcutaneous cyclophosphamide group was 0.5 h. The C_{max} was (8020.35 ± 798.01) ng/mL, AUC_{0t} was (10728±1636)h ng/mL.③ In the subcutaneous testosterone undecanoate group, the male cynomolgus monkey group was administered 20 mg/kg test article, and the blood concentration data was close to the vehicle control group, while the female cynomolgus monkey group was administered 20 mg/kg test article, and the blood concentration was lower than the lower limit of quantitation (LLOQ), so the TK parameters of testosterone were not calculated.
   2) Detection of drug concentration in semen, testicles, and epididymis tissue and drug penetration through the blood–testis barrier: After detection, the concentrations of drugs in semen, testis, and epididymis tissues were all lower than the lower limit of quantification. Considering that the long storage time of semen, testis, and epididymis tissue samples after collection or the absence of stabilizer protection may lead to drug degradation, drug penetration through the blood–testis barrier could not be evaluated.

(11) Histopathological examination: See "Appendix II Pathology Report." 2M04 in the cyclophosphamide group died spontaneously on D_9, and no obvious abnormality was found in gross necropsy and histopathology, and no obvious cause of death was observed. At the end of the administration period, compared with the animals in the vehicle control group, no abnormal changes related to the test article were observed in the organs of the animals in each test group. Histopathological examination showed that no pathological changes related to the test article were observed in each organ.

8.1.14 Conclusion

Under the conditions of this study, cynomolgus monkeys were repeatedly administered cyclophosphamide (15 mg/kg) via subcutaneous injection for 7 days and observed for

60 days. One animal was found dead out of schedule. No significant changes related to the test article were observed in the general condition observation, body weight and weight gain, food consumption, body temperature, testicular volume of male monkey, weight and coefficient of reproductive organs of male and female animals, and microscopic histomorphology of each reproductive organ. The adverse reactions that may be related to the test article were observed in the changes of various indexes in the sperm analysis of male monkeys (D_{43} semen weight, sperm density, motile sperm density, forward motile sperm density, percentage of sperm motility, percentage of rapid motility, sperm motility distribution, etc., were significantly decreased) and menstrual cycle disorders in female monkeys. Due to the lower frequency and long interval of blood collection (blood collection once every 2 weeks) in this test, the changes of hormone indexes could not be well monitored, and whether cyclophosphamide administration had an effect on hormone indexes of male and female animals could not be well judged. It is considered that subcutaneous injection of cyclophosphamide (15 mg/kg) may have harmful effects on the fertility of cynomolgus monkeys under the set conditions of the study. However, the above conclusions should exclude the misjudgment of the test results caused by the problems of the test system. Therefore, it is suggested that sexually mature animals should be selected for the formal test. For female animals, the menstrual cycle pre-dose should be observed, so as to select female animals with regular menstruation for the test; For male animals, semen collection shall be performed pre-dose, and sexually mature animals that can ejaculate normally are selected for the test. Appropriately increase the number of animals and exclude individual differences in the evaluation of the test results.

Under the set conditions of this study, cynomolgus monkeys were repeatedly administered testosterone undecanoate (20 mg/kg) via subcutaneous injection for 7 days and observed for 60 days. No animals died out of schedule. No significant changes related to the test article were observed in the general condition, body weight and weight gain, food consumption, body temperature of all the animals, male monkey spermatozoon analysis, testicular volume of male monkey, weight and coefficient of male and female reproductive organs, and microscopic histomorphology of the reproductive organs. Adverse reactions that may be related to the test article were observed in menstrual cycle disorders in female monkeys. Due to the lower frequency and long interval of blood collection (blood collection once every 2 weeks) in this test, it is not possible to monitor the changes in hormone indexes well, and it is not possible to judge whether the administration of testosterone undecanoate has an effect on the hormone indexes of male and female animals. It is considered that subcutaneous injection of testosterone undecanoate (20 mg/kg) may have harmful effects on the fertility of female cynomolgus monkeys under the conditions set in this study. However, the above conclusions should exclude the misjudgment of the test results caused by the problems of the test system. Therefore, it is suggested that sexually mature animals should be selected for the formal test. For female animals, the menstrual cycle pre-dose should be observed, so as to select female animals with regular menstruation for the test; For male animals, semen collection should be performed pre-dose, and sexually mature animals that can ejaculate normally are selected for the test. Appropriately increase the number of animals and exclude individual differences in the evaluation of the test results.

8.1.15 Record Retention

In addition to the data directly collected by the computer automation instrument, all other actual research data shall be recorded directly, timely, and accurately with a neutral pen on the prepared form or record paper, and be sorted and bound at any time. All data records shall indicate the record date and be signed by the recorder. The amendment to the raw record shall follow the relevant requirement. All data recorded is checked and signed to ensure that the data is reliable. After the end of the study, all the raw data, documents, and other materials will be submitted to the archives for storage when the final report is submitted. The specific management contents, procedures, and methods shall be implemented in accordance with the standard operating procedures formulated by the institution.

8.1.16 Data Archiving Time and Site

(1) Archiving date: December 31, ×××.
(2) Archiving place: Archives Room of ××× Company.
(3) Storage time: 5 years.

8.1.17 Appendix

Appendix 1 Toxicokinetics Analysis Report

8.1.17.1 Purpose

The purpose of the study was to analyze the time dynamic change of drug concentration in the plasma of cynomolgus monkeys by detecting the in vivo plasma concentrations in cynomolgus monkeys and investigate the in vivo TK profile of the drug in the set dose range after the administration of testosterone undecanoate as positive drug for 7 days followed by observation for more than 60 days, so as to provide a reference for the design of subsequent clinical studies.

8.1.17.2 Test Material

(1) Standard: See Table 8.16
(2) Internal standard: See Table 8.17
(3) Major software/data systems: see Table 8.18
(4) Matrix: The plasma of the blank cynomolgus monkey was obtained from the blank matrix bank of our institution and stored in the ultra-low temperature refrigerator for backup. For specific information, see the relevant raw data of the blank matrix bank. Before using, blank plasma was balanced to room temperature. The blank plasma batch numbers of cynomolgus monkeys used in this test are shown in Table 8.19.

Table. 8.16 Standard

Identity	Testosterone	Cyclophosphamide
Batch number	F2206482	100234–201604
Specification	1 g/bottle	100 mg/vial
Content	98%	93.5%
Correction factor	88.78% (content×coefficient of salt) none	None
Stability	Stable under storage conditions and within expiration date	Stable under storage conditions and within expiration date
Expiration date	06/07/xxx	Valid until issued by CCDI
Storage condition	Seal and store at room temperature away from light	Avoid light, sealed, refrigerated at 2°C–8°C
Supplier	XXX	National Institutes for Food and Drug Control

Table. 8.17 Internal standard

Identity	Orinase
Batch number	K2125618
Specification	1 g/bottle
Purity	99.73%
Expiration date	02/09/xxx
Storage condition	−20°C
Stability	Stable under storage condition and within expirarion date
Manufacture/supplier	XXX

Table. 8.18 Software and data system

Software/data system	Version number	Function
Analyst	1.7.2	Blood concentration analysis by LC–MS/MS
WinNonlin	8.3.2	Calculation of TK parameters

Table. 8.19 Cynomolgus monkey blank plasma

Using date	Matrix number
01/31/xxx	Cynomolgus Monkey Plasma-20211027-006
02/02/xxx	Cynomolgus Monkey Plasma-20211027-002
02/03/xxx	Cynomolgus Monkey Plasma-20211027-002

Note: The ID number of the matrix is X–Y–Z, X represents animal species and matrix type, Y represents blood collection date. Z stands for the serial number, and the serial number of the blank matrix after mixing and packaging is named after M, and consists of four digits. M stands for mix, the first two digits represent the batch of mixing, and the last two digits represent the serial number after mixing and packaging

8.1.17.3 Study Design

(1) Group Assignment: In this TK study, the dose of testosterone undecanoate group was 20 mg/kg, and the dose of the cyclophosphamide group was 15 mg/kg. Dosage and grouping information are shown in Table 8.20.

(2) Administration method: The route of administration was subcutaneous injection (sc). Dose volume 1 mL/kg; Administration time: 08:00–12:00.
Administration frequency and duration: ① Male cynomolgus monkey: Cyclophosphamide or testosterone undecanoate were administered once a day and the animals were observed for more than 60 days after continuous administration for 7 days (considering the duration of spermatogenesis and the time of sperm transport through the epididymis of cynomolgus monkeys, the administration period should not be less than 60 days to evaluate the effect on germ cell production, that was, the spermatogenesis time of male cynomolgus monkeys was 40–46 days. The transit time of sperm through the epididymis was 5–10 days.② On the second day after the beginning of menstruation, the female cynomolgus monkeys were administered cyclophosphamide or testosterone undecanoate once a day according to the groups. After 7 days of continuous administration, the female animals were observed for more than two menstrual cycles. ③ Subcutaneous injection was used in this study, and the frequency of administration was repeated, once/day, for a total of seven times. The first day of administration was defined as the first day of the study (D_1), and the male and female animals were administered on 2 days.

(3) Sample collection and processing
   1) Collection time point and collection method: ① Male monkeys: Blood was collected before and 10 min, 30 min, 45 min, 1 h, 2 h, 4 h, 6 h and 24 h after first administration (D_1) and last administration; ② Female monkeys: For the first dose (D_1) and the last dose, blood was collected before and 10 min, 30 min, 45 min, 1 h, 2 h, 4 h, 6 h and 24 h after administration.
   2) Sample handling/storage: No less than 1 mL blood was collected from the limbs veins, whole blood was collected into the collection vessels containing heparin sodium, thoroughly mixed, left for 0.5–1 h, at 2°C–8°C, centrifuged at 1800 × *g* for 10 min, and the upper plasma was absorbed and the solution was packaged and stored in an ultra-low temperature refrigerator at −80°C for testing.
   3) Sample testing: Serum concentrations of cyclophosphamide and testosterone in plasma samples were measured using a methodologically validated method (Study No. ××H19273).

Table. 8.20 Dosage and group assignment

Group	Dosage (mg/kg)	Animal Number	
		♂	♀
Vehicle control group	0	1M01–1M05	1F01–1F05
Cyclophosphamide	15	2M01–2M05	2F01–2F05
Testosterone undecanoate	20	3M01–3M05	3F01–3F05

8.1.17.4 Analysis Method

(1) Sample reception and testing: The samples to be tested began to be tested on January 31, ××××, and the samples were tested on February 03, ××××, with a total of 540 samples to be tested. After the test, the remaining plasma samples were processed according to the relevant SOP regulations of the institution.
(2) System suitability: When the system suitability sample contains analyte and internal standard, the RSD % of the retention time of analyte and internal standard is less than or equal to 5.00%, and the RSD % of the peak area ratio of analyte and internal standard is less than or equal to 15.00%. If the system suitability sample contains only the analyte without an internal standard, the RSD % of the retention time of the analyte is less than or equal to 5.00%, and the RSD % of the peak area of the analyte is less than or equal to 15.00%.
(3) Standard curve: There were two standard curves in each analysis batch, each standard curve contained 8 concentrations, linear regression was performed between nominal concentration and actual response value, linear fitting of standard curve points was performed by least square method, weight factor was 1/*X*2. The accuracy deviation of calibration standard samples (except the LLOQ) should be within ±15.00%, and the accuracy deviation of the LLOQ should be within ±20.00%. At least 75% of calibration standard samples and at least six concentrations of calibration standard samples should meet the correlation r of the standard curve ≥0.9900, the analysis batch should be rejected.
(4) Quality control sample: Quality control samples of low, medium, and high concentrations should be determined, accompanied with each analysis batch. The acceptable standard is that the average relative error (% RE) of each concentration level [average % RE = (average measured concentration − nominal concentration)/nominal concentration × 100] does not exceed ±15.0%. If 67% of the quality control samples pass, it will be considered to meet the acceptance criteria, and the % RE of at least 50% quality control sample at each concentration is within ±15.0%; If there are out-of-limit samples in the analysis batch, dilute quality control samples shall be prepared, and the acceptance criteria is that the accuracy deviation at least 50% dilute quality control samples are within ± 15.00%.
(5) Residue: After the high-concentration sample, the peak area of analyte in the analyte retention time zone of the double-blank sample shall not be higher than 20.00% of the mean peak area of analyte in the LLOQ concentration sample of the calibration sample in the same batch, and the peak area of internal standard in the retention time zone of the internal standard shall not be higher than 5.00% of the mean peak area of the internal standard concentration sample of the calibration sample in the same batch.

8.1.17.5 Bioassay Results

(1)Statistics of analysis batch results: The information of analysis batch is shown in Table 8.21.

Table. 8.21 Summary of analysis batch information

Analysis batch	Analysis time	Content	Note
System Suitability-××××0106-1	01/16/xxx	System suitability	IN-21-09-105
SA-Batch001	01/16/xxx	Cyclophosphamide reserve liquid check	IN-21-09-105
System Suitability-××××0110-1	01/10/xxx	System suitability	IN-21-09-105
SA-Batch002	01/10/xxx	Cyclophosphamide reserve liquid check	IN-21-09-105
System Suitability-××××0131-1	01/31/xxx	System suitability	IN-21-09-105
SA-Batch003	01/31/xxx	Cyclophosphamide sample testing	IN-21-09-105
System Suitability-××××0201-1	02/01/xxx	System suitability	IN-21-09-105
SA-Batch004	02/01/xxx	Testosterone reserve fluid check	IN-21-09-105
System Suitability-××××0202-1	02/02/xxx	System suitability	IN-21-09-105
SA-Batch005	02/02/xxx	Cyclophosphamide sample testing	IN-21-09-105
System Suitability-××××0203-1	02/03/xxx	System suitability	IN-21-09-105
SA-Batch006	02/03/xxx	Testosterone sample testing	IN-21-09-105
SA-Batch007	02/03/xxx	Testosterone sample testing	IN-21-09-105
System Suitability-××××0203-2①	02/03/xxx	System suitability	IN-19-09-057
SA-Batch003②	02/03/xxx	Cyclophosphamide sample testing	IN-19-09-057
SA-Batch005②	02/03/xxx	Cyclophosphamide sample testing	IN-19-09-057

Note: The identity of the analysis batch is the name of the injection sequence table. Due to the saturation of the instrument response, the instrument is replaced and re-sampled for analysis. ① is System Suitability-××××0202-1 reinjection analysis batch, ② is the reinjection analysis batch of SA-Batch003 and SA-Batch005

(2) System suitability: When the system suitability sample contains analyte and internal standard, the RSD% of the peak area ratio of analyte and internal standard is less than or equal to 5.55%, the RSD% of analyte retention time is less than or equal to 0.32%, and RSD% of internal standard retention time is less than or equal to 0.34%. The results are shown in Table 8.22.
(3) Standard curve: The quantitative range of the cyclophosphamide standard curve is 10–10,000 ng/mL, with a total of eight concentrations. The relative error of calibration standard sample concentration on the standard curve is −11.23% to 7.37%, and the correlation coefficient of the standard curve of each analysis

Table. 8.22 System suitability

Analysis batch	SST	Analyte peak area	Peak area of internal standard	Ratio of analyte to internal standard peak area	Analyte retention time (min)	Retention time of internal standard (min)
System Suitability-×××0106-1	1	3.02E+05	N/A	N/A	0.92	N/A
	2	2.99E+05	N/A	N/A	0.92	N/A
	3	3.02E+05	N/A	N/A	0.92	N/A
	4	3.01E+05	N/A	N/A	0.92	N/A
	5	3.01E+05	N/A	N/A	0.92	N/A
	6	2.97E+05	N/A	N/A	0.92	N/A
	Mean	3.00E+05	N/A	N/A	0.92	N/A
	SD	1966.38	N/A	N/A	0.00	N/A
	RSD%	0.65	N/A	N/A	0.14	N/A
System Suitability-×××0110-1	1	2.34E+05	N/A	N/A	1.65	N/A
	2	2.32E+05	N/A	N/A	1.65	N/A
	3	2.38E+05	N/A	N/A	1.65	N/A
	4	2.33E+05	N/A	N/A	1.64	N/A
	5	2.31E+05	N/A	N/A	1.65	N/A
	6	2.30E+05	N/A	N/A	1.64	N/A
	Mean	2.33E+05	N/A	N/A	1.65	N/A
	SD	2828.43	N/A	N/A	0.01	N/A
	RSD%	1.21	N/A	N/A	0.31	N/A
System Suitability-×××0131-1	1	1.36E+04	3.72E+05	3.65E−02	1.99	2.36
	2	1.24E+04	3.78E+05	3.28E−02	1.99	2.36
	3	1.32E+04	3.49E+05	3.78E−02	1.99	2.36
	4	1.25E+04	3.45E+05	3.62E−02	1.99	2.36
	5	1.22E+04	3.68E+05	3.32E−02	2.00	2.36
	6	1.26E+04	3.59E+05	3.52E−02	1.98	2.35
	Mean	1.28E+04	3.62E+05	3.53E−02	1.99	2.36
	SD	535.72	13105.98	0.00	0.01	0.00
	RSD%	4.20	3.62	5.55	0.32	0.17
System Suitability-×××0201-1	1	2.32E+05	N/A	N/A	1.50	N/A
	2	2.31E+05	N/A	N/A	1.50	N/A
	3	2.31E+05	N/A	N/A	1.50	N/A
	4	2.29E+05	N/A	N/A	1.50	N/A
	5	2.31E+05	N/A	N/A	1.50	N/A
	6	2.26E+05	N/A	N/A	1.50	N/A
	Mean	2.30E+05	N/A	N/A	1.50	N/A
	SD	2190.89	N/A	N/A	0.00	N/A

(continued)

Table 8.22 (continued)

System Suitability-xxxx 0202-1	1	1.67E+04	4.17E+05	4.00E−02	1.82	2.22
	2	1.75E+04	4.29E+05	4.07E−02	1.82	2.22
	3	1.69E+04	4.25E+05	3.97E−02	1.82	2.23
	4	1.72E+04	4.35E+05	3.94E−02	1.82	2.22
	5	1.74E+04	4.24E+05	4.11E−02	1.81	2.21
	6	1.67E+04	4.24E+05	3.93E−02	1.81	2.21
	Mean	1.71E+04	4.26E+05	4.00E−02	1.82	2.22
	SD	350.24	5988.88	0.00	0.01	0.01
	RSD%	2.05	1.41	1.81	0.28	0.34
System Suitability-xxxx 0203-1	1	1.89E+04	9.70E+04	1.95E−01	1.45	1.33
	2	1.88E+04	9.86E+04	1.90E−01	1.45	1.33
	3	1.91E+04	9.34E+04	2.05E−01	1.45	1.32
	4	1.85E+04	9.55E+04	1.93E−01	1.45	1.33
	5	1.91E+04	9.68E+04	1.97E−01	1.45	1.33
	6	1.90E+04	9.28E+04	2.05E−01	1.45	1.33
	Mean	1.89E+04	9.57E+04	1.98E−01	1.45	1.33
	SD	228.04	2238.23	0.01	0.00	0.00
	RSD%	1.21	2.34	3.17	0.00	0.31
System Suitability-xxxx 0203-1(Instrument IN-19-09-057)	1	1.43E+04	6.69E+05	2.13E−02	1.60	2.02
	2	1.32E+04	6.56E+05	2.02E−02	1.61	2.03
	3	1.31E+04	6.52E+05	2.01E−02	1.60	2.02
	4	1.30E+04	6.78E+05	1.92E−02	1.60	2.03
	5	1.32E+04	6.81E+05	1.94E−02	1.60	2.03
	6	1.37E+04	6.44E+05	2.12E−02	1.61	2.03
	Mean	1.34E+04	6.63E+05	2.02E−02	1.60	2.03
	SD	495.65	14935.42	0.00	0.01	0.01
	RSD%	3.69	2.25	4.34	0.32	0.25

Note: N/A indicates no relevant data. E+05 means 10 to the fifth, E+04 means 10 to the fourth, e−02 means 10 to the minus second, and E−01 means 10 to the minus first

batch is ≥0.9983. The quantitative range of the testosterone standard curve is 2–80 ng/mL, with a total of eight concentrations. The relative error of calibration standard sample concentration on the standard curve is between −9.91% and 8.34%, and the correlation coefficient of the standard curve of each analysis batch is ≥0.9977. The above results met the passing criteria. The specific results are shown in Tables 8.23 and 8.24.

(4) Quality control sample: The concentrations of low, medium, and high quality control samples were 30, 800, and 8000 ng/mL, respectively. The relative error of concentration accuracy was between −0.72% and 12.23%. The concentrations of low, medium, and high testosterone quality control samples were 5, 12 and 60 ng/mL, respectively, and the relative error of the measured concentration accuracy was between −14.00% and 13.82%. The specific results are shown in Tables 8.25 and 8.26.

Table. 8.23 Determination of cyclophosphamide concentration in the plasma (standard curve)

Analysis batch	Concentration of calibration standard (ng/mL)									Slope	Intercept	r
	Nominal Conc.	C8 (10)	C7 (20)	C6 (100)	C5 (500)	C4 (1 500)	C3 (5 000)	C2 (9 000)	C1 (10 000)			
SA-Batch003	Actual Conc.	9.83	20.73	97.53	529.38	1481.46	5117.45	8523	9882.31	0.00188	0.000628	0.9992
	Accuracy (%)	98.32	103.64	97.53	105.88	98.76	102.35	94.7	98.82			
	RE%	−1.68	3.64	−2.47	5.88	−1.24	2.35	−5.30	−1.18			
SA-Batch005	Actual Conc.	9.8	20.69	100.98	536.85	1529.14	5026.39	7989.02	9893.78	0.00198	0.00227	0.9983
	Accuracy (%)	98.04	103.44	100.98	107.37	101.94	100.53	88.77	98.94			
	RE%	−1.96	3.44	0.98	7.37	1.94	0.53	−11.23	−1.06			

Table. 8.24 Determination of testosterone concentration in the plasma (standard curve)

Analysis batch	Concentration of calibration standard (ng/mL)									Slope	Intercept	r
	Nominal conc.	**C8 (2)**	**C7 (4)**	**C6 (8)**	**C5 (20)**	**C4 (30)**	**C3 (50)**	**C2 (70)**	**C1 (80)**			
SA-Batch006	Actual Conc.	2.01	***3.08***	7.73	20.43	***24.59***	51.09	63.06	86.67	0.0724	0.0404	0.9977
	Accuracy (%)	100.62	***76.99***	96.62	102.16	***81.98***	102.17	90.09	108.34			
	RE%	0.62	***−23.01***	-3.38	2.16	***−18.02***	2.17	−9.91	8.34			
SA-Batch007	Actual Conc.	2.07	3.78	7.81	19.29	29.09	49.81	72.16	86.47	0.0578	0.022	0.9985
	Accuracy (%)	103.60	94.54	97.63	96.46	96.98	99.61	103.09	108.08			
	RE%	3.60	−5.46	−2.37	−3.54	−3.02	−0.39	3.09	8.08			

Note: Italicized bold indicates that it is not within the acceptable range

Table. 8.25 Drug concentration determination in plasma (cyclophosphamide quality control sample)

Analysis batch	Quality control sample concentration (ng/mL)						
	Nominal conc.	LQC (30)		MQC (800)		HQC (8000)	
SA-Batch003	Actual Conc.	***35.41***	32.37	847.92	830.77	8114.90	7942.35
	Accuracy (%)	***118.02***	107.90	105.99	103.85	101.44	99.28
	RE%	***18.02***	7.90	5.99	3.85	1.44	−0.72
SA-Batch005	Actual Conc.	30.47	31.90	870.20	897.82	8499.64	7984.09
	Accuracy (%)	101.58	106.34	108.78	112.23	106.25	99.80
	RE%	1.58	6.34	8.78	12.23	6.25	−0.20

Note: The statistical data is from IN-19-09-05. Italicized bold indicates that it is not within the acceptable range

Table. 8.26 Drug concentration determination in plasma (testosterone quality control sample)

Analysis batch	Quality control sample concentration (ng/mL)						
	Nominal conc.	LQC (5)		MQC (12)		HQC (60)	
SA-Batch006	Actual conc.	5.69	***4.22***	13.57	10.32	***71.29***	54.03
	Accuracy (%)	113.82	***84.37***	113.10	86.00	***118.82***	90.05
	RE%	13.82	***−15.63***	13.10	−14.00	***18.82***	−9.95
SA-Batch007	Actual conc.	N/A	5.21	N/A	12.41	N/A	61.67
	Accuracy (%)	N/A	104.24	N/A	103.45	N/A	102.78
	RE%	N/A	4.24	N/A	3.45	N/A	2.78

Note: "N/A" indicates that the group's quality control has not added a solution, and no sample has been collected. Italicized bold indicates that it is not within the acceptable range

(5) Residue: ① Cyclophosphamide: The peak area of analyte in the retention time zone of double blank sample analyte after the upper limit of quantitation (ULOQ) calibration standard was ≤1.45% of the mean value of analyte peak area in the LLOQ concentration sample of the calibration standard in the same batch, and the peak area of internal standard in the retention time zone was less than 0.00% of the mean value of the internal standard peak area in the LLOQ concentration sample of the calibration standard in the same batch.② Testosterone: The peak area of analyte in the retention time of double blank sample analyte after the ULOQ calibration standard was ≤13.49% of the mean peak area of analyte in the LLOQ concentration sample of the calibration standard in the same batch, and the peak area of internal standard in the retention time zone was less than 0.05% of the mean value of the internal standard peak area in the LLOQ concentration sample of the calibration standard in the same batch. See Tables 8.27 and 8.28 for specific results.

(6) The results of TK and the corresponding TK parameters evaluated after subcutaneous administration of cyclophosphamide in cynomolgus monkeys are shown in Table 8.29. Excel was used to conduct statistical analysis on the data

Table. 8.27 Cyclophosphamide residue

Analysis batch	C8 sample peak area (counts)		Residual percentage (%)	C8 sample peak area (counts)		
	Analyte	Internal standard	Analyte	Internal standard	Analyte	Internal standard
SA-Batch003	1.91E+02	0.00E+00	1.32E+04	6.91E+05	1.45	0.00
SA-Batch005	3.85E+03	0.00E+00	1.25E+07	6.41E+05	0.03	0.00

Note: E+07 means 10 to the seventh, E+05 means 10 to the fifth, E+04 means 10 to the fourth, E+03 means 10 to the third, E+02 means 10 to the second, and E+00 means 10 to the zero

Table. 8.28 Testosterone residue

Analysis batch	C8 sample peak area (counts)		Residual percentage (%)	C8 sample peak area (counts)		
	Analyte	Internal standard	Analyte	Internal standard	Analyte	Internal standard
SA-Batch006	2.55E+03	5.23E+01	1.89E+04	1.01E+05	13.49	0.05
SA-Batch007	2.44E+03	5.95E+01	1.81E+04	1.28E+05	13.48	0.05

Note: E+05 means 10 to the fifth, E+04 means 10 to the fourth, E+03 means 10 to the third, and E+00 means 10 to the first

of accumulation and linear relationship of dose exposure, AUC_{0t}, and the results are shown in Table 8.30.

After D_1 administration, the peak time of blood concentration of cyclophosphamide of the cynomolgus monkeys in subcutaneous cyclophosphamide group was 0.17–0.5 h; The peak concentration C_{max} was (7641.29 ± 1351) ng/mL, AUC_{0t} was (10329 ± 1895) h ng/mL. After D_7 administration, the peak time of blood concentration of cyclophosphamide of the cynomolgus monkeys in subcutaneous cyclophosphamide group was 0.5 h. The peak concentration C_{max} was (8020.35 ± 798.01) ng/mL, AUC_{0t} was (10728 ± 1636) h ng/mL.

In the subcutaneous testosterone undecanoate group, the male cynomolgus monkey group was given a dose of 20 mg/kg, and the blood concentration was close to that of the vehicle control group, while the female cynomolgus monkey group was given a dose of 20 mg/kg, and the blood concentration was lower than the LLOQ, so the TK parameters of testosterone undecanoate were not calculated.

8.1.17.6 Conclusion

The serum concentration of cyclophosphamide reached its peak in cynomolgus monkeys from 0.17 to 0.5 h, and there was no accumulation after 7 days of subcutaneous injection. Before and after the administration of testosterone undecanoate, there was no significant difference in the blood concentration of male animals, and the blood concentration of female animals was lower than the LLOQ.

Table. 8.29 TK parameters and statistical analysis of cyclophosphamide

Animal number	Sex	First dose			Last dose			Accumulation	
		T_{max} (h)	C_{max} (ng/mL)	**$AUC_{0-t\,h}$ (ng h/mL)**	T_{max} (h)	C_{max} (ng/mL)	$AUC_{0-t\,h}$ (ng h/mL)	**Last/first**	
								C_{max}	$AUC_{0-t\,h}$
2F01	Female	0.5	5775.58	7847.36945	0.5	7593.13	10,375.4277	1.31	1.32
2F02	Female	0.5	7592.98	9630.2117	0.5	8521.90	11,537.921	1.12	1.20
2F03	Female	0.5	6571.44	9118.62635	0.5	7678.10	8529.3815	1.17	0.94
2F04	Female	0.5	6866.28	9941.9637	0.5	8473.43	12,452.88095	1.23	1.25
2F05	Female	0.5	6040.23	7724.3217	0.5	7042.05	8467.30075	1.17	1.10
2M01	Male	0.17	9956.35	10,840.2429	0.5	8978.20	11,869.95425	0.90	1.09
2M02	Male	0.5	9028.86	12,316.2769	0.5	9055.59	11,942.59735	1.00	0.97
2M03	Male	0.5	7656.05	10,389.087	0.5	8393.15	10,853.03225	1.10	1.04
2M04	Male	0.5	8440.97	13,594.06505	0.5	6662.66	8676.9189	0.79	0.64
2M05	Male	0.5	8484.19	11,882.87635	0.5	7805.25	12,569.855	0.92	1.06
Female mean		0.5	6569.30	8852.50	0.5	7861.72	10,272.58	1.20	1.16
Female standard deviation		–	715.20	1018.05	–	630.03	1779.27	0.88	1.75
Male		0.17–0.5	8713.28	11,804.51	0.5	8178.97	11,182.47	0.94	0.95
Male standard deviation		–	849.88	1265.29	–	986.40	1529.84	1.16	1.21
Overall mean		0.17–0.5	7641.29	10,328.50	0.5	8020.35	10,727.53	1.05	1.04
Standard deviation		–	1351.00	1895.47	–	798.01	1636.20	0.59	0.86
n		10	10	10	10	10	10	–	–
Male–female ratio		–	0.8	0.7	–	1.0	0.9	–	–

Table. 8.30 Average TK parameters of cyclophosphamide

Administration cycle	Parameter	Unit	Cyclophosphamide 15 mg/kg
First dose	T_{max}	h	0.17–0.5
	C_{max}	ng/mL	7641.29±1351
	$AUC_{0-t\,h}$	ng h/mL	10,329±1895
Last dose	T_{max}	h	0.5
	C_{max}	ng/mL	8020.35±798.01
	$AUC_{0-t\,h}$	ng h/mL	10,728±1636
Accumulation: Last/First	C_{max}		1.07±0.16
	$AUC_{0-72\,h}$		1.06±0.19

8.1.18 Appendix 2 Pathological Examination Report

8.1.18.1 Purpose

Cyclophosphamide and testosterone undecanoate were used as positive drugs, and the effects of cyclophosphamide and testosterone undecanoate on gamete formation, mating behavior, fertility, growth, and development of embryos before and after implantation were observed for more than 60 days after continuous administration for 7 days to identify potential toxic target organs or tissues. This pathology report describes the gross and microscopic pathological changes found in the tests.

8.1.18.2 Material and Method

1) Group assignment: Thirty cynomolgus monkeys were randomly divided into three groups: vehicle control group, cyclophosphamide (15 mg/kg), and testosterone undecanoate (20 mg/kg), with ten animals in each group, half male and half female. The animals were administered via subcutaneous injection and observed for more than 60 days after continuous administration for 7 days. After administration, all animals in each group were euthanized, and gross observation and organ collection were performed. See Table 8.31 for the grouping of laboratory animals at each stage for necropsy.
2) Pathological examination: All animals were systematically dissected by gross necropsy, and abnormal changes in organs and tissues were observed by naked eye, and pathological changes were recorded. The ovaries, uterus, one side testicle, one side epididymis, prostate gland, seminal vesicle gland, levator ani and sphincter, and abnormal organs observed by the naked eye were collected and fixed in 10% formalin. The required tissues were examined by histopathology in the vehicle control group, cyclophosphamide group, and testosterone undecanoate group. After the organs were dehydrated, they were routinely embedded in paraffin, sliced at 3–5 μm, stained by HE, and observed by optical microscope. The results of the microscopic examination were described in two ways, one was "the presence of lesions without classification," and the other was classified into

four levels according to the degree of lesions, namely minimal (+), mild (2+), moderate (3+), and marked (4+).

8.1.18.3 Mortality Test

2M04 in the cyclophosphamide group died spontaneously ON D_9, and no gross abnormalities were found in gross necropsy and histopathological examination.

8.1.18.4 Gross Observation Results

At the end of the administration period, no gross pathological changes related to the test article were observed in the animals scheduled for euthanasia in the administration group, and some common background gross abnormalities were observed in some animals. For example, a small uterine volume was observed in three animals, which may be related to individual development. One animal developed diffuse black spots on the lung surface; Ovarian color changes were observed in two animals, and uterine color changes were observed in one animal. The association between gross abnormalities and histopathology is summarized in Table 8.32.

Table. 8.31 Group assignment for animal necropsy

Pathology number	Test stage	Group	M	F
			Animal number	Animal number
374	End of administration (*n*=5 animal/sex/ group)	1	1M01–1M05	1F01–1F05
		2[1]	2M01–2M03–2M05	2F01–2F05
		3	3M01–3M05	3F01–3F05

[1]Indicates spontaneous death of animals in this Group (animal 2M04 spontaneously died on D_9)

Table. 8.32 Summary of the association between gross abnormal lesions and histological observations

Animal number	Gross abnormality	Observed by optical microscopy
1F02	The fundus of the uterus exhibited a red change	No abnormality
1F05	Small uterine size	No abnormality
2F02	The ovaries exhibited focal red changes	No abnormality
2F05	Small uterine size	Immature
3F02	The surface of the lungs exhibited diffuse small black spots	Moderate diffuse pigmentation was observed in both lungs
3F03	A fleshy-colored change in the ovary measuring 1 cm × 0.5 cm × 0.5 cm. The uterus exhibited a red change	No abnormality
3F05	Small uterine size	No abnormality

Table. 8.33 Description of symbols in the chart of pathological changes

Symbols	Description
1	The group of animals is the vehicle control group
2	The group of animals is test article 1 (cyclophosphamide: 15 mg/kg)
3	The group of animals is test article 2 (testosterone undecanoate: 20 mg/kg)
♀	The sex of the animal is female
♂	The sex of the animal is male
–	No obvious abnormality was found in the animal organs
+	The lesion degree of the animal organ tissue was minimal
2+	The degree of lesion in the animal organ tissue was mild
3+	The lesion degree of animal organ tissue was moderate or obvious
4+	The lesion degree of animal organ tissue was marked or severe
P	Some pathological changes occurred in animal organs and tissues, and the degree of pathological changes was not graded
S, S'	Paired/sampled bilateral organ tissue lesions occurred on one side
B	Bilateral lesions occurred in paired/sampled bilateral organ tissue
/	Animals do not have this organ tissue, or are not suitable for pathological description
×	This organ tissue of the animal was missing during the slide preparation process
T1	Necropsy Time: 11/02/xxx
T2	Necropsy Time: 01/16/xxx
T3	Necropsy Time: 02/27/xxx

8.1.18.5 Histopathological Examination and Discussion

(1) Dose-related pathological changes: At the end of the dosing period, no dose-related changes were observed in animals in the cyclophosphamide or testosterone undecanoate administration groups compared with the vehicle control group (Tables 8.33–8.39).
(2) Spontaneous lesions: At the end of the administration period, common background changes such as inflammatory cell infiltration in the epididymis interstitium, prostate and its interstitium, ovary, uterus and neck of uterus; vacuolation of testis, prostate and sphincter; mineralization of seminal vesicle gland and ovary; atrophy of prostate, diffuse sphincter hemorrhage, diffuse pigmentation in the lungs, and ovarian cysts were observed in the vehicle control group, cyclophosphamide administration group and testosterone undecanoate administration group. There was no significant difference in the severity and incidence of the disease among the groups, which was not related to cyclophosphamide or testosterone undecanoate. The summary of animal spontaneous lesions is shown in Table 8.40.

8.1.18.6 Conclusion

Under the conditions of the study, cynomolgus monkeys were administered cyclophosphamide or testosterone undecanoate via subcutaneous injections for 1 week,

Table. 8.34 Individual data of male animals observed under pathological microscope after administration (vehicle control group, male)

Animal Number		1M01	1M02	1M03	1M04	1M05
Group		1	1	1	1	1
Sex		♂	♂	♂	♂	♂
Necropsy time		T1	T2	T2	T2	T2
Testes	Vacuolization, epithelial, multifocal	–	–	–	–	+
Epididymis		–	–	–	–	–
Prostate	Atrophy	–	–	–	–	3+
	Vacuolated and diffuse	–	–	–	–	2+
	Inflammatory cell infiltration, focal	–	+	–	–	–
	Inflammatory cell infiltration, multifocal	–	–	–	–	+
Seminal vesicle	Mineralized and multifocal	–	2+	2+	–	–
Sphincter		×	–	–	–	–
Levator ani		–	–	–	–	–

Table. 8.35 Individual data of female animals observed under pathological microscope after administration (vehicle control group, female)

Animal number		1F01	1F02	1F03	1F04	1F05
Group		1	1	1	1	1
Sex		♀	♀	♀	♀	♀
Necropsy Time		T1	T3	T3	T3	T3
Ovary	Mineralized, focal, cortical area	×	+, S	–	+, S	–
	Mineralized, multifocal, cortical area	–	–	+, S	+, S	–
	Mineralized, diffuse, cortical area	–	–	+, S	–	–
	Follicular cysts, focal	–	–	+, S	–	–
Uterus	Inflammatory cell infiltration, focal	–	–	+	–	–
Neck of the uterus	Mononuclear inflammatory cell infiltration, focal	–	–	+	+	–

Table. 8.36 Individual data of male animals observed under pathological microscope after administration (Test Article 1 Group, male, cyclophosphamide 15 mg/kg)

Animal number		2M01	2M02	2M03	2M04	2M05
Group		2	2	2	2	2
Sex		♂	♂	♂	♂	♂
Necropsy Time		T1	T2	T2	T2	T2
Testes		–	–	–	–	–
Epididymis	Interstitial multifocal monomorphnuclear cell infiltration	–	+, S	–	–	–
Prostate	Interstitial multifocal monomorphnuclear cell infiltration	–	+	–	–	–
Seminal vesicle		–	–	–	–	–
Sphincter		–	–	–	×	–
Levator ani	Hemorrhage, diffuse	–	–	–	–	–

Table. 8.37 Individual data of female animals observed under pathological microscope after administration (Test Article 1 Group, female, cyclophosphamide 15 mg/kg)

Animal number		2F01	2F02	2F03	2F04	2F05
Group		2	2	2	2	2
Sex		♀	♀	♀	♀	♀
Necropsy Time		T1	T3	T3	T3	T3
Ovary	Mineralization, cortical area, focal	–	–	+, B	+, B	–
	Mineralization, cortical area, focal	–	–	–	–	+, B
	Inflammatory cell infiltration, focal	–	–	+	–	–
Uterus	Inflammatory cell infiltration, multifocal	–	+	+	–	–
Neck of the uterus	Mononuclear inflammatory cell infiltration, focal	–	+	–	–	–

Table. 8.38 Individual data of male animals observed under pathological microscope after administration (Test Article 2 Group, male, testosterone undecanoate 20 mg/kg)

Animal number		3M01	3M02	3M03	3M04	3M05
Group		3	3	3	3	3
Sex		♂	♂	♂	♂	♂
Necropsy Time		T1	T2	T2	T2	T2
Testes	Immature	–	P, B	–	–	–
Epididymis	Immature	–	P, B	–	–	–
Prostate	Inflammatory cell infiltration, multifocal	+	+	+	–	–
Seminal vesicle		–	–	–	–	–
Sphincter		–	–	–	–	–
Levator ani		–	–	–	–	–

Table. 8.39 Individual data of male animals observed under pathological microscope after administration (Test Article 2 Group, female, testosterone undecanoate 20 mg/kg)

Animal number		3F01	3F02	3F03	3F04	3F05
Group		3	3	3	3	3
Sex		♀	♀	♀	♀	♀
Necropsy Time		T1	T3	T3	T3	T3
Lung	Pigmentation, diffuse	–	3+	–	–	–
Overy		–	–	–	–	–
Uterus		–	–	–	–	–

Table. 8.40 Summary of spontaneous lesions

Spontaneous lesion	Degree of lesion	End of administration period (n = 5 animal/sex/group)			End of administration period (n = 5 animal/sex/ group)		
		♂			♀		
		Group 1	Group 2[1]	Group 3	Group 1	Group 2	Group 3
Vacuolization of the testicular epithelium, multifocal	+	1	0	0	0	0	0
Epididymal interstitial multifocal monomorphonuclear cell infiltration	+	0	1	0	0	0	0
Multifocal monomorphonuclear cell infiltration of the prostate stroma	+	0	1	0	0	0	0
Atrophy of the prostate	3+	1	0	0	0	0	0
Diffuse vacuolization of the prostate	2+	1	0	0	0	0	0
Focal/multifocal inflammatory cell infiltration of the prostate	+	1	0	3	0	0	0
Multifocal mineralization of the seminal vesicle glands	2+	2	0	0	0	0	0
Immature testis/epididymis	P	0	0	1	0	0	0
Focal mineralization in the cortical area of the ovary	+	0	0	0	2	2	0
Multifocal mineralization in the cortical area of the ovary	+	0	0	0	2	1	0
Diffuse mineralization in the cortical area of the ovary	+	0	0	0	1	0	0
Ovarian follicular cysts, focal	+	0	0	0	1	0	0
Focal inflammatory cell infiltration in the ovary	+	0	0	0	0	1	0
Focal inflammatory cell infiltration in the uterus	+	0	0	0	1	0	0
Multifocal inflammatory cell infiltration in the uterus	+	0	0	0	0	1	0
Multifocal mononuclear inflammatory cell infiltration in the neck of the uterus	+	0	0	0	0	0	0
Focal mononuclear inflammatory cell infiltration in the neck of the uterus	+	0	0	0	0	1	0
Diffuse pigmentation in the lungs	3+	0	0	0	0	0	1

[1]Indicates spontaneous death of animals occurred in this group (Animal 2M04 was found to have died spontaneously on D_9)

and compared with the vehicle control animals, no pathological changes related to the test article were observed in all test groups.

8.2 A 26-Week Repeated-Dose Study of Monoclonal Antibody AAA Injection in Cynomolgus Monkeys Via Subcutaneous Injection with Combined Fertility Evaluation

8.2.1 Purpose

The purpose of the study was to evaluate the potential effects of the test article on male and female fertility and on the reproductive system (including histopathological evaluation) by observing the possible fertility toxicity of monoclonal antibody AAA injection after repeated subcutaneous injection of monoclonal antibody AAA in cynomolgus monkeys for 26 weeks and the 8-week observation after discontinuation.

8.2.2 Test Article

(1) Identity: AAA injection.
(2) Test Article No.: 2021032.
(3) Batch number: BQ20200802.
(4) Specification: 210 mg(1.75 mL)/bottle.
(5) Content or concentration: 119.0 mg/mL.
(6) Stability: Stable under storage conditions and within the expiration period.
(7) Expiration date: February 23, 2023.
(8) Storage condition: 2°C–8°C, away from light.
(9) Transport environment: 2°C–8°C, away from light, cold chain transport.
(10) Supplier: xxx Limited Company.
(11) Preparation method: No need for preparation.

8.2.3 Excipient Control Article

(1) Identity: AAA placebo.
(2) Batch number: BQ20201004, BQ20211101.
(3) Specification: 1.75 mL/bottle.
(4) Content or concentration: 119.0 mg/mL.
(5) Stability: Stable under storage conditions and within the expiration period.
(6) Expiration date: October 17, 2022, and November 09, 2023.
(7) Storage condition: 2°C–8°C, away from light.
(8) Transport environment: 2°C–8°C, away from light, cold chain transport.
(9) Supplier: xxx Limited Company.
(10) Preparation method: No need for preparation.

8.2.4 Other Main Reagents

(1) Identity: Zoletil 50(Teletamine hydrochloride, Zolazepam hydrochloride for injection).
(2) Batch numbers: 8EZG and 8G4V.
(3) Formula/Components: 125 mg Tiletamine + 125 mg Zolazepam +Excipient (Q.S. 1 bottle).
(4) Concentration in use: 50 mg/mL.
(5) Expiration date: April, ×××× .
(6) Storage condition: Blackout, airtight.
(7) Transport environment: Away from light.
(8) Supplier: ××× Limited Company.
(9) Preparation method: Dissolve the powder in a solid bottle with sterile water for injection in the package (batch numbers 8EZGA and 8G4VA) to a concentration of 50 mg/mL before use.

8.2.5 Test System

(1) Species, strain, and grade: Cynomolgus monkey, conventional.
(2) Sex and quantity: 46 spare animals (half male and half female) were applied, 40 animals (half male and half female) were used in the test, and the extra 6 animals were returned to the Animal Husbandry Department.
(3) Body weight and age range: At reception, male animals weighed 4.025–5.875 kg and female animals weighed 2.160–3.460 kg; before administration, male animals weighed 4.110–5.260 kg and female animals weighed 2.485–3.325 kg. The weight at the time of receiving was for reference only, and the weight during grouping pre-dose was used as the standard. The spare animals on the day of application were 3–5 years old. The animals were 3–5 years old at the time of initiation of administration.
(4) Animal source: Spare animals of the institution were used to carry out the study; spare animals were purchased from ××× company.
(5) Laboratory animal production permission number: SCXK(Gui)2018xxx, issued by the xxx Science and Technology Department.
(6) Laboratory animal use certificate numbers: NO.0005085, NO.0005084, and NO.0005113.
(7) Laboratory animal use permission number: SYXK(E)2021xxx, issued by xxx Science and Technology Department.
(8) Rationale for Study System: Monkeys have a close kinship with humans, and are commonly used nonhuman primate laboratory animals for preclinical studies on biological products, with rich historical background data. According to the *Technical Guidelines for Repeated Dose Toxicity Studies of Drugs* and *General Principles for Technical Review of Nonclinical Safety of Therapeutic Biologics* formulated by National Medical Products Administration (CFDA),

and the *Guidelines for Preclinical Safety Evaluation of Biotechnology-Derived Pharmaceuticals* and *Safety Pharmacology Studies for Human Pharmaceuticals* formulated by the International Council for Harmonization of Technical Requirements for Pharmaceuticals for Human Use (ICH), it is a must to use the relevant animal species in the study. In summary, the cynomolgus monkey is selected for this study, and the sponsor agreed to use this animal.

(9) Animal identification: Animals are numbered in accordance with the SOP of the institution, and the collar and cage card (each animal has its own unique collar number, and the grouped animal number corresponds to the collar number one by one) are used as animal identification marks.

(10) Animal reception date: xxx, xxx,2021.

(11) Feed and Drinking Water ① Feed: The conventional maintenance feed of monkeys was manufactured by xxx, Ltd., batch Nos. 21088211, 21108211, 21128211, etc. Feed nutritional components, microorganism parameters, and chemical contaminants were tested by a supplier entrusted with a qualified unit, and the reports were submitted to the facility. The test parameters referred to GB 14924.32010 and GB 14924.22001. Microorganism parameters and chemical contaminants were tested by a facility entrusted with a qualified unit every year, and the test parameters referred to GB 14924.22001. Feed colony population was tested quarterly by the facility, and the test parameters referred to GB 4789.22016. The above test results of the feed used met the requirements. ② Drinking water: Drinking water for laboratory animals was purified by the facility. Microorganisms, chemical contaminants, and toxic substances in animal drinking water were tested by a facility entrusted to a qualified unit every year, and the testing parameters referred to GB 57492006. Total bacterial colonies were tested once a quarter by the facility, and the test parameters referred to GB 4789.22016. The above test results of the drinking water used met the requirements.

(12) Animal husbandry and environment: Animals were housed in the conventional laboratory. The feeding cages were stainless steel monkey cages, the size was 900 mm × 1000 mm × 2080 mm, and the animals were housed one to two animals per cage during the adaptive training period and were housed individually after grouping with free access to drinking water and feed. The temperature was set at 17.5–24.2°C, humidity was set at 37.4%–91.4%, ventilation rate ≥ 8 times/h, working illuminance ≥200 Lux, animal illuminance 100 Lux–200 Lux, with automatic illumination, on a 12-h alternative cycle of light and darkness. During the study, the above parameters all met the requirements of GB 149252010, except for the deviation of temperature and humidity in some periods (see "Anomalies Causing Study Protocol Deviation" in the main test of this report for details).

(13) Animal welfare: All animal welfare involved in this study was in compliance with the Animals Welfare Guidelines of xxx company. The study was submitted to the Institutional Animal Care and Use Committee (IACUC) for review and approval. The management and use of animals during the study were in line with the *Guide for the Care and Use of Laboratory Animals*

(2011) published by the National Academy Press (NAP) and the *Laboratory Animal Management Regulations* revised in 2017 by the State Scientific and Technological Commission. The management, use, and relevant procedures of the animals involved in this study were reviewed and approved by the Institutional Animal Care and Use Committee (IACUC) of xxx company. Approval No.: IACUC (Approved)2021190.

(14) Veterinary treatment: None of the animals required veterinary treatment/care, or other related conditions during the study.

8.2.6 Group Assignment and Dosage Design

(1) Method for group assignment: Four groups were set up, namely, the excipient control group and the AAA low, medium, and high-dose groups, which were randomly divided according to body weight, with 10 animals in each group (half male and half female) and 40 in total. After grouping, the weight deviation of all animals was between ±20% of the average body weight.

(2) Dosage Setting Basis:

1) Function indications provided by the sponsor: Clinically intended for adults with severe asthma with poor control.
2) Clinical route of administration provided by the sponsor: Subcutaneous injection.
3) Intended clinical dose provided by the sponsor: The proposed single-dose escalation test for healthy subjects in the clinical trial started with a dose of 12 mg/person, and was administered once, followed by dose escalation. The highest dose group was tentatively set at 630 mg/person. If the drug is well tolerated and safe at the highest dose, higher dose groups (>630 mg) test might be carried out.
4) The proposed repeated-dose study dose for healthy subjects in the clinical trial was 420 mg per person each time, administered once every 28 days, for a total of three times. The repeated-dose study in severe asthma patients was designed with three dose groups: low (70 mg/person each time), medium (210 mg/person each time), and high (280 mg/person each time) via subcutaneous injection. In summary, and after consultation with the sponsor, it was determined that the proposed clinical trial dose was 280 mg/person each time, and the average body weight of the person was calculated to be 70 kg, so the proposed clinical dose was 4 mg/kg.
5) The pharmacodynamic test results of the cynomolgus monkey provided by the sponsor: The effective dose is 10 mg/kg.
6) Toxicity test results of single subcutaneous injection in cynomolgus monkey provided by the sponsor: After single subcutaneous injection of 100 and 600 mg/kg, no abnormalities related to the test article were observed

in clinical observation, body weight, food consumption, electrocardiogram, clinicopathology and gross necropsy.

7) Toxicity test results of repeated subcutaneous injection in cynomolgus monkeys provided by the sponsor: Cynomolgus monkeys were given subcutaneous injections of 30, 100, and 300 mg/kg once a week for 5 consecutive weeks, and recovered for 4 weeks after discontinuation. The clinical observation, body weight, food consumption, ophthalmic examination, electrocardiogram, clinical pathology, cytokines, organ coefficient, and histopathology of cynomolgus monkeys were evaluated, and no toxic changes related to administration were found. No antidrug antibody was detected in each dose group. No adverse effect dose (NOAEL) was 300 mg/kg in both male and female animals.
8) Toxicity test results of repeated subcutaneous injection in cynomolgus monkey provided by the sponsor: Cynomolgus monkeys were given subcutaneous injections of 30, 100, and 300 mg/kg once a week for 5 consecutive weeks, and recovered for 4 weeks after discontinuation. After the last dose (D_{29}), C_{max} and $AUC_{0–168\ h}$ were (3384 ± 620) μg/mL and (464198 ± 71861) h μg/mL respectively. There was no significant difference in toxicokinetic parameters between male and female animals. Except that the increase ratio of D_{29} exposure (C_{max} and $AUC_{0–168\ h}$) in 300 mg/kg group was lower than that of dose increase, the increase ratio of D_1 and D_{29} exposure (C_{max} and $AUC_{0–168\ h}$) in other groups was basically consistent with the increase ratio of dose. Compared with the first dose (D_1), the plasma exposure increased after the last dose (D_{29}), and the mean serum elimination half-life $T_{1/2}$ after subcutaneous injection of AAA was 256 h.
9) In summary, the designed doses of this experiment were 15, 50, and 150 mg/kg by subcutaneous injection once a week, which were equivalent to 1.5 times, 5 times, and 15 times of the pharmacodynamic effective dose, respectively.

(3) Dose multiples: 3.0–3.3 times.
(4) Dosage: 15, 50, and 150 mg/kg (Table 8.41).

Table. 8.41 Dosage and group assignment

Group	Dosage (mg/kg)	Multiple of the effective dose	Clinical equivalent dose multiple	Proposed clinical dose multiple	Animal number	
					♀	♂
Vehicle Control	–	–	–	–	1F01–1F05	1M01–1M05
Low-dose	15	1.5	1.25	3.75	2F01–2F05	2M01–2M05
Mid-dose	50	5.0	4.17	12.50	3F01–3F05	3M01–3M05
High-dose	150	15.0	12.50	37.50	4F01–4F05	4M01–4M05

Note: – indicates not applicable. The "pharmacodynamic effective dose multiple" in the table is calculated by 10 mg/kg. The clinical dose is calculated at 4 mg/kg, and the equivalent dose of cynomolgus monkey is 12 mg/kg

8.2.7 Test Method

(1) Administration frequency and duration: A total of 27 doses were administered once a week for 26 weeks, and each dose was divided into 2 days. For any given animal, the first dose was defined as D_1.
(2) Administration route: Subcutaneous injection in the back. The procedure was performed by subcutaneous injection in the middle back in SOP.
(3) Dosage: 0.1–1.3 mL/kg, equal concentration and different volume administration; Excipient control group, low-dose group, medium dose group, and high-dose group were given 150/119, 15/119, 50/119, and 150/119 mL/kg, respectively. Multi-point injection was performed, and the dosage volume at each point was no more than 1 mL. The nominal dosing volume of each animal was accurate to one decimal place (0.1 mL), based on the animal's most recently weighed weight. The actual dosage volume was extracted according to the syringe scale, which was consistent with the nominal dosage volume, and recorded in the raw record of the test.
(4) Administration time: 08:20–13:00.
(5) Description of the administration route of the test article: Consistent with the proposed clinical pathway.
(6) Preparation of the test article and control article: The test article and control article do not need to be prepared. Shake the test article well before use.

8.2.8 Test Method and Observation Indicator

This section shows only the content related to fertility evaluation.

(1) Hormone testing: Commercially available kits were used to detect hormones. The samples were collected from frozen samples of blood biochemical testing in Study No. AAA××××03202. The sample collection time was pre-dose (D_{-9}), middle administration (D_{92}), end of administration period (D_{184}), and end of recovery period (D_{240}). The levels of LH, FSH, E_2, progesterone (P), and testosterone (T) were detected in females. DHT, E_2, and T levels were detected in males.
(2) Staging of spermatogenic cycle: The stages of the spermatogenic cycle of the testicular seminiferous tubule epithelium were stained by the PAS method to describe the toxicological changes of the test article to spermatogenic cells at all levels of the tubule epithelium.
(3) Ovary: The fixed tissues were dehydrated with ethanol, transparented with xylene, embedded with paraffin, sliced continuously (section thickness was 3–5 μ m), baked, and stained with HE, etc. The number of follicles at all levels (including primary follicles, secondary follicles, mature follicles, and corpus luteum) was calculated by observing five consecutive slices under a microscope. Only

the follicles containing oocytes whose nuclei could be observed were counted, and the total was calculated as the number of follicles in the entire ovary.

(4) Endometrial thickness: The fixed uterus was sliced in paraffin and stained with HE. The morphology of the endometrium was observed under a microscope, and the structural characteristics of the endometrium in each stage of estrus were observed by HE staining. The mean value of endometrial thickness at 4 positions of each uterus (12 o′clock, 3 o′clock, 6 o′clock, and 9 o′clock) was measured under a microscope.

(5) Peer review: The staging of the testicular spermatogenesis cycle, ovarian and endometrial thickness were diagnosed by an internal pathologist of the institution, and peer-reviewed by another pathologist of the institution, and a peer-reviewed report was issued.

8.2.9 Statistical Analysis of Data

SPSS (version 17.0 or higher) was used for the input and statistical analysis of hormone data. $P < 0.05$ and $P < 0.01$ indicated a statistical difference. When the sample size was less than or equal to two, only the average or individual data were listed, and no statistics were performed. One-way analysis of variance was used for inter-group comparison, and a paired t-test was used for intra-group comparison. The one-way analysis of variance is as follows:

(1) Firstly, the Shapiro–Wilk test method was used to check whether the data conforms to the normal distribution, $P > 0.05$, the homogeneity test of variance would be used to test the data uniformity; $P \leq 0.05$, the Kruskalwallis test would be used.

(2) If the data were uniform by the homogeneity of variance test (test $P > 0.05$), the analysis of variance test (F-test) would be performed. If the result of the homogeneity of variance test was $P \leq 0.05$, the Kruskal–Wallis test would be performed.

(3) If the result of the ANOVA test was $P \leq 0.05$, the Dunnett parameter test method would be further used for the multiple comparison test. If the result of the variance analysis was $P > 0.05$, statistics would end.

(4) If the result of the Kruskal–Wallis test was $P \leq 0.05$, the multiple comparison test would be further conducted by the Mann–Whitney U two-group nonparametric test. If the result of the Kruskal–Wallis test was $P > 0.05$, the statistics would end.

8.2.10 Results and Discussion

(1) Hormone testing: The summary data of hormone results during administration and recovery period are shown in Tables 8.42 and 8.43.

Androgens and estrogens: Compared with the excipient control group at the same period, the DHT of males in the medium and high-dose groups decreased at the end

Table. 8.42 Summary of hormone data (male, $\overline{X}\pm$SD)

Test indicator	Test stage	Animal number (animal/group)	Vehicle control	AAA		
				Low-dose	Mid-dose	High-dose
DHT (pg/mL)	D_{-9}	5	179.748±46.549	131.923±49.328	168.670±86.806	130.414±33.617
	D_{92}	5[1]	132.765±77.307	126.096±62.834	114.232±72.474	89.403±14.591
	D_{184}	5	174.587±8.778	188.141±86.617	127.943±20.340**	96.080±24.500**
	D_{240}	2	104.864	114.322	117.936	140.500
E_2 (pg/mL)	D_{-9}	5	700.577±402.215	385.218±97.055	487.192±293.046	620.660±276.272
	D_{92}	5	551.706±186.263	584.416±78.337	522.024±167.893	517.843±60.297
	D_{184}	5	851.970±258.682	537.217±62.723	695.296±278.174	528.651±152.182
	D_{240}	2	356.684	337.004	347.739	408.712
T (ng/mL)	D_{-9}	5	1.092±0.146	0.962±0.238	1.271±0.780	1.025±0.479
	D_{92}	5	1.238±0.485	0.818±0.350	0.814±0.370	0.752±0.237
	D_{184}	5	1.453±0.073	1.462±0.650	1.436±0.538	0.981±0.231
	D_{240}	2	0.885	1.268	0.722	0.992

Note: Compared with the vehicle control group, $^{**}P<0.01$ [1]Indicates that 1M04 and 4M03 are not detected due to insufficient sample size

of the administration period (D_{184}) ($P\leq 0.01$), and there were no significant changes in the parameters of each dose group at the other stages, and there was no statistical difference ($P>0.05$).

After analysis, it was considered that: Compared with the same period of the negative control group, DHT in males in mid-dose and high-dose groups decreased by 26.7%–45.0% at the end of the administration period (D184). DHT was converted from T, and no obvious abnormality was observed in T. DHT recovered after the recovery period, and the change of DHT individual data in the excipient control group before administration was about two times (the highest compared with the lowest). The above DHT changes were considered to be normal hormone level fluctuations in animals, and the test article had no correlation with hormones in female and male animals.

(2) Stages of testicular spermatogenesis cycle: The summary data of spermatogenic cell classification and counting results of spermatogenic cycle during administration and recovery period are shown in Table 8.44.

Table 8.43 Summary of hormone data (female, $\overline{X}$±SD)

Test indicator	Test stage	Animal number (animal/group)	Vehicle control	AAA		
				Low-dose	Mid-dose	High-dose
LH (mIU/mL)	D_{-9}	5	27.528±5.203	21.649±12.381	16.985±4.358	25.137±4.942
	D_{92}	5	20.705±2.303	21.403±10.175	21.015±1.550	18.333±7.264
	D_{184}	5	30.763±8.450	29.335±13.618	24.116±5.066	29.139±10.281
	D_{240}	2	23.308	24.724	19.833	28.654
FSH (ng/mL)	D_{-9}	5	263.845±64.753	135.747±27.207	204.591±73.087	188.336±36.216
	D_{92}	5	219.362±78.846	175.542±72.169	232.107±76.313	207.918±30.180
	D_{184}	5	230.576±73.408	222.931±71.982	252.126±79.372	226.509±64.134
	D_{240}	2	364.903	261.144	231.565	243.338
P (ng/mL)	D_{-9}	5	6138.575±4509.387	5167.684±7224.723	6557.194±7346.622	3472.511±3837.113
	D_{92}	5	3314.924±3145.730	6318.366±11982.220	4284.392±5478.669	1337.326±442.592
	D_{184}	5	2936.144±2473.652	4964.419±8724.298	6706.638±5441.406	1989.152±1780.204
	D_{240}	2	4517.391	2330.449	2228.731	8691.292
E_2 (pg/mL)	D_{-9}	5	1125.717±227.710	1012.528±249.302	1169.142±298.267	942.775±206.142
	D_{92}	5	756.396±109.881	858.494±244.162	963.359±307.305	641.164±156.091
	D_{184}	5	915.461±214.973	774.767±157.939	1103.661±279.016	722.536±93.417
	D_{240}	2	933.450	718.501	817.133	785.271
T (ng/mL)	D_{-9}	5	1.007±0.376	1.122±0.376	1.215±0.095	1.076±0.366
	D_{92}	5	0.541±0.073	0.632±0.242	0.783±0.172	0.603±0.124
	D_{184}	5	0.853±0.210	0.813±0.229	1.036±0.251	1.229±0.656
	D_{240}	2	0.594	0.925	0.967	0.969

Twelve morphological stages of the spermatogenic cycle in cross-section of the spermatogenic tubules in cynomolgus monkeys. Sections were stained with PAS/hematoxylin. The numbers I–XII indicate 12 morphological stages.

Compared with the control group at the same period, there was no significant change in the mean number of spermatogenic cells at each stage in the section, and

Table. 8.44 Summary of spermatogenic cycle data ($\overline{X}$±SD)

Test stage	Stages of the spermatogenic cycle	Animal number (animal/group)	Vehicle control	AAA		
				Low-dose	Mid-dose	High-dose
End of administration period (D_{184})	I	3	5.67±1.15	16.00±13.45	12.33±5.03	5.33±3.06
	II	3	4.00±2.00	10.33±8.08	6.67±1.53	4.33±3.51
	III	3	5.33±1.15	5.00±4.58	5.67±2.08	4.33±2.52
	IV	3	5.67±1.53	5.00±4.58	5.33±2.52	5.00±3.61
	V	3	4.33±1.53	4.33±4.04	8.33±4.51	8.67±6.51
	VI	3	6.33±2.08	4.67±1.53	8.67±4.51	12.33±8.62
	VII	3	14.00±1.73	6.67±2.89	8.00±4.00	16.67±4.51
	VIII	3	21.33±1.53	33.00±13.89	27.00±16.09	41.33±11.50
	IX	3	10.33±4.16	15.00±2.65	21.33±4.51	15.33±4.51
	X	3	9.33±2.08	13.00±5.00	12.67±3.06	11.67±3.79
	XI	3	13.00±4.58	16.33±7.64	9.33±2.52	12.33±4.93
	XII	3	9.00±1.73	11.33±4.04	9.00±4.36	9.33±1.15
End of recovery period (D_{240})	I	2	10.00	14.00	13.00	18.50
	II	2	8.00	9.50	9.50	12.00
	III	2	6.50	8.50	8.00	9.50
	IV	2	5.00	7.50	7.00	9.00
	V	2	6.00	9.00	8.00	7.50
	VI	2	10.00	9.50	13.50	12.00
	VII	2	14.00	10.00	12.50	9.50
	VIII	2	32.00	23.00	22.00	24.50
	IX	2	6.50	14.00	26.00	11.00
	X	2	7.50	12.00	11.50	11.50
	XI	2	11.00	12.50	10.00	12.50
	XII	2	4.50	13.50	10.50	7.50

no statistical difference was observed ($P > 0.05$) when each dose group was observed from the center of testicular section in one direction under microscope, and more than five high-power microscope fields were observed continuously at the end of

Table. 8.45 Summary of follicle data at all levels ($\overline{X}\pm$SD)

Test stage	Classification of follicles	Animal number (animal/group)	Vehicle control	AAA		
				Low-dose	Mid-dose	High-dose
End of administration period (D_{184})	Primary follicle	3	1.00±0.53	1.13±0.95	0.67±0.42	0.40±0.35
	Follicle stimulation	3	0.00±0.00	0.20±0.20	0.07±0.12	0.00±0.00
	Mature follicle	3	0.00±0.00	0.00±0.00	0.00±0.00	0.00±0.00
	Corpus luteum	3	3.33±3.51	1.00±1.73	0.87±0.90	0.67±1.15
End of recovery period (D_{240})	Primary follicle	2	1.00	0.50	0.40	1.20
	Follicle stimulation	2	0.00	0.20	0.00	0.20
	Mature follicle	2	0.10	0.40	0.00	0.00
	Corpus luteum	2	3.50	0.60	1.50	2.00

Table. 8.46 Summary of endometrial thickness data ($\overline{X}\pm$SD)

Test stage	Endometrial thickness site	Animal number (animal/group)	Vehicle control	AAA		
				Low-dose	Mid-dose	High-dose
End of administration period (D_{184})	12 points	3	4533.21±1233.12	4155.75±514.63	6258.03±1255.57	2588.81±1220.76
	3 points	3	2254.33±645.57	1964.34±186.60	2739.34±726.41	2683.54±1583.87
	6 points	3	4502.12±1556.30	3680.48±267.74	5730.76±1441.77	2692.21±1132.15
	9 points	3	2351.26±1198.77	1794.73±344.50	3022.36±947.99	2782.52±1510.73
End of recovery period (D_{240})	12 points	2	7725.302	5319.438	5308.63	5840.752
	3 points	2	4232.466	2133.228	3431.615	3712.943
	6 points	2	8409.060	4738.023	5965.927	5915.277
	9 points	2	4555.631	2211.781	3828.949	3684.345

administration period (D_{184}) and recovery period (D_{240}). It was considered that the test article had no correlation with the male testis.

(3) Ovary: Follicles at the administration and recovery stages are summarized in Table 8.45.

Compared with the excipient control group at the same period, there was no significant change in the mean number of follicles (primary follicles, secondary follicles, mature follicles and corpus luteum) in five consecutive sections under the microscope in each dose group at the end of the administration period (D_{184}) and the end of recovery period (D_{240}), and there was no statistical difference ($P > 0.05$), it was considered that the test article had no correlation with the female ovary.

(4) Endometrial thickness: Summary data of endometrial thickness during administration and recovery period are shown in Table 8.46.

Compared with the excipient control group at the same period, there was no significant change in the mean value of endometrial thickness of five consecutive sections (12, 3, 6 and 9 o′clock) under the microscope in each dose group at the end of the administration period (D_{184}) and the end of recovery period (D_{240}), and there was no statistical difference ($P > 0.05$), it was considered that the test article had no correlation with female endometrial thickness.

(5) Peer review: In this study, the raw data of follicle count and uterine cavity thickness of female animals were reviewed and agreed upon. Any differences that arise in the spermatogenic cycle of male animals have been discussed by thematic pathologists and peer-reviewed pathologists, and the raw data have been revised accordingly. The end result is a consistent reflection of the opinions of both thematic pathologists and peer-reviewed pathologists.

8.2.11 Conclusion

The cynomolgus monkeys were injected subcutaneously with 15, 50, and 150 mg/kg monoclonal antibody AAA for 26 consecutive weeks, and a high dose of equal volume placebo was administered subcutaneously as an excipient control. No significant changes were observed in animal sex hormones, testicular spermatogenesis cycle, follicle number, and endometrial thickness in each dose group. In conclusion, the cynomolgus monkeys were given subcutaneous injection of AAA for 26 consecutive weeks, and the NOAEL was 150 mg/kg.

8.3 Fetal Developmental Toxicity with Toxicokinetics Test and Enhanced Perinatal Developmental Toxicity with Toxicokinetics Test in Cynomolgus Monkeys Given Subcutaneous Cyclophosphamide or Thalidomide via Gavage

8.3.1 Purpose

The enhanced perinatal development (ePPND) toxicity test in cynomolgus monkeys is a combination of fetal and perinatal developmental toxicity tests, and according to ICH S5(R3), the dosing cycle is confirmed from pregnancy (about GD_{20}) to delivery, i.e., covering embryo implantation to delivery of the fetus (GD_{20} to PND_0).

This is a systematic validation study with teratogenic positive drugs. Therefore, positive drugs known to have reproductive toxicity were selected [1]: cyclophosphamide and thalidomide. Considering that the toxic effect of positive drugs had a certain teratogenic sensitive period, the administration was only performed in a specific time period.

Using cyclophosphamide and thalidomide as teratogenic positive drugs, they were administered via subcutaneous injection (sc) on GD_{24-28} and gavage (ig) on GD_{24}–GD_{30}, respectively, to evaluate their effects on the development and progeny of pregnant animals, embryos, fetal and fetal development, including the toxicity of pregnant animals, death, growth, development and structural changes of embryos and fetal, prenatal and postnatal death of offspring, changes in growth and development, and functional defects of offspring; Blood concentrations (crossing the placental barrier) were detected at different time points. The main objective was to establish an enhanced perinatal developmental toxicity test method for cynomolgus monkeys, and to provide a reference method for the subsequent study of the effects of drugs on the development of pregnant monkeys, embryos, fetuses, and perinatal development.

8.3.2 Test Article 1

(1) Identity: Cyclophosphamide.
(2) Abbreviation: CP (cyclophosphamide).
(3) Batch number: 602200401.
(4) Component: C7H17Cl2N2O3P.
(5) Content: 97% to 103%.
(6) Supplier: ×××company.
(7) Expiration date: 03/31/xxx.
(8) Storage condition: Ambient temperature.
(9) Preparation method: Prepared with 0.9% sodium chloride injection.

8.3.3 Test Article 2

(1) Identity: Thalidomide.
(2) Abbreviation: 反应停(thalidomide).
(3) Batch number: 20190606.
(4) Component: C13H10N2O4.
(5) Content: Calculated based on the dry product, it should be 98.5%-102.0%.
(6) Supplier: ×××company.
(7) Expiration date: May ×××.
(8) Storage condition: Ambient temperature.
(9) Preparation method: Prepared with olive oil.

8.3.4 Control Article (Saline group)

(1) Identity: Saline.
(2) Batch number: 202127521, 202145971.

(3) Component: The main component of this product is sodium chloride; the excipient is water for injection.
(4) Specification: 100 mL: 0.9 g.
(5) Stability: Stable at ambient temperature.
(6) Supplier: ×××company.
(7) Expiration date: 09/26/xxx.
(8) Storage condition: Sealed storage.
(9) Preparation method: No preparation required.

8.3.5 Laboratory Animal Information

(1) Species, strain, and grade: Cynomolgus monkey, conventional.
(2) Sex and number: 60 female monkeys were applied for this study. There were 15 males (not given the drug) and 35 females who became pregnant during the study.
(3) Age range: Male 6–8 years old, female 4–6 years old, healthy, sexually mature, and unmated cynomolgus monkeys (age at mating).
(4) Weight range: 2.65–3.98 kg for females and 5.8–7.8 kg for males at mating time.
(5) Animal reception: Laboratory animals arrived at our institution in two batches and were transferred to the reserve animal group of our institution after passing quarantine for 14 days. The laboratory animals used in this study were transferred from the reserve animal group of our institution to this study on January 05, ××××.
(6) Animal source: ××× company.
(7) Laboratory animal production permission number: SCXK(Yue) 20××0043, issued by the xxx Science and Technology Department.
(8) Laboratory animal use permission number: SYXK(E)20××0090, issued by xxx Science and Technology Department.
(9) Rationale for Study System: Cynomolgus monkey is one of the recognized standard animals in toxicological reproductive toxicity studies. *Technical Guidelines for Drug Reproductive Toxicity Research* formulated by National Medical Products Administration (NMPA) and ICH S5(R3) recommend the use of this animal, and the sponsor agrees to use this animal, so the cynomolgus monkey is used in this test.
(10) Animal identification: The collar and cage card (each animal has its own unique collar number, and the grouped animal number corresponds to the collar number one by one) are used as animal identification marks. Each animal was assigned a unique animal number during the study.
(11) Feed and Drinking Water
   1) Feed: The maintenance feed of monkeys was manufactured by xxx, Ltd., batch No. 21048211, 21058231, 21078211, etc. The feed supplier provided the inspection report to the facility. The test parameters met GB 14924.32010 and GB 14924.22001. Microorganism, heavy metal, and

chemical contaminants were tested by a facility entrusted with a qualified unit every year, and the test parameters met GB 14924.22001. Feed colony population was tested quarterly by the facility, and the test parameters met GB 4789.22022. The above test results of the feed used met the requirements.

2) Drinking water: Drinking water for laboratory animals was purified by the facility. Microorganisms, chemical contaminants, and toxic substances in animal drinking water were tested by a facility entrusted with a qualified unit every year, and the testing parameters met GB 57492022. Total bacterial colonies were tested once a quarter by the facility, and the test parameters met GB 4789.22022. The above test results of the drinking water used met the requirements during the study.

(12) Animal husbandry and environment: Animals were housed in the monkey observation room. The monkeys were housed in 900 mm×1000 mm×2080 mm or 4200 mm × 2400 mm × 2200 mm cages or group cages, one animal per cage before mating or several animals per cage at mating time (one male, one to three females). After successful mating, pregnant monkeys could be housed in a single cage during pregnancy with free access to drinking water and feed. The temperature was set at 19.12°C–25.15°C, humidity was set at 42%–68%, ventilation rate ≥8 times/h, working illuminance ≥200 Lux, animal illuminance 100 Lux–200 Lux, with automatic illumination, on a 12-h alternative cycle of light and darkness.

(13) Animal welfare: All animal welfare involved in this study was in compliance with the Animals Welfare Guidelines of xxx company. The management and use of animals during the study were in line with the Guide for the Care and Use of Laboratory Animals (2011) published by the National Academy Press (NAP) and the Laboratory Animal Management Regulations revised in 2017 by the State Scientific and Technological Commission. The management, use, and relevant procedures of the animals involved in this study were reviewed and approved by the Institutional Animal Care and Use Committee (IACUC) of xxx company. Approval No.: IACUC (Approved) 20××165.

8.3.6 Group Assignment and Dosage Design

(1) Grouping

1) The females were randomly divided into three groups according to the sequence of pregnancy and random numbers: Group 1 (saline group), cyclophosphamide group, and thalidomide group, respectively.

2) Ensure that there were no fewer than six pregnant monkeys in the saline group, and no fewer than 12 pregnant monkeys in each group of cyclophosphamide and thalidomide.

(2) Dosage setting basis: According to the preliminary test results and domestic and foreign literature reports, thalidomide and cyclophosphamide, which are commonly used in reproductive test and have teratogenic effects, were selected as

test article, and the doses of thalidomide gavage group and cyclophosphamide subcutaneous injection group were selected according to the preliminary test results, with doses of 20 and 15 mg/kg, respectively.

(3) Dosage: See Table 8.47 for specific dosage.

8.3.7 Administration Method

(1) Administration route: Gavage (ig) and subcutaneous injection (sc).
(2) Administration volume: Gavage or subcutaneous injection at 1 mL/kg. The administration volume was accurate to one decimal place (0.1 mL) for each animal and calculated according to the animal's most recently weighed weight.
(3) Administration time: 08:50–09:42.
(4) Administration frequency and duration
   1) Saline group: Pregnant monkeys were administered from GD_{24} for 7 consecutive days and ended on GD_{30}.
   2) Cyclophosphamide subcutaneous group: Pregnant monkeys were administered from GD_{24} for 5 days and ended on GD_{28}.
   3) Thalidomide gavage group: Pregnant monkeys were administered from GD_{24} for 7 consecutive days and ended on GD_{30}.
(5) Description of the route of administration: The same as the clinical proposed route, the clinical proposed route of cyclophosphamide is oral or intravenous injection, and subcutaneous injection is added to investigate the teratogenic effects of different routes of administration.
(6) Preparation method of test article and control article: On the day of administration, test articles were prepared with animal drinking water (cyclophosphamide) and olive oil (thalidomide) in different concentrations according to the preparation requirements of the test article. The formulation was prepared every day before immediate use. The specific preparation method is shown in Table 8.48. The remaining test article formulations were confirmed by the experimenter and returned to the test article preparation room for unified disposal by the institution.

Table. 8.47 Group information and dose design

Group	Route of administration	Dose (mg/kg)	Number of pregnant monkeys (embryo–fetus)	Number of pregnant monkeys (perinatal)
Group 1 (Saline)	Gavage	–	6	3
Group 2 (Cyclophosphamide)	Subcutaneous	20	7	6
Group 3 (Thalidomide)	Gavage	15	7	6

Table. 8.48 Preparation method of test articles

Group number (group)		Route of administration	Dose (mg/kg/day)	Amount of test article (mg)	Solution volume (mL)	Target concentration (mg/mL)
1	Saline	Gavage	–	–	–	–
2	Cyclophosphamide	Subcutaneous	20	1000	50	20
3	Thalidomide	Gavage	15	750	50	15

Note: "–" indicates not applicable; the total amount of the drug prepared for each dose group changes accordingly with the increase in animal weight. The table above represents an example of the preparation method for the first administration

(7) Administration Method of the Test Article and Control Article
  1) Gavage: In accordance with the SOP requirements of the institution, a gastric tube was used through the nose for gavage. Before taking out the gastric tube, about 5 mL of drinking water was taken into the gastric tube to ensure that all the liquid in the gastric tube entered the body of the animal.
  2) Subcutaneous administration: Shave the hair of the back administration area one day before administration, and inject the drug into the shoulder blade area of the animal's back according to the SOP requirements of the institution. After the injection, pull out the needle and gently press the pinhole with a dry cotton ball for about 5 s to prevent drug discharge.

8.3.8 Test Method [3]

(1) Animal quarantine: This test was applied to spare animals of the institution for testing. The spare animals had been quarantined for 14 days before entering the study, and all of them had passed the quarantine.
(2) Adaptive feeding: From entering the study to successful mating, all animals were observed for adaptive feeding, and general symptoms were observed twice a day (once in the morning and once in the afternoon).
(3) Blood collection
  1) A comprehensive hormone assay was performed before mating, and at each stage of pregnancy, i.e., blood was collected before mating, on GD20, GD50, GD100, and GD150.
  2) Method of blood collection: About 2 mL of blood was collected from the limb veins, serum was separated, and frozen at −80°C for hormone detection.
  3) Euthanasia of pregnant monkeys: The gestation period for females is about 160 days. This study was divided into two parts. The first part mainly investigated the fetal development test. The pregnant monkeys were euthanized on GD_{100}, the abdomen was cut open to expose the uterus and internal organs,

and any internal abnormalities were recorded, all abnormal tissues were sampled, marked and fixed in 10% formalin, and histopathological examination was carried out. The second part mainly investigated the perinatal development test and did not euthanize the pregnant monkeys.

(4) Animal mating
   1) Male and female monkeys (1:3 or 1:4) were placed in group cages with monitoring, and the female animals mated with the male animals continuously for 3–7 days during the menstrual cycle D_{12} to D_{14} (ovulation period).
   2) An ultrasound examination (Mindray, M7Vet) was performed 18–20 days after mating to determine pregnancy. If a black gap in the uterine cavity was found on the ultrasound examination, the pregnant monkey would be considered pregnant. When an animal was confirmed pregnant, day 2 of the mating date would be designated as day 0 of gestation (GD_0). After confirming the pregnancy of the animals, B-ultrasonography was performed at irregular intervals every month to confirm the survival and development of the fetus (Fig. 8.2).

(5) Administration: Once pregnancy was confirmed, females would be assigned to each dose group using a random number table. The specific administration time was as follows: ① Saline group: Pregnant monkeys were administered via gavage during GD24_GD30 for 7 consecutive days. ② Cyclophosphamide subcutaneous group: Pregnant monkeys were administered via subcutaneous injection from GD24 to GD28 for 5 days. ③ Thalidomide gavage group: Pregnant monkeys were administered via gavage from GD24 to GD30 for 7 days.

(6) Body weight and food consumption: Weigh regularly and observe food consumption.

(7) Uterine necropsy of pregnant monkeys [4]: ① Take out the fetus and examine the fetal weight (including uterus), placenta weight, fetal survival, fetal sex, weight, crown-rump length, tail length and appearance, internal organs and bones. ② The fetal organs were fixed in 10% formalin solution and underwent examination on the internal organs. The fetus whose internal organs were removed was subjected to skeletal examination.

(8) Preparation of bone specimens: The crown–rump length and tail length were measured. After skin, fat, and gut removal, the fetal monkeys were put into 95% ethanol, and the bone specimens were further stained with Alzin blue and alizarin red dye for 2–7 days (depending on the color depth), and the transparent liquid I and transparent liquid II were applied for transparency for about 30 days (depending on the color depth).

(9) Observe the female monkeys: Whether the female monkeys had abnormal birth or lactation.

(10) Toxicokinetics: Blood concentration detection and the detection method established in the preliminary test in the laboratory. It was intended to use glutamic acid and phosphamide as the internal standard to establish the monkey TK detection method and conduct methodological verification.

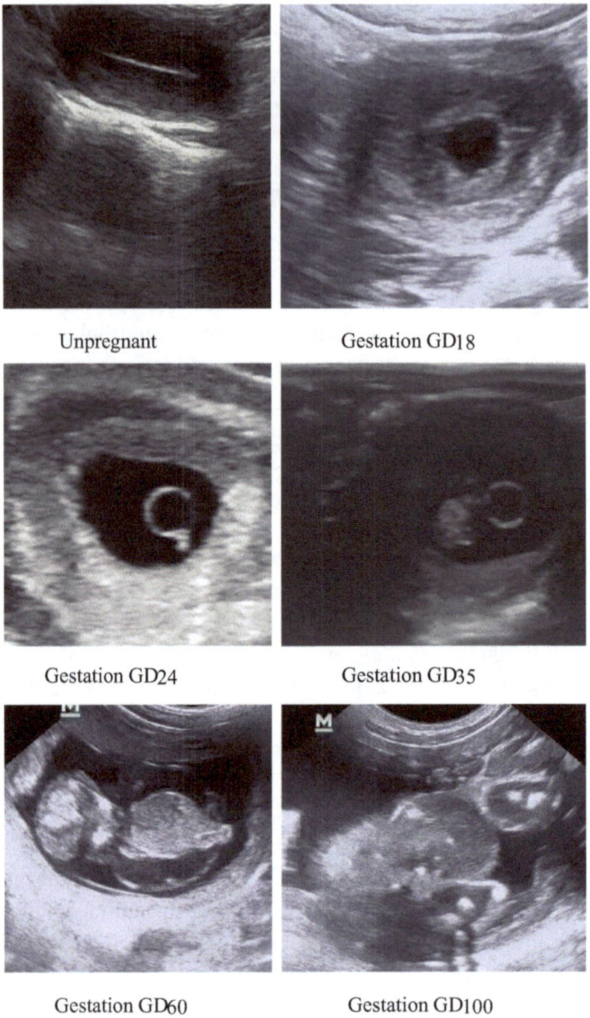

Fig. 8.2 Ultrasound results during gestation

1) Blood collection: TK blood samples of pregnant monkeys in the cyclophosphamide group and the thalidomide group were collected from the upper limb vein (cephalic vein), about 1.5 mL of blood was collected, and whole blood was collected into the collection vessel of EDTA-K_2. The specific collection time was shown in Tables 8.49 and 8.50.
2) Blood sample processing: About 1 mL blood was collected from the veins of the upper limbs, and the blood samples were collected using an anticoagulant tube containing heparin sodium, thoroughly mixed, left for 0.5–1 h, centrifuged at 3000 r/min at 4°C for 10 min, then the upper plasma was absorbed,

Table. 8.49 Toxicokinetic blood sampling time points

Day	Group	Time points[1]
GD_{24}	2, 3	Pre-dose, 0.5 h post-dose, 1, 2, 4, 8, and 24 h
GD_{28}/GD_{30}	2, 3	Pre-dose, 0.5 h post-dose, 1, 2, 4, 8, and 24 h

[1]The acceptable time range for each blood sampling point as shown in 8.50; TK blood sampling time starts after the end of dosing

Table. 8.50 Acceptable time ranges for blood sampling time point

Time point	Acceptable time range	Time point	Acceptable time range
0–2 h	Within ±1 min	4–8 h	Within ±2 min
24 h and above	Within ±30 min	–	–

divided and put into EP tubes, and frozen at −80°C to store the samples for testing.

8.3.9 Observation Indicators

(1) General condition observation: Observe the general condition of animals twice a day (once in the morning and once in the afternoon), record the appearance, behavior, or abnormal signs of animals; Cesarean section of found dead, or moribund animals was performed in time.
(2) Body weight and food consumption: After successful mating, the weight of pregnant monkeys was measured on GD_0, GD_{20}, GD_{28}, GD_{42}, GD_{56}, GD_{70}, GD_{84}, GD_{98}, GD_{112}, GD_{126}, GD_{140}, and GD_{154}. The feeding situation of pregnant monkeys was observed every morning (qualitative), that is, the animal diet was recorded daily, and the feed residue of less than one-third was acceptable, the feed residue of one-third to two-third was borderline, and the feed residue of more than two-third was poor.
(3) Hysterectomy: Cut the uterus of GD100 pregnant monkey from the neck of the uterus, take out the fetus, check the fetal weight (including uterus), placenta weight, fetal survival, fetal sex, weight, crown-rump length, tail length and appearance, internal organs, and bones.
(4) Examination of Fetal Malformations
    1) Appearance examination: Each fetus was inspected by the naked eye first, and if the naked eye could not determine a certain deformity, the fetus would be further examined under a stereo microscope.
    2) Head deformity examination: Whether there was hydrocephalus, open brain, cerebral hernia, meningocele, anophthalmia, microphthalmia, anotia, and cleft palate.

3) Deformity examination of limbs: Whether there was polydactyly, syndactyly, oligodactyly, strephenopodia, and brachydactylia.
4) Trunk deformity examination: Whether there was an umbilical hernia, gastroschisis, myelocele, spina bifida, and scoliosis.
5) Tail deformity examination: Whether there were short tails, curly tails, taillessness, and tail bifurcation.
6) Anal malformation examination: Whether there was anal atresia.
7) Bone deformity examination: The integrity of the skull and the degree of ossification; Whether there were sternal nodes missing, incomplete ossification, double ossification points, sternal node dislocation, multiple ribs, few ribs, rib bifurcation, rib fusion, and undulating ribs. Whether there were four limbs of bone ossification, stubbiness, deformity, polydactyly, and oligodactyly.
8) Examination for organ malformations: Whether there was cleft palate, abnormal tongue, enlarged nasal passage, single nasal passage, brain edema, and hydronephrosis; Whether the eyeballs were normal; Whether the size and position of the heart, liver, spleen, lungs, kidneys, and uterus were abnormal.

(5) Hormone testing: The levels of anti -mullerian hormone (AMH), FSH, LH, progesterone (P), E2, prolactin (PRL), testosterone (T), and DHT in pregnant monkeys were determined by ELISA. According to the testing instructions of the kit, absorbance (OD value) was measured at 450 nm wavelength by using the microplate reader, and the concentration of the hormone to be measured in the sample was calculated by the standard curve.

(6) Toxicokinetics
1) The blood concentrations of pregnant monkeys in the cyclophosphamide group and the thalidomide group were detected at each blood sampling point, and the amniotic fluid and placenta of pregnant monkeys at GD100 were detected in each group.
2) C_{max}, T_{max}, and AUC values of blood drug concentration; toxicokinetic data were described by descriptive statistics such as mean, standard deviation, and sample size.

(7) Evaluation Indicators of Young Monkeys
1) Observe general signs twice a day.
2) Measure the body weight of the animals once a week or once a month.
3) Appearance examinations were performed on the animals on PND_1, PND_{21}, PND_{58}, PND_{88}, and PND_{178}. Tibia length, head circumference, tail length, crown–rump length, and anogenital distance were measured.
4) Grip strength was evaluated on PND_1, PND_{14}, and PND_{28} after birth, and the ability of newborn monkeys to grasp the rope for at least 30 s was measured.
5) Neurobehavioral evaluation of newborn monkeys: Monkeys in each group were evaluated on PND_{100}, PND_{125}, PND_{150}, and PND_{178}, and the evaluation criteria were shown in Table 8.51.
6) Ophthalmic examination was performed on PND_{100}, PND_{150}, and PND_{178}, including macroscopic observation, ophthalmoscope examination (fundus) and slit lamp examination.

(8) Clinical pathology: On PND_7, PND_{30}, PND_{60}, PND_{120}, PND_{150}, and PND_{178}, the blood samples of each group were collected from the young monkeys after fasting for 12–18 h before collection. The blood samples were collected through the femoral vein/limb vein and placed in the transfer box/test tube rack at ambient temperature and sent to the clinical laboratory of the institution for processing and analysis at room temperature.

Table. 8.51 Operation methods and scoring criteria for behavioral and neurological function evaluation on newborn cynomolgus monkeys

Category	Item	Standard Score	Definition
Locomotion ability	Visual orient	1	Eyes orient toward an object held in four positions in an infant's periphery (0 = no contact; 1 = direct brief contact; 2 = direct prolonged contact)
	Visual follow	1	Eyes follow a moving object in both horizontal and vertical directions (0 = contact but no following; 1 = starts to follow then stops; 2 =complete follow).
	Duration of looking	1	Length of looks on visual orient and follow (0=no looking; 1 = brief looks; 2 = 1- to 2-s looks)
	Attention	1	Rating of attention on visual orienting items (0 = no attention; 1 = slight attention 25% of time; 2 = definite attention 75% of time).
	Reach and grasp	2	Attempts to grasp toy from orientation items (0 = no attempts to grasp; 1 = swat, no finger flexion; 2 = intentional grasp with finger flexion)
Status assessment	Irritability	1	Amount of distress during examination (0 = extreme, constant distress; 1 = slight, distress few times; 2 = none, no distress)
	Vocalizations	3–5 times	Number of "whoo" vocalizations during a 1-min period in which the infant is placed alone in an enclosed Plexiglas area, approximately
	Struggle during the test	2	Amount of squirming during examination (0 = little, 25% of time; 1 = moderate, when appropriate; 2 = difficult, continuous squirming)
	Consolability	2	Ease of consoling infant during examination (0 = cannot console, nothing works; 1 = consoles with difficulty, pick up, rock and talk; 2 = easy to console, pick up only)
	Soothability	1	Necessity and frequency of soothing infant during examination (0 = less than average, intervention seldom necessary; 1 = moderate, intervention often necessary; 2 = harder than average, continuous intervention necessary)
	Predominant state	0	State of infant during examination (0 = alert, awake, and aware; 1 = alert but somewhat agitated; 2 = extreme agitation, body jerks and screams)

Table 8.51 (Continued)

Category	Item	Standard Score	Definition
	Response intensity	0	Quality of vocal reactions during 1-min vocalizations test (0 = low, "laid back"; 1 = moderate; 2 = high distress, intense in expression)
	Motor activity	1	Observation of motor activity during 1-min vocalizations test (0 = slight, 25% of time moving; 1 = normal, 50% of time moving; 2 = excessive, in continuous movement)
	Coordination	2	Quality of movement rated (0 = poor, clumsy; 1 = adequate; 2 = excellent, agile)
Activity	Spontaneous crawl	2	Quality of crawl locomotion (0 = absent, no crawl; 1 = weak try, uncoordinated; 2 = coordinated crawl).
	Passive resistance	2	Degree of resistance to passive flexion and extension of limbs (0 = barely discernible resistance; 1 = moderate resistance; 2 = strong resistance)
	Balance	2	Infant is held in the sitting position and support is withdrawn (0 = infant falls; 1 = places arms out but falls; 2 = uses arms for support, no fall)

(Adapted from Laughlin NK, Lasky RE, Giles NL et al (1999) Lead effects on neurobehavioral development in the neonatal rhesus monkey (Macaca mulatta). Neurotoxicol Teratol 21(6):627–638)

The blood vessel of blood samples for hematology and coagulation tests was gently turned upside down several times after blood collection to ensure that the blood was fully mixed with the anticoagulant. Blood samples for blood biochemical/immune indicators and hemagglutination detection were centrifuged at room temperature for 10 min at 3500 r/min to obtain serum and plasma samples, respectively. Specific detection indicators are shown in Tables 8.52–8.54.

8.3.10 Statistical Analysis of Data

SPSS software was used for data entry and statistical analysis. The experimental data were expressed as Mean±SD. The mean weight, mean food consumption, mean number of live births, mean live birth weight, maternal weight gain, weight of young monkeys, physiological development indicators, reflection development indicators, and hormone levels were analyzed by one-way ANOVA using SPSS statistical software. Data such as live birth rate, stillbirth rate, monstra rate, and mating rate are expressed by percentages.

Table. 8.52 Hematology

Item	Unit	Method
White blood cell (WBC) count	$\times 10^9$/L	Flow cytometry
Differential leukocyte count (NEU#, LYM#, MONO#, EO#, BASO#)	$\times 10^9$/L	Flow cytometry
Differential leukocyte count percentage (NEU%, LYM%, MONO%, EO%, BASO%)	%	Flow cytometry
Red blood cell (RBC) count	$\times 10^{12}$/L	DC sheath flow detection method
Hemoglobin (HGB)	g/L	SLS hemoglobin detection method
Hematocrit (HCT)	%	RBC cumulative pulse height detection method
Mean corpuscular volume (MCV)	fL	Calculated from RBC and HCT
Mean corpuscular hemoglobin (MCH)	pg	Calculated from RBC and HGB
Mean corpuscular hemoglobin concentration (MCHC)	g/L	Calculated from HCT and HGB
Reticulocyte count (RET)	$\times 10^9$/L	Flow cytometry
Reticulocyte count percentage (RET%)	%	Flow cytometry
Platelet count (PLT)	$\times 10^9$/L	Scepter DC detection method

Table. 8.53 Hematological biochemistry and immunological indices

Item	Unit	Method
Alanine aminotransferase (ALT)	U/L	IFCC recommended method
Aspartate aminotransferase (AST)	U/L	IFCC recommended method
Alkaline phosphatase (ALP)	U/L	AMP as substrate IFCC optimized method
Urea (UREA)	mmol/L	Urease dynamic UV method
Creatinine (CREA)	μmol/L	Enzymatic method
Albumin (ALB)	g/L	Bromocresol green method
Total protein (TP)	g/L	Biuret method
Total bilirubin (TBIL)	μmol/L	Modified diazo method
Glucose (GLU)	mmol/L	Hexokinase method
Triglycerides (TRIG)	mmol/L	GPO-PAP method
Cholesterol (TCHO)	mmol/L	CHOD-PAP method
Gamma-glutamyl transferase (GGT)	U/L	IFCC enzymatic method
Creatine kinase (CK)	U/L	Enzymatic method
Lactate dehydrogenase (LDH)	U/L	Enzymatic method
Globulin (GLO)	g/L	Calculation
Albumin/globulin ratio (A/G)	N/A	Calculation
Sodium (Na+)	mmol/L	Ion-selective electrode method
Potassium (K+)	mmol/L	Ion-selective electrode method
Chloride (Cl-)	mmol/L	Ion-selective electrode method
Immunoglobulins (IgA, IgG, and IgM)	mg/dL	Immunoturbidimetry
Complement (C3 and C4)	mg/dL	Immunoturbidimetry
Circulating immune complexes (CIC)	μg/mL	ELISA method

Table. 8.54 Coagulation function

Item	Unit	Method
Prothrombin time (PT)	s	Coagulation method
Partial thromboplastin time (APTT)	s	Coagulation method
Fibrinogen (FIB)	g/L	Coagulation method

8.3.11 Conclusion

8.3.12 Mating of Female Monkeys

A total of 60 female monkeys were mated, and 47 pregnant animals were confirmed by B-ultrasound. There were 11 pregnant monkeys in the saline group, 20 in the cyclophosphamide group, and 16 in the thalidomide group. The success rate of mating was 78% (47/60).

8.3.13 Overall Situation of Pregnant Monkeys (Gestation Period GD_0–GD_{178})

(1) General Condition Observation
  1) Cyclophosphamide: During the whole gestation period, except for seven pregnant monkeys (7/20) who developed vaginal bleeding and/or abortion successively after the administration (GD_{32}–GD_{56}), there were no abnormalities observed in the appearance, physical signs, behavioral activities, animal posture, diet, hair, irritation response, glandular secretions, and respiration of other pregnant monkeys.
  2) Thalidomide: During the whole gestation period, except for three pregnant monkeys (3/16) who developed vaginal bleeding and/or abortion successively after the administration (GD_{41}–GD_{53}), there were no abnormalities observed in the appearance, physical signs, behavioral activities, animal posture, diet, hair, irritation response, glandular secretions, and respiration of other pregnant monkeys.
  3) Regarding abortion in pregnant monkeys during pregnancy: Two pregnant monkeys in the saline group (2/11) had abortions, seven pregnant monkeys in the cyclophosphamide group (7/20) had abortions, and three pregnant monkeys in the thalidomide group (3/16) had abortions, with abortion rates of 18% in saline, 35% in cyclophosphamide, and 19% in thalidomide (Table 8.55 and Figs. 8.3 and 8.4).

(2) Body weight and extrauterine weight gain
  1) Cyclophosphamide ① Body weight: During gestation ($GD_{0\text{–}156}$), compared with the saline group, the body weight of cyclophosphamide group decreased

Table. 8.55 Abortion conditions in pregnant monkeys during pregnancy (GD_{0-168})

Group		Animal number	Abortion rate (%)	Gestational day	Cause
Group 1 (saline group)	Embryonic–fetal development toxicity	1F06	18% (2/11)	GD_{37}	Vaginal hemorrhage (small amount), abortion, pregnant monkey survived
	Perinatal development toxicity	1F10		GD_{134}	Abortion, a pregnant monkey survived
Group 2 (cyclophosphamide group)	Embryonic–fetal development toxicity	2F03	35% (7/20)	GD_{32}	Vaginal hemorrhage (large amount), abortion, pregnant monkey survived
		2F07		GD_{34}	Abortion, a pregnant monkey survived
		2F09		GD_{47}	Abortion, a pregnant monkey survived
	Perinatal development toxicity	2F14		GD_{42}	Vaginal hemorrhage (large amount), abortion, pregnant monkey survived
		2F18		GD_{46}	Abortion, a pregnant monkey survived
		2F13		GD_{38}	Abortion, a pregnant monkey survived
		2F17		GD_{56}	Abortion, a pregnant monkey survived
Group 3 (thalidomide group)	Embryonic–fetal development toxicity	3F02	19% (3/16)	GD_{41}	Abortion, a pregnant monkey survived
	Perinatal development toxicity	3F13		GD_{47}	Vaginal hemorrhage (small amount), abortion, pregnant monkey survived
		3F16		GD_{53}	Abortion, a pregnant monkey survived

from GD_{44} to GD_{156}, with a statistical difference ($P \leq 0.05$). Therefore, it was considered that cyclophosphamide had an effect on the weight of pregnant monkeys during gestation (Table 8.56 and Fig. 8.5). ② Extrauterine weight gain: During gestation (GD_{0-100})), there was a statistically significant decrease in extrauterine weight gain in the cyclophosphamide group compared with the saline group ($P \leq 0.01$). The results showed that cyclophosphamide could decrease extrauterine weight gain in pregnant monkeys (Table 8.57 and Fig. 8.6).

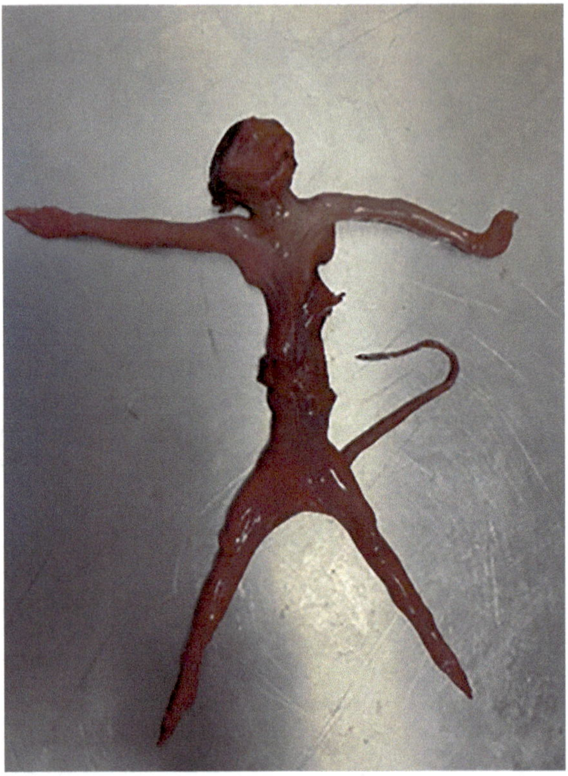

Fig. 8.3 Abortion of animal 1F14 in Group 1 (Saline Group) on GD_{134}

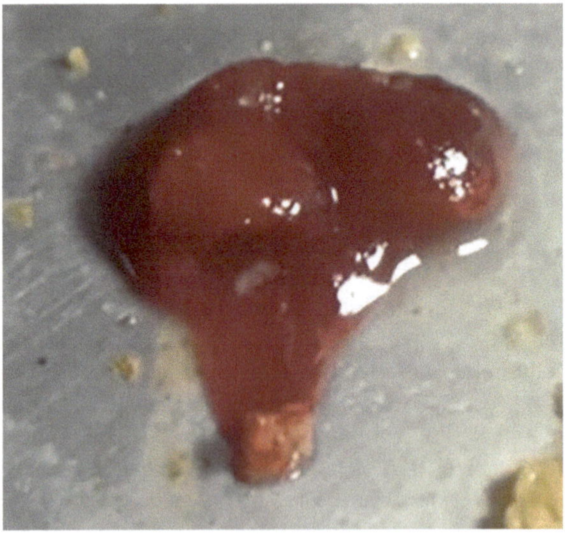

Fig. 8.4 Abortion of animal 2F07 in group 2 (cyclophosphamide group) on GD_{34}

Table. 8.56 Body weight of pregnant monkeys during pregnancy (kg, GD_{0-156})

Day	Group 1 (saline)	Group 2 (cyclophosphamide)	Group 3 (thalidomide)
Number of pregnant mo nkeys (n)	9	13	13
GD_0	3.08±0.26	3.13±0.25	3.00±0.35
GD_{20}	3.22±0.32	3.19±0.25	3.08±0.37
GD_{36}	3.29±0.29	3.24±0.25	3.13±0.35
GD_{44}	3.40±0.32	3.28±0.30*	3.36±0.40
GD_{52}	3.52±0.34	3.32±0.30*	3.46±0.34
GD_{60}	3.64±0.24	3.35±0.31*	3.52±0.35
GD_{68}	3.73±0.26	3.38±0.35*	3.61±0.37
GD_{76}	3.85±0.23	3.44±0.40*	3.67±0.35
GD_{84}	3.90±0.19	3.50±0.38*	3.89±0.36
GD_{100}	3.99±0.23	3.60±0.41*	3.86±0.37
GD_{132}[1]	3.98±0.13	3.40±0.39*	3.89±0.22
GD_{156}[1]	4.05±0.16	3.41±0.37*	3.93±0.18

[1]Only includes animals with perinatal developmental toxicity (Group 1: 3; Group 2: 6; Group 3: 6).
*Compared to the saline group, $P \leq 0.05$

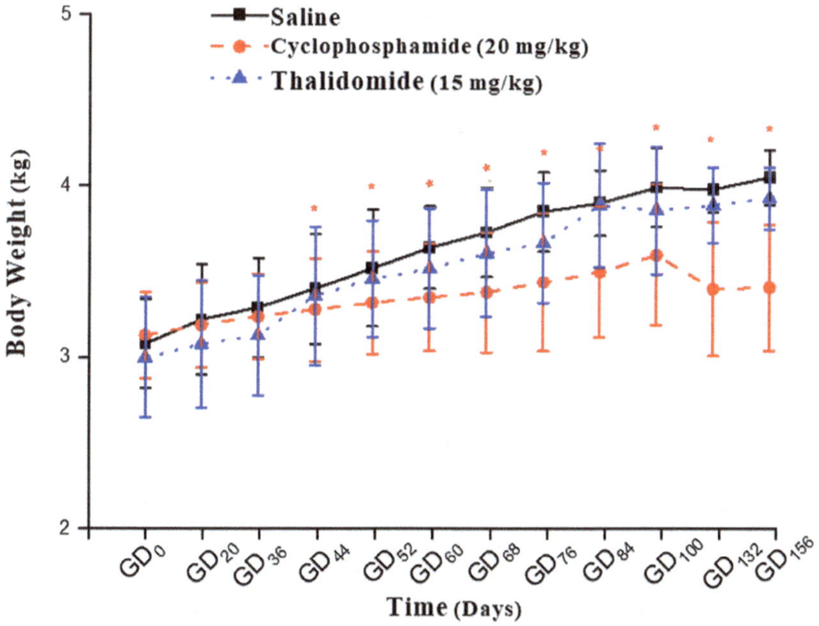

Fig. 8.5 Body weight of pregnant monkeys during pregnancy (GD_{0-156})

Table. 8.57 Extrauterine weight gain of pregnant monkeys during pregnancy (kg, GD_{0-100})

Day	Group 1 (saline)	Group 2 (cyclophosphamide)	Group 3 (thalidomide)
Number of pregnant m onkeys (*n*)	6	7	7
GD_0	3.08±0.26	3.13±0.25	3.00±0.35
GD_{100}	3.99±0.23	3.60±0.41	3.86±0.37
Extrauterine weight gain	0.54±0.17	0.28±0.29**	0.50±0.27

Note: Extrauterine weight gain calculation method: GD_{100}–GD_{20}–Uterus with fetus weight.
**Compared to the saline group, $P \leq 0.01$

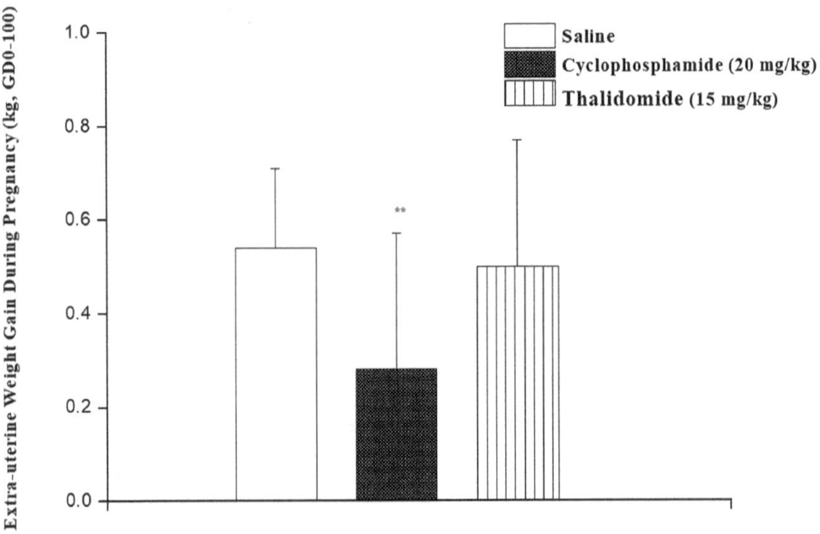

Fig. 8.6 Extrauterine weight gain during pregnancy (GD_{0-100})

2) Thalidomide: ① Body weight: During gestation (GD_{0-156}), compared with the saline group, there was no significant change in body weight in the thalidomide group with no statistical difference ($P > 0.05$). It was considered that thalidomide had no significant effect on the weight of pregnant monkeys (Table 8.56 and Fig. 8.5). ② Extrauterine weight gain: During gestation (GD_{0-100}), there was no significant change in extrauterine weight gain in the thalidomide group compared with the saline group ($P > 0.05$). It was considered that thalidomide had no significant effect on extrauterine weight gain in pregnant monkeys (Table 8.57 and Fig. 8.6).

(3) Assessment of food consumption: Throughout gestation (GD_{20}–GD_{178}), the animals in the saline, cyclophosphamide, and thalidomide groups were assessed

Table. 8.58 Pregnancy outcomes in each group (GD_{100})

Group	Number of pregnant monkeys (n)	Number of live fetus (n)	Live fetus rate (%)	Number of dead fetus (n)	Dead fetus rate (%)
Saline group	6	6	100	0	0
Cyclophosphamide group	7	6	86	1	14
Thalidomide group	7	7	100	0	0

as "acceptable" (less than one-third of the feed residue daily). No abnormality was observed in the food consumption assessment in all groups.

3. Pregnancy outcome (GD_{100}) On the 100th day of gestation (GD_{100}), the first half of pregnant monkeys in each group were necropsied, including six pregnant monkeys in the saline group, seven pregnant monkeys in the cyclophosphamide group, and seven pregnant monkeys in the thalidomide group (Table 8.58).

(1) In the saline group, there were six live births and zero stillbirths; the live birth rate was 100%, and the stillbirth rate was 0%.
(2) Cyclophosphamide group: There were six live births and one stillbirth, the live birth rate was 86%, the stillbirth rate was 14%.
(3) Thalidomide group: There were seven live births, zero stillbirths; the live birth rate was 100%, and the stillbirth rate was 0%.

8.3.14 Hysteroscopy (GD_{100})

(1) Fetal weight and physical development examination: The indicators are summarized in Tables 8.59 and 8.60.
   1) Cyclophosphamide: The fetal weight, chest circumference, tibia, and forearm length in cyclophosphamide group were lower than those in the saline group ($P \leq 0.05$).
   2) Thalidomide: Fetal body weight, chest circumference, tail length, tibia, and forearm length in thalidomide group were lower than those saline group ($P \leq 0.05$ or $P \leq 0.01$).
(2) Fetal organ weight: The summary of fetal organ weight is shown in Table 8.61.
   1) Cyclophosphamide: Compared with the saline group, the weight of major organs (heart, liver, spleen, lung, kidney, ovary, and testis) in the cyclophosphamide group had no significant changes ($P > 0.05$).
   2) Thalidomide: Compared with the normal saline group, the weight of major organs (heart, liver, spleen, lung, kidney, ovary, and testis) in the cyclophosphamide group had no significant changes ($P > 0.05$).

Table. 8.59 Fetal physical development indicators in cesarean section (GD_{100}, $\overline{X}$±SD)

Day		Group 1(saline)n=6	Group 2(cyclophosphamide)n=7	Group 3(thalidomide)n=7
Weight (g)		134.12±13.25	125.12±15.23*	119.95±9.23*
Crown–rump length (mm)		168±11	163±5	162±7
Chest circumference (mm)		123±23	112±14*	115±9*
Tail length (mm)		229±18	211±12	175±23*
Femur length (mm)		45±18	39±6*	13±2*
Forearm length (mm)		43±16	34±12	9±3*
Anogenital distance (mm)	Male[1]	23–33	19–31	23–37
	Female[1]	6–13	8–12	9–11

[1]Due to the number of animals in some groups being less than three, individual value ranges are used for statistics. *Compared to the saline group, * $P \le 0.05$; ** $P \le 0.01$

Table. 8.60 Fetal body weight and organ weights (GD_{100}, g, $\overline{X}$±SD)

Day	Group 1(saline)n=6	Group 2(cyclophosphamide)n=7	Group 3(thalidomide)n=7
Sex	3 F/3 M	3 F/4 M	3 F/4 M
Brain	15.831±32.15	14.461±52.15	15.231±24.15
Heart	0.72±0.11	0.56±0.25	0.67±0.41
Liver	4.03±0.88	4.21±1.49	3.93±0.67
Spleen	0.31±0.55	0.33±0.51	0.32±0.45
Lungs	3.25±0.77	2.86±1.20	3.01±0.34
Kidneys	0.82±0.64	0.73±0.41	0.75±0.42
Ovaries	0.027±0.027	0.023±0.017	0.022±0.005
Testes	0.029±0.057	0.024±0.061	0.026±0.035

Note: *F* female, *M* male

8.3.15 Deformity Examination (GD_{100})

(1) Appearance examination
   1) Cyclophosphamide: Three (3/7) of the fetuses had facial deformities (mouth and nose cleft), so it was considered that cyclophosphamide had an effect on the appearance of the fetuses (Fig. 8.7).
   2) Thalidomide: Five (5/7) of the fetuses had developmental deformities of the limbs (missing, undeveloped, or shortened front/rear limbs), so it was considered that thalidomide had an effect on the appearance of the fetus (Fig. 8.8).

Table. 8.61 Fetal skeletal examination results

Examination item	Saline group(Group 1)	Cyclophosphamide group(Group 2)	Thalidomide group(Group 3)
Number of fetuses examined	6	7	7
Osteogenesis imperfecta			
Parietal bone	0/6	2/7	0/7
Frontal bone	0/6	4/7	0/7
Occipital bone	0/6	1/7	0/7
Mandible	1/6	0/7	0/7
Sternum (manubrium)	0/6	1/7	0/7
2nd Sternum	1/6	2/7	1/7
5th Sternum	0/6	1/7	0/7
6th Sternum	0/6	3/7	1/7
Bilateral humerus	0/6	0/7	1/7
Bilateral ulna	0/6	0/7	1/7
Bilateral radius	0/6	0/7	1/7
Bilateral tarsal bones	0/6	0/7	1/7
Bilateral femur (hind limbs)	0/6	0/7	2/7
Bilateral femur (hind limbs)	0/6	0/7	1/7
Bilateral tibia	0/6	0/7	3/7
Bilateral fibula	0/6	0/7	4/7
Bilateral tarsal bones	0/6	0/7	5/7
Right hind limb femur	0/6	0/7	3/7
Right 2nd metatarsal	0/6	0/7	1/7
Right 1st phalanx (counting from left to right)	0/6	0/7	1/7
Tail vertebrae curvature/deformity			
Incomplete ossification and disordered arrangement of tail vertebrae 9–17	0/6	0/7	1/7
Curvature of tail vertebrae 10–14	0/6	0/7	2/7
Deformity of the shape of the tail vertebrae	0/6	0/7	1/7
Missing phalanges			
Left hind limb 4th phalanx missing (counting from left to right)	0/6	0/7	1/7

Examination item	Saline Group (Group 1)	Cyclophosphamide group (Group 2)	Thalidomide group (Group 3)
Right hind limb 2nd phalanx missing (counting from left to right)	0/6	1/7	1/7
Polydactyly (phalanges)			
Polydactyly (6 digits) in left and right hind limbs	0/6	3/7	0/7

Table 8.61 (Continued)

Ossification points			
3–4 Sternum	0/6	1/7	0/7
5–6 Sternum	0/6	6/7	2/7
7–9 Sternum	6/6	0/7	5/7
Ribs (short ribs)			
Left side 14th rib	0/6	2/7	4/7
Right side 12th rib	0/6	1/7	3/7
Ribs/costal cartilage (fusion)			
3rd and 4th Ribs (bilateral)	0/6	1/7	0/7
1st and 2nd Costal cartilage are fused at 1st sternum (bilateral)	0/6	1/7	0/7
1st and 2nd Costal cartilage are fused on left side at sternum (bilateral)	0/6	0/7	1/7
6th and 7th Ribs, right costal cartilage are fused	0/6	0/7	1/7
7th Costal cartilage not fused with sternum (bilateral)	0/6	0/7	1/7
8th Costal cartilage is fused with sternum (bilateral)	0/6	1/7	5/7
1st and 2nd Costal cartilage are fused at sternum (bilateral)	0/6	0/7	3/7
3rd and 4th Costal cartilage asymmetrical dislocation (bilateral)	0/6	1/7	0/7
1st, 2nd, 4th, and 5th Costal cartilage are fused (left side)	0/6	1/7	0/7
Bone fusion			
Fusion of 2nd and 3rd sacral vertebrae	0/6	1/7	0/7
Examination item	Saline Group (Group 1)	Cyclophosphamide group (Group 2)	Thalidomide group (Group 3)
Fusion of 2nd, 3rd, and 4th sacral vertebrae	0/6	2/7	1/7
Fusion of 1st and 2nd lumbar vertebrae, fusion of 5th and 6th lumbar vertebrae	0/6	1/7	0/7
Fusion of 7th lumbar vertebra and 1st, 2nd, 3rd sacral vertebrae	0/6	1/7	0/7
Fusion of 13th and 14th caudal vertebrae	0/6	3/7	3/7
Fusion of 11th and 12th caudal vertebrae	0/6	2/7	3/7
Fusion of 7th and 8th caudal vertebrae	0/6	3/7	2/7
Bone deficiency			
Radius	0/6	0/7	5/7
Metacarpal bones	0/6	0/7	5/7
Phalanges	0/6	0/7	5/7
Femur	0/6	0/7	5/7
Tibia	0/6	0/7	5/7
Long bone irregularities			
	0/6	0/7	3/7

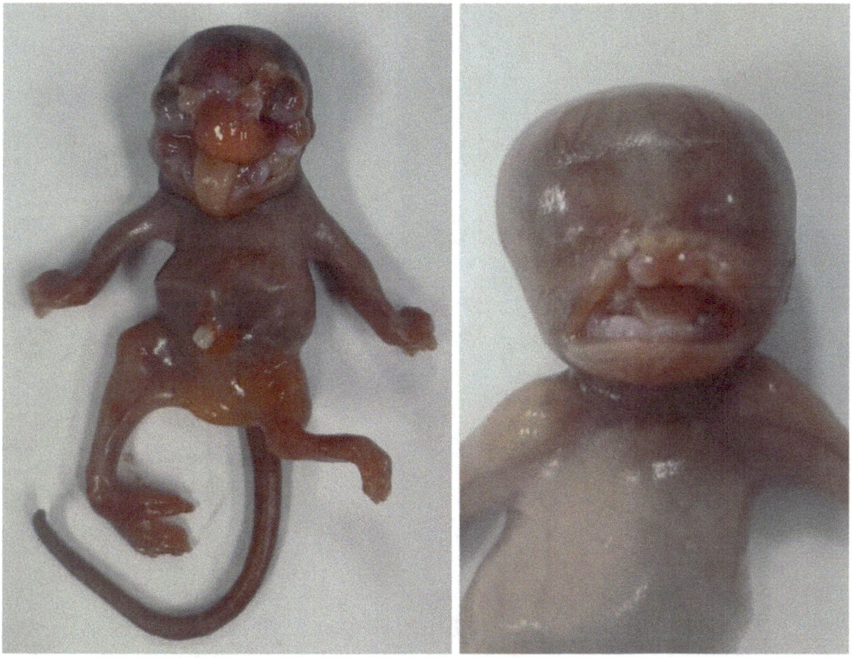

Fig. 8.7 Cesarean section examination—cyclophosphamide group (facial malformations)

(2) Bone examination: Bone examination was performed on 20 fetuses necropsied on GD_{100} (6 in the saline group, 7 in the cyclophosphamide group, and 7 in the thalidomide group). The specific examination results were shown in Table 8.61 and Fig. 8.9.
   1) Cyclophosphamide: Seven fetal bones were examined, among which ossification was not complete: Skull (four cases), sternum (three cases), and occipital bone (one case). The incidence of sternal ossification decreased (seven cases), rib (one case with short rib), phalanx (three cases with polydactyly), rib/costal cartilage (fusion, one case) and other bone malformations increased significantly.
   2) Thalidomide: Seven fetal bones were examined, mainly with an increased rate of skeletal deformity of limbs, including curvature/deformity of the tail vertebra (four cases), absence of radius, metacarpal, phalanges, femur, and tibia (five cases each), and irregular long bones (three cases).

(3) Visceral examination: A total of 20 fetuses were examined, of which 6 were negative, 7 in the cyclophosphamide group, and 7 in the thalidomide group. Compared with the saline group, there were no obvious abnormal changes in fetal viscera in each group.

6. Hormone tests include AMH, FSH, LH, progesterone (P), E_2, prolactin (PRL), testosterone (T), and DHT. The summary results of hormones are shown in Table 8.62.

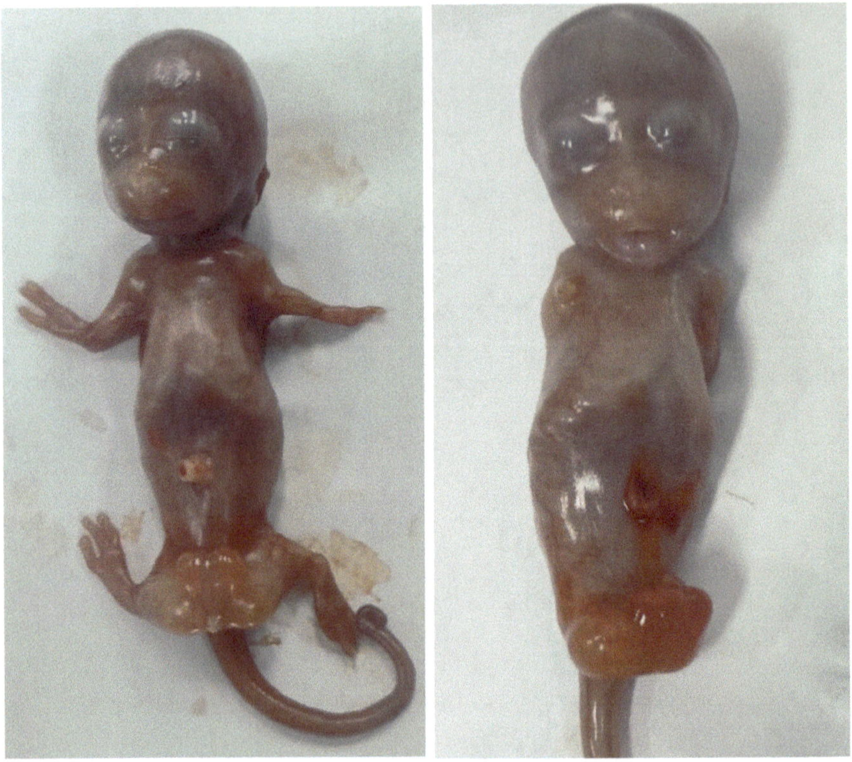

Fig. 8.8 Cesarean section examination—thalidomide group (limb malformations)

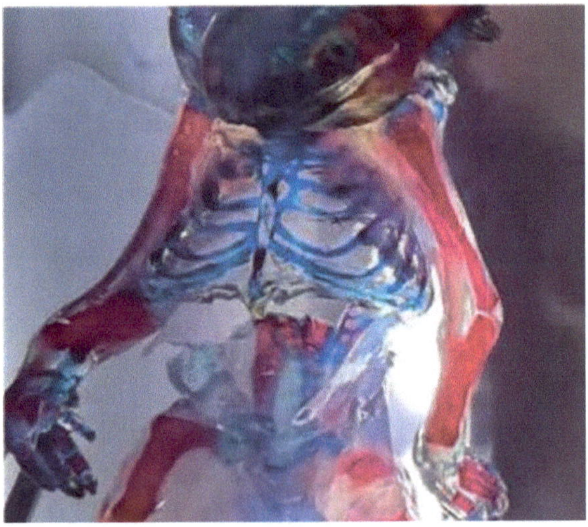

Fig. 8.9 Rib skeletal anomalies induced by cyclophosphamide (disorder, fusion, dislocation, and abnormal shape)

Table. 8.62 Hormone levels in pregnant monkeys during pregnancy

Test indicator	Time	Sodium chloride group	Cyclophosphamide group	Thalidomide group
Animal number (n)	-	9	13	13
AMH (pg/mL)	GD_{0}	1589.861±412.373	2381.674±399.142	1625.401±318.028
	GD_{20}	1581.783±609.309	1983.567±431.762	1521.829±312.772
	GD_{50}	1463.788±419.458	2071.674±399.142	1581.829±312.772
	GD_{100}	1440.453±267.690	1878.786±392.645	1484.657±285.332
	GD_{150}[a]	1317.574±278.949	1778.786±392.645	1284.657±285.332
FSH (IU/L)	GD_{0}	11.537±1.615	12.015±1.616	10.015±1.575
	GD_{20}	9.71±3.570	9.364±1.957	8.061±2.619
	GD_{50}	6.687±1.156	6.293±2.036	7.714±4.916
GD_{150}[a]	3.615±1.489	5.118±3.840	3.840±2.587	
LH (ng/L)	GD_{0}	50.764±8.940	42.827±17.594	32.298±12.617
	GD_{20}	65.173±10.361	53.278±18.566	45.583±8.360
	GD_{50}	100.768±8.615	80.962±17.231	75.973±13.878
	GD_{100}	42.827±17.594	61.741±30.424	65.173±10.361
	GD_{150}[a]	32.298±12.617	49.852±32.398	33.165±14.982
Progesterone (pmol/L)	GD_{0}	723.535±81.757	753.463±209.504	886.502±108.500
	GD_{20}	999.270±169.628	831.164±202.831	1000.808±218.226
	GD_{50}	965.605±128.170	902.347±187.088	1271.255±146.228
	GD_{100}	1199.980±144.003	1283.420±202.146	1157.874±106.506
	GD_{150}[a]	1330.390±112.016	1271.074±228.208	1240.817±90.398
E_2 (ng/L)	GD_{0}	84.596±22.946	78.607±23.267	66.955±16.334
	GD_{20}	250.330±10.011	198.387±23.048	234.450±18.421
	GD_{50}	380.221±8.059	345.785±22.459	367.104±31.799
	GD_{100}	328.522±22.522	367.413±13.260	323.128±16.030
	GD_{150}[a]	299.031±10.265	310.201±25.440	303.501±24.021
PRL (ng/L)	GD_{0}	923.542±131.997	926.677±179.270	802.476±73.432
	GD_{20}	897.998±329.205	716.127±250.579	794.755±97.784
	GD_{50}	778.601±165.581	922.934±159.411	685.409±100.316
	GD_{100}	1398.984±281.239	1447.939±320.725	1365.005±92.714
	GD_{150}[a]	1494.102±190.857	1542.076±150.759	1412.521±87.462
Testosterone (nmol/L)	GD_{0}	20.905±1.396	17.421±5.304	23.911±7.846
	GD_{20}	19.083±3.824	19.723±4.762	26.146±2.903
	GD_{50}	24.054±4.236	23.286±2.853	23.277±5.971
	GD_{100}	10.152±9.789	15.823±6.382	14.199±7.165
	GD_{150}[a]	14.573±11.637	16.490±12.195	11.914±9.651
HDT (nmol/L)	GD_{0}	8.743±0.421	7.879±0.977	6.861±0.704
	GD_{20}	8.385±4.419	7.890±0.986	6.546±1.154
	GD_{50}	7.487±3.439	7.815±1.087	6.729±0.921
	GD_{100}	8.272±0.783	7.901±0.643	6.867±0.565
	GD_{150}[a]	8.089±3.267	7.698±4.272	6.221±3.103

(1) AMH: From GD_0 to GD_{150}, AMH levels in the normal saline group, cyclophosphamide group, and thalidomide group showed a slow decreasing trend. The change trend and amplitude of the cyclophosphamide group and the thalidomide group were basically the same as that of the saline group.
(2) FSH: From GD_0 to GD_{150}, the levels of FSH in the normal saline group, cyclophosphamide group, and thalidomide group showed a slow decrease trend. The change trend and amplitude of the cyclophosphamide group and the thalidomide group were basically the same as that of the saline group.
(3) LH: From GD_0 to GD_{50}, LH hormone levels in the saline group, cyclophosphamide group, and thalidomide group showed an overall increasing trend and a decreasing trend from GD_{50} to GD_{150}. The overall change law showed an increasing trend in the first trimester and a decreasing trend in the later trimester. The change trend and amplitude of the cyclophosphamide group and the thalidomide group were basically the same as that of the saline group.
(4) Progesterone: From GD_0 to $GD1_{50}$, the hormone levels of progesterone in the saline group, cyclophosphamide group, and thalidomide group showed an overall increasing trend and increased slowly from GD_0 to GD_{50}, and obviously from GD_{100} to GD_{150}. The change trend and amplitude of the cyclophosphamide group and the thalidomide group were basically the same as that of the saline group.
(5) E_2: From GD_0 to GD_{150}, estradiol levels in the saline group, cyclophosphamide group, and thalidomide group showed an overall increasing trend. The increasing trend was obvious from GD_0 to $GD5_0$, and the increasing trend slowed down from GD_{100} to GD_{150}, but the overall level was higher than GD_0. The change trend and amplitude of the cyclophosphamide group and the thalidomide group were basically the same as that of the saline group.
(6) PRL: From GD0 to GD150, the levels of prolactin in the normal saline group, the cyclophosphamide group, and the thalidomide group showed an overall increasing trend. The increasing trend was obvious from GD_0 to GD_{50}, and the increasing trend slowed down from GD_{100} to GD_{150}, but the overall level was higher than GD_0. The change trend and amplitude of the cyclophosphamide group and the thalidomide group were basically the same as that of the saline group.
(7) Testosterone: From GD_0 to GD_{150}, the levels of testosterone in the saline group, cyclophosphamide group, and thalidomide group were stable at first and then decreased slightly. The levels of testosterone in all groups showed a slight downward trend from GD_{100} to GD_{150}. The change trend and amplitude of the cyclophosphamide group and the thalidomide group were basically the same as that of the saline group.
(8) DHT: From GD_0 to GD_{150}, there was no significant change in DHT levels in the saline group, cyclophosphamide group, and thalidomide group. Compared with the saline group, the change trend and amplitude of DHT in the cyclophosphamide group and the thalidomide group were basically the same as those of the saline group.

8.3.16 Toxicokinetics

(1) Analysis batch

1) Cyclophosphamide: There were five analysis batches, four sample analysis batches, and one ISR analysis batch in TK plasma sample detection. Five analysis batches met the requirements.

2) Thalidomide: There were a total of three analysis batches, two sample analysis batches, one ISR analysis batch in TK plasma sample detection, and three analysis batches met the requirements.

(2) Standard curve

1) Cyclophosphamide: The standard curve quantification range was 10.00–10,000.00 ng/mL, a total of 8 concentrations. The accuracy deviation of cyclophosphamide standard curve back-calculated concentration ranged from −9.84% to 10.06%, and the linear coefficient of standard curve of each analysis batch was $R^2 \geq 0.9928$ (Table 8.63).

2) Thalidomide: The quantitative range of the standard curve was 50.00–10,000.00 ng/mL, with a total of 8 concentrations. The accuracy deviation of thalidomide standard curve back-calculated concentration ranged from − 9.68% to 9.21%, and the linear coefficient R^2 of standard curve of each analysis batch was ≥0.9950 (Table 8.64).

(3) Quality Control Sample

1) Cyclophosphamide: The concentrations of low, medium, and high quality control samples were 30, 800, and 8000 ng/mL, respectively. The accuracy of three quality control samples with different concentrations ranged from −8.72% to 14.77% (Table 8.65).

2) Thalidomide: The concentrations of low, medium and high quality control samples were 150 ng/mL, 1200 ng/mL and 8000 ng/mL, respectively. The accuracy of three quality control samples with different concentrations ranged from −7.03% to 14.27% (Table 8.66).

(4) TK results (Table 8.67)

1) Cyclophosphamide: ① After the first dose (GD_{24}), the peak time of blood concentration of cynomolgus monkeys was 0.5 h. The C_{max} was (5160.91 ± 960.02) ng/mL and AUC_{0-t} was (6167.46 ± 1161.82)h ng/mL, respectively. (2) After the fifth dose (GD_{28}), the peak time of blood concentration of cynomolgus monkeys was 0–0.5 h. The C_{max} was (4822.83 ± 1837.59) ng/mL and AUC_{0-t} was (6065.23 ± 2307.81) h ng/mL, respectively.

2) Thalidomide: ① After the first dose (GD_{24}), the peak time of blood concentration of cynomolgus monkeys was 4–24 h. The C_{max} was (1231.86 ± 389.07) ng/mL, and AUC_{0-t} was (19601.53 ± 7243.93) h·ng/mL, respectively. ② After the seventh dose (GD_{30}), the peak time of blood concentration in the thalidomide group was 2–24 h. The C_{max} was (2277.09 ± 826.98) ng/mL, and AUC_{0-t} was (37949.53 ± 13612.97) h ng/mL, respectively.

Table. 8.63 Cyclophosphamide standard curve results

Analysis batch	Standard curve concentration (ng/mL)									Slope	Intercept	R^2
	Nominal concentration	C8 (10. 00)	C7 (20. 00)	C6 (100. 00)	C5 (500. 00)	C4 (1 500. 00)	C3 (5 000. 00)	C2 (9 000. 00)	C1 (10 000. 00)			
SA-Batch001	Actual concentration	9.65	21.32	99.95	547.58	1 405.44	5 502.94	8 114.54	9 345.56	0.001 930	−0.001 940	0.992 8
	Accuracy (%)	96.55	106.62	99.95	109.52	93.70	110.06	90.16	93.46			
	RE%	−3.45	6.62	−0.05	9.52	−6.30	10.06	−9.84	−6.54			
SA-Batch002	Actual concentration	9.72	10 064.90	101.25	517.54	5 299.08	21.07	1 387.16	8 424.04	0.001 9	−0.000 664	0.996 8
	Accuracy (%)	97.16	100.65	101.25	103.51	105.98	105.37	92.48	93.60			
	RE%	−2.84	0.65	1.25	3.51	5.98	5.37	−7.52	−6.40			
ISR-Batch001-r2-Reinjection-1	Actual concentration	9.85	10 074.13	97.67	527.18	5 340.64	20.67	1 400.38	8 473.56	0.001 85	0.000 164	0.997 0
	Accuracy (%)	98.49	100.74	97.67	105.44	106.81	103.34	93.36	94.15			
	RE%	−1.51	0.74	−2.33	5.44	6.81	3.34	−6.64	−5.85			
SA-Batch004	Actual concentration	10.1	19.5	100.98	542.87	1 536.36	4 933.47	8 497.82	9 645.13	0.003 71	0.000 749	0.997 8
	Accuracy (%)	100.97	97.51	100.98	108.57	102.42	98.67	94.42	96.45			
	RE%	0.97	−2.49	0.98	8.57	2.42	−1.33	−5.58	−3.55			
SA-Batch005	Actual concentration	10.08	19.75	97.12	526.61	1 510.41	5 161.06	8 584.41	9 872.35	0.003 34	0.001 73	0.998 8
	Accuracy (%)	100.81	98.73	97.12	105.32	100.69	103.22	95.38	98.72			
	RE%	0.81	−1.27	−2.88	5.32	0.69	3.22	−4.62	−1.28			
SA-Batch006	Actual concentration	9.91	20.51	95.18	530.66	1 488.33	5 036.97	8 844.78	9 881.88	0.0032 2	−0.002 04	0.998 8
	Accuracy (%)	99.1	102.53	95.18	106.13	99.22	100.74	98.28	98.82			
	RE%	−0.90	2.53	−4.82	6.13	−0.78	0.74	−1.72	−1.18			
ISR-Batch002	Actual concentration	9.91	20.43	96.97	524.16	1 442.14	5 241.63	8 770.58	9 846.2	0.003 2	−0.001 02	0.998 6
	Accuracy (%)	99.14	102.16	96.97	104.83	96.14	104.83	97.45	98.46			
	RE%	−0.86	2.16	−3.03	4.83	−3.86	4.83	−2.55	−1.54			

Table. 8.64 Thalidomide standard curve results

Analysis batch name	Standard curve concentration (ng/mL)									Slope	Intercept	R^2
	Nominal concentration	C8 (50.00)	C7 (100.00)	C6 (400.00)	C5 (1 000.00)	C4 (3 000.00)	C3 (6 000.00)	C2 (9 000.00)	C1 (1 0000.00)			
SA-Batch001-r1	Actual concentration	48.27	106.41	418.73	956.46	2 856.46	5 419.40	9 350.73	10 729.78	0.001 100	−0.009 430	0.995 2
	Accuracy (%)	96.53	106.41	104.68	95.65	95.22	90.32	103.90	107.30			
	RE%	−3.47	6.41	4.68	−4.35	−4.78	−9.68	3.90	7.30			
SA-Batch002-r2	Actual concentration	50.93	96.25	404.75	977.88	2 953.91	5 497.19	9 590.62	10 626.29	0.001 0	0.008 580	0.996 8
	Accuracy (%)	101.86	96.25	101.19	97.79	98.46	91.62	106.56	106.26			
	RE%	1.86	−3.75	1.19	−2.21	−1.54	−8.38	6.56	6.26			
ISR-Batch001-r1	Actual concentration	52.21	92.75	366.33	1 038.62	3 081.36	6 020.86	8 959.37	10 478.46	0.001 16	−0.003 530	0.996 6
	Accuracy (%)	104.41	92.75	91.58	103.86	102.71	100.34	99.55	104.78			
	RE%	4.41	−7.25	−8.42	3.86	2.71	0.34	−0.45	4.78			
SA-Batch004	Actual concentration	47.87	107.19	411.79	1 092.15	2847.77	5 504.01	9 275.37	9 519.21	0.001 21	0.007 48	0.995 0
	Accuracy (%)	95.74	107.19	102.95	109.21	94.93	91.73	103.06	95.19			
	RE%	−4.26	7.19	2.95	9.21	−5.07	−8.27	3.06	−4.81			
ISR-Batch002	Actual concentration	48.13	105.68	432.22	982.67	3 091.34	6 005.09	8 234.62	9 712.46	0.001 57	0.011 2	0.996 4
	Accuracy (%)	96.25	105.68	108.05	98.27	103.04	100.08	91.5	97.12			
	RE%	−3.75	5.68	8.05	−1.73	3.04	0.08	−8.50	−2.88			

Table. 8.65 Cyclophosphamide quality control sample results

Analysis batch	Quality control sample concentration (ng/mL)						
	Nominal concentration	LQC (30. 00)		MQC (800. 00)		HQC (8000. 00)	
SA-Batch001	Actual concentration	32.54	34.43	772.75	853.33	8 591.26	8 631.07
	Accuracy (%)	108.46	114.77	96.59	106.67	107.39	107.89
	RE%	8.46	14.77	−3.41	6.67	7.39	7.89
SA-Batch002	Actual concentration	35.08	34.09	778.86	730.25	8 178.48	8264.88
	Accuracy (%)	*116.92*	113.62	97.36	91.28	102.23	103.31
	RE%	*16.92*	13.62	−2.64	−8.72	2.23	3.31
RE%	11.88	*17.66*	3.72	−1.96	5.70	3.68	
SA-Batch004	Actual concentration	31.63	30.22	833.75	813.14	7968.17	7731.53
	Accuracy (%)	105.44	100.74	104.22	101.64	99.6	96.64
	RE%	5.44	0.74	4.22	1.64	−0.40	−3.36
SA-Batch005	Actual concentration	31.5	28.36	868.73	802.25	8164.33	7625.21
	Accuracy (%)	105.01	94.54	108.59	100.28	102.05	95.32
	RE%	5.01	−5.46	8.59	0.28	2.05	−4.68
SA-Batch006	Actual concentration	30.95	30.75	844.64	820.74	7 965.45	7 888.29
	Accuracy (%)	103.16	102.51	105.58	102.59	99.57	98.6
	RE%	3.16	2.51	5.58	2.59	−0.43	−1.40
ISR-Batch002	Actual concentration	30.5	30.37	875.27	783.48	8385.36	7566.44
	Accuracy (%)	101.68	101.23	109.41	97.94	104.82	94.58
	RE%	1.68	1.23	9.41	−2.06	4.82	−5.42

Note: "Bold type" indicates not within the acceptable standard range.

3) Tissue samples (amniotic fluid, placenta): ① Cyclophosphamide: The concentration of the drug in amniotic fluid and placenta in all animals was lower than the LLOQ concentration (Table 8.68). ② Thalidomide: The concentration of the drug in amniotic fluid and placenta in all animals was lower than the LLOQ concentration (Table 8.69).

8.3.17 Evaluation of Young Monkeys (Perinatal Developmental Toxicity)

(1) Appearance morphological examination of young monkeys: The other half of pregnant monkeys in each group gave birth from GD_{160} to GD_{178}. A total of 15 live monkeys were born, including 3 in the saline group, 6 in the cyclophosphamide group, and 6 in the thalidomide group. No fetus was found dead.
   1) No abnormality was found in the appearance of all animals in the saline group.

Table. 8.66 Thalidomide quality control sample results

Analysis batch	Quality control sample concentration (ng/mL)						
	Nominal concentration	LQC (150.00)		MQC (1200.00)		HQC6 (8000.00)	
SA-Batch001-r1	Actual concentration	156.22	147.10	1226.14	1 133.81	9 141.45	9 951.93
	Accuracy (%)	104.15	98.06	102.18	94.48	114.27	*124.40*
	RE%	4.15	−1.94	2.18	−5.52	14.27	*24.40*
SA-Batch002-r2	Actual concentration	151.02	141.40	1 191.58	1 145.92	8 597.44	9 715.82
	Accuracy (%)	100.68	94.27	99.30	95.49	107.47	*121.45*
	RE%	0.68	−5.73	−0.70	−4.51	7.47	*21.45*
ISR-Batch001-r1	Actual concentration	155.03	158.90	1141.26	1119.18	8491.30	8469.47
	Accuracy (%)	103.35	105.93	95.10	93.27	106.14	105.87
	RE%	3.35	5.93	−4.90	−6.73	6.14	5.87
SA-Batch004	Actual concentration	150.24	144.99	1123.69	1121.65	8341.29	8164.78
	Accuracy (%)	100.16	96.66	93.64	93.47	104.27	102.06
	RE%	0.16	−3.34	−6.36	−6.53	4.27	2.06
ISR-Batch002	Actual concentration	140.47	164.08	1115.66	1301.41	8655.31	9352.84
	Accuracy (%)	93.64	109.39	92.97	108.45	108.19	116.91
	RE%	−6.36	9.39	−7.03	8.45	8.19	16.91

Note: "Bold type" indicates not within the acceptable standard range

Table. 8.67 Toxicokinetic parameters of each group

Days of administration	TK parameters (units)	Cyclophosphamide (Group 2)	Thalidomid (Group 3)
	Number of animals	n=13	n=13
GD_{24}	T_{max} (h)	0.5	4–24
	C_{max} (ng/mL)	5 160.91± 960.02	1 231.86± 389.07
	$AUC_{0-24\,h}$ (h*ng/mL)	6 167.46± 1 161.82	19 601.53± 7 243.93
GD_{28}/ GD_{30}	T_{max} (h)	0–0.5	2–24
	C_{max} (ng/mL)	4 822.83± 1 837.59	2 277.09± 826.98
	$AUC_{0-24\,h}$ (h*ng/mL)	6 065.23± 2 307.81	37 949.53± 13 612.97

Note: The last administration day for Group 2 is GD_{28}, and for Group 3 is GD_{30}

Table. 8.68 Concentration of cyclophosphamide in cynomolgus monkeys tissues (ng/mL)

Animal number	Amniotic fluid	Placenta	Within placenta	Edge of placenta
2F01	BLQ	BLQ	BLQ	BLQ
2F02	BLQ	BLQ	BLQ	BLQ
2F03	BLQ	BLQ	BLQ	BLQ
2F04	BLQ	BLQ	BLQ	BLQ
2F05	BLQ	BLQ	BLQ	BLQ
2F06	BLQ	BLQ	BLQ	BLQ
2F07	BLQ	BLQ	BLQ	BLQ

Note: "BLQ" indicates below the lower limit of quantification

Table. 8.69 Concentration of thalidomide in cynomolgus monkeys tissues (ng/mL)

Animal number	Amniotic fluid	Placenta	Within placenta	Edge of placenta
3F01	BLQ	BLQ	BLQ	BLQ
3F02	BLQ	BLQ	BLQ	BLQ
3F03	BLQ	BLQ	BLQ	BLQ
3F04	BLQ	BLQ	BLQ	BLQ
3F05	BLQ	BLQ	BLQ	BLQ
3F06	BLQ	BLQ	BLQ	BLQ
3F07	BLQ	BLQ	BLQ	BLQ

Note: "BLQ" indicates below the lower limit of quantification

2) Cyclophosphamide: Three (3/6) of the fetuses had facial deformities (mouth cleft, nose cleft), 1 (1/6) of the fetus had syndactyly and short toes of hind limbs, and 1 (1/6) of the fetus had naturally closed external ear canal (Figs. 8.10–8.12).

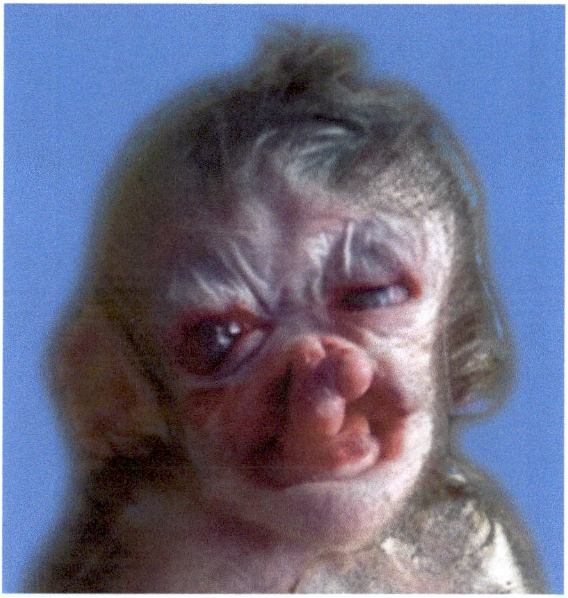

Fig. 8.10 Facial malformations (cleft lip, cleft palate) of the animal in cyclophosphamide group after birth

3) Thalidomide: Five (5/6) of the fetuses had dysplasia of the limbs (missing, undeveloped, or shortened front/rear limbs) (Fig. 8.13).

(2) Body weight: The body weight data of the young monkeys in each group are shown in Table 8.70 and Fig. 8.14.

1) Cyclophosphamide: The fetal monkeys in the cyclophosphamide group began to gain weight slowly from PND_0 and continued to PND_{182} after lactating; Compared with the saline group, the weight of the fetus decreased from PND_{28} to PND_{182}, and there was statistical difference ($P \leq 0.05$ or $P \leq 0.01$). ($P \leq 0.05$ or $P \leq 0.01$).

2) Thalidomide: The fetal monkeys in the cyclophosphamide group began to gain weight slowly from PND_{84} and continued to PND_{182} after lactating. Compared with the saline group, the weight of the fetus decreased from PND_{133} to PND_{182}, and there was a statistical difference ($P \leq 0.05$).

(3) Physical development: The physical development data of the young monkeys in each group are summarized in Table 8.71 and Figs. 8.15–8.18.

1) In the cyclophosphamide group: Compared with saline group, tibia length, head circumference, tail length and crown-rump length at PND_1, PND_{21}, PND_{58}, PND_{88} and PND_{178} showed a decreasing trend, and there was a statistical difference in above changes ($P \leq 0.01$).

2) In the thalidomide group: Compared with the saline group, tibia length and tail length at PND_1, PND_{21}, PND_{58}, PND_{88}, and PND_{178} showed a decreasing trend, and there was a statistical difference in the above changes ($P \leq 0.05$).

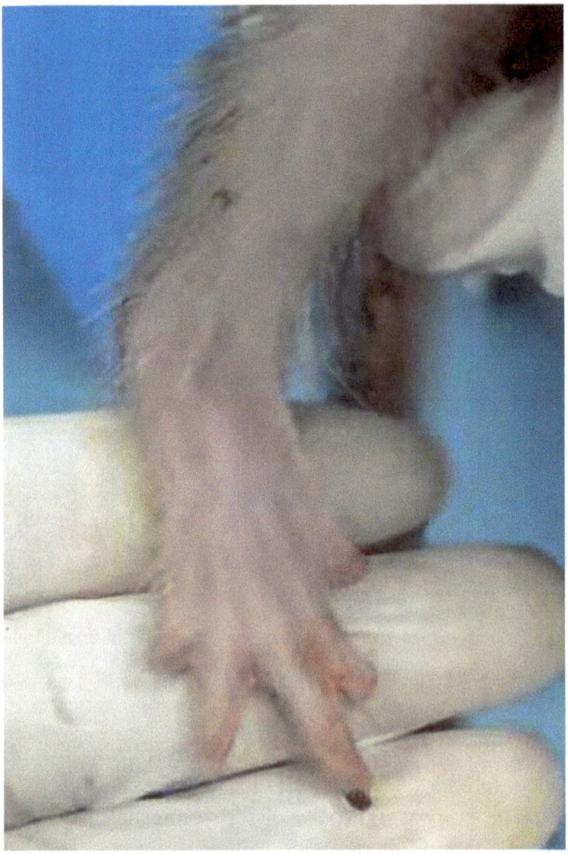

Fig. 8.11 Toe malformations (syndactyly, short toes) of the animal in cyclophosphamide group after birth

(4) Grip strength test: The time of holding the rope of the young monkeys was tested, and the retention of 30 s was qualified. The summary results of grip strength of each group were shown in Table 8.72.
   1) Cyclophosphamide group: Compared with the saline group, there was no significant difference in the gripping strength test of the cyclophosphamide group at PND_1, PND_{14}, and PND_{28}, and all the monkeys could hold for 30 s.
   2) Thalidomide group: Compared with the saline group, the grasping time of young monkeys in the thalidomide group decreased at PND_1, PND_{14}, and PND_{28}, and there was a statistical difference ($P \leq 0.05$ or $P \leq 0.01$).
(5) Behavioral and neurological function evaluation: The neurobehavioral evaluation results of animals in each group are shown in Tables 8.73–8.76.
   1) Cyclophosphamide group: Compared with the saline group, six/six young monkeys (four females and two males) in the cyclophosphamide group failed the animal coordination and balance scores at PND_{100}, PND_{125}, and

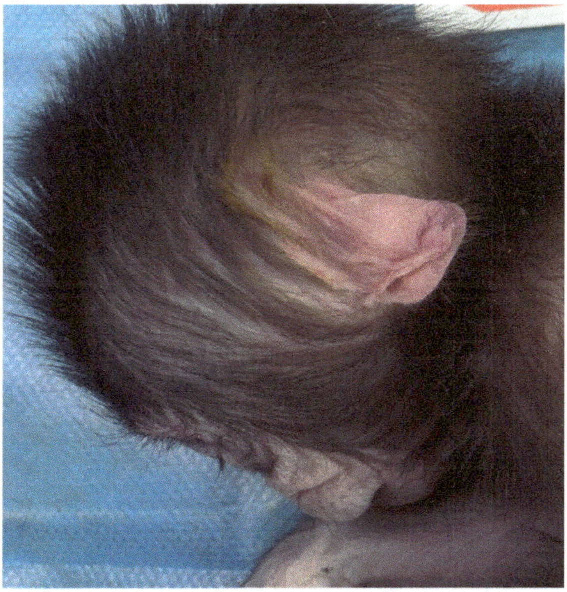

Fig. 8.12 Natural closure of external auditory canal of the animal in cyclophosphamide group after birth

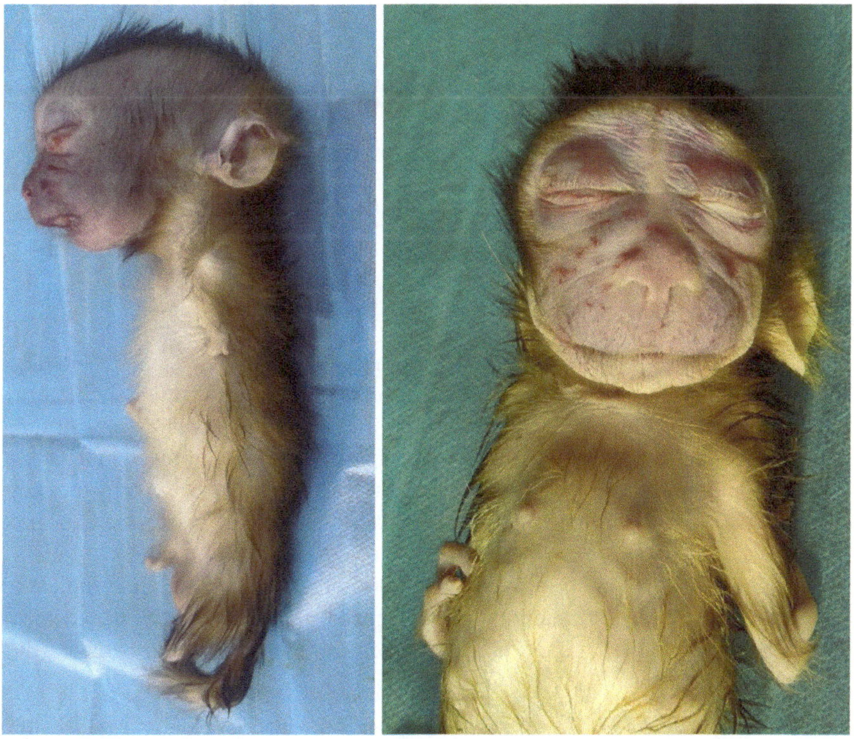

Fig. 8.13 Limb development malformations of the animal in thalidomide group after birth

Table 8.70 Changes in infant monkey weight (kg, $\overline{X}\pm$SD, PND_{0-182})

Day	Group 1 (saline)	Group 2 (cyclophosphamide)	Group 3 (thalidomide)
Number of pregnant monkeys	3	6	6
PND_0	0.39±0.02	0.24±0.05	0.34±0.05
PND_7	0.40±0.02	0.26±0.06	0.36±0.08
PND_{14}	0.39±0.06	0.30±0.07	0.38±0.06
PND_{28}	0.44±0.06	0.34±0.07*	0.42±0.07
PND_{35}	0.42±0.04	0.35±0.06*	0.44±0.07
PND_{42}	0.49±0.06	0.37±0.05*	0.46±0.06
PND_{49}	0.53±0.05	0.39±0.05*	0.49±0.08
PND_{56}	0.54±0.04	0.40±0.05*	0.51±0.09
PND_{63}	0.55±0.02	0.43±0.06*	0.52±0.09
PND_{70}	0.58±0.03	0.44±0.07*	0.55±0.09
PND_{77}	0.61±0.02	0.44±0.06*	0.57±0.09
PND_{84}	0.64±0.03	0.47±0.08*	0.58±0.10
PND_{91}	0.64±0.03	0.49±0.07*	0.59±0.08
PND_{98}	0.68±0.03	0.52±0.07*	0.61±0.07
PND_{105}	0.70±0.03	0.53±0.07*	0.61±0.07
PND_{112}	0.71±0.03	0.54±0.07**	0.62±0.07
PND_{119}	0.75±0.03	0.53±0.05**	0.62±0.04
PND_{126}	0.79±0.03	0.54±0.04**	0.62±0.06
PND_{133}	0.81±0.03	0.53±0.05**	0.62±0.05*
PND_{140}	0.83±0.03	0.54±0.04**	0.64±0.05*
PND_{147}	0.86±0.04	0.54±0.05**	0.66±0.05*
PND_{154}	0.88±0.06	0.57±0.04**	0.68±0.05*
PND_{161}	0.90±0.07	0.56±0.05**	0.69±0.06*
PND_{175}	0.91±0.04	0.58±0.04**	0.71±0.07*
PND_{182}	0.93±0.04	0.59±0.05**	0.72±0.07*

Note: Compared to the saline group, $^*P\leq0.05$; $^{**}P\leq0.01$

PND_{150}, and passed the animal coordination and balance scores at PND_{178}. No abnormalities were observed in the evaluation indicators such as orientation, attention, reaching and grasping, irritability, vocalization, struggle during the test, appeasement, activity, and motor behavior during the test.

2) Thalidomide group: Compared with the saline group, 6/6 young monkeys (two females and four males) in the thalidomide group failed the coordination, spontaneous crawling and balance scores at PND_{100}, PND_{125}, PND_{150}, and PND_{178}. No abnormalities were observed in other evaluation indicators such as orientation, attention, reaching and grasping, irritability, vocalization, struggle during the test, appeasement, activity, and motor behavior during the test.

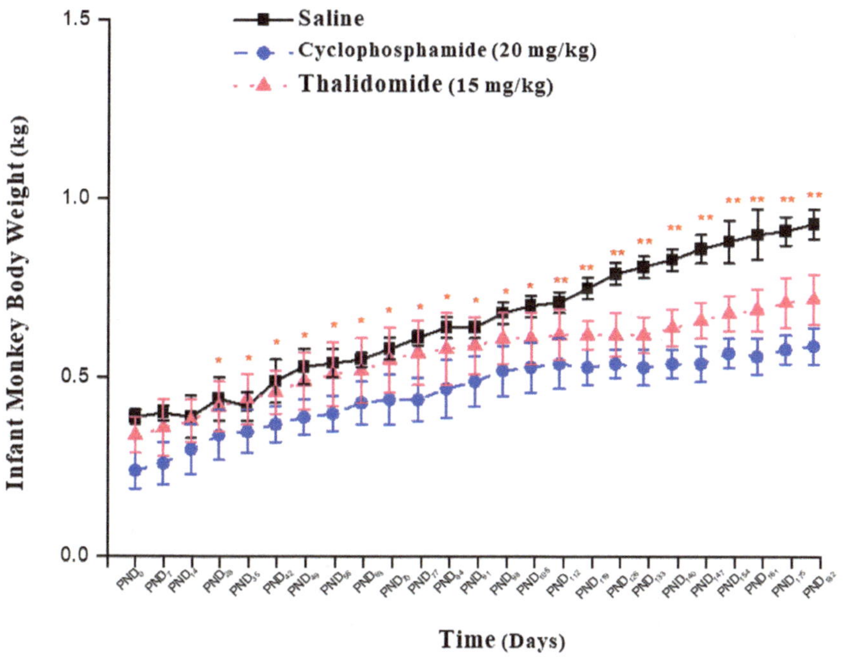

Fig. 8.14 Changes in infant monkey weight (PND_0–PND_{182})

(6) Ophthalmic testing: The animals in each group underwent ophthalmic testing at PND100, PND150, and PND178. Compared with the saline group, no abnormality was observed in the eyelid, conjunctiva, cornea, pupil, iris, and fundus in the cyclophosphamide group and thalidomide group.

(7) Clinical pathology: At PND7, PND30, PND60, PND120, PND150, and PND178. There were no significant differences in clinicopathological indicators (hematology, blood biochemistry, coagulation indicators, and immune indicators) between the cyclophosphamide group and the thalidomide group (Tables 8.77–8.80).

8.3.18 Discussion

8.3.18.1 General Situation of Pregnant Monkeys (Gestation Period)

(1) General observation: During gestation ($GD_{0\text{-}168}$), the main abnormalities were vaginal hemorrhage and fetal abortion. Compared with the saline group, the pregnancy miscarriage rate was higher in the cyclophosphamide group (18% in the saline group vs. 35% in the cyclophosphamide group) and was comparable

Table. 8.71 Physical development indicators of infant monkeys (PND_1–PND_{178}, $\overline{X}\pm SD$)

Parameter	Day	Group 1 (saline)	Group 2 (cyclophosphamide)	Group 3 (thalidomide)
Tibia length (cm)	PND_1	5.33±0.76	4.00±0.18*	0.53±0.21**
	PND_{21}	6.03±0.74	3.87±0.52*	1.28±0.15**
	PND_{58}	6.50±0.70	4.32±0.55*	1.57±0.21**
	PND_{88}	6.90±0.61	4.70±0.58*	1.87±0.26**
	PND_{178}	7.63±0.64	5.28±0.45*	2.63±0.22**
Head circumference (cm)	PND_1	18.17±1.53	12.47±0.65**	16.17±1.34
	PND_{21}	18.90±1.40	13.05±0.53**	16.60±1.31
	PND_{58}	19.43±1.27	14.00±0.45**	16.87±1.00
	PND_{88}	19.87±1.40	14.52±0.43**	17.35±1.03
	PND_{178}	20.87±1.44	15.58±0.39**	18.05±1.03
Tail length (cm)	PND_1	23.50±0.89	17.08±2.61**	20.93±1.23
	PND_{21}	26.07±2.35	17.82±2.49**	21.78±1.44*
	PND_{58}	26.40±2.31	18.33±2.40**	22.45±1.36*
	PND_{88}	26.80±2.17	18.70±2.26**	23.02±1.44*
	PND_{178}	27.23±2.12	19.28±2.36**	23.73±1.21*
Crown–rump length (cm)	PND_1	17.80±0.78	15.02±1.22*	17.37±1.68
	PND_{21}	18.73±0.68	15.68±1.09*	18.00±1.68
	PND_{58}	19.13±0.58	16.27±1.14*	18.52±1.59
	PND_{88}	19.73±0.49	16.83±1.11*	19.17±1.69
	PND_{178}	20.50±0.26	17.60±0.96*	19.97±1.74
Anogenital distance[1] (cm)	PND_1	M:3.2 F:1.8–1.9	M:2.9–3.0 F:1.8–2.3	M:3.1–3.3 F:2.0–2.1
	PND_{21}	M:4.2 F:2.3–2.9	M:3.9 F:2.3–2.9	M:3.9–4.2 F:2.3–2.7
	PND_{58}	M:4.7 F:2.7–2.8	M:4.2–4.3 F:2.7–3.1	M:4.3–4.8 F:2.7–3.1
	PND_{88}	M:5.3 F:3.1–3.2	M:4.9–5.1 F:3.2–3.9	M:5.1–5.6 F:3.3–3.5
	PND_{178}	M:5.6 F:3.3–3.4	M:5.1–5.6 F:3.5–4.0	M:5.6–6.1 F:3.4–3.6

[1]Due to the number of animals in some groups being three or less, individual value ranges are used for statistics; M stands for male; F stands for female. Compared to the saline group, *$P \leq 0.05$; **$P \leq 0.01$.

in the thalidomide group (18% in the control group vs. 19% in the thalidomide group). In conclusion, it is possible that cyclophosphamide can lead to increased abortion rate in pregnant monkeys, while thalidomide group has no significant effect.

(2) Body weight and extrauterine weight gain
   1) Cyclophosphamide: During gestation (GD_{0-168}), both body weight and extrauterine weight gain decreased in cyclophosphamide group compared with saline group ($P \leq 0.05$ or $P \leq 0.01$), so it was considered that

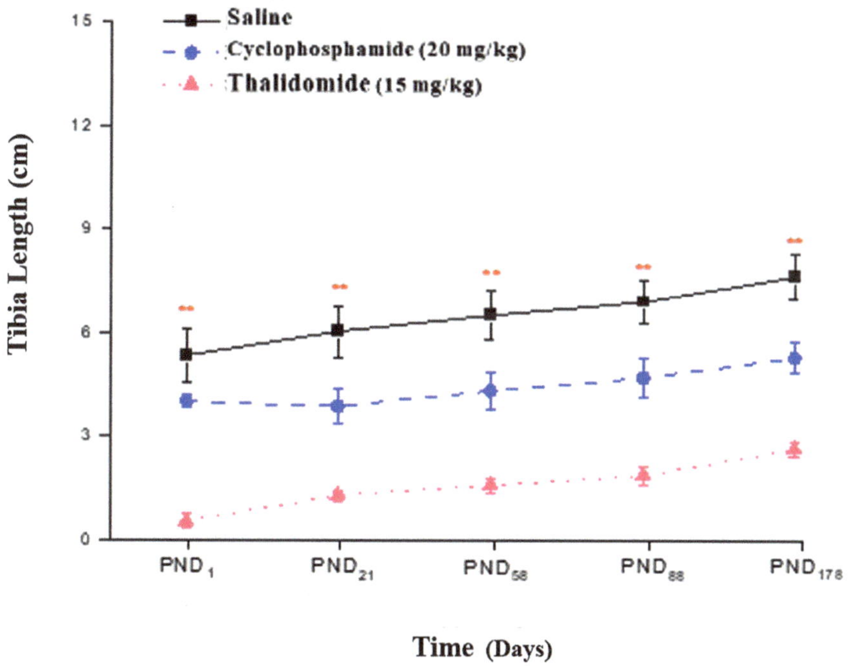

Fig. 8.15 Tibia length of infant monkey

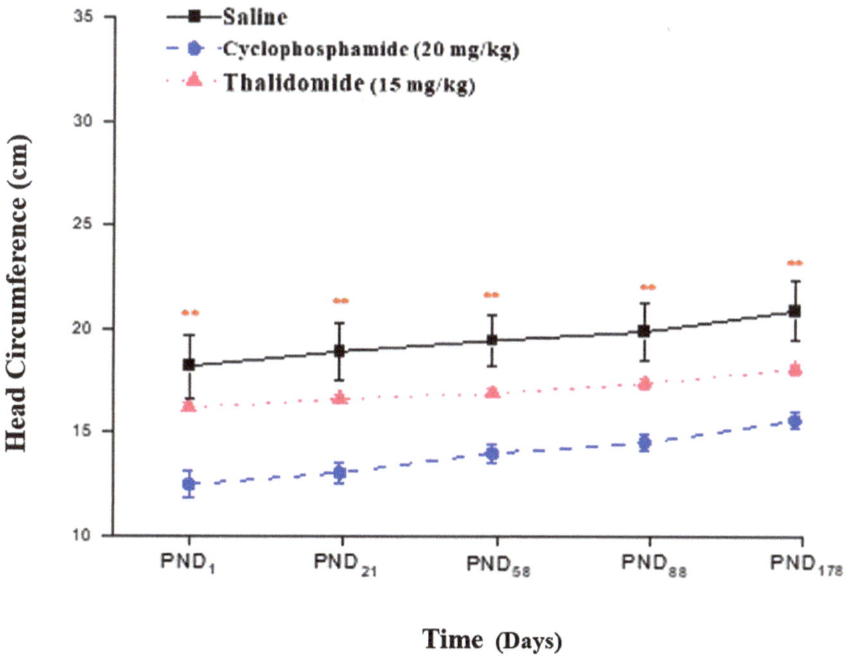

Fig. 8.16 Head circumference of infant monkeys

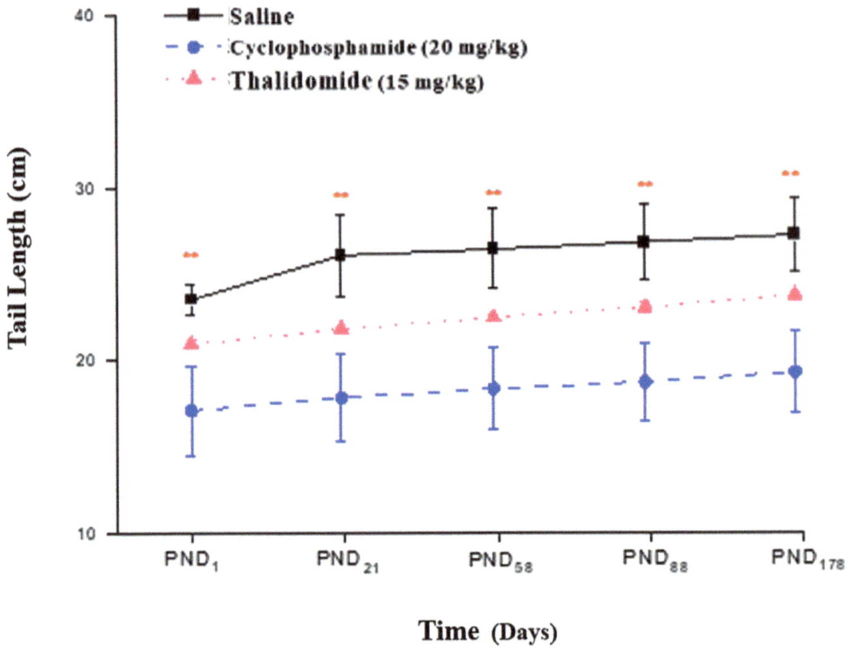

Fig. 8.17 Tibia length of infant monkeys

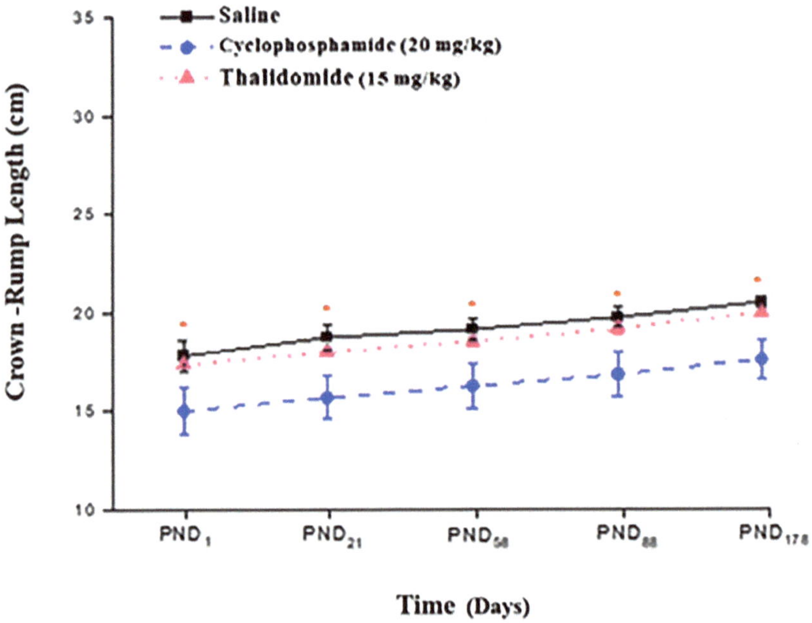

Fig. 8.18 Head circumference of infant monkeys

Table. 8.72 Summary table of infant monkey's grip strength (s, $\overline{X}\pm$SD)

Time	Indicator	Group 1(saline)n=3	Group 2(cyclophosphamide)n=6	Group 3(thalidomide)n=6
PND_1	Grasp time (s)	30.0±0.0	29.5±1.2	3.5±0.5**
	Fall rate (%)	0% (0/3)	83% (5/6)	100% (6/6)
PND_{14}	Grasp time (s)	30.0±0.0	30.0±0.0	17.0±7.2**
	Fall rate (%)	0% (0/3)	0% (0/6)	83% (5/6)
PND_{28}	Grasp time (s)	30.0±0.0	30.0±0.0	20.5±6.9*
	Fall rate (%)	0% (0/3)	0% (0/6)	67% (4/6)

Note: Compared to the saline group, *$P\leq0.05$; **$P\leq0.01$

cyclophosphamide could lead to a decrease in weight and extrauterine weight gain in pregnant monkeys.

2) Thalidomide: During gestation (GD_{0-168}), the weight and extrauterine gain of pregnant monkeys in the thalidomide group were basically the same as those in the saline group, so it was considered that thalidomide had no significant effect on the weight and extrauterine gain of pregnant monkeys.

(3) Assessment on food consumption: During gestation (GD_{0-168}), the assessment on the food consumption of pregnant monkeys in the cyclophosphamide and thalidomide groups was basically the same as that in the saline group. The results showed that cyclophosphamide/thalidomide had no significant effect on the food consumption of pregnant monkeys.

8.3.18.2 Pregnancy Outcome (GD_{100})

(1) Cyclophosphamide: Seven pregnant monkeys were necropsied, of which six fetuses were alive, and one was stillborn, with a live birth rate of 86% and a stillbirth rate of 14%. The live birth rate of cyclophosphamide was lower than that of the saline group (100%), so it was considered that cyclophosphamide had an effect on the pregnancy outcome of pregnant monkeys.

(2) Thalidomide: Seven pregnant monkeys were necropsied, of which seven fetuses were alive without stillbirth, with a live rate of 100% and a stillbirth rate of zero. The live birth rate of the phosphamide and saline group was 100%, so it was considered that thalidomide had no effect on the pregnancy outcome of pregnant monkeys.

8.3.18.3 Hysteroscopy (GD_{100})

(1) Fetal weight, physical development, and morphological examination: Compared with the saline group, fetal weight, top hip length, chest circumference, tail length, tibia length, and forearm length in the cyclophosphamide group and the thalidomide group were lower than those in the saline group. In addition, three

Table. 8.73 Summary of behavioral and neurological function scores (PND_{100}; Unit: Points)

Category	Test indicator	Observer	Standard score	Group 1(saline)n=3	Group 2(cyclophosphamide)n=6	Group 3(thalidomide)n=6
Locomotion ability	Visual orient	1	1	1	1	1
		2		1	1	1
	Visual follow	1	1	1	1	1
		2		1	1	1
	Duration of looking	1	1	1	1	1
		2		1	1	1
	Attention	1	1	1	1	1
		2		1	1	1
	Reach and grasp	1	2	2	2	1
		2		2	2	1
Status assessment	Irritability	1	1	1	1	1
		2		1	1	1
	Vocalizations	1	3–5 times/min	4	3	4
		2		3	4	4
	Struggle during the test	1	2	2	2	2
		2		2	2	2
	Consolability	1	2	2	2	2
		2		2	2	2
	Soothability	1	1	1	1	1
		2		1	1	1
	Predominant state	1	0	0	0	0
		2		0	0	0
Activity	Response intensity	1	0	0	0	0
		2		0	0	0
	Motor activity	1	1	1	1	1
		2		1	1	1
	Coordination	1	2	2	1	1
		2		2	1	1
	Spontaneous crawl	1	2	2	2	1
		2		2	2	1
	Passive resistance	1	2	2	2	2
		2		2	2	2
	Balance	1	2	2	1	1
		2		2	1	1

Note: *n* represents the number of animals

(three/seven) fetuses in the cyclophosphamide group were found to have facial deformities (mouth cleft, nose cleft). In the thalidomide group, five (five/seven) young monkeys had developmental deformity of limbs, and the incidence of appearance deformity was higher. Therefore, it was considered that cyclophosphamide/thalidomide has a teratogenic effect on the fetus.

Table. 8.74 Summary of behavioral and neurological function scores (PND_{125}; Unit: Points)

Category	Test indicator	Observer	Standard score	Group 1(saline)n=3	Group 2(cyclophosphamide)n=6	Group 3(thalidomide)n=6
Locomotion ability	Visual orient	1	1	1	1	1
		2		1	1	1
	Visual follow	1	1	1	1	1
		2		1	1	1
	Duration of looking	1	1	1	1	1
		2		1	1	1
	Attention	1	1	1	1	1
		2		1	1	1
	Reach and grasp	1	2	2	2	1
		2		2	2	1
Status assessment	Irritability	1	1	1	1	1
		2		1	1	1
	Vocalizations	1	3–5 times/min	3	4	3
		2		3	3	5
	Struggle during the test	1	2	2	2	2
		2		2	2	2
	Consolability	1	2	2	2	2
		2		2	2	2
	Soothability	1	1	1	1	1
		2		1	1	1
	Predominant state	1	0	0	0	0
		2		0	0	0
Activity	Response intensity	1	0	0	0	0
		2		0	0	0
	Motor activity	1	1	1	1	1
		2		1	1	1
	Coordination	1	2	2	1	1
		2		2	1	1
	Spontaneous crawl	1	2	2	2	1
		2		2	2	1
	Passive resistance	1	2	2	2	2
		2		2	2	2
	Balance	1	2	2	1	1
		2		2	1	1

Note: *n* represents the number of animals

(2) Organ weight: Compared with the saline group, the weight of major organs (heart, liver, spleen, lung, kidney, ovary, and testis) in the cyclophosphamide group and the thalidomide group had no significant changes ($P > 0.05$), so it was considered that cyclophosphamide/thalidomide had no significant effect on fetal organ weight.

Table. 8.75 Summary of behavioral and neurological function scores (PND_{150}; Unit: Points)

Category	Test indicator	Observer	Standard score	Group 1(saline)n=3	Group 2 (cyclophosphamide) n=6	Group 3 (thalidomide) n=6
Locomotion ability	Visual orient	1	1	1	1	1
		2		1	1	1
	Visual follow	1	1	1	1	1
		2		1	1	1
	Duration of looking	1	1	1	1	1
		2		1	1	1
	Attention	1	1	1	1	1
		2		1	1	1
	Reach and grasp	1	2	2	2	1
		2		2	2	1
Status assessment	Irritability	1	1	1	1	1
		2		1	1	1
	Vocalizations	1	3–5 times/min	3	5	3
		2		4	3	4
	Struggle during the test	1	2	2	2	2
		2		2	2	2
	Consolability	1	2	2	2	2
		2		2	2	2
	Soothability	1	1	1	1	1
		2		1	1	1
	Predominant state	1	0	0	0	0
		2		0	0	0
Activity	Response intensity	1	0	0	0	0
		2		0	0	0
	Motor activity	1	1	1	1	1
		2		1	1	1
	Coordination	1	2	2	1	1
		2		2	1	1
	Spontaneous crawl	1	2	2	2	1
		2		2	2	1
	Passive resistance	1	2	2	2	2
		2		2	2	2
	Balance	1	2	2	1	1
		2		2	1	1

Note: *n* represents the number of animals

8.3.18.4 Deformity Examination

(1) Bone examination

1) Cyclophosphamide: Seven fetal bones were examined, among which ossification was not complete: skull (four cases), sternum (three cases), and occipital bone (one case). The incidence of sternal ossification decreased (seven cases), rib (one case with short rib), phalanx (three cases with polydactyly),

Table. 8.76 Summary of behavioral and neurological function scores (PND_{178}; Unit: Points)

Category	Test indicator	Observer	Standard score	Group 1(saline)n=3	Group 2(cyclophosphamide) n=6	Group 3(thalidomide) n=6
Locomotion ability	Visual orient	1	1	1	1	1
		2		1	1	1
	Visual follow	1	1	1	1	1
		2		1	1	1
	Duration of looking	1	1	1	1	1
		2		1	1	1
	Attention	1	1	1	1	1
		2		1	1	1
	Reach and grasp	1	2	2	2	1
		2		2	2	1
Status assessment	Irritability	1	1	1	1	1
		2		1	1	1
	Vocalizations	1	3–5 times/min	5	4	5
		2		3	4	5
	Struggle during the test	1	2	2	2	2
		2		2	2	2
	Consolability	1	2	2	2	2
		2		2	2	2
	Soothability	1	1	1	1	1
		2		1	1	1
	Predominant state	1	0	0	0	0
		2		0	0	0
Activity	Response intensity	1	0	0	0	0
		2		0	0	0
	Motor activity	1	1	1	1	1
		2		1	1	1
	Coordination	1	2	2	2	1
		2		2	2	1
	Spontaneous crawl	1	2	2	2	1
		2		2	2	1
	Passive resistance	1	2	2	2	2
		2		2	2	2
	Balance	1	2	2	2	1
		2		2	2	1

Note: *n* represents the number of animals

rib/costal cartilage (fusion, one case), and other bone malformations increased significantly. Therefore, it was considered that cyclophosphamide might cause fetal skeletal retardation and deformity.

2) Thalidomide: Seven fetal bones were examined, mainly with an increased rate of skeletal deformity of limbs, including curvature/deformity of the tail vertebrae (four cases), absence of radius, metacarpal, phalanx, femur, tibia

Table. 8.77 Summary of biochemical indicators ($\overline{X}$±SD, males)

Test indicators	Test stage	Group 1(saline)n=3	Group 2(cyclophosphamide)n=6	Group 3(thalidomide)n=6
ALB (g/L)	PND$_{7}$	46.8±2.5	46.2±4.8	47.1±2.1
	PND$_{30}$	43.9±3.1	41.4±4.7	44.7±3.5
	PND$_{60}$	44.3±2.8	44.4±4.9	45.8±3.1
	PND$_{120}$	44.2±2.7	46.9±2.9	45.7±2.3
	PND$_{150}$	43.3±7.1	46.7±2.9	44.7±2.7
	PND$_{178}$	43.4±6.5	43.4±7.3	45.9±2.4
ALT (U/L)	PND$_{7}$	57±13	71±40	76±41
	PND$_{30}$	66±18	81±42	90±23
	PND$_{60}$	35±4	47±19	46±10
	PND$_{120}$	47±20	51±24	53±11
	PND$_{150}$	35±11	35±10	36±7
	PND$_{178}$	36±7	32±33	41±11
CK (U/L)	PND$_{7}$	320±52	345±70	238±17
	PND$_{30}$	236±51	464±49	276±82
	PND$_{60}$	180±57	271±60	244±15
	PND$_{120}$	230±11	252±15	275±61
	PND$_{150}$	337±15	331±76	315±67
	PND$_{178}$	195±46	254±74	225±83
GGT (U/L)	PND$_{7}$	69±22	81±12	69±24
	PND$_{30}$	60±18	68±3	63±23
	PND$_{60}$	57±15	70±5	61±25
	PND$_{120}$	53±14	68±8	55±21
	PND$_{150}$	62±25	79±7	61±21
	PND$_{178}$	68±29	84±34	61±17
PND$_{178}$	45±15	75±57	45±7	
ALP (U/L)	PND$_{7}$	572±65	522±142	618±243
	PND$_{30}$	652±60	669±152	671±184
	PND$_{60}$	605±78	569±144	651±228
	PND$_{120}$	595±91	561±115	619±191
	PND$_{150}$	718±205	528±173	646±154
	PND$_{178}$	735±200	705±270	669±209
TCHO (mmol/L)	PND$_{7}$	2.54±0.53	2.84±0.86	2.70±0.45
	PND$_{30}$	2.93±0.54	3.12±0.76	2.73±0.22
	PND$_{60}$	3.10±0.81	3.07±0.88	3.00±0.20
	PND$_{120}$	3.08±0.99	3.23±0.76	2.93±0.43
	PND$_{150}$	3.21±0.60	3.30±0.90	3.04±0.53
	PND$_{178}$	2.84±0.35	3.44±1.57	2.84±0.71

Table 8.77 (continued)

TG (mmol/L)	PND_7	0.3±0.1	0.3±0.1	0.3±0.1
	PND_{30}	0.5±0.2	0.4±0.1	0.4±0.1
	PND_{60}	0.4±0.1	0.3±0.2	0.3±0.1
	PND_{120}	0.4±0.1	0.4±0.1	0.4±0.1
	PND_{150}	0.5±0.1	0.4±0.1	0.5±0.1
	PND_{178}	0.4±0.1	0.6±0.4	0.3±0.1
CREA (μ mol/L)	PND_7	73±11	69±6	77±11
	PND_{30}	66±12	62±10	64±11
	PND_{60}	65±11	65±6	67±11
	PND_{120}	64±10	63±11	67±10
	PND_{150}	73±14	77±11	77±17
	PND_{178}	66±15	73±15	72±12
PND_{178}	5.57±0.96	7.19±0.58	6.01±0.45	
T-BIL (μ mol/L)	PND_7	3.3±1.7	3.2±1.0	4.2±2.6
	PND_{30}	3.3±1.7	2.3±1.0	3.6±3.0
	PND_{60}	2.1±0.3	2.3±0.6	2.3±0.9
	PND_{120}	2.1±0.6	1.8±0.4	2.1±0.5
	PND_{150}	1.9±0.4	2.1±0.9	2.3±0.6
	PND_{178}	3.3±0.8	3.0±2.6	2.8±1.2
TP (g/L)	PND_7	74.4±2.0	75.3±7.0	72.8±2.7
	PND_{30}	73.4±2.9	71.1±6.2	71.8±1.7
	PND_{60}	74.8±4.1	75.2±4.5	74.2±2.3
	PND_{120}	74.2±4.8	76.1±2.6	73.0±4.0
	PND_{150}	76.9±4.0	74.1±5.2	70.5±3.8
	PND_{178}	80.2±5.9	75.3±5.1	75.8±1.7
GLU (mmol/L)	PND_7	4.72±0.52	4.25±0.73	4.18±0.56
	PND_{30}	3.46±0.46	3.47±0.39	3.39±0.46
	PND_{60}	4.01±0.64	3.59±0.25	4.02±0.43
	PND_{120}	3.30±0.60	2.98±0.55	3.31±0.53
	PND_{150}	3.58±0.77	3.77±0.85	3.72±0.79
	PND_{178}	3.48±0.42	3.19±0.33	4.01±0.25
LDH (μ mol/L)	PND_7	385±96	384±76	519±274
	PND_{30}	522±116	535±191	533±74
	PND_{60}	327±60	356±65	309±65
	PND_{120}	685±180	773±160	697±163
	PND_{150}	425±87	469±96	375±63
	PND_{178}	347±57	538±146	365±58

(continued)

Table 8.77 (continued)

	PND_{178}	148.9±2.8	150.3±4.2	150.3±1.4
K^+ (mmol/L)	PND_7	5.11±0.38	5.31±0.62	4.58±0.59
	PND_{30}	4.55±0.33	4.99±0.30	4.57±0.54
	PND_{60}	4.91±0.49	5.24±0.37	4.94±0.28
	PND_{120}	5.50±0.54	4.91±0.43	4.77±0.31
	PND_{150}	4.87±0.57	4.64±0.57	4.41±0.48
	PND_{178}	5.37±0.68	5.71±0.56	5.48±0.68
Cl-(mmol/L)	PND_7	107.9±1.0	106.1±0.9	107.0±2.5
	PND_{30}	107.2±1.2	105.6±1.3	106.7±2.2
	PND_{60}	105.7±1.4	103.3±1.2	105.0±2.0
	PND_{120}	106.7±1.9	103.0±2.3	106.1±1.7
	PND_{150}	103.9±1.0	103.5±1.6	105.0±1.9
	PND_{178}	108.1±0.6	106.9±1.6	108.7±1.7
GLO (g/L)	PND_7	27.6±2.9	29.0±5.6	25.7±1.1
	PND_{30}	29.5±3.7	29.7±6.9	27.1±2.7
	PND_{60}	30.5±3.3	30.8±5.0	28.4±2.5
	PND_{120}	30.0±5.5	29.3±4.3	27.3±3.1
	PND_{150}	33.5±7.1	27.4±4.8	25.8±2.7
	PND_{178}	36.8±11.7	31.9±7.2	29.8±2.4
A/G	PND_7	1.71±0.24	1.65±0.45	1.84±0.09
	PND_{30}	1.51±0.30	1.47±0.45	1.67±0.27
	PND_{60}	1.47±0.20	1.49±0.42	1.63±0.25
	PND_{120}	1.53±0.38	1.64±0.38	1.69±0.20
	PND_{150}	1.38±0.51	1.75±0.34	1.75±0.20
	PND_{178}	1.29±0.44	1.44±0.44	1.55±0.19

(five cases), and long bone irregularity (three cases). Therefore, it was considered that thalidomide could cause fetal limb deformity.

(2) Visceral examination: Compared with the saline group, there were no significant abnormalities in the visceral development of the fetuses in the cyclophosphamide and thalidomide groups. Therefore, it was considered that cyclophosphamide/thalidomide had no significant effect on fetal visceral development.

During gestation, compared with the saline group, estrogen and sex hormones of pregnant monkeys in the cyclophosphamide group and the thalidomide group occasionally fluctuated, but there was no significant difference between groups, which was considered as normal physiological fluctuations of animals. The results showed that cyclophosphamide/thalidomide had no significant effects on estrogen and sex hormones in pregnant monkeys.

Table. 8.78 Summary of hematological indicators ($\overline{X}$±SD)

Test indicators	Test stage	Group 1(saline)n=3	Group 2(cyclophosphamide)n=6	Group 3(thalidomide)n=6
xWBC (× 10^9/L)	PND_{7}	13.05±1.92	12.60±5.18	14.89±3.57
	PND_{30}	15.24±2.21	12.71±4.40	13.94±3.82
	PND_{60}	12.95±4.10	12.01±5.01	11.87±1.69
	PND_{120}	13.69±5.34	16.38±6.64	15.15±2.88
	PND_{150}	16.94±4.47	19.41±4.11	20.42±6.10
	PND_{178}	14.19±1.92	11.23±3.56	12.95±2.90
RBC (× 10^{12}/L)	PND_{7}	5.98±0.55	6.14±0.27	5.88±0.30
	PND_{30}	5.49±0.51	5.51±0.35	5.55±0.43
	PND_{60}	5.50±0.44	5.66±0.32	5.65±0.37
	PND_{120}	5.11±0.53	5.29±0.66	5.12±0.21
	PND_{150}	5.47±0.66	5.71±0.45	5.47±0.16
	PND_{178}	5.21±0.22	5.46±0.73	5.08±0.25
HGB (g/L)	PND_{7}	144±9	141±14	137±6
	PND_{30}	131±9	126±7	128±9
	PND_{60}	130±7	129±10	130±7
	PND_{120}	123±11	121±6	121±5
	PND_{150}	130±16	131±5	129±7
	PND_{178}	120±11	121±13	115±6
HCT (%)	PND_{7}	45.2±2.2	45.7±2.3	44.1±1.8
	PND_{30}	41.9±2.6	41.6±0.7	42.0±2.2
	PND_{60}	42.6±2.3	43.0±0.9	43.2±2.1
	PND_{120}	40.4±2.5	41.0±2.7	40.2±1.0
	PND_{150}	42.0±4.2	43.2±1.0	41.6±1.5
	PND_{178}	39.8±3.0	41.5±4.0	39.2±1.4
MCV (fL)	PND_{7}	75.8±3.5	74.5±4.3	74.9±1.7
	PND_{30}	76.5±2.8	75.7±4.4	75.7±2.3
	PND_{60}	77.5±2.5	76.1±4.6	76.6±2.2
	PND_{120}	79.3±3.5	77.9±4.8	78.6±2.6
	PND_{150}	76.9±3.4	75.9±4.5	76.1±2.5
	PND_{178}	76.4±3.5	76.4±4.4	77.4±3.1
PND_{178}	22.9±1.3	22.3±2.0	22.6±1.1	
MCHC (g/L)	PND_{7}	319±11	309±17	311±7
	PND_{30}	312±8	303±14	306±6
	PND_{60}	307±9	300±18	300±4
	PND_{120}	305±12	297±12	300±6
	PND_{150}	308±11	303±14	309±6
	PND_{178}	300±11	292±14	292±9

(continued)

Table 8.78 (continued)

PLT (× 10^9/L)	PND_7	332±82	305±84	293±51
	PND_{30}	397±96	400±88	402±120
	PND_{60}	489±130	492±105	475±133
	PND_{120}	427±56	439±115	451±86
	PND_{150}	413±148	392±101	405±121
	PND_{178}	396±146	445±69	424±182
NEU# (× 10^9/L)	PND_7	6.63±1.01	5.16±2.55	9.24±3.60
	PND_{30}	9.83±2.30	5.49±1.84	8.23±4.13
	PND_{60}	6.18±3.91	4.16±1.29	4.93±1.91
	PND_{120}	7.49±3.46	9.12±7.12	8.68±3.90
	PND_{150}	10.83±5.25	14.04±2.32	15.75±7.00
	PND_{178}	6.78±1.93	6.23±1.92	8.01±3.09
LYM# (× 10^9/L)	PND_7	5.46±2.05	6.31±3.06	4.60±1.33
	PND_{30}	4.24±1.71	6.04±3.83	4.59±1.51
	PND_{60}	5.69±1.71	6.70±3.67	5.96±1.97
	PND_{120}	4.81±1.24	6.02±3.14	5.53±2.61
	PND_{150}	4.73±1.56	3.83±2.06	3.58±1.34
	PND_{178}	6.29±1.45	3.86±3.06	4.09±2.39
PND_{178}	1.03± 0.37	1.03±0.28	0.78±0.35	
EO# (×10^9/L)	PND_7	0.10±0.08	0.20±0.15	0.17±0.09
	PND_{30}	0.14±0.15	0.19±0.13	0.11±0.05
	PND_{60}	0.15±0.09	0.22±0.13	0.14±0.11
	PND_{120}	0.15±0.08	0.18±0.14	0.11±0.06
	PND_{150}	0.12±0.11	0.17±0.15	0.09±0.08
	PND_{178}	0.08±0.03	0.11±0.10	0.06±0.04
BASO# (× 10^9/L)	PND_7	0.01±0.01	0.01±0.01	0.01±0.01
	PND_{30}	0.02±0.02	0.02±0.01	0.01±0.00
	PND_{60}	0.02±0.02	0.01±0.01	0.01±0.01
	PND_{120}	0.02±0.01	0.02±0.01	0.01±0.01
	PND_{150}	0.02±0.01	0.02±0.01	0.02±0.01
	PND_{178}	0.01±0.01	0.00±0.01	0.01±0.00
NEU%	PND_7	52.1±12.0	41.2±9.8	60.8±12.5
	PND_{30}	64.6±13.3	45.1±15.0	57.1±16.7
	PND_{60}	45.6±16.7	36.9±11.1	41.7±16.1
	PND_{120}	53.3±6.2	50.8±20.1	56.2±21.9
	PND_{150}	60.6±17.1	73.2±9.7	73.4±17.6
	PND_{178}	47.6±10.8	58.0±17.6	62.1±20.6
LYM%	PND_7	40.8±10.8	49.2±10.4	31.8±11.0
	PND_{30}	27.9±11.5	45.5±16.8	34.9±15.4
	PND_{60}	45.8±13.8	53.2±10.9	50.1±16.4
	PND_{120}	36.9±6.4	39.9±17.6	37.6±21.2
	PND_{150}	31.0±16.4	19.1±7.2	20.9±16.2
	PND_{178}	44.5±10.3	31.5±16.7	31.5±19.8

Table 8.78 (continued)

PND_{178}	7.2±2.1	9.5±2.4	5.9±1.6	
EO%	PND_{7}	0.7±0.6	1.8±1.8	1.2±0.6
	PND_{30}	0.9±0.9	1.5±0.9	0.8±0.4
	PND_{60}	1.2±0.8	1.9±1.0	1.1±0.8
	PND_{120}	1.1±0.3	1.5±1.7	0.7±0.4
	PND_{150}	0.9±0.9	0.9±0.8	0.5±0.5
	PND_{178}	0.5±0.2	1.0±0.7	0.4±0.3
BASO%	PND_{7}	0.1±0.0	0.1±0.0	0.1±0.0
	PND_{30}	0.2±0.1	0.1±0.1	0.1±0.0
	PND_{60}	0.2±0.1	0.1±0.1.	0.1±0.0
	PND_{120}	0.1±0.0	0.1±0.0	0.1±0.0
	PND_{150}	0.1±0.0	0.1±0.0	0.1±0.0
	PND_{178}	0.1±0.0	0.0±0.1	0.1±0.0
RET ($\times 10^9$/L)	PND_{7}	28.2±7.2	31.5±13.3	40.4±30.9
	PND_{30}	81.8±30.0	94.3±39.3	107.1±63.9
	PND_{60}	70.1±13.3	80.8±22.9	95.3±44.9
	PND_{120}	154.8±60.1	151.7±31.1	160.2±62.5
	PND_{150}	55.7±14.8	43.9±21.4	56.6±11.6
	PND_{178}	67.5±13.3	89.9±43.5	108.3±47.4
RET%	PND_{7}	0.48±0.16	0.52±0.22	0.68±0.50
	PND_{30}	1.54±0.67	1.69±0.60	1.98±1.34
	PND_{60}	1.29±0.31	1.42±0.34	1.72±0.91
	PND_{120}	3.09±1.29	2.87±0.50	3.15±1.29
	PND_{150}	1.03±0.29	0.75±0.31	1.04±0.22
	PND_{178}	1.29±0.21	1.73±0.99	2.16±1.00

8.3.18.5 Toxicokinetics

During gestation, the blood concentration of cyclophosphamide in pregnant monkeys quickly reached a peak, and there was no accumulation after repeated subcutaneous administration for 5 days. The blood concentration of thalidomide reached a peak slowly in pregnant monkeys, and there was accumulation after 7 days of repeated gavage. The concentrations of cyclophosphamide or thalidomide in amniotic fluid and placenta were lower than the LLOQ concentration. Considering that cyclophosphamide or thalidomide were small-molecule compounds with short half-lives (less than 24 h), the administration cycle of the two drugs was GD_{24}–GD_{30}, and the amniotic fluid and placenta were collected on GD_{100}, the drug concentration at this time point was lower than the LLOQ concentration.

Table. 8.79 Summary of coagulation indicators ($\overline{X}$±SD)

Test indicators	Test stage	Group 1(saline)n=3	Group 2(cyclophosphamide)n=6	Group 3(thalidomide)n=6
APTT (s)	PND_7	19.0±1.3	18.6±1.6	17.5±1.9
	PND_{30}	19.1±1.9	18.4±1.8	17.3±2.4
	PND_{60}	18.7±1.4	18.6±1.9	17.7±1.8
	PND_{120}	20.0±2.0	19.8±1.5	18.2±2.3
	PND_{150}	20.0±3.1	18.8±1.9	17.5±1.3
	PND_{178}	20.7±2.5	21.0±2.9	18.6±2.3
FIB (g/L)	PND_7	2.07±0.59	1.96±0.25	1.95±0.22
	PND_{30}	2.92±1.00	2.29±2.17	2.33±0.31
	PND_{60}	2.07±0.59	2.01±0.29	1.80±0.28
	PND_{120}	2.34±0.83	2.44±0.42	2.18±0.24
	PND_{150}	2.45±1.77	2.34±0.18	1.74±0.13
	PND_{178}	2.55±1.07	2.13±2.16	1.86±0.42
PT (s)	PND_7	9.0±0.4	9.0±0.2	9.4±0.2
	PND_{30}	8.8±0.5	9.1±0.6	8.8±0.3
	PND_{60}	9.0±0.3	9.3±0.1	9.1±0.4
	PND_{120}	8.6±0.6	9.0±0.3	8.8±0.3
	PND_{150}	8.6±0.4	8.9±0.3	9.0±0.4
	PND_{178}	9.0±0.3	9.3±0.9	8.9±0.5

8.3.18.6 Evaluation of Fetal Monkeys (Perinatal Period)

(1) Appearance examination: In the cyclophosphamide group, three (three/six) fetuses had facial deformities (mouth cleft, nose cleft), one fetus had syndactyly and short toes on the hind limbs, and one fetus had a naturally closed external auditory canal. In the thalidomide group, five (five/six) of the fetuses had dysplasia of the limbs (missing, undeveloped, or short front/rear limbs). Therefore, it was considered that cyclophosphamide/thalidomide could cause deformity in young monkeys.

(2) Body weight and physical development: Compared with the saline group, the body weight, tibia length, head circumference, tail length, and crown and hip length in the cyclophosphamide and thalidomide groups were lower than those in the saline group. There were statistical differences at some time points ($P \leq 0.05$ or $P \leq 0.01$), so it was considered that cyclophosphamide/thalidomide had an effect on weight gain and physical development of young monkeys.

(3) Grip strength test: Compared with the saline group, the cyclophosphamide group and thalidomide group did not reach the standard at PND_1 (the standard

Table. 8.80 Summary of Immunological Indicators($\overline{X}$±SD)

Test indicators	Test stage	Group 1(saline)n=3	Group 2(cyclophosphamide)n=6	Group 3(thalidomide)n=6
C3 (mg/dL)	PND_7	141.4±23.6	130.8±32.8	132.9±7.0
	PND_{30}	135.2±28.4	122.6±12.7	132.7±8.5
	PND_{60}	143.7±22.4	130.6±8.2	130.5±8.9
	PND_{120}	149.8±36.2	119.2±6.5	120.0±9.6
	PND_{150}	144.4±42.9	146.4±42.0	142.2±21.8
C4 (mg/dL)	PND_{178}	23.5±5.2	20.2±3.2	19.0±6.4
	PND_7	21.8±5.1	19.1±2.7	19.6±6.0
	PND_{30}	23.6±4.6	23.9±2.1	20.6±5.5
	PND_{60}	25.6±6.9	18.9±4.0	17.2±5.0
	PND_{120}	24.5±6.9	28.2±11.6	25.1±8.0
IgG (mg/dL)	PND_{150}	969.6±233.1	991.6±269.0	921.6±55.8
	PND_{178}	1057.1±249.8	1069.9±216.0	994.6±53.1
	PND_7	1101.4±267.0	1140.8±202.3	1027.1±85.1
	PND_{30}	1273.5±212.7	980.3±216.8	956.2±56.1
	PND_{60}	1306.2±456.6	943.3±156.0	1090.0±123.6
IgA (mg/dL)	PND_{120}	137.6±78.5	180.8±79.7	141.7±53.6
	PND_{150}	139.8±79.1	197.6±95.2	140.3±50.9
	PND_{178}	141.9±78.1	180.8±104.1	136.1±53.6
	PND_7	157.0±85.8	168.1±101.6	129.9±57.5
	PND_{30}	166.7±115.3	148.0±83.6	127.7±51.3
IgM (mg/dL)	PND_{60}	149.1±25.5	152.8±75.2	118.0±38.2
	PND_{120}	144.5±21.3	176.5±122.1	120.3±45.0
	PND_{150}	156.2±21.3	173.2±117.9	121.0±42.0
	PND_{178}	190.8±45.9	167.1±94.3	124.0±43.2
	PND_7	184.2±107.3	163.6±113.0	125.5±36.2
CIC (μg/mL)	PND_{30}	20.056±8.836	18.620±9.092	14.012±10.873
	PND_{60}	18.651±9.730	15.520±2.322	11.734±5.209
	PND_{120}	10.274±5.261	12.472±3.178	10.438±4.109
	PND_{150}	16.016±11.166	16.553±3.189	11.599±4.877
	PND_{178}	17.003±7.333	20.588±5.727	11.159±1.802

was reached by persisting in grasping for 30 s), and the young monkeys in the cyclophosphamide group could reach the standard at PND_{14}. Animals in the thalidomide group did not reach the standard at PND_{28}. Cyclophosphamide/thalidomide had no direct effect on the grasping ability of the young monkeys, considering that the malformed limbs of the young monkeys in the thalidomide group were unable to complete the grasping movements normally due to the dysplasia of the forelimbs. Due to the early impact on the physical development of young monkeys, it indirectly led to the temporary substandard grip strength.

(4) Behavioral and neurological evaluation

1) Cyclophosphamide: Compared with the saline group, coordination (rating: clumsy movement) and balance (rating: falling) were temporarily not up to standard at PND_{100} and PND_{150}, and the above indicators were up to standard at PND_{178}. Therefore, it was considered that cyclophosphamide had a certain effect on the coordination and balance of young monkeys.
2) Thalidomide: Coordination (rating: clumsy movement), spontaneous crawling (rating: no crawling), and balance (rating: falling) were all subpar at PND_{100}, PND_{150}, and PND_{178} compared to the saline group. Coordination, spontaneous crawling, and balance could not be evaluated in the thalidomide group due to congenital limb deformity.

(1) Ophthalmic examination: Ophthalmic examination was performed at PND_{100}, PND_{150}, and PND_{178}. No abnormalities were observed in the eyelids, conjunctiva, cornea, pupil, iris, and fundus. The results showed that cyclophosphamide/thalidomide had no significant effect on the eye development of newborn monkeys.
(2) Clinical pathology (hematology, blood biochemistry, coagulation): Compared with the normal saline group, the clinicopathological parameters of the cyclophosphamide group and thalidomide group fluctuated occasionally, but the range of changes was small, and all fluctuated within or near the background range of adult cynomolgus monkeys in the institution. It was considered that cyclophosphamide/thalidomide had no significant effect on the clinicopathological indicators of newborn monkeys.

8.3.19 Conclusion

Under the conditions of this study, the pregnant cynomolgus monkeys were given a dose of 20 mg/kg cyclophosphamide per day by subcutaneous injection or 15 mg/kg thalidomide per day via gavage. The test results showed that: (1) cyclophosphamide had obvious toxicity in pregnant monkeys, embryos, fetuses and monkeys. Resulting in higher abortion rates, lower live birth rates, appearance and skeletal deformities of the fetus/young monkeys, and developmental delays of young monkeys. (2) Thalidomide: No maternal or fetal toxicity had been observed, but it could lead to reduced fetal weight, chest circumference, tail length, shin and forearm length, as well as appearance and skeletal deformity.

In conclusion, both cyclophosphamide and thalidomide have teratogenic effects.

The results of accompanying toxokinetics during GD_{24}–GD_{30} administration showed that there was no accumulation after 5 days of continuous subcutaneous injection of cyclophosphamide during the first and last administration. There was an accumulation after 7 days of continuous gavage of thalidomide, and the concentrations of cyclophosphamide or thalidomide in amniotic fluid and placenta were lower than the LLOQ concentration.

8.3.19.1 Record Retention

Except for the data collected by the computer-automated instrument, all other data of the study were directly, timely, and accurately recorded on the prepared forms or record papers, and could be sorted at any time. All the data records were indicated with dates and signed by the recorder. Upon completion of the study and submission of the final report, all raw records and materials were stored in the archive room. The specific management contents, procedures, and methods were performed according to the SOP formulated by the facility.

8.3.19.2 Data Archiving Time and Site

(1) Archiving time: December, ××××.
(2) Archiving site: ×××archive room.
(3) Archiving period: 5 years after the completion of the study.

Ethical Approval

All animal experiments conducted in this study complied with the Guide for the Care and Use of Laboratory Animals (2011) published by the US National Academy Press and the Regulations for the Administration of Laboratory Animals (revised in 2017) issued by the National Science and Technology Commission of China. The management, use, and related procedures involving animals were reviewed and approved by the Institutional Animal Care and Use Committee (IACUC).

References

1. Yanjun C, Yichao T, Li Z (2021) Selection of teratogenic drug for reproductive and developmental toxicity test in non-human primates. Chin J New Drugs 30(14):12661273
3. Sun Z, Zhou L (2015) Drug reproductive and developmental toxicology. Shanghai Scientific & Technical Publishers, Shanghai
4. Zhou L, Sun Z (2015) Atlas of common malformations in laboratory rabbits and rats. Shanghai Scientific & Technical Publishers, Shanghai

Advances in Reproductive and Developmental Toxicology Studies in Cynomolgus Monkeys

9

Wang Chun, Zhou Li and Sun Zuyue

Abstract

This chapter reviews advances in reproductive and developmental toxicology studies in cynomolgus monkeys, with emphasis on the regulatory background, scientific considerations, and practical strategies for developmental and reproductive toxicity (DART) testing of biopharmaceuticals. It summarizes the key recommendations of ICH S5(R3) and related guidelines, the advantages and limitations of nonhuman primates (NHPs) in DART studies, and the current status of NHP DART research institutions in Europe, the United States, Southeast Asia, and multinational pharmaceutical companies. The chapter discusses critical considerations for fertility and early embryonic development (FEED), embryo-fetal development (EFD), and pre- and postnatal development (PPND)/enhanced PPND (ePPND) studies in cynomolgus monkeys, including pregnancy confirmation, mating strategies, placental transfer, study design, group size, and postnatal evaluation. It also addresses juvenile toxicity testing, histological determination of sexual maturity, and DART evaluation strategies for different drug modalities, such as monoclonal antibodies, oligonucleotide therapeutics, and pediatric anesthetic neurotoxicity research. Furthermore, the chapter highlights the weight-of-evidence approach, the 3Rs principles, and alternative methods including the embryonic stem cell test, whole embryo culture, and zebrafish

W. Chun (✉) · Z. Li
Hubei Topgene Biotechnology Co., Ltd., Wuhan, China
e-mail: wangchun@topgenebio.com

S. Zuyue
The GBA National Institute for Nanotechnology Innovation, Guangdong Canosafe Pharmtech Co., Ltd, Guangdong, China

L. Zhou and Z. Sun (eds.), *Reproductive and Developmental Toxicology on Macaca Fascicularis*, https://doi.org/10.1007/978-981-92-3834-7_9

embryotoxicity test, as well as the emerging role of artificial intelligence in predicting developmental toxicity. Overall, the chapter provides a comprehensive reference for designing and interpreting NHP DART studies, promoting scientific, ethical, and regulatory soundness in drug development.

Keywords

Cynomolgus monkey · Developmental and reproductive toxicity · Nonhuman primate · Enhanced pre- and postnatal development · Monoclonal antibody · Oligonucleotide · Weight of evidence · 3Rs · Alternative methods

The International Council for Harmonization of Technical Requirements for Pharmaceuticals for Human Use (ICH) released the guidelines of "S5 (R3): Detection of Reproductive and Developmental Toxicity for Human Pharmaceuticals" in 2020, which provided requirements or recommendations for animal species used in developmental and reproductive toxicity (DART) studies. The preferred species for fertility and early embryonic development (FEED) studies and pre and postnatal development (PPND) studies were rats, while embryo fetal development (EFD) studies should include at least two types of animals: rodents and non-rodents, with rats and rabbits being recommended. As the most commonly used species in DART evaluation, rats and rabbits can meet the evaluation requirements for most small-molecule chemical drugs. However, due to the species specificity, immunogenicity, and ADME differences of large molecule biotech drugs such as proteins and peptides, most cannot be directly designed using the species recommended by traditional DART evaluation methods. It was clearly stated in "S6(R1): Preclinical safety evaluation of biotechnology-derived pharmaceuticals" that the species in the safety evaluation plan should include relevant species that can produce pharmacological activity. Therefore, when the test substance has pharmacological activity only in nonhuman primates (NHPs), the reproductive and developmental toxicity test in NHPs is the preferred choice [1].

Although ICH S5 (R3) has not brought fundamental changes to the DART test in biopharmaceuticals, the update incorporates relevant recommendations on DART trials from other latest ICH guidelines (such as ICH M3, S6, and S9):

(1) Whether pregnancy will alter the toxicokinetic properties of drugs should be determined.
(2) Although it is strongly recommended to measure drug levels in infant monkeys in enhanced PPND (ePPND) studies on NHPs, it is still not mandatory to measure drug levels in embryos or newborn fetuses.
(3) When necessary, the evidence of the excretion in breast milk can be obtained by sampling milk or proving exposure of offspring before weaning.
(4) It is generally believed that mating research is not feasible in NHPs.
(5) If fertility evaluation is based on histopathological examination of reproductive organs in repeated-dosing studies, the application of sexually mature animals in the study is particularly important, unless a biological product is used to treat

advanced cancer. Specialized fertility studies are needed for biopharmaceuticals with pharmacological activity in rodents.

(6) For biopharmaceuticals exhibiting pharmacological activity solely in NHPs, conducting DART trials in NHPs should be considered only as a final recourse. The use of alternative molecular or transgenic animal models for DART studies in rodents is encouraged. If biopharmaceuticals have consistent pharmacological activity in rodents (rats or mice) and non-rodents (rabbits or miniature pigs), EFD studies are required, and PPND studies are conducted on rodents. Biological products intended for use in the treatment of advanced cancers usually only need to be evaluated in a single pharmacologically relevant species.

(7) ePPND studies can replace EFD and PPND studies for biopharmaceuticals with NHPs as the only relevant species. However, it should only be conducted when there is a potential impact on hazard identification.

(8) Determining the exposure level and duration of drugs, and incorporating toxicity endpoints for juvenile animals in ePPND studies, can eliminate the need for specialized juvenile studies.

(9) All recommendations regarding vaccine trials follow the guidelines of the Considerations for Developmental Toxicity Studies for Preventive and Therapeutic Vaccines for Infectious Disease, approved by the Food and Drug Administration (FDA).

(10) The high-dose design of DART trials in biopharmaceuticals can be limited to ten times the clinically recommended maximum exposure (based on AUC or C_{max}), provided that it can cause maximum biological effects. The Risk Assessment section suggests a diminished concern regarding developmental toxicity reactions occurring at exposures exceeding ten times the maximum recommended dose. It emphasizes that transient findings, such as fetal variations, are of lesser significance compared to fetal death or malformation.

In comparison to S5 (R2), S5 (R3) introduces a plethora of novel evaluation concepts and technical prerequisites, offering more precise directives for drug registration applicants and researchers. Furthermore, it presents a set of challenges in devising trial strategies, formulating technical methodologies, conducting risk assessments, and various other facets of the developmental process. The new guiding principles have significantly influenced drug reproductive toxicity studies, and the emergence of new ideas, concepts, methodologies, and challenges will also markedly promote the development of reproductive and developmental toxicity studies in China.

In recent years, the development of small-molecule drugs has been limited by the discovery of new targets. In addition, the decreasing growth rate of diversity in small molecule libraries has posed some challenges to the development of small molecule drugs. Furthermore, the global biopharmaceutical market is experiencing robust growth. With the rapid development of biotechnology, the variety and scope of treatment of biopharmaceuticals have been continuously optimized, their advantages in safety, effectiveness, and wide applications have been highlighted, and the market size and share have rapidly expanded. Antibody drugs now dominate the global pharmaceutical market, boasting the highest sales and fastest growth rates. Other innovative biotherapies, such as antibody–drug conjugates (ADCs), CAR T-cell therapy, gene therapy, RNA therapeutics, and oncolytic viruses, are rapidly proliferating. The global demand for NHP research has risen due to the growing need for novel biopharmaceuticals and the impact of COVID-19. While in vitro and computational models offer alternatives to animal research, their limitations in capturing the complex interplay of living systems prevent them from fully replacing NHPs. For monoclonal antibodies specifically, the Cynomolgus monkey species is used in 76% (13 out of 17) of the studied cases during nonclinical development. With deepening research in areas such as neuroscience, neurodegenerative diseases, infectious diseases, immunotherapy, reproduction, aging, and chronic inflammatory diseases, coupled with the continued rapid development of biopharmaceuticals, the demand for using NHP to evaluate the efficacy and safety of new drugs is anticipated to rise in the future. The reproductive characteristics of rhesus macaques and marmosets hinder their widespread application in DART studies, despite their suitability as models in some cases [2].

9.1 Benefits of Using NHPs in DART Drug Research

Beyond test substance-specific considerations for species selection, NHPs provide further advantages over rodents and rabbits in DART studies owing to their greater physiological and phylogenetic similarity to humans. There are also some limitations (Table 9.1), such as those related to endocrinology (including testicular and ovarian function), the endocrinology of early pregnancy, placental morphology and physiology, implantation timing, embryonic development rate, and the response to some known human teratogens (e.g., thalidomide and vitamin A). However, there are also ethical and practical constraints associated with the use of NHPs. Macaca mulatta offspring are typically singletons. Twin pregnancies/births are extremely rare, with an overall live birth rate of approximately 0.1%. Macaca mulatta have a fertility rate well below 100% (around 60% per animal, with a 35%–45% chance per menstrual cycle), and experience approximately 25% preimplantation loss. In addition, compared to DART studies using rodents or rabbits, NHP studies have an overall duration of three to five times longer, resulting in higher costs. To address these concerns, the sample size within each group in DART studies using NHPs was reduced to the minimum necessary for valid data interpretation, in contrast to studies using rodent/rabbit models [2].

Currently, only a very limited number of NHP species are suitable for establishing drug testing models, with macaca mulatta being the most commonly used NHP strain in toxicology research. Of the species within this family, macaca mulatta (rhesus macaques) and Cynomolgus monkeys represent the most extensively utilized and characterized NHP models in contemporary research. The reproductive physiology and embryonic development characteristics of Cynomolgus monkeys and Rhesus macaques are very similar to those of humans. Their embryonic and fetal development

Table. 9.1 Principle advantages and disadvantages of NHPs for developmental and reproductive toxicity testing

NHPs advantages	NHPs disadvantages	Rodent/rabbit
• Generally more phylogenetically and physiologically similar to humans than other species • More likely than rodents to show similar pharmacology to humans • Placentation similar to human • Placentation similar to human • Transfer of antibodies across the placenta similar to humans	• Small number of test facilities • Less historical control data and laboratory experience/capability • Limited supply of sexually mature animals • Long menstrual cycle (30 days) and gestation (165 days) • Impractical for fertility (mating) studies • F1 reproduction function not practical to evaluate due to late sexual maturity (around 3–6 years of age) Smaller group sizes, therefore lower statistical power and higher inter-group variability. Phase I: 5–8 per group ePPND: 16–20 per group, 16 per group as in ICH S5 (R3) • Single offspring • High abortion rate (usually 10%–20% but can be as high as 40%) • Low fertility rate (35%–45% per cycle; –60% per female) • Small number of fetuses/infants for evaluation (10–16/group) • Long-duration studies (12–30 months) • Sexual maturity cannot be determined by age and body weight • Ethical considerations • Highly variable age, weight, and pregnancy history at the start	• Large number of test facilities • Vast historical database • Sexually mature animals readily available • Sexual maturity 2–3 months • The group sizes for the following phases can be easily achieved: Phase I: 20–25 animals/group Phase II: 18–20 animals/group Phase III: 20–25 animals/group • High fertility rate (>90%) • Low abortion/resorption rate (<1%) • Multiple offspring (8–12/litter) • Large number of fetuses/pups for evaluation(200+/group) • Short-duration studies (4–6 months)

processes also share many similarities, and background data can be cross-referenced. However, rhesus macaques can reach a maximum weight of 20 kg, have a long breeding cycle and low fertility, and are now rarely used. In addition, marmosets can also be used for animal experiments. However, it has a too small body size (with a weight range of 250–500 g), a large upper limit of blood volume, and significant differences from human reproductive physiology, so it is rarely used in toxicology research. Therefore, Cynomolgus monkeys are the most suitable nonhuman primate models for DART studies.

In general, the reproductive parameters and feedback mechanisms of Cynomolgus monkeys are very similar to those of humans (Table 9.2). Cynomolgus monkeys provide a robust model for the study of numerous reproductive physiological characteristics. Cynomolgus monkeys exhibit a reproductive endocrinology highly similar to that of both human males and females. For example, in females, the principles of endocrine control of the human menstrual cycle were initially described using animal

Table. 9.2 Comparison of female reproductive systems between humans and Cynomolgus monkeys

Chronology of reproduction	*Cynomolgus*	*Human*
Lifespan	25–30 years	Human 75–80 years
Puberty/sexual maturity	2.5–4 years	10–18 years
Menopause	20–25 years	50 years
Seasonality	All year—no seasonality	All year—no seasonality
Menstrual cycle length	28–32 days	28–30 days
Ovulation	Day 11–14 of the Menstrual cycle	Day 13–15 of the Menstrual cycle
Implantation window	Day 9–15 of pregnancy	Day 6–13 of pregnancy
Gestation time (normal)	160 days (range [observed extremes]: 134–184)	280 days (range: 259–294)
Organogenesis	Gestational weeks 3–7 (Days 20–50)	Gestational weeks 3–8 (Days 20–57)
Average weight of offspring at term	Mean: 350 g (325–375 g)	Mean: 3.4 kg
Number of offspring	Uniparous (twinning 0.1%)	Uniparous (twinning 1%)
Ovary		
Average size (per ovary)	1.0 × 0.8 × 0.8 cm	2 × 1.5 × 0.5–4 × 2 × 1 cm
Average weight (paired)	0.42 g ± 0.14 g	10–16 g
Average weight (per ovary)	Right ovary weight: 0.21 g right (min: 0.02, max: 0.57, $n = 100$); Left ovary weight: 0.21 g left (min: 0.08, max: 0.94, $n = 100$)	Single ovary: 5–8 g
Total number of oocytes	Fetal: 5–7 million; Birth: 1–2 million; Menarche: 200–450 thousand	Fetal: 6–7 million (at 20 weeks); Birth: 1–2 million; Menarche: 300–500 thousand
Developmental time (initial recruitment to Graafian follicle)	215 days (30 weeks, 7 cycles)	195 days (28 weeks, 7 cycles)
Follicular size	Primordial: 30–40 μm; Primary: 70–100 μm; Early secondary: 150 μm; Advanced secondary: 250 μm; Early tertiary: 400–500 μm; Advanced tertiary: 1–2 mm; Preovulatory: 3–5 mm	Primordial: 40–60 μm; Primary: 90–130 μm; Secondary: <300 μm; Early tertiary: 2–5 mm; Advanced tertiary: 3–8 mm; Preovulatory: 16–25 mm
Ovulation	Mono-ovulatory	Mono-ovulatory
Corpus luteum size	Maximum diameter: 10 mm	Maximum diameter: 20 mm
Microscopic appearance	The luteal body is composed of uniformly large luteal cells	The luteal body is composed of a majority of centrally located large luteal cells and a minority of peripherally located small luteal cells
Corpus luteum life span	14 ± 2 days	14 ± 2 days
Common pathologic conditions	Ovarian cysts; Granulosa cell tumors; Cortical (follicular) mineralization, multiple	Ovarian cysts; Surface/stromal tumors

Table 9.2 (Continued)

Uterus		
Anatomic classification	Uterus simplex	Uterus simplex
Average size	40 mm in length (incl. cervix) × 20 mm	75 mm in length, 50 mm in diameter at its upper part, and nearly 25 mm thick
Average weight/weight range	7.42 ± 2.98 g (range: 2.83–16.37 g)	40–80 g
Gland morphology	Onset of subnuclear (glycogen) vacuolation in the glands of the functionalis is preovulatory; Postovulatory intensification of the epithelial proliferation in the zona basalis	Onset of subnuclear (glycogen) vacuolation in the glands of the functionalis is definitely postovulatory; Postovulatory, a quiescent zona basalis
Stroma morphology	Pseudodecidualization: not present—very poor	Pseudodecidualization: moderate
Stroma estrogen receptor (Er) expression	Er is downregulated in stromal cells during the luteal phase	Stromal cells express the estrogen receptor throughout the whole luteal phase
Common pathologic conditions	Adenomyosis, endometriosis, endometrial polyps, leiomyoma	Adenomyosis, endometriosis, endometrial polyps, leiomyoma, endometrium hyperplasia, endometrium carcinoma
Placenta		
Average placental weight at term	150 g	540 g ± 100 g
Placenta classification	Shape: Bidiscoid (70%) or discoid; Structure: Villous placenta; Maternal relationship: Deciduate hemochorial placenta	Shape: Discoid; Structure: Villous placenta; Maternal relationship: Deciduate hemochorial placenta
Early placentation	Medium-grade stromal decidualization; Temporary epithelial plaque	Prominent stromal decidualization; No epithelial plaque
Implantation site	Divided into primary and secondary implantation sites	Single implantation site
Blastocyst	Luminal (part of the blastocyst exposed to the lumen)	Interstitial (blastocyts embedded within the endometrium)
Trophoblast invasion	Endometrial: Superficial; Arterial: Aggressive	Endometrial: Deeper in the endometrium: Arterial: Less aggressive
Trophoblastic shell	Regular, continuous, relatively thick, and sharply delineated from the underlying endometrium with a relatively small number of loose trophoblasts	Irregular with many extravillous, invading trophoblasts
Functional uteroplacental circulation	Established in the 3rd week postconception	Established in the 6th week postconception

Table 9.2 (Continued)

Persistent maternal vascular changes in the myometrium	Common, can persist for months or even years	Not described
Common pathologic conditions	Epithelial plaque in the absence of pregnancy	Extrauterine pregnancy
Cervix		
Average size	15 mm long; −18 mm in diameter	25–30 mm long and 20–25 mm in diameter
Shape the cervical canal	Sigmoid; transvaginal endometrial biopsy not possible	Straight
Transformation zone	Distinct	Distinct
Common pathologic conditions	Squamous cell metaplasia; CIN (cervical intraepithelial neoplasia) (papilloma virus [MPV]-related)	Reserve cell & squamous cell metaplasia; CIN (human papilloma virus [HPV]-related); squamous cell carcinoma
Mammary gland		
Thelarche	1.5–2.5 years	10–14 years
Common pathologic conditions	Ductal hyperplasia and carcinoma; Focal lobular hyperplasia	Ductal hyperplasia and carcinoma

models of Macaca. In males, the hormonal dependence of spermatogonial proliferation (at the cellular level) is the same in Cynomolgus monkeys and humans [3].

The sperm production cycle of male Cynomolgus monkeys is 40–46 days, while that of humans is 64–74 days. Both take 5–10 days to transport sperm through the epididymis. The spermatogonial proliferation of Cynomolgus Monkeys is hormone-dependent, similar to that of humans, and insufficient endocrine hormones at an early stage have a direct impact on the differentiation of spermatogonia in both humans and Cynomolgus monkeys. Cynomolgus monkeys represent a suitable animal model for investigating prostate growth and function.

9.2 Current Status of NHP DART Research Institutions

9.2.1 Current Status of International Cynomolgus Monkeys DART Research Institutions

Wild NHPs are absent from European and American countries. Consequently, a 2019 US study utilized NHPs sourced 60% from China, while the EU's NHP supply was derived almost entirely from imports originating in China, Indonesia, Vietnam, Cambodia, the Philippines, and Mauritius. NHPs have always been a scarce resource due to inherent physiological characteristics, such as the large inter-individual variation in the onset and development of puberty and age at sexual maturity (2.5–5 years), and low fecundity resulting from high rates of abortion, stillbirth, and post-natal mortality (<1 offspring/female per year). Due to the impact of the COVID-19 pandemic, the supply of NHPs available for nonclinical toxicity evaluation of new drugs in Europe and America has further decreased. Driven by these factors, both the industry and the FDA are strongly pushing for reduced reliance on NHPs in nonclinical drug safety evaluations. The 2021 annual meeting of the FDA, the preclinical safety leadership group (DruSafe), and the nonclinical Safety expert group of the Biotechnology Innovation Organization (BioSafe) focused on identifying ways to improve the use of NHPs under current regulations. Collaboration between pharmaceutical companies and regulators to develop alternative methods is encouraged, but the progress will be slow.

With an early start and strong emphasis on NHP research, Developed countries such as Europe and America have achieved a significant lead in medical research and biotechnology. Rapid progress in the early 2000s solidified their dominance in areas such as NHP gene modification, gene knockout, epigenetics, precise genome editing, and the precise regulation of local gene expression in experimental primates. Refinement of methodologies and guidelines for the evaluation of reproductive and developmental toxicity in Cynomolgus monkeys is an active area of research, resulting in enhanced reliability and translational potential. Specific advancements include optimized perinatal study design, sampling time, and data analysis strategies. Currently, institutions with mature and extensive experience in conducting NHP reproductive and developmental toxicity evaluation are still primarily located overseas.

9.2.1.1 Current Status of NHP Reproductive and Developmental Research in the United States

Although the US has no wild nonhuman primate (NHP) populations, it hosts several leading primate research facilities. Notably, publicly available information indicates that this includes seven National Primate Research Centers (NPRCs) funded by the National Institutes of Health (NIH). These centers develop NHP models for both basic and applied research aimed at advancing human health. These seven NPRCs maintain more than 20 distinct species of NHPs, with a combined population ranging from 18,000 to 20,000 individuals. A substantial proportion of this population consists of macaques, which are primarily selected for their utility in practical applications and research settings [4].

Investments have grown significantly with the advancement of research techniques and methodologies using primate models. Between the fiscal years 2018 and 2022, the funding for NHP research by the U.S. Federal Government increased by 12%. Concurrently, the total number of NHPs at the seven NPRCs rose from 26,181 to 27,067. Other institutions with a strong focus on NHP research also receive federal and state funding. Even some private NHP breeding facilities also receive government grants to sustain the overall capacity for NHP research in the United States. Research institutions in Europe and the United States that conduct studies related to NHP reproduction and development are listed in Table 9.3.

Table. 9.3 NHP reproductive and developmental research facilities in Europe and the United States

Facility	Research direction	Link
California National Primate Research Center	All developmental stages (embryo, fetus, newborn, infant), juveniles, young adults, premenopausal/ transitional reproductive stages	https://cnprc.ucdavis.edu/
Oregon National Primate Research Center)	Reproduction and controlling reproductive disorders and fertility	https://www.ohsu.edu/onprc
Southwest National Primate Research Center	Animal reproduction	https://snprc.org/
Tulane National Primate Research Center	Infectious and chronic diseases	https://tnprc.tulane.edu/
Emory/Yerkes National Primate Research Center	Neural development	https://www.enprc.emory.edu/
Washington National Primate Research Center	Neurobiological sciences, AIDS-related research, reproductive and developmental sciences, genomics, etc	https://www.washington.edu/
Wisconsin National Primate Research Center	Regenerative and reproductive medicine, neuroscience	https://primate.wisc.edu/
Karolinska Institutet	Developmental biology, reproductive medicine	https://ki.se/
Centre of Reproductive Medicine and Andrology/ Westfälische Wilhelms-Universität Münster	The function of testicular stem and germ cells, the regulation of spermatogenesis, sperm physiology, and embryonic development.	https://www.medizin.uni-muenster.de/en/cera/

9.2.1.2 Current Status of NHP Reproductive and Developmental Research in Europe

In Europe, around 10,000 NHPs are used each year for evaluating the safety of pharmaceuticals and medical devices, and for basic biological research and the development of medical products and devices. The EU-funded EUPRIM-Net (European Primate Network) connects nine European primate centers to support their broad biological and biomedical research and development activities. From 2011 to 2015, the EU invested over €9 million in the EUPRIM-Net project, significantly contributing to NHP breeding and scientific research, particularly advancing and refining the 3Rs principles for NHPs [4].

The EU imposes rigorous restrictions on the employment of NHPs, allowing their use exclusively in specific areas of research. In nonclinical safety assessments for novel drugs, substances, and medical devices intended primarily for human use, NHPs are employed in approximately 67% of the tests. Nearly all of these primate studies are mandatory and required by nonclinical safety assessment regulations. Of all NHPs used for safety assessments, approximately half are involved in medium-and long-term repeated-dose toxicity studies, which require repeated administration of the tested drug. One-third are utilized for single-dose studies, and the remaining are used for research on reproductive and developmental effects or other experiments. Additionally, primates are also used in basic biological research (approximately 14% of all NHPs used) and in the research and development of human medical and dental products and devices (approximately 13% of all NHPs used).

9.2.1.3 Current Status of NHP Reproductive and Developmental Research in Southeast Asia

Despite the prominence of the United States and Europe in NHP research, Southeast Asian countries, which host native populations of such primates, are increasingly directing attention to these important resources. Southeast Asia has witnessed a notable enhancement in its NHP research infrastructure in recent years, resulting in the establishment of multiple research institutions and breeding facilities. Notably, some of these breeding facilities have obtained accreditation from the Association for Assessment and Accreditation of Laboratory Animal Care (AAALAC). With these facilities and their attendant resources, the capacity for investigations utilizing NHPs has been substantially improved across the region.

9.2.1.4 Current Status of NHP Reproductive and Developmental Research in Multinational Pharmaceutical Companies

Apart from government or non-government public sectors, global pharmaceutical giants and their respective contract research organizations (CROs) hold a more prominent position in NHP DART research and its practical applications. According to current reports, the primary organizations conducting NHP reproductive and developmental toxicity research are top-tier global pharmaceutical companies. CROs, specialized scientific institutions offering outsourced services to pharmaceutical companies in drug development, have become a cornerstone of the global pharmaceutical R&D value chain. Indispensable to multinational pharmaceutical corporations, large-scale pharmaceutical enterprises, and biotechnology firms in early-stage product development and clinical trials, CROs leverage their extensive project experience to achieve significant cost savings (30%–70%) and accelerate new drug development timelines (by 1/4–1/3), thereby playing a crucial role in drug R&D. An analysis of the global drug safety evaluation market reveals that in 2017, the market size for nonclinical safety evaluation was $4.08 billion, which subsequently increased to $6.64 billion in 2021. Projections suggest that by 2026, this market will expand significantly to $16.06 billion. Table 9.4 lists some examples of biologics for which reproductive and developmental toxicity studies were conducted in NHPs.

(1) Covance Laboratories (currently LabCorp) partnered with AstraZeneca to undertake a study examining background pregnancy outcome data in Cynomolgus Monkeys, particularly focusing on the period surrounding the ICH guidance that suggested the use of ePPND study designs in NHP testing. This study utilized practical modeling techniques to analyze and interpret perinatal loss data in NHP developmental toxicity studies, and it facilitated the optimization of group sizes and research design for ePPND trials in Cynomolgus Monkeys. In 2020, the enhanced prototype normograms (e-normograms) for pregnant long-tailed

Table. 9.4 Examples of reproductive and developmental toxicity studies in NHPs

Generic name	Study type	CRO	Reference
Brolucizumab	ePPND	Labcorp (Germany)	Reprod Toxicol. 2023
Ofatumumab	PPND	Labcorp (Germany)	Reprod Toxicol. 2022
^{125}iodinated humanizedimmunoglobulin G2Δα	Mechanism of humanized IgG placental transfer	Covance (Germany)	Birth Defects Res. 2020
Satralizumab	ePPND	Covance (Germany)	Birth Defects Res. 2017
Daclizumab	FEED, EFD, PPND	/	Neurol Ther. 2016
Tanezumab	ePPND, EFD	SNBL (USA)	Reprod Toxicol. 2015
Taltz (ixekizumab)	FEED, EFD, PPND	Charles River (USA)	Reprod Toxicol. 2015
Denosumab	EFD, PPND	Charles River (USA)	Reprod Toxicol. 2013 Bone. 2014
AMG ZX.41	FEED	/	Regul Toxicol Pharmacol. 2013
Briakinumab	FEED, PPND	Covance (Germany)	Birth Defects Res B Dev Reprod Toxicol. 2012
Rituximab	EFD, PPND	Covance (Germany)	Toxicol Sci. 2011
Ustekinumab	EFD, ePPND	SNBL (Japan)	Birth Defects Res B Dev Reprod Toxicol. 2010
Pegylated Interferon Alpha-2b	Menstrual cycles and ovarian hormones	/	Birth Defects Res B Dev Reprod Toxicol. 2009
Golimumab	EFD (GD20–GD50), PPND (GD50–PND33)	SNBL (USA)	Am J Reprod Immunol. 2007
Onartuzumab (Phase III, failures)	ePPND	SNBL (Japan)	Toxicol Sci. 2018
MAGE-A3 (Phase III, failures)	FEED	Citoxlab (France)	Reprod Toxicol. 2015
Tabalumab (Phase III, failures)	ePPND	Charles River (USA)	Birth Defects Res B Dev Reprod Toxicol. 2015

Note: "/" indicates data is unknown or not applicable

macaques were rereleased in regulated ePPND studies to support the design and control of animal numbers in the latest ePPND research. The new normograms have higher resolution in late-term pregnancy and interbirth intervals, enabling more accurate evaluation of whether the duration of pregnancy is within the expected range. In recent years, Covance has made significant contributions to the development and pathology of male and female reproductive organs, as well as to the optimization of 3Rs in NHPs. Currently, they have completed over 120 NHPDART studies in pregnancy models and conducted more than 25 ePPND/PPND studies.

(2) Charles River Laboratories: Charles River has conducted extensive work on specialized pathophysiological changes in NHPs, as well as perinatal eye development. They have completed over 100 complex DART studies. Charles River also curates a substantial database of DART study background data, which encompasses a wide spectrum of reproductive, developmental, and juvenile toxicology information across various species, including mice, rats, rabbits, hamsters, guinea pigs, miniature pigs, and large animals (canines, NHPs). The database is intended to serve as a resource for DART investigators.

(3) SNBL Laboratories: SNBL Laboratories represents one of the select few institutions worldwide with the capacity to execute reproductive and developmental toxicity studies utilizing NHP models. They can conduct EFD, PPND, and ePPND toxicity studies for biotechnology-derived drugs. They also perform juvenile toxicity and testicular toxicity studies. Furthermore, SNBL has published numerous findings concerning NHP genetic polymorphisms, biomolecular profiling, and genetic mutations.

9.2.2 Current Status of Domestic Cynomolgus Monkeys DART Research Institutions

Compared to the United States and Europe, China possesses abundant NHP resources, with over 24 species identified. It represents approximately 6% of the world's primate species. In particular, Yunnan Province possesses the most abundant NHP resources and undertakes the majority of early and current NHP research. Despite being a leading source of NHP resources, China is behind other nations in the development of innovative long-acting NHP models. Conversely, while reproductive and developmental toxicology research in China started relatively late, it has demonstrated remarkably rapid progress.

The economic crises and resulting "austerity" budgets in the US and developed European countries have led to a decline or standstill in funding for NHP research. Moreover, mounting criticism from animal rights activists and the intense pressure from animal welfare have forced some research institutions to restrict, or even cease, NHP research. Conscious of the significant advantages and benefits gained from NHP research, an increasing number of researchers from developed countries are actively seeking partnerships with primate research institutions in China and other Southeast Asian developing countries. Such collaborations could potentially bring to China unprecedented opportunities and substantial challenges in the fields of life science and biomedical research.

To foster China's shift from being a producer of NHP resources to a nation leading in NHP research, the Chinese government has increased its investment considerably in experimental primates and new drug development. Since 2010, significant advancements have been made in research and innovation involving experimental primates.

Currently, several universities and research institutions in China have established dedicated experimental animal centers, reproductive toxicology research teams, or laboratories specifically for studying the reproductive and developmental toxicity of Cynomolgus Monkeys. Breeding and rearing facilities for Cynomolgus monkeys have been established, guaranteeing a large and consistent supply of experimental animals to satisfy research requirements. The technical expertise of researchers in reproductive and developmental toxicology studies using Cynomolgus Monkeys is also continuously advancing. By learning from international peers, innovating independently, adopting new detection technologies, and standardizing experimental designs, the reliability and precision of NHP reproductive and developmental toxicity research have been substantially enhanced. It must be recognized that the use of Cynomolgus monkeys and other primates is rigorously regulated by laws and regulations due to concerns about bioethics and animal conservation. Therefore, when conducting research in this area, it is imperative to adhere to relevant ethical and animal welfare guidelines and obtain the necessary regulatory approvals. Overall, both domestic and international efforts are continuously advancing the progress of Cynomolgus monkeys' reproductive and developmental toxicity research, with the aim of enhancing the safety assessment of pharmaceuticals and chemicals and contributing to human health and environmental protection.

In 2018, under the auspices of China's "13th Five-Year Plan" for the National Major New Drug Innovation Program, the Shanghai Institute of Planned Parenthood Research, now known as the Shanghai Institute of Biomedical and Pharmaceutical Technologies (Chinese National Evaluation Center for the Toxicology of Fertility Regulating Drugs), along with the Hubei Nonhuman Primate Reproductive and Developmental Toxicity Research Platform, successfully applied for and received approval for the project titled "Establishment and Application of Key Technologies in Nonclinical Reproductive and Developmental Toxicology of Drugs" (Project Number: 2018ZX09201017002). This initiative included a sub-task aimed at "Establishing and Enhancing the Reproductive and Developmental Toxicology Technology System for Experimental Monkeys and Promoting Its Application," which has now been completed to satisfaction. Under the auspices of the National Major Program, the Hubei Nonhuman Primate Reproductive and Developmental Toxicity Research Platform has successfully completed the construction and validation of a reproductive and developmental toxicity platform for Cynomolgus monkeys. This includes multiple fertility assessments accompanying repeated-dose toxicity tests (sexual maturity) in Cynomolgus monkeys, as well as EFD and ePPND studies on the blood–testis barrier, placental barrier, and blood–milk barrier following the administration of a monoclonal antibody. Presently, the platform is engaged in conducting GLP-compliant reproductive and developmental toxicity tests aimed at new drug registration. Moreover, multiple CROs are considering the establishment of NHP platforms dedicated to reproductive and developmental toxicity studies. Besides CROs, research institutions such as the Kunming Institute of Zoology, Chinese Academy of Sciences, and the NHP Research Platform of the Excellence in Brain Science and Intelligence Technology, Chinese Academy of Sciences are also actively advancing the progress of NHP research in China, particularly in areas like development, physiology, and neuroscience.

9.3 Key Considerations for NHP Reproductive and Developmental Toxicity Testing

9.3.1 Key Considerations for NHP in FEED Studies

The purpose of FEED toxicity studies is to determine the toxicological effects of dosing during the period from pre-mating (both males and females) up to mating and implantation. The research has further investigated possible changes in the estrous cycle of females and evaluated potential functional impairments, which might be missed in single and repeat dose toxicity assessments, by histologically examining the reproductive organs of males.

(1) Clinical pathological indicators for assessing fertility in NHPs

For NHPs, fertility is typically not assessed through cohabitation mating. ICH S5 (R3) guidelines identify histopathological evaluation of reproductive organs, performed in repeat-dose toxicity studies with a dosing period of not less than 3 months, as an alternative method for fertility assessment. This methodology must include a complete histopathologic assessment of the reproductive organs in both male and female subjects.

Furthermore, the criteria for infertility diagnosis employed by gynecologists and andrologists are applied to NHPs in order to evaluate influences on both male and female fertility. Thus, numerous parameters are available for consideration (as shown in Table 9.5). The fertility of NHPs can be assessed in targeted studies of male and female reproductive function, as well as in the context of standard toxicity evaluations. Evaluation of the reproductive tract (organ weights and histopathological assessment) is performed in repeat-dose toxicity studies lasting at least 3 months, provided sexually mature animals are used, and no adverse findings are observed. In the event of significant negative outcomes or specific concerns, a more comprehensive examination of fertility is warranted, employing more sophisticated parameters including testicular volumetry, semen analysis, and evaluation of spermatogenesis [5].

It is particularly important that proper sampling and processing procedures are utilized for the testes and epididymides to maintain the integrity of the seminiferous epithelium. A thorough microscopic qualitative assessment of the spermatogenic cycle offers a sensitive means of detecting alterations in spermatogenesis. Additional endpoints, like immunohistochemistry, homogenization-resistant sperm counts, flow cytometry, and quantitative analysis of testicular staging, while often not crucial, can be employed in the experimental design to provide further characterization of any identified impacts. For female animals, a thorough microscopic qualitative assessment of the ovaries (including follicles, corpora lutea, stroma, interstitium, and vasculature),

Table. 9.5 Clinical parameters for evaluating male and female NHP fertility

Male	Females
Spermatogenesis Histology Spermatogenic stages	*Oogenesis* Histology
Sperm maturation Epididymis	*Ovarian cyclicity* Swabs Hormone levels
Semen parameters	
Testis size Caliper Ultrasound	*Endometrial changes* Biopsies Ultrasound
Testis biopsy	*Ultrasound examination* Follicular growth Cysts
Endocrinology luteinizing hormone, LH follicle-stimulating hormone, FSH prolactin, PRL estrogen, E progesterone, P androgen, A Inhibin B, INH B Sex hormone binding globulin (SHBG)	*Endocrinology* LH FSH chorionic gonadotropin, CG Prolactin Estrogens Estrogens Androgens Inhibin A/B, INH A/B
Prostate status Volume Uroflow	
Fertility (mating)	*Fertility (mating)*

uterus, and vagina is required, alongside consideration of the reproductive cycle and the presence of primordial and primary follicles.

The following data can serve as a reference for the physiological parameters of reproductive organs in Cynomolgus monkeys [5].

Testes: For adult animals, the mean weight of the left testis is 21.18 g ± 6.69 g, and the right is 20.98 g ± 5.47 g. No statistically significant difference is found between the weights of the left and right testes. Testicular weight as a percentage of body weight increases significantly from juvenile to adult stages ($P = 0.0001$), with a marked increase in the percentage of total body weight represented by the combined weight of both testes in adults. In sexually mature animals, the testis weight accounts for more than 0.25% of their body weight. In aged animals, the testicular weight as a proportion of body weight does not exhibit a decline.

Prostate: In adult animals, the mean absolute prostate weight is 5.30 g ± 1.66 g, representing approximately 0.08% of body weight. Juvenile and peripubertal animals exhibit a significantly lower percentage of prostate weight relative to body weight compared to young, adult, and aged animals ($P < 0.0001$). There is no further increase in prostate weight relative to body weight in aged animals compared to adult animals.

Ovaries: The mean weight of the left ovary in adult animals is 0.26 g ± 0.12 g, and the right is 0.24 g ± 0.12 g. The percentage of ovarian weight relative to body weight increases significantly from the juvenile to the adult stage of life ($P < 0.001$). From early adulthood, the percentage of body weight accounted for by the combined weight of both ovaries tends to stabilize.

Uterus: In ovary-intact females, juvenile animals have a lower uterine weight of 0.25 g ± 0.13 g, while adult animals have a weight of 5.41 g ± 2.82 g ($P < 0.0218$). Following adulthood, ovariectomized animals have a mean uterine weight of 1.60 g ± 1.25 g, compared to 5.41 g ± 2.82 g in adult non-ovariectomized uterine. Uterine weight in juveniles is approximately 0.2%–0.3% of body weight, while it is 0.05% in ovariectomized animals ($P < 0.0001$).

9.3.2 Key Considerations for Sperm Assessment

Male fertility study design in clinical research constantly faces a dilemma, which highlights the unique and irreplaceable role of NHPs in evaluating male fertility. Specifically, the ethical acceptability of using young male volunteers in trials is called into question whenever there is any residual doubt concerning the reversibility of a drug's effects as observed in pre-clinical studies with rats. Clearly, aged male volunteers offer minimal benefit in fertility assessments, thereby emphasizing the unique importance of NHPs.

Within the framework of nonclinical safety evaluations, the histopathological analysis of reproductive organs plays a pivotal role in evaluating reproductive outcomes for both males and females. The age and reproductive status of animals in these investigations play a critical role in assessing the reproductive system, interpreting the potential findings associated with the test substances, and ultimately influencing the risk assessment outcomes. Nonclinical safety trials employ animals of varying ages based on research design, species, institutional conventions, and/or animal availability. In both inter-and intra-study settings, animals may present to toxicological pathologists at various stages of age and reproductive system development. This variability necessitates a thorough understanding of the normal anatomy, physiology, and histology of the reproductive system across different ages and species [6].

The most common adverse reactions to drugs are a decrease in sperm count (reduced spermatogenesis or death of developing and developed sperm), followed by reduced sperm viability, abnormal sperm morphology, testicular atrophy, and tumorigenesis (most commonly benign interstitial cell tumors in rodents). Some of these drugs have also been observed to produce similar results in humans, including reduced sperm count, decreased viability, and abnormal sperm morphology. The DailyMed database, established by the National Library of Medicine (NLM), contains up-to-date drug labeling information for over 85% of FDA-approved drugs. A statistical analysis of this database identified 235 FDA-approved drugs (17%; 235/1318) containing active ingredients that may cause a reduction in sperm count/concentration or a decrease in sperm quality, viability, or fertility, based on data from at least one animal model. Rats are the most commonly used animal model in reproductive toxicity studies (184 out of 235), while only 34 out of 235 drugs affect spermatogenesis in primates. While established methods used to evaluate reproductive toxicity are useful for informing clinical decisions and have been refined through automation and advanced analysis (such as of sperm viability subtypes), they were initially developed in the 1960s and 1970s, and may not fully capture current needs.

Studies estimate that sperm or semen abnormalities (affecting parameters such as sperm count, morphology, and viability, or semen volume, composition, and viscosity) contribute to infertility in 5%–10% of men in developed countries. In systematic reviews of infertile men, medication is a frequently identified exogenous factor. However, the effects of most drugs on male reproductive function (spermatogenesis, sperm parameters, and sexual function) are generally unclear, except for a few prescription drugs that have undergone rigorous reproductive toxicity tests [7].

Numerous studies on spermatotoxicity indicate that the predictive value of animal models for human toxicity may be lower than anticipated. Of the drugs with documented adverse effects in animals, only 27% (63/235) are reported (in drug labels or the literature) to have negative impacts on human sperm. Further research indicates that less than half of the drug labels reporting adverse effects on human sperm also indicate similar findings in animals. For over half of the drugs with adverse effects on animal spermatogenesis or sperm, the impact on humans remains unclear due to a lack of testing, monitoring, or reporting of results (Table 9.6). Even in cases with clear reports of the type of human sperm toxicity and a number of affected individuals, the data are often insufficient to determine the reversibility of these effects or the time required for recovery.

9.3.3 Key Considerations for Ovarian Assessment

Ovarian development and function in females are highly susceptible to toxicant-induced damage, which can be triggered via direct exposure, endocrine disruption, and transgenerational epigenetic inheritance. Given that mating assessments are often infeasible in NHPs, comprehensive histopathological examination of female reproductive organs represents a crucial approach for evaluating potential drug effects on female reproductive function. Assessment of ovarian toxicity relies on the established cyclical morphology of the reproductive tract, including the ovaries. This allows for the identification of pathological signs such as follicular depletion, increased follicular atresia, and an increased incidence of currently formed corpora lutea. This assessment can provide valuable insights into the effects on female reproductive performance, as manifested by irregularities of the estrous cycle and preimplantation loss. If previous research has revealed pharmacological activity or identified alterations suggestive of reproductive system damage, including histopathological changes with potential implications for female fertility, further in-depth evaluation, such as menstrual cycle analysis or hormone monitoring in repeat-dose toxicology studies, may be required [8].

Precise assessment of follicle counts across various developmental phases is an essential indicator of folliculogenesis, intimately associated with endocrine signaling and paracrine/autocrine pathways that regulate the development and maturation

Table. 9.6 FDA-approved drugs with adverse effects on sperm (NHP vs. human)

Main category	Generic name	Effect(s) in animals	Species	Human toxicity	Reported effect(s) in humans (PubMed)
Antihyperlipidemic agent	Rosuvastatin calcium	Testicular spermatidic giant cells are visible, with vacuolization of the epididymal epithelium	Dogs, NHPs	Yes	Reversible azoospermia
Antineoplastic agent	Abiraterone acetate	Testicular atrophy, aspermia/hypospermia, reduced sperm counts and motility, altered morphology	Rats, NHPs	No/uncertain	Decreased testosterone and decreased weights of androgen-responsive organs in a xenograft fetal testis model
	Ado-trastuzumab emtansine	Degeneration of seminiferous tubules with hemorrhage in the testes, decreased weights of the epididymides, prostate, and seminal vesicles	Rats, NHPs	Uncertain	No studies identified
	Cladribine	Testicular degeneration	NHPs	Uncertain	No studies identified
	Ponatinib	Degeneration of the epithelium of the testes	Rats, NHPs	No/uncertain	No studies identified
	Ziv-aflibercept	Decreased sperm motility, alterations in sperm morphology	NHPs	Uncertain	No studies identified
Antituberculosis agent/ anti-infectious	Rifabutin	Testicular atrophy	Rats, NHPs	Uncertain	No studies identified
Antiviral agent	Cidofovir	Inhibition of spermatogenesis	Rats, NHPs	Uncertain	No studies identified
Cardiovascular agent	Propafenone hydrochloride	Decreased spermatogenesis	Rabbits, dogs, and NHPs	Uncertain	No studies identified
Immunological factor	ACTIMMUNE® (Interferon gamma-1b)	Decreased spermatogenesis and sperm counts, increased abnormal sperm (very high doses), and monkeys	Mice, NHPs	Uncertain	Effect of local or systemic treatment unclear, but no effect on sperm treated in vitro
Ophthalmic drug	Aflibercept	Changes in sperm morphology and motility	NHPs	Uncertain	No studies identified
Antibacterial agent	Clarithromycin	Testicular atrophy	Rats, NHPs	No	Improves motility(Seminal Helicobacter pylori treatment improves sperm motility in infertile asthenozoospermic men)

of both the oocyte and its surrounding follicular cells. Ovarian histopathology can serve as a valuable assessment tool in fertility research to evaluate the development of follicles within the ovaries. Ovarian changes are strictly regulated by hormones and growth factors. The stimulation of follicular growth, along with the majority of follicular development stagnation, leads to the periodic changes in female reproduction in mammals, ultimately resulting in the release of viable oocytes. The development of follicles within the ovary relies on and is supplemented by a pool of non-growing immature primordial follicles. These follicles synchronize their transition into the growth phase while managing the depletion rate of the follicle reserve.

Ovarian assessment is an important endpoint in toxicological evaluation, as the loss of oogonia, oocytes, or supporting cells may adversely affect reproduction. Accurate follicle counting can complement the qualitative assessment of the ovaries to identify the characteristics of ovarian toxicants, understand their sites of action, and evaluate the integrity of primordial follicles when ovarian lesions are minimal. Nonetheless, it is important to acknowledge that the data obtained from counting follicles may exhibit significant variability, which can complicate their interpretation. When a reduction or damage of small follicles is clearly observed in qualitative histological examinations, follicle counting may provide little or no additional information for identifying chemical hazards. The evaluation of ovarian toxicity should employ a weight-of-evidence approach, taking into account qualitative histopathological data and other available information, such as fertility data, clinical observations, organ weights, and male reproductive toxicity data. Inspections should be carried out by a toxicologic pathologist who is knowledgeable about the normal reproductive cycle of the species, and should encompass an evaluation of all major ovarian components (follicles, corpora lutea, stroma, interstitium, and vasculature), with special emphasis on the qualitative evaluation of primordial and primary follicles. Ovarian qualitative assessments should be integrated with a microscopic examination of the entire reproductive tract, considering all supplementary reproductive data, including organ weights and estrous cycles [9].

Moreover, similar to the toxicity research on sperm in male fertility, the effects of drugs that have been shown to adversely affect ovarian development and function in animals are also not clearly defined in humans (Table 9.7).

9.3.4 Evaluation Methods for the Menstrual Cycle in Cynomolgus Monkeys

The menstrual cycle of Cynomolgus Monkeys consists of a follicular phase lasting 12–14 days, an ovulatory phase lasting 3 days, and a luteal phase lasting 14–16 days. The lengths of the ovulatory and luteal phases are consistent between Cynomolgus monkeys and humans. However, the duration of the follicular phase is more variable. The common method for confirming the menstrual cycle in Cynomolgus monkeys involves gently collecting vaginal bleeding samples using a cotton swab. In accordance with the established subjective grading standards, the blood volume observed on the swab can be divided into four to five classes: ① No bleeding; ② Mild bleeding;

Table. 9.7 Some FDA-approved drugs have negative effects on the ovaries (NHP vs. human)

Main category	Generic name	Effect(s) in animals	Species	Human toxicity	Reported effect(s) in humans (DailyMed/PubMed)
Hormone modulators	Ospemifene	Decreases in ovarian and uterine weights, decreased corpora lutea number, increased ovarian cysts, uterine atrophy, and disrupted cycles were observed	Rats, NHPs	Yes	Vaginal discharge, Endometrial thickening, Endometrial Cancer
	Toremifene citrate	Cystic ovaries and reduction in endometrial stromal cellularity	Mice, Rats, dogs, NHPs	Yes	Endometrial cancer, endometrial hypertrophy, hyperplasia, and uterine polyps
Antineoplastic agent/ estrogen antagonists	Elacestrant	Atrophy of the vagina, cervix, and uterus, and follicular cysts in the ovary	Rats, NHPs	Uncertain	No studies identified
Antineoplastic agent	Lenvatinib	Follicular atresia of the ovaries, decreased incidence of menstruation	Rats, NHPs	Uncertain	No studies identified
	Sacituzumab govitecan-hziy	Endometrial atrophy, uterine hemorrhage, increased follicular atresia of the ovary, and atrophy of vaginal epithelial cells	NHPs	Uncertain	No studies identified
	Dasatinib	Uterine inflammation and mineralization	Rats, NHPs	Uncertain	Uterine hemorrhage, and vaginal hemorrhage
	Ramucirumab	Increased duration of the follicular cycle, dose-dependent increases in follicular mineralization of the ovary	NHPs	Uncertain	No studies identified
	Trastuzumab	Decreases in the weight of the uterus	Rats, NHPs	Uncertain	No studies identified
	Ziv-aflibercept	Inhibited ovarian function and follicular development: decreased ovary weight, decreased amount of luteal tissue, decreased number of maturing follicles, atrophy of uterine endometrium and myometrium, vaginal atrophy, abrogation of progesterone peaks and menstrual bleeding	NHPs	Uncertain	No studies identified
Hypoglycemic agent	Rosiglitazone	Diminished the follicular phase rise in serum estradiol with consequential reduction in the luteinizing hormone surge, lower luteal phase progesterone levels, and amenorrhea	Rats, NHPs	Uncertain	May be present Ovulation abnormalities

③ Moderate bleeding; ④ Excessive bleeding; and ⑤ Extremely excessive (visible) bleeding. The first day of menstrual bleeding is designated as the first day of the menstrual cycle, while the day before the start of the next cycle is designated as the last day of the current cycle [5].

The menstrual cycle of Cynomolgus Monkeys ranges from 1 to 8 days, with 85% of cycles averaging 3–5 days. The menarche typically begins at 2–3 years of age, with the earliest occurrence of vaginal bleeding observed at 18 months of age. The cycle length typically ranges from 28 to 32 days, with a mean duration of 30.4 ± 4.7 days (a median of 30.0 days and a range of 19–69 days). No synchronization of cycles is observed among paired female animals. For female animals that have been housed individually for a long period, a prolonged menstrual cycle may occur after transitioning to group housing or following transportation. It is recommended to allow a 3- to 6-month acclimatization period to help the female animals adjust to the new housing and social environment, thereby forming a stable menstrual cycle [5, 10].

Studies have shown that there is a lack of consensus among researchers from different institutions regarding the methods used to calculate the menstrual cycle. Researchers must be trained on the standards for ascertaining the beginning and end of a menstrual cycle. Personnel tasked with determining cycle length require rigorous instruction to enable accurate and consistent interpretation of any irregular or spotting episodes occurring during the menstrual cycle. For example, a heavy menstrual flow lasting 2–3 consecutive days can easily indicate the start of the menstrual cycle. The interpretation of menstrual cycle data becomes intricate when there is a single day of light bleeding, or a day of mild bleeding succeeded by 1 or 2 days of no bleeding, followed by an additional day of light bleeding. In such cases, it becomes challenging to pinpoint the exact onset of the cycle. If all researchers use consistent standards to interpret menstrual data, it can significantly reduce data variability [11].

9.3.5 Single Housing or Group Housing

NHPs are typically social animals. The transition from single housing (Fig. 9.1) to group housing is significant for animal compatibility in both general and specific toxicity studies, particularly for sexually mature animals, as it pertains to the evaluation of reproductive toxicity endpoints. Given these considerations, certain guidelines mandate group housing for NHPs, where feasible. Group housing notably changes the body weight and testicular size of male animals, and these suppressive effects typically normalize within about 26 weeks. These effects on reproductive parameters and body weight can largely be avoided if a period of at least 26 weeks of social interaction is allowed prior to experimentation. These findings should be considered in the group housing of mature animals in toxicity research [12].

Specifically, the group housing of male animals can temporarily inhibit weight gain in comparison to single housing. This weight effect is considered to be the result of physical activity related to establishing and maintaining social status. In animals of lower status, testicular volume drops to approximately 45% of baseline levels within 13 weeks, and then recovers to baseline levels between 21 and 26 weeks. However, the

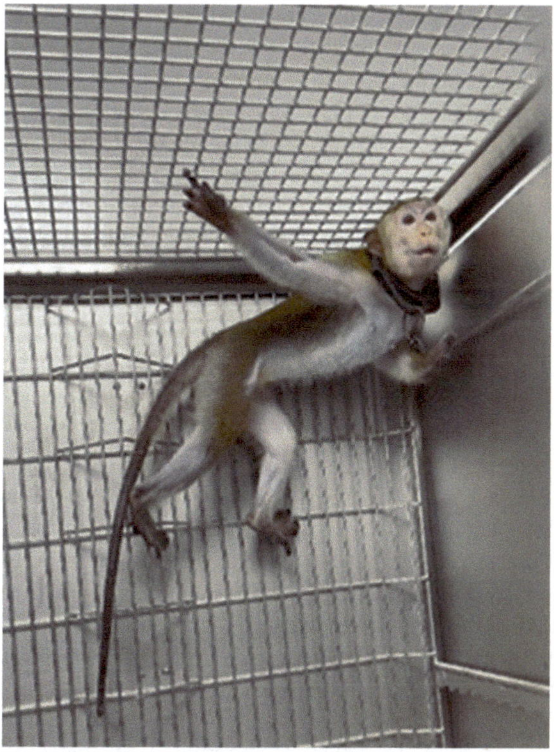

Fig. 9.1 Individual housing mode in single cage

parameters related to ejaculation and endocrine function do not exhibit corresponding changes. Grouping animals that have had prior contact and familiarity with each other can help mitigate the impacts on body weight and testicular size. For female Cynomolgus monkeys, the average duration of the menstrual cycle is prolonged during periods of group housing. The duration of the cycle rose from 31 to 46 days for about 6 months, after which it began to revert to baseline duration from the sixth cycle onward. The prolongation of the duration of the menstrual cycle corresponds to the absence or reduction of the preovulatory estradiol peak in the third cycle, along with the loss of the normal progesterone elevation. However, from the sixth cycle onward, the hormonal profile appears to return to normal. Interestingly, the effects on the menstrual cycle are also evident in pair-housed animals.

9.3.6 Key Considerations for NHP in EFD Studies

The EFD toxicity test is intended to detect adverse effects on pregnant monkeys and their fetuses following intrauterine exposure, primarily concentrating on the period between implantation and the closure of the hard palate. However, NHP pregnancies can not be diagnosed until gestational days (GD) 18–20, which means that only part of the time frame between implantation and the closure of the hard palate can be assessed (approximately until GD50 in Cynomolgus monkeys). Animals are subjected to drug administration on GD20–GD50, followed by cesarean section to retrieve and examine the fetuses. There is considerable evidence that Cynomolgus monkeys are a relevant model for detecting the effects of drugs on EFD.

9.3.6.1 Considerations for Acquiring Pregnant Female Cynomolgus Monkeys

The breeding system comprising multiple females and a single male (Fig. 9.2), referred to as the "harem" system, is the most frequently employed breeding strategy. This housing mode offers the benefit of addressing the social needs of monkeys and potentially reducing pregnancy loss. However, it also presents limitations, such as the inability to ascertain the precise gestational age or expected delivery date of fetuses. In the mating mode where one female and one male are placed in the same cage around the expected ovulation date, it is easier to estimate the age of the fetuses and the expected delivery date. However, the lack of social interaction during this process can lead to physiological changes in the animals, potentially affecting conception and embryonic survival. Additionally, this mode may not meet the animal welfare requirements for NHPs. Regardless of the mating mode used, estimating the ovulation date is necessary. However, the details of ovulation in Cynomolgus monkeys remain unclear. Historically, the estimation of ovulation dates in Cynomolgus monkeys has relied on recording menstrual cycles prior to drug administration, predicting the length of the next cycle, and selecting the midcycle as the optimal mating day (potential ovulation day). However, the midcycle can be affected by fluctuations in cycle length, leading to potential misjudgments and reduced conception rates.

Research has demonstrated that the serum levels of follicle-stimulating hormone (FSH) in Cynomolgus monkeys increase significantly between 8 and 15 days after menstruation, with ovulation occurring in the last 1–2 days. Consequently, the optimal

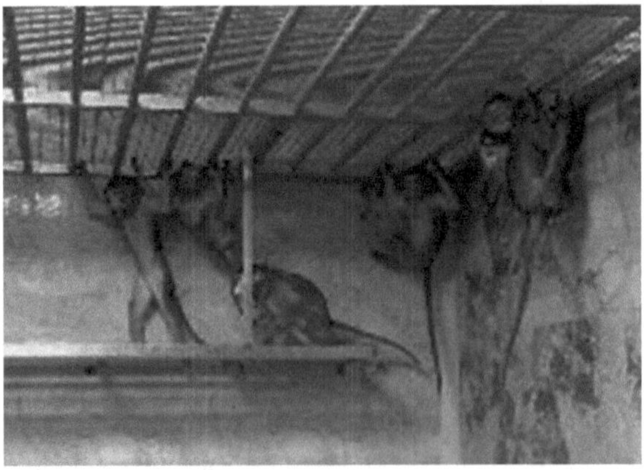

Fig. 9.2 Social group housing mode

mating period is typically regarded as being approximately 12 days following menstruation. The hormone levels in Cynomolgus monkeys are easily influenced by external stimuli. For instance, moving from single housing to group housing can significantly change the body weight and testicular size of males, and may temporarily extend or suppress the menstrual cycle of females (recovering after about 26 weeks). Therefore, developing a background database of hormone levels and monitoring them daily can enhance the success rate of ovulation predictions.

In a study focused on the reproductive efficiency of Cynomolgus monkeys and the simplification of mating systems, the differences between a 3-day timed mating system and a 7-day timed mating system, as well as the impact of age on fertility, were compared (Table 9.8). The 3-day timed mating system involved placing one male and one female in interconnected cages starting from 11 days after menstruation for 3 days, while the 7-day timed mating system began on day 9 after menstruation and lasted for 7 days. The findings showed that no statistically significant difference was found in pregnancy rates between the two mating systems ($P > 0.05$) [9].

Animals over 20 years of age are considered to have lost their reproductive capacity. Female animals under 6 years old have regular menstrual cycles, but their pregnancy rates are lower than those of older animals.

Table. 9.8 The impact of two mating strategies and female age on pregnancy rates (number of pregnancies/number of pairings)

Age	3-Day pairing system		7-Day pairing system		Number of animals	Relative pregnancy rate (%)
	Pregnancy ratio[a]	Relative pregnancy rate (%)	Pregnancy ratio[a]	Relative pregnancy rate (%)		
20–24	0/21	0	0/17	0	12	0
19	0/13	0	1/2	50.0	5	20.0
18	3/4	75.0	3/8	37.5	5	80.0
17	3/45	6.7	5/26	19.2	22	36.0
16	4/20	20.0	2/30	6.7	14	43.0
15	9/37	24.3	6/46	12.2	30	53.0
14	9/57	15.8	4/34	11.8	28	46.0
13	9/48	18.8	6/36	16.7	33	45.0
12	5/26	19.2	8/37	21.6	26	54.0
11	7/33	21.2	6/32	18.8	27	48.0
10	6/36	16.7	6/34	17.6	23	52.0
9	7/43	16.3	15/44	34.1	37	54.0
8	4/24	16.7	6/32	18.8	23	43.0
7	2/46	4.2	11/56	19.6	40	33.0
6	5/44	11.4	12/48	25.0	44	36.0
5	2/43	4.7	1/47	2.1	35	9.0
4	4/57	7.0	4/43	9.3	51	16.0
Total	78/597	13.10	95/575	16.5	455	38.0 (173/455)

Table. 9.9 Number of matings required to achieve pregnancy in animals

Number of mating times	3-Day pairing system	7-Day pairing system
1st	41 (0.53)	55 (0.58)
2nd	17 (0.22)	21 (0.21)
3rd	10 (0.13)	13 (0.13)
4th	5 (0.06)	4 (0.04)
5th	5 (0.06)	0 (0.00)
6th	0 (0.00)	2 (0.02)
Total	78	95

Moreover, regardless of the mating system or the age group of the animals, at least 50% of the animals are expected to become pregnant after their initial mating. As the number of mating pairs in a cyclical mating system increases, the pregnancy rate gradually declines, with approximately 90% of the animals becoming pregnant after three matings. The probability of pregnancy following the 6th mating is negligibly low. Therefore, if female Cynomolgus monkeys have not become pregnant after six matings, it can be considered to have lost its reproductive capacity (with a misclassification rate of less than 5%) (Table 9.9).

Given the low natural fertility rate and high incidence of spontaneous abortion in NHPs, only a small percentage of matings may lead to successful pregnancies. Thus, it is crucial to confirm pregnancy via ultrasound, which serves as the gold standard for pregnancy assessment. To avoid administering drugs to non-pregnant animals and exceeding the required animal numbers, it is best to initiate drug administration only after pregnancy is confirmed via ultrasound. Currently, there are two known methods for confirming pregnancy: through ultrasound examination or by measuring serum monkey chorionic gonadotropin (mCG ≥ 1 ng/mL) 3 days after implantation. Using ultrasound to determine pregnancy has the benefit of providing immediate results, but it cannot definitively identify false pregnancies. This is because ultrasound may reveal uterine changes similar to those observed after implantation in animals that have not achieved confirmed pregnancy. Retrospective measurement of mCG serum concentration (i.e., failure to observe pregnancy through continuous ultrasound after treatment) can clarify whether the non-pregnancy after treatment is due to an ultrasound misdiagnosis or an early pregnancy loss caused by the test substance.

9.3.6.2 Considerations for Placental Transfer

The primary endpoints of EFD studies in NHPs are the neonate and offspring, not the intrauterine fetuses. The reduced placental transfer of immunoglobulin G (IgG) during organogenesis in primates negates the requirement for specific EFD studies. Therefore, taking IgG-based monoclonal antibody as an example, administration during the entire organogenesis period (GD20–50) is not expected to result in significant embryonic exposure. Classic EFD study designs are no longer applicable for clearly defining the potential impact of biological products on EFD. Specifically, based on the biology of placental transfer, it is improbable that monoclonal antibodies would directly affect embryonic organ development.

In primates, high molecular weight proteins (greater than 5000 Da) cannot pass through the placenta via simple diffusion. For monoclonal antibodies with molecular weights up to 150,000 Da, placental transfer is a complex process that develops in synchrony with the dynamic anatomical and physiological changes of the placenta throughout the embryogenesis phase. For placental transfer, antibodies must possess the Fc domain, which is mediated by the neonatal Fc receptor (FcRn) and FcγRIIIb. Antibodies that lack the Fc region (such as IgA) do not cross the placenta, whereas IgM- and IgG-based antibodies are actively transported. The majority of monoclonal antibodies developed for therapeutic purposes are IgG, and the efficiency of IgG transfer across the human placenta varies by subclass (with IgG1 being the most efficient, followed by IgG4, IgG3, and IgG2). In humans and NHPs, biologically significant antibody transfer does not occur during the organogenesis period but peaks in the third trimester of pregnancy. Specifically, the placental transfer rate is very low during organogenesis, begins to increase in early mid-pregnancy, and reaches its highest level in the late stage of the third trimester of pregnancy [13].

Biopharmaceuticals containing the Fc region of IgG, such as monoclonal antibodies and antibody-based biopharmaceuticals, represent a specific class of drugs known to cross the placenta in a manner that is specific to the molecule, species, and stage of pregnancy. Antibodies are a class of naturally occurring proteins in maternal animals that enter the developing offspring through specialized transfer mechanisms, thereby providing protection against numerous diseases during the early vulnerable days to months of the infant's life. The mechanisms of uptake and transport for maternal and therapeutic monoclonal antibodies to the developing offspring differ entirely from those of small-molecule drugs. Understanding the patterns and timing of placental transfer is vital, as biopharmaceuticals such as monoclonal antibodies, which are engineered to target mammalian proteins, have the potential to disrupt or impair critical developmental processes.

Despite considerable interspecies diversity in placental morphology and potential temporal variations, placental transfer of IgG is a common physiological process. At present, the assessment of reproductive and developmental toxicity of Fc-containing biopharmaceuticals in experimental animals, as well as the predictive value of various models for humans, is still limited. Critical clinical data from pregnant women typically take a long time to become available after drug approval, leading to the current human risk assessment for Fc-containing biopharmaceuticals during pregnancy and development being largely based on experiences [14, 15].

Given ethical considerations regarding animal testing, a standalone EFD study is not recommended in NHPs, which are the only relevant species, and the ePPND toxicity study is proposed as an alternative to the EFD study.

9.3.7 Considerations for NHPs in PPND/ePPND Studies

The standalone/enhanced pre and postnatal development (PPND/ePPND) toxicity studies, along with traditional EFD and PPND studies, require two groups of pregnant animals to be exposed to the test monoclonal antibodies. In essence, the currently recommended ePPND study design combines the endpoints of both EFD and PPND studies into a single developmental toxicity study in NHPs.

In general, the ePPND study evaluates fetal survival and growth at specific time points during pregnancy using ultrasound examinations in early gestation. Following birth, infant monkeys undergo detailed appearance inspections at predetermined intervals, which include basic measurements of limb length, head circumference, and chest circumference. Skeletal examinations may also be conducted on all offspring, and morphological changes in the visceral organs are assessed at the endpoint. This ePPND design allows for the observation of the effects of gestational exposure on the offspring's appearance, morphology, and various functions, all within a single animal. Therefore, even though fetal morphology is not assessed via cesarean, morphological abnormalities in each F1 animal can still be evaluated, including late miscarriages and stillbirths. Unlike rodents, Cynomolgus monkeys species do not exhibit the behavior of consuming stillborn offspring, allowing for the preservation of carcasses for morphological examination. Currently, ePPND studies have become the preferred type of developmental toxicity research for the development of monoclonal antibodies.

The gestation period for Cynomolgus Monkeys is approximately 160 days, with pregnancy typically confirmed around $GD_{18–20}$. As a result, the administration of the test substance usually begins on GD_{20} and continues until GD_{50}, by which time hard palate closure is complete and major organogenesis is finished in the Cynomolgus monkeys. In classic EFD studies, animals are administered the test substance from GD_{20} to GD_{50} to cover the organogenesis phase, followed by cesarean and examination of the fetuses at a later stage. In traditional PPND studies, dosing generally starts at GD_{20} and continues until delivery, primarily to achieve placental transfer/equilibrium of drug concentrations by late gestation. Consequently, some PPND studies also involve dosing between GD_{120} and GD_{150}. In ePPND studies, the dosing schedule is fixed from GD_{20} until delivery (Table 9.10). This design not only covers standard EFD and PPND studies but also includes the basic functional development of the immune system starting from GD_{80}, greatly reducing the number of animals required while fulfilling reproductive toxicity data collection needs.

In ePPND studies, the endpoint of "practicability" is the offspring and their postnatal development. EFD studies are conducted via visual examination of offspring, skeletal imaging evaluations (e.g., X-ray), and specific visceral inspection during necropsy, providing data typical of EFD studies.

Another key point of the ePPND study design is the postnatal observation period. The parameters and duration of monitoring required for infant monkeys after birth depend on the clinical indications of the test substance. Body weight and clinical pathology are standard postnatal parameters and should be evaluated regularly. A postnatal observation period of 3–6 months is typically established to evaluate basic immune system function. In specific cases, this period may be extended to 12–18 months. A modified Brazelton Behavioral Assessment Scale designed for NHPs is applicable for early evaluation of the central nervous system (CNS). In some cases, learning and memory tests need to be conducted on infant monkeys. Since only animals older than 6 months can be successfully trained and cooperate in such tests, the postnatal observation period must be extended to at least 9 months, and in some

Table. 9.10 Design of ePPND toxicity tests: cynomolgus monkeys

Parameter	
Group size	Approximately 16 pregnant females
Number of dose groups	At least 2 (including 1 control)
Administration period	From confirmation of pregnancy (approximately GD 20) to parturition
F0 females	
Clinical observations/mortality	At least once daily
Body weight	At least weekly
Parturition observations	Document the day of completion
Placenta	Collect and preserve if possible
Necropsy and tissue evaluation	Only as warranted
Exposure Assessment	TK profiles and/or systemic drug levels should be measured, as appropriate
F1	
Clinical observations/mortality	Daily from PND 0
Body weights	Weekly
Morphometry/physical and/or functional assessment	At regular intervals, as appropriate
Neurobehavioural test battery	At least 1 interval during the first 2 weeks postpartum
Grip strength	PND 28
Mother-infant interaction	Minimally in the early postnatal period to confirm nursing, as appropriate thereafter
Exposure assessment	Systemic drug levels should be measured, as appropriate
External evaluation	At regular intervals
Skeletal evaluation	Approximately PND 28 or later
Approximately PND 28 or later	At necropsy
Necropsy	At a minimum of 1 month, depending on the aim of the evaluations. Preserve and retain tissues for possible histological evaluation

cases, up to 12 months. In practical research settings, these learning tests require Cynomolgus monkeys aged 9 months or older to ensure testing of animals at comparable developmental stages. Therefore, this assessment is currently not recommended. Over the past few years, classical standard toxicological evaluation parameters have been increasingly included in postnatal evaluation parameters, such as ophthalmic examinations and cardiovascular checks. Furthermore, body composition analysis and skeletal growth assessments may also be included (Fig. 9.3) [12].

Compared to rodents and rabbits, the failure rate of natural pregnancy in the macaque population is relatively high. Consequently, in developmental toxicity studies, the number of successful pregnancies and the quantity of fetuses/infant monkeys available for evaluation are notably lower than the number of pregnant animals initially enrolled in the study. In the breeding populations of macaques, the pre-birth loss rate

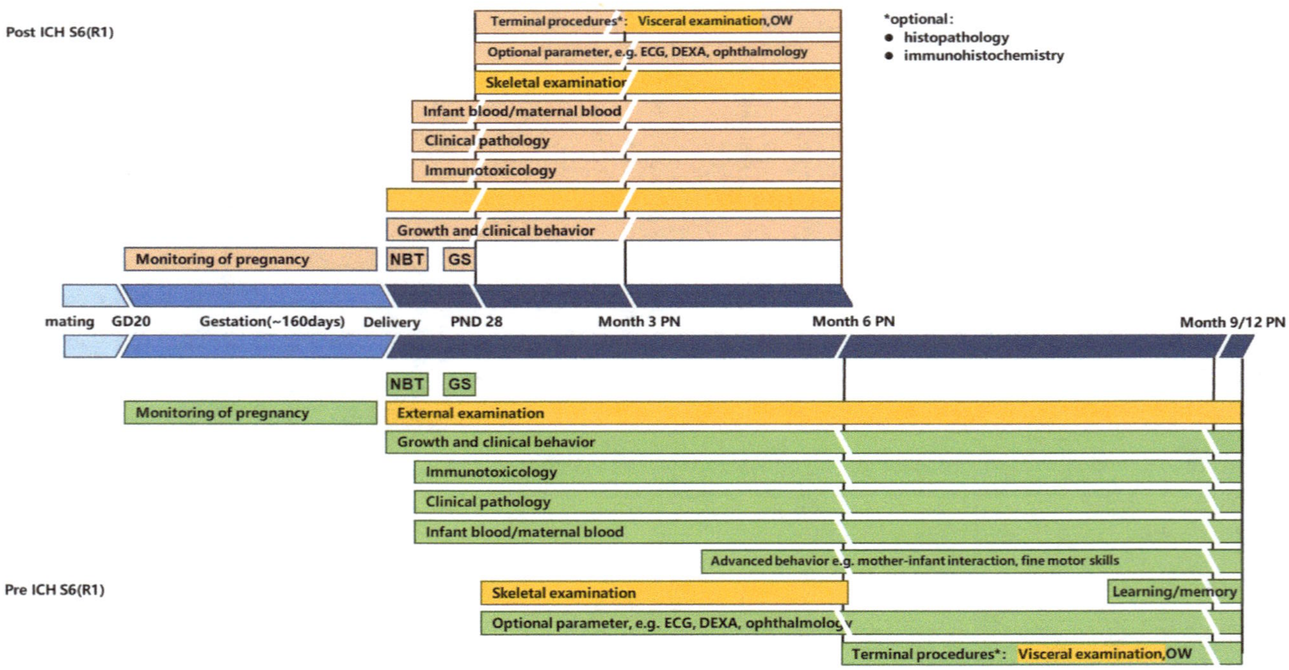

Fig. 9.3 Schematic diagram of the "standardized" design for the ICH S6(R1)ePPND study. Note that according to ICH S6(R1), instrumental learning tests are not required anymore. The minimal postnatal observation period is 1 month. For most instances, a postnatal observation period of 6 months might be sufficient as laid out in the ICH S6(R1). *ECG* electrocardiography, *DEXA* dual-energy X-ray absorptiometry, *NBT* neurobehavioral test battery (Brazelton test), *GS* grip strength, *OW* organ weight, *pc* postcoital, *pn* postnatal. Yellow-boxed parameters are derived from embryofetal development studies ("enhanced")

for rhesus macaques (seasonal breeding) ranges from 13% to 23% annually, while for Cynomolgus monkeys (nonseasonal breeding), the pre-birth loss rate ranges from 8.6% to 28%. In contrast to overall loss rates, the pre-birth loss rate for the solvent control group in developmental toxicity assessments can vary significantly, ranging from 0% to 40%. Additionally, NHPs may experience infant mortality both at term and afterward. The stillbirth rate for Cynomolgus Monkeys is reported to be between 12% and 22%, with an overall developmental loss rate (both pre-birth and post-birth) of approximately 30%, which may reach up to 50% in some studies [16].

An enhanced nomogram (e-nomogram) developed by Jarvis, Heiko, and colleagues for the ePPND study is utilized to predict and monitor the number of pregnancies maintained during gestation and the survival of infants from birth to postnatal day 7 (PND7). The nomogram for the 16 animals within the group is presented in Fig. 9.4. The nomogram resembles a survival curve, displaying confidence intervals for both the pre-birth and post-birth phases. Birth data are collected at gestational days (GD) 126–150, 151–160, 161–170, and >170. These time points are grouped into prenatal (gestational) and delivery stages in a nomogram, with two separate recordings made. Regarding the post-birth phase, the intervals are PND 0, 1, 2–7, 8–50, and 51–90, with insufficient data for infants observed beyond 90 days to generate a nomogram.

Table 9.11 illustrates the correlation of the probability of achieving at least 6–8 live births by PND7 and PND50 with the number of pregnant animals at the beginning of the study. Based on these probabilities, the number of animals in the ePPND study can be reduced from 16–24 to 14–16, while still meeting the ICH S6(R1) requirement of achieving 6–8 live infant monkeys on PND7. Moreover, the practical experience reported in the literature regarding ePPND studies supports this view: 14–24 maternal animals per group have consistently delivered more than 6–8 live infants on PND7. Accordingly, a group size of 14 animals can be recommended. The ICH S5 (R3) reproductive toxicity guidelines suggest that each group should include at least 16 maternal animals [17].

In DART evaluations, NHP models are frequently utilized in the study of biologics (such as monoclonal antibodies and peptides) due to their capacity to exhibit cross-reactivity with human targets for which these therapeutics are designed. This is in contrast to rodents or rabbits, which often lack this crucial cross-reactivity. Since 2016, the FDA has approved a total of 278 new drugs, of which approximately 80% have undergone EFD/ePPND (Table 9.12) studies, while only about 10% of DART studies have utilized NHP (Table 9.13). Except for small-molecule compounds like Empaveli, which exhibit negligible pharmacological activity in rodents or rabbits, NHPs are seldom used in DART assessments for small molecules [18–21].

The new drugs selected for EFD/ePPND studies using NHP are primarily biological products. In the biologics license application (BLA), two-thirds of the DART evaluations have not utilized EFD or ePPND data from NHP. The details are as follows.

(1) EFD/PPND studies in rodents and rabbits with active pharmaceutical ingredients (API) (28%).
(2) Weight of evidence (WoE) methods based on the mechanism of action, indicating risk (23%).

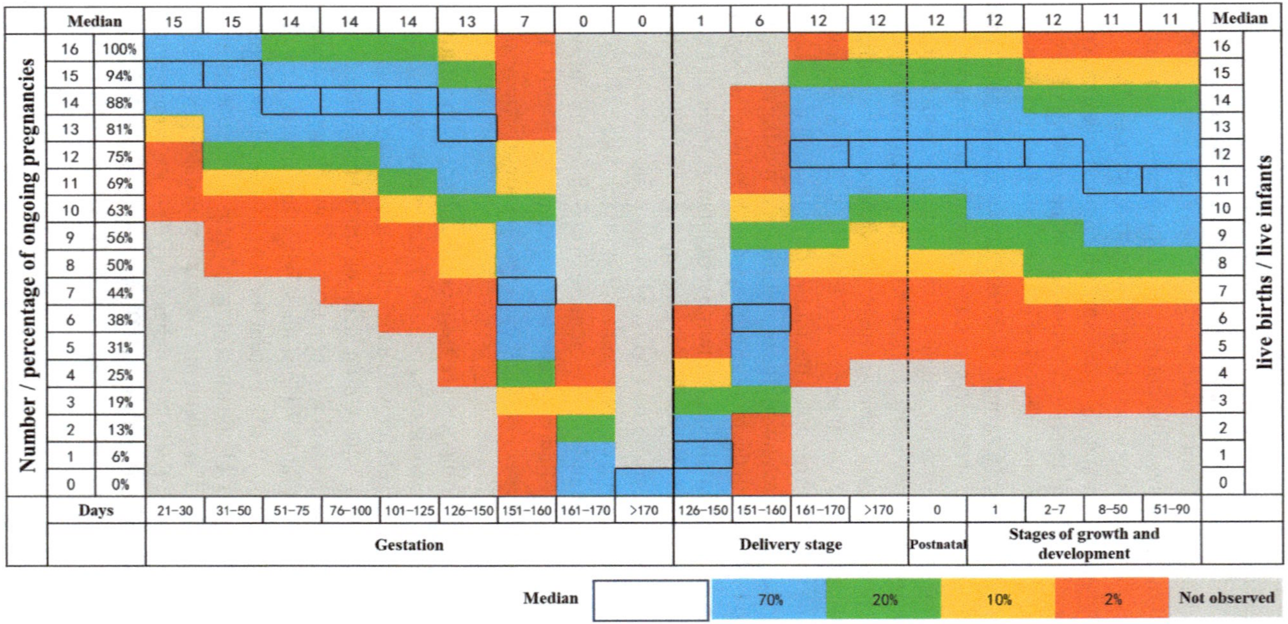

Fig. 9.4 Enhanced normogram for a group size of 16 pregnant long-tailed macaques. Note: The corresponding number of births in the "birth" stage is the cumulative number of births. The two vertical columns on the left represent the number of pregnant animals and the corresponding percentage, and the vertical columns on the right represent the number of live baby monkeys. The hollow rectangle at the top of the graph is the median distribution, with five color-coded categories, including "Possible" (70%), "Likely to Happen" (20%), "Unusual" (10%), "Unlikely" (2%), and "Not Observed"

Table. 9.11 Estimated probabilities (%) of achieving at least 6, 7, or 8 live infant monkeys on PND2–7 and PND51–90, based on the number of pregnant animals at study start

Number of pregnant animals	PND 2–7			PND 51–90		
	Number live infants			Number live infants		
	6	7	8	6	7	8
10	87	69	43	86	67	40
12	97	91	77	96	89	74
14	99	97	93	99	97	91
16	99	99	98	99	99	97
18	99	99	99	99	99	99
20	100	100	100	100	100	100

Table. 9.12 Drug therapy categories approved by the FDA from 2016 to 2021 (with or without EFD studies)

	2016–2017		2018–2019		2020–2021	
	Number of drugs	Approvals with EFD studies	Number of drugs	Approvals with EFD studies	Number of drugs	Approvals with EFD studies
Total approvals	68	54	107	88	103	78
Small molecule, non-oncology	36	28	58	51	55	45
Small molecule, oncology	13	12	22	18	21	17
Biopharmaceutical, non-oncology	14	11	19	16	16	13
Biopharmaceutical, oncology	5	3	8	3	11	4

Table. 9.13 Species selection for drugs approved by the FDA from 2016 to 2021

	2016–2017	2018–2019	2020–2021
Total of EFD	78	88	54
Rats/rabbits	68	81	47
NHPs	10	7	7

(3) WoE methods based on the mechanism of action (such as enzyme replacement therapy) or therapeutic population, indicating negligible risk (10%).
(4) EFD/PPND studies using alternatives that are active in rodents (3%).
(5) Genetically modified rodents (modified to respond to API or knock out targets for API) (3%).

Additionally, in the context of BLAs, DART studies in NHPs are more frequently used for non-oncology products to inform developmental toxicity risk labeling. Specifically, the BLAs of non-oncology products account for 87% of the instances where DART data from NHPs are crucial for labeling decisions. Among the approved BLAs for oncological products, the majority employed WoE evaluations (75%), while only 16% of non-oncological BLAs used this method. The DART study is evaluating non-oncology drugs approved for new indications, including adbury, enspryng, saphnelo, and tezspire, alongside the oncology biologic, margenza.

The WoE method has been successfully utilized in the majority of BLAs for oncology drugs approved for the treatment of advanced cancer. The reason is that these products are frequently anticipated to induce embryonic death and/or exhibit teratogenic effects, and the determination of a therapeutic safety window is often not mandated. For non-oncological indications, the WoE method is applied based on the patient population (treating X-linked disorders) or mechanism of action, concluding with an integrated assessment that developmental toxicity risks are negligible. Additionally, a WoE assessment of reproductive toxicity risk for a specific non-oncology product is based on prior reproductive toxicity data from similar agents targeting the same target.

In recent years, the use of NHP species in the safety evaluation of developmental toxicity has decreased, while the number of biologics tested in rodents and/or rabbits has correspondingly increased. The COVID-19 pandemic has led to a severe shortage of mature NHP available for laboratory use. Consequently, the demand for alternative strategies to replace NHP studies for developmental toxicity tests of biopharmaceutics has become more urgent. In 2022, the FDA released guidance on "Nonclinical Considerations for Mitigating Nonhuman Primate Supply Constraints Arising from the COVID-19 Pandemic." This guidance largely reiterates the recommendations originally presented in the ICH S5(R3) guideline, as follows [22].

(1) The FDA considers NHPs to be an unconventional test species for DART assessment of small-molecule drugs. The FDA strongly advises applicants not to use NHPs to evaluate the DART endpoints of their small-molecule drug development programs.
(2) NHPs should only be used for the DART evaluation of biologics, provided they are the only relevant species.
(3) The use of alternative methods, including species-specific surrogate molecules and genetically modified rodents, is actively promoted.
(4) A WoE method can be used to substitute for nonclinical studies when there is sufficient scientific justification, such as strong evidence linking developmental hazards to the drug's mechanism of action.
(5) For products other than vaccines for noninfectious disease indications, applicants are encouraged to conduct a well-designed ePPND study in NHPs. A reduced number of experimental groups (e.g., one control group and one treatment group) may be considered sufficient for risk evaluation, provided that the treatment group achieves target saturation (i.e., maximum exposure at complete inhibition or target activation), maximum pharmacological effect, and/or a sufficient clinical safety window.

Additionally, it is recommended that applicants discuss the proposed methods and schedule for evaluating DART endpoints with the relevant regulatory authorities before initiating any alternative DART evaluations. Table 9.14 lists the drugs for which PPND/ ePPND studies in NHPs have been publicly disclosed from 2007 to 2023.

Table. 9.14 Drugs with publicly disclosed PPND/ePPND studies in NHPs from 2007 to 2023

Generic name	Mechanism	Study type	Animal toxicity	Human toxicity	Reference
Brolucizumab	VEGF-A inhibitors	ePPND	No test article-related maternal toxicity or adverse effects on fetuses or infants	Uncertain	Reprod Toxicol. 2023
Ofatumumab	CD20 inhibitors	ePPND	A reversible depletion of CD20 + B cells in maternal animals and their infants, Potentially secondary to pharmacologically induced immunosuppression	Limited data, but the FDA does not recommend use during pregnancy	Reprod Toxicol. 2022
Satralizumab	IL-6 receptor family antagonists	ePPND	No test article-related maternal toxicity or adverse effects on fetuses or infants	Uncertain	Birth Defects Res. 2017
Pateclizumab	targeting lymphotoxin-alpha	ePPND	A decreased fetal inguinal lymph node-to-body weight ratio was present in the high-dose group without microscopic abnormalities	Unclear, poor efficacy, clinical trial terminated	Reprod Toxicol. 2016
Daclizumab	IL-2 receptor α chain antagonists	FEED+EFD + PPND	No test article-related maternal toxicity or adverse effects on fetuses or infants	Unclear, discontinued	Neurol Ther. 2016
Tanezumab	NGFB inhibitors	ePPND+EFD	Test article-related increased stillbirths, neuropathology, and reduced postnatal survival, growth, and immune function	Unclear, rejected for marketing authorization	Reprod Toxicol. 2015
Ixekizumab	Inhibitor of interleukin-17A	FEED+EFD + PPND	No test article-related maternal toxicity or adverse effects on fetuses or infants	Uncertain	Reprod Toxicol. 2015
Human IgG2 mAb (IgG2X)	Bound human and cynomolgus monkey neonatal Fc-receptor, FcRn, with similar high affinity	ePPND	Male-mediated mab drug transfer via seminal fluid does not present a health risk to the female partner and is not bioavailable to the developing conceptus.	Mechanism study, no clinical data	Reprod Toxicol. 2014

Table 9.14 (Continued)

Generic name	Mechanism	Study type	Animal toxicity	Human toxicity	Reference
Denosumab	RANKL inhibitors	EFD+PPND	PPND: Pharmacological effects observed in both mother and infant; increased stillbirth and postnatal mortality, effects on growth, development, bones, and lymph nodes in infant monkeys	Contraindicated for use in pregnant women, contraception at least 5 months after the last dose	Reprod Toxicol. 2013 Bone. 2014
Briakinumab	Against the p40 subunit of IL-12/IL-23	FEED+PPND	No test article-related maternal toxicity or adverse effects on fetuses or infants	Uncertain, clinical trial terminated	Birth Defects Res B Dev Reprod Toxicol. 2012
Rituximab	CD20 inhibitors	EFD+PPND	Depletion of B cells in the lymphoid tissues of fetuses recovered in infancy	B-cell lymphocytopenia in infants	Toxicol Sci. 2011
Ustekinumab	against the p40 subunit of IL-12/IL-23	EFD*2+ePPND	No maternal toxicity and no toxicity in the fetuses or infants, including no effects on the TDAR or DTH responses	Uncertain	Birth Defects Res B Dev Reprod Toxicol. 2010
Golimumab	TNF-α inhibitors	EFD (GD20–GD50)+PPND (GD50~PND33)	No test article-related maternal toxicity or adverse effects on fetuses or infants	Crosses the placenta during pregnancy, increasing the risk of infection	Am J Reprod Immunol. 2007
Onartuzumab	c-Met inhibitors	ePPND	Shortened gestation, reduced birth weight, increased fetal and perinatal mortality, induced placental damage, delayed offspring development, and changes like dilated hepatic sinusoids.	Uncertain, clinical trial terminated	Toxicol Sci. 2018
Tabalumab	BAFF inhibitors	ePPND	Placental and mammary transfer	Uncertain, clinical trial terminated	Birth Defects Res B Dev Reprod Toxicol. 2015

Table 9.14 (Continued)

Generic name	Mechanism	Study type	Animal toxicity	Human toxicity	Reference
Belimumab	BAFF inhibitors	EFD+ePPND	Limited to the expected pharmacology, primarily decreased numbers of B-lymphocytes in the peripheral blood of Mothers and infants, and in fetal lymphoid tissues, Infants demonstrated full recovery	Limited data, no birth defects found	Reprod Toxicol. 2009
Thiamazole	Thyroperoxidase inhibitors	Late gestational period PPND (GD120–deliver)	Oral administration of thiamazole to maternal animals during the late gestational period induced retardation of behavioral development in their infants	Treatment in the late gestational period may lead to hypothyroidism in infants	Congenit Anom (Kyoto). 2013
Natalizumab	CD49d (α4β 1 integrin) antagonists	PPND	Elevated lymphocyte and nucleated red blood cell counts, consistent with the pharmacological effect in infants	Neonatal thrombocytopenia	Birth Defects Res B Dev Reprod Toxicol. 2009
Soluble IL-4R	IL-4R homologous protein	EFD+PPND	Increase in abortion/embryo–fetal death	Uncertain	Regul Toxicol Pharmacol. 2009
Barusiban	OXTR antagonists	PPND	No test article-related maternal toxicity or adverse effects on fetuses or infants	No adverse maternal or fetal effects found; clinical trial terminated	Reprod Toxicol. 2007

Therefore, it is crucial for each study on monoclonal antibodies or individual toxicity to leverage existing flexibility and best practices, adhering to the principles of Reduction, Replacement, and Refinement (the 3Rs) to minimize the use of animals.

9.4 Juvenile Toxicity Testing and Considerations for Pediatric Medication Design

Data from studies on fertility and EFD typically cannot be directly applied to the pediatric population prior to puberty, as the primary objectives of these studies often do not focus on this population. However, such research may assist in identifying critical developmental windows. In PPND studies, exposures during late pregnancy or early lactation may provide a "worst-case scenario" for potential impacts on newborns. These studies could be particularly beneficial for supporting pediatric medications with long half-life periods. Understanding the transport mechanisms across the placenta and during lactation, as well as the exposure of offspring following maternal drug administration, is also crucial.

Due to their precocious development and behavior at birth and their vulnerability to certain prenatal exposures, NHPs may serve as appropriate models for the human perinatal/neonatal period. For example, their lungs, gastrointestinal tract, kidneys, and skeletal systems are relatively well-developed at birth, and their central nervous system functions better than that of humans at the same stage. Fc-containing biopharmaceutics and related therapeutics undergo active placental transfer in late gestation, and their extended half-life results in significant exposure of offspring, with this exposure continuing after birth. Even basic evaluations of pharmacological and toxicological effects on offspring can significantly contribute to pediatric medication risk identification.

While standard DART studies and specialized juvenile toxicity studies both assess potential developmental effects, the former is based on maternal dosing, whereas the latter involves direct dosing after birth. Juvenile toxicity studies are intended to support the clinical application of drugs and typically include typical, standardized, and pathological indicators for general toxicity studies. In studies involving the administration of drugs to pregnant animals, the focus is primarily on pregnancy outcomes and overall growth and development, providing essential information for human reproductive risk assessment. According to the scope of nonclinical trial plans for drugs, if the research data is also adapted to support pediatric clinical applications, it may be crucial to include anatomical and pathological indicators of offspring in PPND studies to assess potential developmental impacts.

Overall, information from general toxicology studies and/or DART trials can help avoid unnecessary duplication of studies in juvenile animals to support pediatric clinical medication. Numerous technical and feasibility hurdles are encountered when designing studies to support the administration of therapeutics to neonates and infants. A fundamental understanding of species-specific developmental physiology is essential for success in this, as in many aspects of drug development. Current literature on developmental toxicity primarily focuses on functional endpoints; however, this may not adequately correspond to the key developmental stages in histology for animals of different ages. Nonclinical assessment of toxicity in juvenile animals should consider information from various sources, including adult clinical toxicity programs (if available), mechanisms of action, the nonclinical toxicity profile, and developmental information from both juvenile humans and animal experiences. This requires an analysis of case-specific characteristics to determine areas of focus, which may necessitate additional studies or endpoints. For instance, supplementary assessments of immune function or extended neuropathological studies may be warranted. Caution should be exercised when interpreting isolated results of endpoints, especially in the presence of individual variability or limited historical control data [23].

Normal body and organ weights of Cynomolgus monkeys across different age groups serve as important background and reference values in toxicology research. In Cynomolgus monkeys, the percentage of body weight accounted for by the adrenals, brain, kidneys, lungs, liver, thymus, and thyroid decreases from infancy to early adulthood. The brain, in particular, exhibits a substantially higher relative weight during infancy compared to adulthood. In contrast, the percentage of body weight attributed to the pancreas, prostate, testes, and uterus increases [24].

9.5 Histological Determination of Sexual Maturity in Cynomolgus Monkeys

Overall, the onset of sexual maturity in Cynomolgus Monkeys is difficult to predict and exhibits considerable individual variability. The timing of sexual maturity is influenced by various factors, including genetics, environmental conditions, nutritional status, and individual experiences. Therefore, to more accurately predict the onset of sexual maturity in Cynomolgus Monkeys, it is essential to consider these factors comprehensively and conduct further in-depth research.

9.5.1 Males

In most general toxicity studies, the rodents at the end of the study are typically sexually mature, while non-rodents may still be sexually immature or may present a mix of immature, peripubertal, and/or mature individuals (Tables 9.15 and 9.16). Therefore, when studying non-rodent species, it is often necessary to document the sexual maturity status. Additionally, recording the reproductive maturity of rodents aids in the analysis of toxicity studies involving juvenile animals and/or early mortality outcomes prior to the anticipated study termination. In these studies, the sexual maturity status of the animals is usually assessed by toxicologic pathologists based on the appearance of the reproductive organs and microscopic observations. However, depending on the endpoints required by the study design and protocol, other research parameters may also be considered, such as age, body weight, semen analysis, testicular volume, estrous/menstrual cycles, and/or hormone measurements [25].

Table. 9.15 General features of male reproductive system development

General physiological features	Rat	Mouse	Rabbit	Dog	Minipig	NHPs
Testicular descent completed	~PND_{21}	~PND_{19}	12–16 weeks	5–6 weeks	At birth	~36 months[1]
Preputial separation	$PND_{39–45}$	$PND_{27–34}$	~PND_{72}	−7 weeks	Not determined	2.5 years
blood–testis barrier formation	$PND_{15–20}$	$PND_{15–25}$	9–10 weeks	20 weeks	Not determined	−3 years
Initial spermatogonial proliferation	$PND_{4–12}$	$PND_{4–8}$	7–8 weeks	16 weeks	<4 weeks	~3 years
Mature spermatids present	~PND_{46}	~PND_{30}	14–15 weeks	8–12 months	As early as 8 weeks	~3.5–5 years
Total duration of spermatogenesis (days)	51.6	34.5	44–52	54.4	35–40	42
Epididymal transit time (days)	8–11	5	10–14	10	9–11	11

[1]Indicates a brief descent at birth, followed by movement near the inguinal region shortly after birth, and finally, complete descent during puberty

Before spermatogenesis, males are typically considered sexually immature, with the onset of spermatogenesis being considered to be the beginning of peripuberty. During the initial wave of spermatogenesis, pathologists can observe the onset of mitotic activity in spermatogonia, the first appearance of primary spermatocytes, and the formation of the lumen within the seminiferous tubules. This period of puberty generally lasts until spermatogenesis is complete (with the presence of mature spermatozoa and residual bodies), and extends through most of the seminiferous tubules. At this stage, fully developed sperm are observed in the epididymal tail, and the accessory glands are fully developed, indicating sexual maturity in males (Tables 9.15 and 9.16).

In assessing the sexual maturity of male macaques, internal parameters are critical reference points. Generally, male macaques weighing over 4.5 kg and aged 4–5 years are likely to have reached sexual maturity. Additionally, a testicular volume greater than 10 mL, serum testosterone concentrations between 15 and 20 nmol/L, and the presence of spermatozoa in the ejaculate are important criteria for assessing maturity. However, it is important to note that, aside from the presence of sperm in the ejaculate, the aforementioned standards do not fully guarantee the sexual maturity status of the macaque [8].

Testicular volume is also one of the commonly used parameters in nonclinical toxicology to help identify sexually mature male Cynomolgus monkeys when semen evaluation is not feasible. Due to the variability in testicular volume during the peripubertal phase, it is indeed challenging to distinguish between adult males and those before and after puberty with similar confidence. The method of measuring testicular volume is practical for distinguishing between immature (testicular

Table. 9.16 General microscopic features of male reproductive system immaturity, puberty, and maturity

Reproductive organs/tissues	Immaturity	Peripubertal period	Sexual maturity
Testis	No spermatogenesis; seminiferous tubules lack a lumen and contain only Sertoli cells and spermatogonia	*Early*: Spermatogonial proliferation is evident; formation of a lumen within the seminiferous tubules *Middle*: Spermatocytes present; meiotic division present with formation of early round spermatids; apoptotic and sloughed germ cells commonly observed within the seminiferous tubules *Late*: Round and elongated spermatids present; residual bodies present; apoptotic and sloughed germ cells present within the seminiferous tubules The above early, middle, and late features begin in some tubules with intervening areas of immature tubules	Active spermatogenesis across all seminiferous tubules with the presence of mature spermatids and residual bodies
Epididymis	No sperm present in the head, body, or tail; low cuboidal epithelium	Variable amounts of sperm and/or cellular debris present; overall increase in epithelial height and size of lumen	Abundant sperm present in the tail
Prostate	Small inactive glands, no secretory activity	Increase in epithelial height, extent of lobulation, and secretory activity; timing may occur slightly before or after testicular development	Full size with secretory activity
Seminal vesicles	Small inactive glands, no secretory activity	Increase in epithelial height and secretory activity; timing may occur slightly before or after testicular development	Full size with secretory activity
Mammary gland	Some ducts present extending from the nipple into the fat pad	Transient mammary gland development may occur	Limited numbers of ducts

volume ≥ serum testosterone > body weight > age) and peripubertal (testicular volume ≥ body weight > serum testosterone > age) animals (Fig. 9.5). A testicular volume exceeding 10 mL can also indicate sexual maturity to some extent. Some literature recommends a total testicular volume of 10–25 mL as a criterion for identifying sexually mature male Cynomolgus monkeys. In vitro measurements of testicular weight and the diameter of testicular sections also aid in differentiating mature animals from immature or peripubertal animals.

Due to the high sensitivity of hormone secretion and its short half-life, there is significant variability in hormone levels within the same individual at different physiological stages and between different individuals. Reliable biological markers for

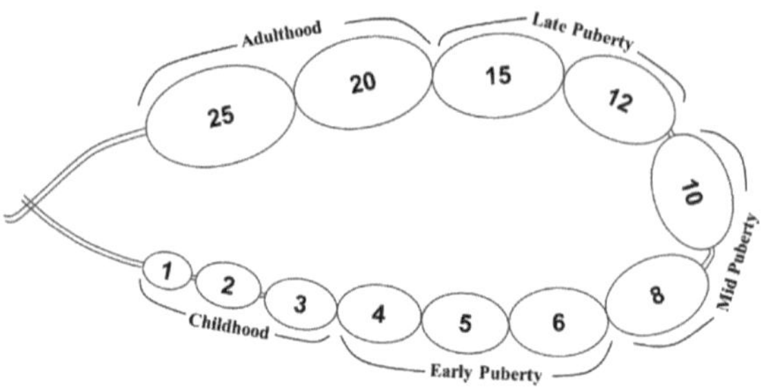

Fig. 9.5 Relationship between testicular volume measured using an orchidometer and sexual maturity. The numbers represent the measured testicular volume (mL)

sexual maturity are not based on single measurements of hormones such as luteinizing hormone (LH), FSH, testosterone, or inhibin B. It is also considered that inhibin B is not valuable for distinguishing sexually mature animals from those in early sexual development. However, when testosterone levels exceed 20 nmol/L, it typically reflects the sexual maturity status of Cynomolgus monkeys [25].

9.5.2 Females

When there is no microscopic evidence of ovulation (absence of corpus luteum) and no evidence of cyclical glandular/epithelial development in the reproductive tract, females are typically considered sexually immature. During the peripubertal phase, it can be challenging to determine histological characteristics, and these may overlap between immature and mature animals, making it impossible to record peripubertal parameters in all cases. There may be the presence of corpus luteum or remnants of the corpus luteum and/or development of glandular and epithelial components in the tubules, but these features can be variable and may not obviously correlate with physiological markers of sexual development in individual animals, such as the appearance of the vaginal opening or the onset of menarche. After the first ovulation, there is a variable period during which the estrous/menstrual cycle is irregular, complicating the evaluation of the reproductive tract. This irregularity during the peripubertal phase is found across all species, but the duration and type of variations vary by species and individual animals (Table 9.17).

Changes in NHPs during the peripubertal phase are particularly pronounced and prolonged, with extended periods of anovulation (Table 9.18). Ideally, key histological characteristics for determining sexual maturity in females include evidence of ovulation over multiple menstrual cycles (preferably the corpus luteum from the current or previous cycle) and complete development of the reproductive tract; however, not all species exhibit recognition of both characteristics. Due to the lack of a clear distinction between peripubertal and mature females, the presence of any corpus luteum

Table. 9.17 General features of estrous or menstrual cycles in female animals

General physiological features	Rat	Mouse	Rabbit	Dog	Minipig	NHPs
Vaginal opening	$PND_{31–36}$	$PND_{25–32}$	PND 29	PND 21	Prenatal	Prenatal
Age at first ovulation	$PND_{33–46}$	$PND_{35–45}$	Not applicable (due to induced ovulation; can reproduce at 4–5 months)	8–14 months	5–7.5 months (varies with housing practices and presence of a mature boar)	2.5–3 years
Age at onset of regular cycles	$\sim PND_{65}$	$\sim PND_{49}$	Not applicable (due to induced ovulation)	Not applicable (due to variable anestrus period)	Within 1–2 initial cycles (based on domestic swine)	-4 years
Cycle type	Estrous cycle; Spontaneous ovulation; polyovulatory	Estrous cycle; Spontaneous ovulation; polyovulatory	Estrous cycle; Induced ovulation; polyovulatory	Estrous cycle; Spontaneous ovulation; polyovulatory	Estrous cycle; Spontaneous ovulation; polyovulatory	Menstrual cycle; Spontaneous ovulation; monovulatory
Cycle length	4–5 days	4–5 days	Not applicable (due to induced ovulation)	5–12 months	17–22 days	28–32 days
Total duration of folliculogenesis (days)	At least 60	At least 47	~100	~170	–100 (based on domestic swine)	~215

Table 9.18 General microscopic features of female reproductive system immaturity, puberty, and sexual maturity

Reproductive organs/tissues	Immaturity	Peripubertal period	Sexual maturity
Ovary	Small to medium-sized variably atretic follicles and no corpora lutea	Corpus luteum (current and/or regressing) from at least one cycle	Corpus luteum (current and/or regressing) from multiple cycles
Uterus	Small and with limited glandular development; thin epithelium, compact stroma	May see evidence of cyclic changes, but animals may have an inactive endometrium and a maturity designation based on the presence of the corpus luteum	May see evidence of cyclic changes, but anovulatory animals may have an inactive endometrium and maturity designation based on the presence of corpus luteum
Cervix	Thin inactive epithelium, limited mucous production, squamocolumnar junction within the internal cervical canal	Squamocolumnar junction everted to the external cervical os	Squamocolumnar junction everted to the external cervical os
Vagina	Thin epithelium, nonkeratinized	Thickened and heavily keratinized	Thickened and heavily keratinized
Mammary gland	Ducts present within the mammary fat pad, with limited lobular development	Ducts and lobules present	Ducts and lobules present

(as observed microscopically) is typically regarded as the sole definitive criterion for sexual maturity. Therefore, for the practical purposes of most nonclinical safety studies, it is recommended to consider females as immature in the absence of a corpus luteum and as sexually mature when there is clear evidence of ovulation and the presence of a corpus luteum [8].

Microscopic examination of reproductive tissues during anatomy is the principal method for assessing sexual maturity. Nevertheless, factors such as age, body weight, in vivo observations, breed/genetic sources, macroscopic inspection, organ weight, and other unconventional techniques (like semen analysis, testicular volume detection, estrous/menstrual cycles, or hormone measurements) should be regarded as contributing evidence. The method of determining sexual maturity under the microscope differs from traditional histopathological recording practices. Initially, sexual maturity reports are records of normal tissue characteristics rather than abnormalities or changes associated with the subjects. Therefore, these data should be kept distinct from histopathological results, although they can be formatted into tables or queried. Additionally, the microscopic evaluation of sexual maturity in males and females is based on a comprehensive assessment of multiple tissues in the entire reproductive system, rather than isolated evaluations of individual reproductive organs. To report comprehensive results for multiple organs, it is recommended to include a summary tissue in the data collection system. This summary tissue is an extra entry in the "pathological tissue list" of the data entry system, intended to assist in documenting the overall evaluation results of sexual maturity across various tissues. The concept of summary tissue can be viewed as a "virtual tissue (or pseudo tissue)."

When recording sexual maturity based on microscopic observations of male and female reproductive organs, it is advisable to use "reproductive system, maturity" (or a similar term) as the "summary tissue" for all animals in the study and to record using one of the following terms: immature, before and after puberty (or peripubertal), mature, or uncertain. It is essential to differentiate the pathological diagnoses of individual reproductive organs from the records of sexual maturity assessments. For example, if there is inadequate sexual development without any pathological changes, macro-level observations such as smaller testicles may be noted. In this case, the testicular tissue should be recorded as "normal," while the "summary tissue" should be "immature."

The application of "summary tissue" for recording is particularly important during puberty, as various reproductive organs may not develop from immaturity to maturity at the same rate, leading to potentially contradictory and unclear records if each tissue's maturity is documented separately. Nonetheless, it should be acknowledged that using "summary tissue" may pose challenges regarding the traceability of individual reproductive tissues.

In studies evaluating reproductive maturity under microscopic examination, most entries do not need to be summarized or described in a pathology report because the documentation of sexual maturity represents a sign of normal characteristics rather than a histopathological diagnosis. However, in some cases, the results and/or discussion sections of the pathology report may need to include more detailed information to explain any potential impact of the maturity status on the ability to detect and/or interpret potential findings in the reproductive system.

In studies requiring sexually mature animals, the study protocol should provide sufficient detail so that researchers and pathologists can clearly understand how to determine and document sexual maturity.

Study data and/or reports should contain clear documentation of sexual maturity, including in vivo checks before the study begins and/or microscopic examinations conducted by the pathologist in any study where histopathological evaluation of the reproductive system is part of the study design.

In NHPs, the assessment of sexual maturity of Cynomolgus monkeys should be a comprehensive evaluation based on multiple indicators, not solely determined by a single phenomenon or factor. Relying solely on age and/or body weight to determine sexual maturity is generally not reliable; therefore, when sexually mature animals are required, confirmation of maturity should be included as part of the baseline parameter evaluation prior to research and/or as part of the pathologist's microscopic examination evaluation.

9.6 Strategies for NHP in DART Evaluation of Different Types of Drugs

9.6.1 Strategy for Nonclinical Safety Evaluation of Monoclonal Antibodies

Since the twenty-first century, biologics, primarily monoclonal antibodies (mAb) and recombinant proteins, have increasingly been approved for human use. These novel therapies offer new treatment options and significantly improve patients' quality of life, thus bringing substantial hope to those suffering from severe and refractory diseases such as cancer, autoimmune/inflammatory diseases, and many other diseases. Particularly, the clinical success of mAbs implies that in the future, more mAbs targeting the same or new targets and pathways will enter clinical development or be approved for human use.

Understanding the potential mechanisms by which monoclonal antibodies might affect EFD is fundamental to their nonclinical safety assessment. These studies are fundamentally focused on investigating the potential for embryos to be exposed to pharmacological concentrations of a drug during key developmental periods. In general, small molecular chemical drugs (with the molecular weight <500 Da) are passively transported to the placenta, thus it can be assumed that the systemic exposure of the embryo throughout pregnancy is aligned with the maternal blood concentration. However, for monoclonal antibodies with a high molecular weight of up to 150 kDa, there exists a specialized transport mechanism primarily mediated by the binding of antibodies to surface antigens on target cells, facilitating endocytosis of the antibodies and enabling their transport into the cell. Studies have shown that the amount of large-molecule drugs entering the embryo through maternal circulation during pregnancy is significantly lower than their content in maternal plasma.

The mechanism by which the embryo is exposed to monoclonal antibodies is similar to the placental transfer of endogenous maternal IgG. In most mammalian species, including humans, maternal IgG antibodies cross the placenta, providing passive immune protection to the developing embryo. The Fc region of maternal IgG binds to the neonatal Fc receptor (FcRn) in an acid-dependent manner. At physiologic pH levels, the affinity between FcRn and IgG is low. The drug binds IgG in the bloodstream to FcRn via endocytosis (either fluid-phase or receptor-mediated) by vascular endothelial cells and/or monocytes in the circulation, and enters the cells through the formation of endosomes. The acidic environment within these endosomes increases the affinity between IgG and FcRn. Once bound, the FcRn–IgG complex is transported to the cell surface, where it is exposed to physiologic pH levels, causing IgG to be released back into the bloodstream. This process prevents IgG and FcRn from being degraded by lysosomes within the cell and facilitates their transmembrane transport into the embryo.

Monoclonal antibodies and other Fc-containing biopharmaceutics can cross the placenta via FcRn. Altering the Fc region can reduce its binding to human FcRn, thus minimizing placental transfer. Except for albumin, large molecule biopharmaceuticals without Fc fragments do not typically undergo FcRn-mediated transfer.

For small molecules with short half-life periods, traditional EFD studies, with dosing limited to the period of organogenesis, can provide a basis for risk assessment of unintended exposures during early pregnancy. As per ICH M3 (R2), large-scale clinical trials in women of reproductive potential can be permitted based on EFD data alone (without additional PPND research information), in cases where unintended pregnancy exposure is statistically possible. Postponing PPND studies may also occur due to market approval. However, this approach of delaying PPND may not be the best for all long half-life monoclonal antibodies, as the risk of fetal harm post-organogenesis is crucial information for clinical dosing in pregnant women exposed unintentionally during large-scale phase III trials. Therefore, whether during clinical trials or post-market, pharmaceutical companies are responsible for considering the need for PPND data before large-scale, long-term exposure to monoclonal antibodies in women of childbearing age. This need will vary depending on the disease condition.

Given the limited possibility of fetal exposure to monoclonal antibodies during early pregnancy, the incidence of malformations caused by direct fetal exposure during organogenesis is lower than the concerns raised by small molecules. However, even with limited direct contact of the embryo, monoclonal antibodies in the maternal body may still have adverse effects on pregnancy, potentially leading to miscarriage. For example, the anti-epidermal growth factor receptor (EGFR) monoclonal antibody, panitumumab, not only causes expected menstrual cycle irregularities in nonpregnant monkeys but can also lead to miscarriage. Based on existing literature regarding the role of EGFR in ovarian physiology and EFD, studies on the anti-EGFR monoclonal antibody panitumumab in primates can be regarded as a confirmation of existing toxicity evidence.

The safety of mAbs is primarily driven by the drug's highly specific pharmacology and mechanism of action. Given that mAbs are comprised of natural amino acids, and they exhibit exceptional affinity and specificity for their targets, the occurrence of off-target toxicities, which are commonly seen in new chemical entities (NCEs), is rare. To best predict potential adverse reactions in humans, pharmacologically relevant animal species must be used, where the monoclonal antibody binds its target and exhibits pharmacodynamic effects similar to those anticipated in humans. Due to the high specificity of monoclonal antibodies for humans, NHPs are typically the only pharmacologically relevant species, with Cynomolgus monkeys or other macaques (such as rhesus macaques) being the most commonly selected for safety evaluations. If a second relevant species (such as rodents) is available, ICH S6 (R1) recommends conducting long-term repeated-dose toxicity studies in rodents (rather than NHPs), provided that short-term toxicity studies get similar results. However, rodents are often limited in their use for long-term repeated-dose toxicity studies due to their higher immunogenicity [26].

This raises questions about the value of NHPs in nonclinical safety assessments of drugs. Particularly for mAbs, some believe that nearly all adverse events can be predicted, as these events are either mediated by the pharmacology of the drug (potentially amplified by dose escalation) or caused by immune responses to the drug. Others argue that in many cases, the immunogenicity of humanized or fully human monoclonal antibodies in NHPs hinders a thorough safety assessment. For example, the severe adverse reactions observed in humans with the superagonistic anti-CD28 monoclonal antibody, TGN1412, emphasize the importance of clearly identifying toxicologically and pharmacologically relevant sensitive species. These reactions were not predicted in NHP studies due to insufficient investigation of the target's biology prior to clinical trials. It is now known that CD28 is not expressed on effector memory T cells in Cynomolgus Monkeys to the same extent as in humans. Therefore, TGN1412 does not induce widespread T cell activation in NHPs as it does in humans.

Indeed, for standard IgG-class monoclonal antibodies targeting well-characterized pharmacological and safety targets in both animals and humans, such as mAbs targeting soluble cytokines (e.g., TNF, IL-6, and IL-17) or anti-CD20 B-cell depleting mAbs, next-generation "me-too" "me-better" drugs, or biosimilars are unlikely to provide any significant benefit for human risk assessment from extensive nonclinical studies in NHPs. In these cases, unnecessary nonclinical study programs should be reduced, thereby minimizing the use of NHPs [27].

However, for mAbs targeting novel targets or with novel pharmacological mechanisms, as well as for new mAb scaffolds and constructs (e.g., bi/trispecific mAbs and other constructs), where much of the pharmacology is not well understood, and adverse reactions are unpredictable, evaluating the impact of pharmacological modulation on safety in NHPs is critical (provided that pharmacological relevance to humans has been clearly demonstrated).

Several cases highlight that while knockout (KO) mice can be valuable in identifying potential toxicities for further investigation, the complete absence of the target protein in these mice across their lifespan, including developmental stages, could lead to an overestimation of human toxicity. KO animals may also underestimate human risk, as observed with anti-FGF19 mAb, due to their development in the absence of the target, potentially leading to the evolution of compensatory pathways that differ from those in adult humans. Consequently, they may not accurately reflect the risks associated with administering a mAb to adult humans. The following case studies will illustrate the important role of NHPs in mAb reproductive and developmental toxicity studies.

BIO5, an IgG4 monoclonal antibody targeting a cytokine, is under development for inflammatory diseases. Cynomolgus monkeys have been identified as the sole pharmacologically relevant species for nonclinical safety assessment based on studies showing similar downstream signaling pathway activity to humans, in vivo efficacy in disease models, and literature evidence of comparable target distribution and function. In contrast, BIO5 is inactive in rodents. Furthermore, no adverse outcomes were observed in KO mouse studies or mouse dosing trials, injecting a homologous mAb. Monoclonal antibodies intended for clinical use did not exhibit adverse effects in general toxicity studies in healthy adult monkeys. Given that the treated population will include women of childbearing potential and children, it is necessary to evaluate toxicity during pregnancy. In ePPND toxicity studies, pregnant monkeys were subjected to drug administration from GD20 until delivery, with a 9-month monitoring period for the offspring. BIO5 administration was well-tolerated during pregnancy and did not increase the incidence of spontaneous abortions. However, a significant prolongation of the gestation period was observed in all treated pregnant animals, and some animals experienced mortality at parturition without prior signs of abnormality. Pathological findings indicated that dystocia was primarily caused by retained placenta, with some cases involving excessive bleeding of the reproductive system. Secondary pup mortality resulting from dystocia was also observed. Infant monkeys that survived dystocia developed normally, including their immune systems. Due to physiological differences in parturition between rodents and higher mammals, none of the findings from the ePPND study were observed in KO mice or in pregnant mice treated with anti-mouse cytokine receptor mAb [28].

Based on these observations and an in-depth review of relevant literature on parturition mechanisms, it was hypothesized that the target molecule could be one of many factors related to inflammation, cervical ripening, and the disappearance of the gap between the placenta and uterus during labor in humans and higher mammals. Indeed, this cytokine has been demonstrated to be essential for normal parturition. This study was the first to demonstrate that this factor plays a more crucial role in parturition in NHPs than previously understood. It also revealed that pregnant individuals may face risks of dystocia, hemorrhage, and infant loss if administered BIO5.

The research indicated that BIO5, through a previously unknown mechanism of cytokine inhibition, elicited a profound and deleterious impact on the health of pregnant mothers. These effects were not observed in either KO mice or mice injected with the homologous mAb. Previously, an increased rate of abortion was observed with an IL4Ra fusion protein (which inhibits IL4 through a different pathway than BIO5) in NHPs but not in mice. Following the results of the monkey ePPND study, the BIO5 clinical trial in patients with autoimmune diseases has continued without the identification of any unexpected safety risks. However, the informed consent specifically cautions against the use of BIO5 during pregnancy and directs that women who become pregnant while receiving BIO5 must immediately discontinue the treatment.

In conclusion, the Cynomolgus monkeys is the only appropriate species for evaluating reproductive and developmental toxicity. This study identified life-threatening risks to women and infants in late pregnancy that were not predicted by prior literature or mouse models (either KO or administration of mAb).

9.6.2 Application in Pediatric Anesthesia Neurotoxicity Research

General anesthetics (GAs) exert their effects primarily by inhibiting excitability or enhancing inhibitory synaptic transmission. Over the past three decades, extensive research involving rats, mice, and NHPs has confirmed that prolonged exposure to clinically relevant GAs during critical periods of brain development can induce neurotoxicity in the immature brain. Evidence of neurodevelopmental toxicity found in animal studies has raised public health concerns about the safety of pediatric GA. Retrospective and prospective studies in human patients indicate that a single brief exposure to GAs in children under three years old is unlikely to be associated with negative long-term neurodevelopmental outcomes. The link between extended or frequent use of GAs during pediatric surgeries and neurodevelopmental impairments in children is still highly debated, primarily due to the numerous confounding variables that can influence a child's neurological development. With advancements in anesthetic support and intraoperative monitoring, there are now more surgical interventions available for pediatric patients, including intrauterine fetuses, all performed using a range of anesthetic or sedative techniques. This has led to an increased likelihood of immature brains being exposed to GAs for extended periods. Additionally, some life-threatening patients require complex surgical treatments and prolonged anesthetic exposure before the age of three [29].

The results from NHP models are crucial for understanding the risks associated with anesthesia during early life. However, due to species differences and variations in GA exposure among animals, the GA-induced neurodevelopmental toxicity results obtained from animal studies may not fully predict the effects on human patients. Nevertheless, considering the ethical issues surrounding pediatric clinical research, the use of animal models to explore GA-induced neurodevelopmental toxicity remains irreplaceable. Although translating the findings from animal studies on GA-induced neurotoxicity into clinical management for pediatric anesthesia presents challenges, animal models remain a powerful tool for exploring the neurodevelopmental impacts of GAs on humans. Various animal models have been used to investigate the toxic effects of GAs on neurodevelopment, including nematodes, zebrafish, rodents, and NHPs. Although various animal models have been used in research reports, the age of animals exposed to anesthetics is strictly defined to coincide with critical periods of brain development, most commonly during synaptogenesis. This period marks a key stage in brain development, characterized by vigorous synaptic formation and heightened neuronal sensitivity to neurotoxic drugs. In studies using neonatal rats, compared to control animals, there is a significant increase in neuronal cell death in the cerebral cortex and thalamic nuclei from PND3 to PND14, with the highest number of apoptotic neurons observed at PND7. This suggests that the severity of GA-induced apoptotic neurodegeneration may be related to the rapid pace of synaptogenesis. Although rodent models are widely used in preclinical anesthesia research, there are practical challenges in using rats for pediatric anesthesia studies due to anesthetic states, difficulties in monitoring physical health, and the collection of biological fluids such as blood and cerebrospinal fluid. The peak of synaptogenesis in rhesus macaques occurs from GD122 to PND5, with a sharp decline by PND35. Among animal models used to assess the neurotoxic potential of GAs and other substances (such as methamphetamine, nicotine, cocaine, and cannabis), NHP models are considered to have superior predictive value because of their close similarities to humans in genetics, reproduction, development, neuroanatomy, and cognitive abilities. For GA research, the unique benefits of NHP models include the feasibility of controlled anesthetic procedures, the capacity for real-time monitoring of physiological parameters during exposure, and the opportunity to obtain sufficient blood and/or cerebrospinal fluid specimens for analysis. No other commonly used animal models can match humans in terms of functional placental units, the tendency for single offspring births, and the fetal-to-maternal weight ratio [30].

Numerous nonclinical in vivo and in vitro studies have demonstrated that GA can induce neuronal cell death during both single administration and continuous exposure, and this effect involves, but is not limited to, N-methyl-D-aspartate receptor (NMDAR) antagonists (such as ketamine and nitrous oxide) and gamma aminobutyric acid (GABA) receptor agonists (such as sevoflurane and propofol). Exposure of developing mammals to NMDAR agonists or antagonists disrupts the endogenous NMDAR system and leads to increased neuronal cell death. The early stages of life and the growth spurt period are critical for synaptic remodeling and myelination. It is hypothesized that excessive inhibition and/or stimulation of neuronal activity during synaptogenesis may activate an internal signal, inducing programmed cell death in developing neurons. Research has shown that 24-h exposure to ketamine (a noncompetitive NMDA receptor antagonist) significantly increases cortical neuronal death, as evidenced by elevated caspase-3 expression, increased degenerated neuron staining, and more silver-stained positive neurons in newborn monkeys (PND5) and early-stage fetal macaques (GD122). These changes have not been observed in PND35 macaques. Another study found that 8-h exposure to sevoflurane anesthesia did not cause brain damage or neuroinflammatory responses in adult monkeys. These findings suggest that the brains of relatively mature and/or adult monkeys may have some resistance to the neurotoxic effects of GAs, while the developing macaque brain is more susceptible to damage from GA. Moreover, the data indicate that neuronal cell death does not result from the suppression of cardiac and respiratory functions during GA, but rather from the heightened sensitivity of the developing brain to GAs. Additionally, physiological stimulation of NMDAR during development is essential for synaptogenesis, differentiation, and survival of neurons, and interfering with NMDAR activation may reduce synaptogenesis and cellular interactions.

Preclinical research has shown that extended or repeated exposure to GAs during early development results in widespread apoptotic neurodegeneration within cortical and subcortical brain regions. This subsequently leads to delayed and persistent behavior disorders, particularly in memory and learning. Other components of psychological processes, such as motivation and inhibition, sequence learning, and counting mediated by the prefrontal cortex and striatal circuitry, have also been evaluated in neonatal animal models under anesthesia. Because of the shared complexities in behavior and cognition between NHPs and humans, NHP models of GA-induced cognitive impairments are highly valuable for translational investigations into the developmental neurotoxicity of anesthetics. The National Center for Toxicological Research (NCTR) Operant Test Battery (OTB), an operant behavioral assessment tool employed to measure cognitive abilities in NHPs following exposures to toxins or pharmaceutical agents, is adaptable for juvenile animals. Rhesus macaques at PND5 (or PND6), after 24-h anesthesia with ketamine, showed considerably reduced OTB scores when compared with control groups. They presented distinct impairments in color and location discrimination, motivation, sequence learning, and concept formation. In a separate experiment with rhesus macaques, animals exposed to 1% isoflurane combined with 70% nitrous oxide for 8 h exhibited significantly reduced response rates (defined as the rate at which a button is pressed to obtain a reward) compared to controls, suggesting impairment in both response and incentive learning. *Rhesus macaques* share similarities with humans in social interaction, basic emotions, and behavioral complexity, making them a valuable model for assessing the impact of GA exposure on socio-emotional maturity and motor skill development. The study results revealed that group-housed rhesus macaques exposed to isoflurane (0.7%–1.5% for 5 h, repeated on PND6, 9, and 12) presented motor reflex deficits and elevated anxiety levels at one year old. Similarly, neonatal rhesus macaques receiving repeated sevoflurane administration (2.5% for 4 h, on PND6, PND14, and PND28) exhibited increased anxiety-related behaviors in response to intruders. Across diverse animal models, NHP models are viewed as superior for translational research concerning cognitive impairments related to pediatric anesthesia.

While preclinical neurotoxicity studies often involve animal models, including NHPs, the use of NHPs in translational research presents both significant challenges and opportunities. The strength of NHP models lies in their closer genetic, physiological, and behavioral resemblance to humans. Conversely, challenges inherent in translational research must be recognized, as complete replication of human conditions in any animal model is impossible, including pharmacokinetic variations between humans and NHPs. Moreover, the numerous human-like characteristics of NHPs, compared to other models such as rodents, raise significant ethical concerns regarding their use in research.

It is plausible that prolonged exposure of infants to commonly used anesthetics/analgesics may lead to impaired cognitive development. However, it remains unclear whether neurodevelopmental deficits are caused by GA or by the surgical procedures/underlying conditions necessitating its use. There is a growing recognition that genetic variations and other factors, such as social interactions between individual rhesus macaques or Cynomolgus monkeys, can potentially influence experimental outcomes. Furthermore, it is impractical (slow and costly) to compare or implement multiple drug/dosing regimens or high-throughput approaches due to the substantial cost associated with each animal in NHP research and the potential difficulty in obtaining a sufficient number of female, neonatal, or juvenile animals.

It is difficult to study critical dose–response and time-course data regarding anesthetic/analgesic-induced neurotoxicity in humans. In vitro models have overcome many limitations and yielded greater data output due to their capacity for enhanced investigation of specific mechanisms and their greater amenability to novel technologies that are difficult to implement in in vivo studies. For example, neural stem cell (NSC) models derived from NHPs can recapitulate key developmental processes (including proliferation and differentiation) and serve as an effective alternative for evaluating anesthetic-induced neurotoxicity. To develop new and improved testing methods for better predicting human responses to drugs and/or environmental chemicals, the NSC cultivation system for NHPs can assist in conducting mechanism research that is difficult to achieve in animal models (due to the scarcity of newborn monkeys), such as anesthetic neurotoxicity. However, the understanding and prevention of the harmful effects of perinatal anesthetic exposure should not be neglected.

Recently, the NCTR Pediatric Anesthetic Research Team has successfully established an NHP NSC model using embryonic Cynomolgus Monkeys. In this preliminary study, cortical and hippocampal neural stem cells were successfully extracted from the fetal brain of Cynomolgus Monkeys at GD80, creating NHP neural stem cells that simulate in vivo cell development. These NSC models can infinitely yield high quantities of differentiated neurons, astrocytes, and oligodendrocytes. Consequently, cultured NSCs and/or cells derived from them can be exposed to GAs at selected concentrations (including both lower and higher doses with thresholds) and for different durations (short-term and long-term exposure). This may aid in establishing detection limits for analysis and predicting response thresholds for potential in vivo toxicity. Therefore, the availability of robust NHP-based NSC culture models will bring biologically relevant models closely mimicking human conditions into the laboratory. The application of these NHP in vitro models will not only minimize the use of animals in developmental neurotoxicity studies but also provide models that meet the needs of human-focused scientific and regulatory inquiries, allowing for deeper exploration into the cellular and molecular mechanisms behind anesthesia-induced neurotoxicity. Another critical and consistent element in the field of anesthesia research is conducting nonclinical studies using clinically relevant doses of anesthetics, such as ketamine, to mimic the clinical conditions of neonatal animals under surgical stress. Data have been accumulated supporting the correlation between surgery and subsequent physiological changes; however, whether neurodevelopmental deficits are directly caused by GA remains uncertain. Due to the difficulty in distinguishing the effects of anesthesia from those of surgery or pre-existing conditions, continued research on neonatal NHP is necessary to gain valuable information on the potential neuroprotective effects of anesthetics (such as ketamine) or ketamine-induced neurodegeneration. Importantly, the physiological similarities between NHPs and humans provide an opportunity to test this theory.

9.6.3 Considerations for Evaluating the Reproductive and Developmental Toxicity of Oligonucleotide Drugs

The fundamental principles of toxicology apply to all therapeutic drugs and products. However, the rationale for developing a specific toxicology testing strategy depends on the unique properties of the product. Chemically synthesized small molecules or NCEs (drugs, pharmaceutical products) and biomacromolecules or new biological entities (NBEs) (biologics, biopharmaceutical products) inherently possess distinct product attributes (Table 9.19). The difference between drugs and biopharmaceutical products can be characterized as a distinction based on the molecular size and complexity of the products. Oligonucleotide-based therapeutics exhibit characteristics of both NCEs and NBEs (Table 9.19). Historically, the nonclinical safety evaluation of oligonucleotides (ONs) follows the guidelines for small molecule nonclinical safety evaluation, as they are chemically synthesized and typically contain chemical components not present in biological systems. However, the attributes of certain ON products are more akin to biologics, including species specificity, structural similarity to endogenous molecules (i.e., DNA and RNA), and longer half-life periods and/or pharmacodynamic effects. Therefore, considering that oligonucleotide drugs exhibit both on-target toxicity due to pharmacologic amplification and off-target toxicity arising from binding to homologous

Table. 9.19 Comparison of attributes across different product categories

	New chemical entities	Oligonucleotides	New biological entities
Molecular weight	Low (<1 kDa)	Mid (>6 kDa)	High (>30 kDa)
Manufacture	Chemical synthesis	Chemical synthesis	Biologically derived
Manufacture	Single entity	Single entity	Heterogeneous
Tissue distribution	Intra- and extracellular Wide distribution	Intra- and extracellular Selected distribution	Largely extracellular Limited distribution
PK/ADME	Species-specific metabolites Short half-life	Catabolized to nucleotides Long acting	Catabolized to amino acids Long half-life
Species specificity	Less likely	More likely	Often
Off-target toxicity	Often	Sometimes	Rarely

RNA sequences or their inherent physicochemical properties, the evaluation of ON reproductive toxicity considers both their unique product attributes and the perspectives outlined in current drug and biologic evaluation guidelines. Product attributes are key to supporting a case-by-case approach for the nonclinical safety evaluation of biologics, which is the recommended approach for ON developmental and reproductive toxicity (DART) assessment. To date, experience with reproductive evaluations has primarily been derived from phosphothioate (PS)-modified oligonucleotides in a simple saline solution, ranging from 18 to 22 nucleotides in length, some with alkyl modifications at position 2 in the ribose. Consequently, toxicological findings can be attributed to the structure of the ON. However, the principles discussed are also applicable to ON drug products incorporating delivery formulations or conjugates/linkers. Therefore, evaluation is recommended for all such drug products [31].

For ONs, there are many different structural subclasses and biological mechanisms that may require specialized adjustments in the design of reproductive toxicity studies. Structural subclasses include platforms based on single-stranded DNA and double-stranded RNA (dsRNA), which possess varying degrees of PS, 2′-O-alkyl, 2′-fluoro, or other modifications that can modify the ribose, such as using synthetic morpholino rings or modifying internucleotide phosphodiester linkages by substituting with PS or phosphoramidate moieties. These chemical structure differences can have a significant impact on pharmacokinetics (PK), metabolic stability, nonspecific interactions, and the potential needs for complex formulations. The main mechanisms of action rely on interactions with nucleic acid targets, including antisense inhibition (involving complementary base pairing with mRNA targets and subsequent RNase H-mediated degradation of the double-stranded target), RNA interference (dependent on the binding of RNA-induced silencing complexes to target mRNA), pre-mRNA splicing and control, and regulation of transcriptional activity of multiple mRNAs through microRNA pathways. Additionally, ON drugs can also exert their pharmacological effects through interactions with specific proteins. Most molecular modifications are designed to minimize immune responses, but there are exceptions, such as CpG modifications, which aim to enhance immune stimulation. Therefore, similar to biologics, a single study design may not be suitable for all ON subtypes.

Instead, the product attributes of each ON subtype will determine the most scientifically effective method.

In designing reproductive toxicity assessments, careful consideration should be given to the special effects of pharmacological targets, as they may be related to reproductive function and could potentially have enhanced pharmacological effects on pregnancy or fetal development. For the majority of ONs, this assessment usually concentrates on the effects on the expression or function of the target protein. For microRNAs, the focus may be on the impact of increased expression of the RNA family. Therefore, if the pharmacological target of the ON is not well conserved between humans and the standard species used in reproductive studies, the evaluation may be challenging. It is of great benefit when the function of the specific target is established, and when literature is available regarding reproductive function in relevant knockout or transgenic mouse models, and in human populations with either a deficiency or excess expression of the target. If this evaluation is feasible, it should take into account the functional changes that occur across different developmental stages, including both systemic effects and those specific to reproductive tissues. In the absence of such data, alternative approaches should be explored.

Knowing the expression profile of the specific target is crucial to gauge the level of concern. Typically, exposure of the testes to ON is lower. With low fetal exposure to ON, opportunities for direct target effects on the embryo or fetus might be restricted. For instance, the placental transfer of phosphorothioate ONs is minimal. However, in several investigations concerning phosphorothioate ONs, measurable ON concentrations have been found, as seen in the regulation of target expression in the fetus. Furthermore, while it remains unclear whether and to what extent ON reaches the fetus to exert any direct effect, or an effect at the appropriate time during development, pharmacologically relevant changes in maternal physiology can impact not only embryo implantation and pregnancy maintenance, but also potentially lead to fetal abnormalities (e.g., angiogenesis inhibitors or compounds inducing hypoglycemia through their pharmacological action). The application of pharmacologically relevant models is especially important when reproductive or developmental effects are anticipated.

Animal models ought to closely resemble humans with respect to pharmacokinetics, metabolism, toxicological sensitivity, and pharmacological actions. Aptamers and ONs containing CpG are designed to exert their function through direct interaction with proteins, typically exhibiting cross-species potency. Therefore, they may be active in at least one of the commonly used species for EFD research (mice and rabbits). In contrast, human antisense oligonucleotides (ASOs) are typically inactive in rodents and rabbits due to species differences in mRNA target sequences. In such cases, it may be necessary to use an analog (alternative molecule) that is active in that species for reproductive toxicity studies.

The selection of animal species should primarily consider whether the clinical candidate demonstrates pharmacological activity in rodents and/or rabbits. For clinical candidates that exhibit pharmacological activity in rodents and/or rabbits, or those with targets not endogenous to any animal species (e.g., antimicrobial ONs), standard rodent and rabbit studies may be performed, as commonly done for small molecules. According to the recommendations of the Exaggerated Pharmacology (EP) Subcommittee of the Oligonucleotide Safety Working Group (OSWG) for general toxicology studies, reproductive toxicity studies conducted in a pharmacologically relevant species are deemed acceptable. If a clinical candidate demonstrates positive findings in a standard species (rat or rabbit) used in EFD studies, another EFD study in a second species is still required to thoroughly evaluate the effects of the chemical. If a clinical candidate is not pharmacologically active in either rodents or rabbits, it would still be deemed valuable to conduct reproductive toxicity studies in these standard species, as the chemical structure has not yet been evaluated in reproductive toxicity studies. However, in cases where a clinical candidate drug exhibits a lack of activity in rats or rabbits, applicants should contemplate additional study designs to assess reproductive and developmental effects potentially magnified by the pharmacological mechanism.

Overall, in assessing reproductive toxicity, DART studies using NHPs should only be considered when there are clear reasons for concern and NHPs are the sole relevant species for the clinical candidate drug. Although this method enables assessment of clinical candidate drug effects stemming from nucleotide sequence, chemical modifications, and pharmacodynamics, variations in target sequence will still constrain the absolute extent of drug cross-reactivity. In addition, NHP studies are often limited by the small number of animals, which can reduce the ability to detect risks. If the study goal is to delineate the reproductive toxicity profile of a relatively well-established agent, it is advisable to conduct DART studies in NHPs. For example, such studies may be necessary when an RNA target has specific reproductive concerns that cannot be investigated using rodents or special indicators within general toxicology studies.

9.6.3.1 Case Study 1: Antisense ON Administered Orally

In an antisense ON program targeting an inflammatory pathway for the treatment of inflammatory bowel disease (IBD), the ON demonstrated good pharmacological activity in mice (but not in rats) and NHPs. The drug is formulated in a specific enteric-coated capsule that delivers the drug directly to the lower gastrointestinal tract (the target site of the disease), thus minimizing systemic absorption. In general, toxicology studies using the clinical formulation, systemic exposure is very low after repeated oral intragastric administration at high dose levels. The applicant focused the reproductive toxicity evaluation on EFD studies and requested a waiver for FEED and PPND studies. To ensure adequate systemic exposure, intravenous (IV) administration was chosen for EFD studies.

Given the pharmacological activity data in mice (and previous experience with this species in general toxicology studies), the mice (instead of the rats) were chosen as the primary pharmacologically relevant species. While the pharmacological relevance of the rabbit was uncertain (considered unlikely and not further investigated), the rabbit was used as a second species in the EFD studies to examine the effects of the test substance on reproduction and development. A study in NHP (a pharmacologically relevant species) was considered uninformative, as all observed toxicities in both mouse and NHP toxicity studies were consistent with known "class effects" of phosphorothioate ONs, with no adverse effects related to pharmacology. Daily dosing was employed to mimic the clinical regimen; the ON was a first-generation PS structure with limited stability. Routine dose-ranging EFD studies were conducted in both species, with maternal toxicity meticulously characterized based on clinical signs, reduced body weight gain, decreased food consumption, and macroscopic lesions in the neck (observed post-necropsy). Toxicokinetic (TK) sampling was not included in the dose-ranging studies, but was included in the mouse EFD study (using satellite animals) and followed by a dedicated PK study in pregnant rabbits to obtain exposure data in the second species. Sample analysis in rabbits was limited to plasma from animals at the no-observed-adverse-effect level (NOAEL). This analysis indicated very high multiples of exposure for the intravenous route compared to human PK data from oral administration, barely detectable using sensitive hybrid assays. In mice, adverse developmental effects were observed, characterized by increased post-implantation loss (embryo fetal mortality) and decreased fetal weight, concomitant with severe maternal toxicity.

9.6.3.2 Case Study 2: Intravitreal Administration of Nucleic Acid Aptamers

Pegaptanib, a pegylated aptamer that binds to VEGF, has been approved for the treatment of wet age-related macular degeneration (AMD). It exhibits pharmacological activity in mice, rats, rabbits, canines, and NHPs. Clinically, Macugen is administered via intravitreal injection (IVT). In nonclinical studies, IVT administration has demonstrated that the drug slowly enters the systemic circulation from the vitreous humor, resulting in minimal systemic exposure. Nonclinical PK and general toxicity studies of Macugen were conducted using subcutaneous (SC), intravenous (IV), and IVT routes. The safety of IVT and IV administration of Macugen was evaluated in acute, subchronic, and chronic studies across mice, rats, rabbits, canines, and NHPs. Macugen showed very high tolerability after systemic and IVT administration, with the maximum tolerated dose yet to be determined.

Due to the advanced age (with the median age over 70 years) and limited reproductive potential of the patients, restricted reproductive toxicity studies were performed for the AMD indication (dose-ranging EFD studies were conducted in rabbits and mice, and formal EFD studies were conducted via intravenous administration in mice). In addition to the initial indication for AMD, diabetic macular edema (DME) was subsequently investigated as an indication, which would entail treatment of a younger patient population. Based on the two potential indications (AMD and DME), reproductive toxicity study designs were discussed with the FDA. A consensus was reached that studies focusing on fertility, reproductive toxicity, teratogenicity, and PPND can be postponed until the commencement of Phase III clinical trials for the DME indication. Furthermore, the possibility of waiving a second species study based on the results of the EFD study was also discussed. Based on discussions with other regulatory agencies, prior to Phase III clinical trials, dose-ranging in mice via IV administration, formal EFD and fertility studies, as well as dose-ranging EFD studies in rabbits via IVT administration were conducted.

The properties of ONs are akin to those of NCEs and NBEs, and guidelines for both drug classes can be referred to when planning reproductive toxicity studies. Testing strategies in DART studies must account for both the potential effects of the chemical structure and the expected pharmacological action of the drug. Standard reproductive toxicology species (rodents/rabbits) can generally be used, as most toxicities are related to the chemical structure. Alternative molecules (analogs active in the test species) can be evaluated for potential reproductive effects related to either the chemical structure or pharmacology. The selection of relevant animal species, dosing regimen, and whether to use the clinical candidate drug or an alternative molecule must be carefully considered based on the specific properties of the ON product. Information from general toxicity studies and previous experience with similar ONs will further contribute to the decision-making process. For the aforementioned reasons, NHP studies should be conducted only when required to answer particular questions or when no other suitable alternatives are available. A tailored dosing strategy is necessary to guarantee sufficient drug exposure during the organogenesis phase, while maintaining the ability to accurately assess PD and PK parameters.

9.6.4 Failure Cases of NHP in DART

The routine use of NHP models in DART studies may not be entirely predictive of clinical toxicities. Artemisinin combination therapy (ACT), a first-line treatment for uncomplicated malaria in adults and children, is recommended by the World Health Organization (WHO). While considered safe during the second and third trimesters of pregnancy, animal studies have shown that artemisinin derivatives can cause fetal death and congenital malformations during a narrow window of time in early embryonic development. During this specific period, artemisinin derivatives have been observed to induce defective erythropoiesis and vasculogenesis/angiogenesis in experimental models. However, clinical data on the safety of ACT in pregnant women have not shown an increased risk of miscarriage, stillbirth, or congenital malformations associated with artemisinin exposure in early pregnancy, nor an increased risk of low birth weight.

In vivo developmental toxicity studies have revealed that artemisinin can only induce fetal death and congenital malformations in rodents when the embryo is exposed within a narrow window of early embryogenesis. For instance, embryo death and malformations are observed in rats following a single gavage administration of artesunate between GD10 and GD14. The same dose at GD9, or even a higher dose at GD16 or GD17, does not induce embryotoxicity. Therefore, GD10–14 is identified as the developmental period more sensitive to artemisinin, with GD10 being the most sensitive period for inducing malformations (mainly cardiovascular defects and bone abnormalities) and GD11 being the most sensitive for inducing embryonic lethality. In other studies, administering different artemisinin derivatives such as dihydroartemisinin (DHA), artesunate, arteether, and artemether to rats at GD10 resulted in similar teratogenic patterns. This suggests that embryonic lethality and malformations might be associated with the endoperoxide bridge, a structural feature characteristic of this drug class and responsible for its antimalarial activity. Therefore, developing an artemisinin derivative that maintains antimalarial efficacy while reducing embryotoxicity is not feasible. However, artefenomel (OZ439), which also contains a peroxide group structure, demonstrates a higher safety margin compared to artesunate. Assuming that the embryotoxicity of artemisinin is due to the reduction in heme biosynthesis, artefenomel might have lower toxicity due to its structural differences. Another approach to reducing the embryotoxicity of artemisinin is to combine it with other drugs that can prevent or mitigate toxicity. For example, folic acid administration in mice can prevent the detrimental effects of artesunate on cardiac development, specifically the induction of ventricular septal defects and alterations in the thickness of the ventricular and atrial septa. Pharmacokinetic extrapolation from animal studies to human treatment demonstrates that the drug concentrations observed in these animals fall within the exposure range targeted in human therapy [32].

To better evaluate the pathogenic mechanisms associated with the embryotoxic effects of artemisinin, researchers using the WEC method have shown that the yolk sac is the primary site of high sensitivity to artemisinin compounds: During the entire culture period (GD9.5–11.5), exposure to DHA (an unsaturated fatty acid) in rat embryos resulted in severe depletion of circulating erythrocytes. When the embryos were exposed for 1.5 h at the beginning of culture (GD9.5), similar results were observed. However, at the end of the culture period (GD11.5), exposure for 1.5 h only affected the morphology of the red blood cells. The test concentrations were within the range of maximum plasma concentrations detected in patients post-treatment (0.01–2 µg/mL). Considering that the WEC method covers the critical period of yolk sac hematopoiesis (primary hematopoiesis), which occurs between GD9 and GD14 in rats and corresponds to GD15 to the sixth week of gestation in humans, a single exposure to DHA (administered to pregnant rats at 7.5 or 15 mg/kg) in utero showed that primitive erythroblasts from yolk sac hematopoiesis were affected at GD9.5 and GD10.5, leading to anemia and subsequent hypoxia. At GD11.5, notable cellular damage within the embryo was observed, followed by embryo–fetal death. In another study, the WEC model was used to analyze the mechanism of inducing erythroblastic depletion in embryos. Following DHA administration, embryonic erythrocytes exhibited abnormal cell division and apoptosis, manifested as increased symmetrical and asymmetrical binucleated cells, TUNEL (terminal deoxynucleotidyl transferase dUTP nick end labeling) positive cells, Caspase3-positive cells, and embryonic erythrocytes with fragmented nuclei.

While most studies on the developmental effects of artemisinins have focused on rodents, alternative animal models such as FETAX (Frog Embryo Teratogenesis Assay–Xenopus) have also been used. Exposure of Xenopus embryos to DHA (0.01–5 µg/mL) at early developmental stages (24 h post-fertilization) resulted in a reduction of primitive erythrocytes, whereas erythrocytes in late-stage *Xenopus larvae* were only minimally affected. In this study, no embryonic lethality occurred, and congenital malformations were only induced at the highest dose levels (0.1–0.5 µg/mL).

The zebrafish model was also utilized to test the potential embryotoxicity of DHA. Exposure to DHA (1–10 µg/mL) during primitive hematopoiesis and hematopoietic stem cell differentiation resulted in abnormal embryonic phenotypes similar to those observed in other animal models (pericardial effusion, trunk axis abnormalities, and dyspigmentation), developmental delays, or death. However, in contrast to other animal models, DHA increased angiogenesis and vasculogenesis in zebrafish. These discrepancies may arise from differences in breeding conditions and drug delivery routes between zebrafish and mammals, but could also indicate distinct mechanisms of action. The difference in hematopoietic sites between zebrafish and mammals must also be considered.

Another study in primates, administering artesunate to pregnant Cynomolgus monkeys (15 monkeys/group) at different durations (3, 7, or 30 days) from GD20–50, demonstrated dose-and time-dependent developmental toxicity. Artesunate administration at the onset of organogenesis, at doses ≥12 mg/kg for more than 12 days, resulted in embryolethality, while shorter periods of administration did not (3–7 days). It is noteworthy that, although ACTs are the recommended treatment for uncomplicated malaria, developmental toxicity studies are rarely conducted in vitro for ACTs, compared to artemisinin derivatives alone.

The results of multiple animal experiments, including those involving NHPs, clearly indicate that artemisinin has clear teratogenic effects. However, a meta-analysis of a prospective observational study involving 30,000 human pregnancies has concluded that artemisinin treatment in the first trimester is not associated with an increased risk of miscarriage or stillbirth, and the incidence of congenital birth defects is similar to that of other WHO-approved antimalarial therapies during pregnancy. The available human and animal data, as summarized in the artesunate label, far exceeds the amount of data generated in EFD-specific studies aligned with ICH S5 guidelines.

The observed discrepancies between animal studies and human data regarding the safety of artemisinin derivatives during pregnancy are difficult to reconcile and may be attributed to various reasons.

Animal studies are conducted in healthy subjects, while drug-exposed women are often infected with Plasmodium parasites. Underlying physiological conditions, pregnancy, and malaria have the potential to influence the pharmacokinetic characteristics of various drugs, including antimalarial agents. Following oral administration of artemisinin, plasma concentrations of the parent drug and its primary metabolite, DHA, are higher in pregnant women with malaria compared to the same women in a healthy state (i.e., postpartum). The absorption of artesunate and its conversion to DHA also differ between malaria patients and healthy volunteers. Moreover, the stability of endoperoxides may vary under different physiological conditions. In vitro, DHA degradation is influenced by assay conditions (pH, temperature, and hemolysis), suggesting that clinical conditions associated with malaria severity, such as fever, hemolysis, or acidosis, may contribute to unstable artemisinin. Pregnancy can further exacerbate variability.

In malaria patients, artemisinins primarily concentrate in infected erythrocytes. It has been suggested that during malaria infection, limited transfer of artemisinins to the embryo occurs because more of the drug is activated, leading to degradation and the formation of carbon-centered free radicals, which then bind to parasite proteins.

In rat and monkey embryos, the targets of artemisinin toxicity are circulating primitive erythroblasts. Since primitive erythroid precursors form in the yolk sac during weeks 3–6 of gestation and circulate in the embryo during weeks 4–9, this period is considered the most sensitive to artemisinin derivative toxicity in humans. However, the duration of ACT treatment in humans is very short (3–7 days). If these primitive erythroblasts, which are sensitive to artemisinin derivatives, are generated over a longer period, then damaged cells would be replaced by newly formed cells, and the consequences might be less severe. Therefore, the duration of drug exposure appears critical. Differences in exposure duration may lead to discrepancies between human safety data and embryotoxicity data from animal models.

9.7 Trends in the Advancement of Reproductive and Developmental Toxicity Studies in NHPs

Currently, toxicologists are gradually combining toxicogenomics, high-tech non-invasive diagnostics and analyses, immunotoxicology, alternative models, and other specialized disciplines in DART research.

Many large pharmaceutical companies are conducting research in genomics, proteomics, and toxicogenomics, aiming to develop solutions that truly replace traditional in vivo testing. Today, anyone can use toxicogenomic tools to generate data, but we know that this requires a larger volume of data and the involvement of researchers from different disciplines to validate and interpret it. Furthermore, it is impossible to explain in vivo results of test articles through in vitro studies, or predict pre-existing pathological changes in vitro, until databases can identify normal genetic variation and associated typical variation patterns with sufficient accuracy. Although the foundational research required for this will take years, preliminary and promising results have already emerged.

Even at this stage, institutions with long-standing experience in nonhuman primate drug toxicology research can make significant contributions to the development of new technologies, such as toxicogenomics. Once conventional drug toxicology tests are completed, minimal additional work is needed to obtain tissue samples from different organs of the test animals, then isolate mRNA from these samples and store it in a nucleic acid repository for future validation and comparison. Currently, although only mice and rats have preliminary toxicology chip databases, the advent of nonhuman primate chips is just a matter of time. Institutions with large toxicology datasets for various compounds can integrate toxicological data with gene modulation data, which will offer a significant research advantage in the field of toxicogenomics.

9.7.1 The 3 R strategy for NHPs

The shortage of NHPs has severely limited the availability of NHPs for reproductive toxicity studies requiring EFD or PPND, especially considering the already limited supply of sexually mature NHPs. Against this backdrop, the development plan for each drug should be assessed to determine whether the WoE (weight of evidence) approach can adequately assess and communicate risks, rather than automatically defaulting to developmental toxicity evaluation in NHPs. It is important to recognize that the use of the WoE approach is inevitably limited when evaluating novel targets or new therapies. Currently, feasible directions can be broadly divided into three: ①

Reducing the number of dose groups in studies; ② using alternative molecules; and ③ applying alternative methods [33].

Since developmental toxicity studies conducted in NHPs are intended solely for risk identification, these studies can be performed with one control group and one dose group, provided that a scientifically reasonable justification is presented for the selected dose levels. An example of an appropriate scientific justification is that under the clinical dosing regimen, a monoclonal antibody's binding to a soluble target is expected to reach saturation. If it can be demonstrated in the selected animal species that target binding has reached saturation and exposure exceeds ten times the therapeutic drug level, a single-dose group and control group design would be sufficient to provide adequate evidence for potential embryonic and fetal development hazards.

It is encouraged to reuse maternal NHPs from vehicle control groups. Additionally, if there are concerns regarding mechanisms of action that may affect EFD or lead to miscarriage, testing can be conducted in a limited number of animals to confirm potential hazards.

Another alternative method for NHPs is to use alternative molecules that are active in rodents or rabbits, or to use animal models expressing human targets (e.g., genetically modified mice expressing human targets). Both approaches require pharmacological relevance to be demonstrated before they can be used for DART evaluations (i.e., well-characterized models). Several examples of alternative molecules have already been generated and used in DART studies. Specifically, Wakefield et al. used polyethylene glycol (PEG)-conjugated Fab and anti-rat TNFα antibody as alternatives to evaluate the developmental and reproductive toxicity potential of certolizumab pegol, a PEG-conjugated Fab fragment of a humanized IgG1 antibody targeting human TNFα. Additionally, Clarke et al. used an anti-mouse CD11a monoclonal antibody to characterize placental transfer in mice as an alternative for evaluating the safety of adalimumab. These examples demonstrate the feasibility of using alternative molecules in rodents for DART evaluations. As for the use of genetically engineered rodent models, this approach is less commonly used due to the time and resources required to generate viable, well-characterized models. An example of this method is the use of a humanized CD4 transgenic mouse model by Bugelski et al. to characterize the safety of kalevalizumab in general toxicology and DART studies. To utilize alternative molecules or genetically modified rodent models, drug development teams need to identify suitable alternatives and/or generate appropriate animal models early in the process, as these methods are challenging to develop and difficult to justify scientifically for safety evaluation.

Alternative methods for reproductive toxicity assessment, such as rat whole embryo culture, embryonic stem cells, and zebrafish models, are worth considering. It is generally believed that these tests are more useful in candidate selection or exploratory studies of small molecules, rather than as direct substitutes for in vivo testing. As experience with common mechanisms/pathways leading to adverse pregnancy outcomes accumulates, the value of in vitro methods may increase.

9.7.1.1 Embryonic Stem Cell Test (EST)

The embryonic stem cell test (EST), described by the European Reference Laboratory for Alternative Methods to Animal Testing, is widely used for in vitro screening of potential embryotoxic effects of chemicals and drug candidates. Mouse embryonic stem cells (mESC) are cultured with leukemia inhibitory factor (LIF) to maintain growth in a pluripotent state. The test measures the cytotoxicity of 3T3A31 fibroblasts and ESCs, evaluating whether ESCs exposed to test substances can differentiate into functional contractile cardiomyocytes. It further assesses the ability of stem cells to differentiate into all embryonic components in vitro. This model summarizes the process of establishing the three germ layers (ectoderm, mesoderm, and endoderm) and the subsequent differentiation of these embryonic cells. Thus, the model has the capability to evaluate many events related to embryogenesis. One potential future development is the use of molecular markers to assess phenotypic differentiation. Another advantage of this system is the direct comparison it enables between differentiation and cytotoxicity/proliferation, which may aid in eventually classifying exogenous substances as in vivo developmental toxicants. Due to the nature of embryonic stem cells, they are easily subjected to relatively high-throughput culture modifications (automation, scale-down) and point-by-point visual assessment of physical structures, facilitating morphological evaluation (such as cellular contraction, significant lipid droplet changes, etc.). Additionally, once obtained, mESCs do not require animal use, which is a significant advantage in some cases. In contrast, maintaining pluripotency for some human ESC lines does require the use of mouse embryonic fibroblasts as feeder layers, necessitating additional animals. Progress has been made with xenogeneic human ESC cultures that do not require animal use.

Embryotoxicity of test substances is typically evaluated using three endpoints: ① Inhibition of differentiation into beating cardiomyocytes; ② byproducts of cytotoxic effects on stem cells; and ③ differentiation of T3 fibroblasts.

Extensive studies using 20 known embryotoxic test substances have been conducted to validate various variants of this test.

The EST is relatively simple to implement, and its primary endpoint (beating score) does not require an in-depth understanding of phenotypic and morphological development. The evaluation of proliferation and cytotoxicity relies on standard, well-established assays already used in many laboratories. Therefore, laboratories proficient in cell culture only require limited additional training to perform the EST described in the EURLECVAM protocol. This analysis is more suited for relatively high-throughput modifications (automation, scale-down). EST appears to be most effective at both ends of the activity spectrum: If a compound is classified as non-developmental toxic, it is very likely (>90%) to be true. For strong developmental toxicants, these assays can detect all of them, but they may also classify some weak nontoxic substances as strong developmental toxicants. Currently, predictive models for EST largely depend on the absolute concentrations of various toxicities. If a compound produces cytotoxicity at very low concentrations, even if its activity in vivo is weak or low, the model will classify the compound as "strongly toxic." Like in vitro whole embryo culture (WEC), this test lacks maternal components and has limited metabolic capacity (although the S9 fraction can be used to add this component when necessary), which is both an advantage and a disadvantage. The advantage is that metabolites and parent compounds can be tested separately, identifying true active agents. In contrast, identifying and obtaining metabolites can also be a challenge.

The EST also has limitations. The lack of meaningful maternal components means that these tests currently have limited ability to simulate the direct effects of compounds on the developmental system and predict dose-limiting maternal toxicity. Predicting developmental effects from changes in maternal physiology, such as acidosis, is not impossible, and these changes may, in turn, alter in vivo development. Current EST models tend to be overly sensitive, leading to many non-toxic developmental substances being classified as toxic. Effectively distinguishing between non-toxic and weakly toxic compounds is one of the major challenges faced by these assays. Another potential drawback of EST is its reliance on a differentiated outcome in the evaluation. Identifying beating cells as markers of cardiomyocyte differentiation may be influenced by the test substance's effect on myocardial cell contraction (e.g., altered energy production) or may be confused with direct cardiotoxicity. Furthermore, there is no distinction between 10 beating cells per well and 10,000 beating cells per well in evaluating differentiation, so the lack of specific features to distinguish "differentiation" may reduce the assay's specificity. Additionally, the random differentiation of pre-embryos and the production of unknown growth/protective factors and cell types by differentiated cells add another layer of uncertainty. Generally, this type of test does not produce cell types seen in late-stage differentiation, such as those found in teratomas.

The use of molecular markers to evaluate multiple differentiation phenotypes in mESCs after undirected differentiation is a promising direction for the future. Quantitative methods can be employed to assess the relative mRNA levels of specific molecular markers (e.g., αMHC for cardiomyocytes) to determine differentiation for each phenotype and the relative differentiation across multiple phenotypes (such as comparing ectoderm and mesoderm). The use of lineage-specific markers may also aid in predicting the target tissue effects of a test substance as a developmental toxicant.

9.7.1.2 Whole Embryo Culture (WEC)

Whole embryo culture (WEC) has a long history in evaluating embryotoxicity in developing rodent embryos. For rats, embryos with yolk sacs are typically extracted on gestation day (GD) 9.5 or 10. The embryos are then cultured in a mixture of serum, medium, and the test substance (if applicable) for 44–48 h while rotating, with an increased oxygen concentration in the gas overlay. At the end of the culture period, various developmental endpoints of the embryos are evaluated, such as the number of somites, visual development, forelimb development, and neural tube development. Each of these endpoints is given a score, and the scores for each concentration of the test substance are summed. The presence and types of malformations are also recorded. The test outcomes can include: ① The concentration at which malformation signs first become apparent; ② a comparison of malformation types and severity among different compounds at a given concentration; and ③ the results from the linear judgment analysis formula when using the EURLECVAM version.

Rodent WEC has been included in the EURLECVAM validation study for embryotoxicity testing. According to predefined performance criteria, the repeatability of the WEC assay and the consistency between in vitro data and in vivo data for embryotoxicity potential are good. The predictive model correctly classified 80% of the

20 test compounds across all embryotoxicity categories (non-embryotoxic, weakly embryotoxic, and strongly embryotoxic). For more information on the validation study, including the comprehensive protocol for the method, the EURLECVAM website can be accessed. Using techniques similar to those developed for rat and mouse WEC, rabbit embryos can be relatively easily cultured. Typically, one rabbit embryo is assigned per test substance concentration, and rotating culture chambers with continuous gas flow are used. The evaluated endpoints include survival rate, growth, morphological scoring, and biochemical measurements (total protein and DNA). A key difference between rat and rabbit embryos lies in the yolk sac: GD_9 rat embryos rely on inverted visceral yolk sac-dependent tissue nutrition, with the embryo encased in the yolk sac, while rabbit embryos lack the inverted yolk sac and are located outside of it around GD_{13}. However, yolk sac-mediated tissue nutrition is specific to rodents and may not be as relevant to humans (which rely on blood nutrition). For the future, similar to rat and mouse WEC, it is expected that functional endpoints (e.g., phagocytosis and proteolysis), gene expression (e.g., yolk sac transport proteins), and imaging technologies (e.g., micro-CT, MRI, morphological measurements of embryo volume, or specific developmental markers) will become useful endpoints in rabbit WEC analysis. Rabbit WEC may also help address species differences in developmental toxicity responses.

For many laboratories, growth parameters (such as crown–rump length, protein content) are good predictors of potential embryotoxicity, with the added advantage of being continuous variables (unlike morphology-based parameters). Therefore, it is recommended to modify the standard WEC approach for evaluating embryotoxicity so that it does not rely solely on morphological scoring. The no-observed-adverse-effect concentration (NOAEC) for a compound may be related to the overall morphological score, but there is typically a steep dose–response curve, leading to a rapid transition from non-embryotoxic to strongly embryotoxic effects. In these cases, the maximum inhibitory concentration (ICmax) corresponds to the concentration that produces the highest rate of malformation. Additionally, embryos from different species provide different predictions, as is the case in vivo. Currently, WEC should not be used for human risk assessment purposes, partly due to the lack of maternal components and the very limited exposure window. Compound-class-specific predictive models can enhance the ability to predict the toxicity of drugs or chemical classes.

The species used for WEC (mouse, rat, and rabbit) are the same as those most commonly used in overall animal reproductive toxicity studies, allowing for a direct correlation between in vitro and in vivo findings, and comparison with mouse embryonic stem cell data. WEC can reproduce up to 48 h of in vivo embryonic development. Embryos can be treated in an environment isolated from maternal effects, but if necessary, some maternal influences can be introduced into the culture system (such as using cultured serum from treated animals, adding known maternal metabolites to the culture medium, or introducing high temperatures). WEC can be used for mechanistic studies, compound prioritization/screening, studying species-specific differences, providing supporting information for regulatory/risk assessment purposes, or further investigating in vivo findings to increase data credibility while minimizing animal use.

Currently, WEC cannot replace in vivo developmental toxicity studies because it cannot encompass the maternal–fetal interaction nor expose embryos to the critical pregnancy period (from implantation to full term). WEC also cannot isolate maternal influences (such as metabolism and toxicity), which may only have effects in vivo. Additionally, the relatively narrow developmental time window of WEC may fail to capture certain manifestations of developmental toxicity, and differences between serum samples or collection methods also exist. As WEC has not been validated, it is not used by U.S. regulatory agencies (FDA, EPA) for regulatory decision-making.

9.7.1.3 Zebrafish Embryotoxicity Test (ZET)

The Zebrafish Embryotoxicity Test (ZET) has been developed as a screening tool, and its ability to predict the teratogenic potential of chemicals and candidate drugs has been validated. This test holds great promise for the screening and evaluation of teratogenic potential in compounds. Most of the signaling pathways identified in both zebrafish and mammalian embryos are similar, and the heart development in both rodents and zebrafish may follow the same pattern. Zebrafish is an in vivo developmental model with many advantages over in vitro systems and holds great potential to meet the requirements for simple, cost-effective, and rapid screening of teratogenicity. Zebrafish are easy to culture and breed, relatively low in cost, and their developmental processes are similar to those in humans. Many molecular pathways are evolutionarily conserved between zebrafish and humans. It has been demonstrated that zebrafish share homologous genes for most human drug targets (86%). Toxicologists have been using zebrafish embryos for years to identify endpoints and elucidate the developmental toxicity mechanisms of various chemicals. Additionally, due to zebrafish's rapid external development, they provide a unique advantage for testing the effects of compounds during the entire organogenesis process. This crucial feature is not achievable in other commonly used teratogenicity screening assays, such as EST or rodent whole-embryo culture (WEC). Furthermore, the transparency of the surrounding egg membrane (chorion) and embryonic tissues allows direct observation of the developmental process throughout embryogenesis.

Recent studies on the "Zebrafish Developmental Toxicity (DarT)" assay have demonstrated the widespread utility of zebrafish in screening potential teratogenic compounds. Brannen et al. conducted a retrospective study aimed at developing a zebrafish teratogenicity screening method capable of describing teratogenicity related to specific abnormalities and concentration–response relationships, as well as evaluating the consistency and predictability of this assay. This review included 34 substances, both exploratory and marketed drugs, that were known teratogens or non-teratogens in vivo. The study developed a morphological scoring system and described the characteristics of the assessment. The results indicate that using zebrafish embryos to predict in vivo mammalian teratogenicity has a high success rate.

A total of 34 compounds, including those validated by EURLECVAM and drugs with in vivo teratogenic potential, were evaluated using the ZET testing protocol. The basic experimental design involved treating chorion-free zebrafish embryos with the compound 24 h after fertilization, during which the embryos are rapidly undergoing organogenesis. The classic exposure time was 48 h, with morphological evaluation conducted around 120 h after fertilization (approximately 4 days post-fertilization). Two general toxicity measurements were included in the predictive model. The first measurement followed the approach used in previous EURLECVAM predictive modeling for rat whole embryo culture and mouse embryonic stem cell assays, where the corresponding compounds were evaluated within a dose range in NIH3T3 fibroblasts. The second general toxicity measurement involved assessing the compounds within a zebrafish embryo concentration range, determining the general toxicity concentration based on the 25% lethal dose (LC25). The study developed a morphological scoring system, evaluating various structures and organs in the zebrafish larvae on day 5, including a severity score for the malformations. Each compound's predictive model classification involved calculating the toxicity concentration based on overall morphology and the ratio of toxicity concentration to the no observed adverse-effect concentration (NOAEC). The results of the comparative review by Brannen et al. showed that the predictive model results were consistent with the accumulated in vivo teratogenicity data with an accuracy of 92%. The success rates for clearly identifying in vivo teratogens and non-teratogens were both 94%, while the success rate for clearly identifying in vivo morphological outcomes (such as the absence of fetal morphological adverse effects or the clear identification of at least one affected structure/organ system associated with compound exposure) was 87.5%. Additionally, the in vivo morphological outcomes could be successfully described positively.

Although this work highlights the overall utility and predictability of zebrafish assays in evaluating developmental toxicity, several unresolved issues remain regarding the broader application of zebrafish in predicting teratogenicity. There is limited knowledge about the pharmacokinetics and metabolism of water-soluble compounds in zebrafish embryos and larvae, and exploring these characteristics was not the aim of this study. A better understanding of zebrafish exposure, pharmacokinetics, and metabolism mechanisms, as well as their correlation with mammals, would be valuable for interpreting the relationship between zebrafish test results and teratogenicity in humans and other mammals. Additionally, in these experiments, to increase the exposure of the embryos to the compound, the chorion was removed from each embryo.

As a teratogenic screening tool, zebrafish offers the concept of a whole organism at all developmental stages, rather than limited developmental parts or isolated cells in cell culture. This complete model allows for the normal interaction of all cells and tissue layers, providing a level of integrity that other models lack. The small size of the embryos also means minimal compound requirements, which is particularly beneficial for evaluation studies that require the synthesis of new compounds. Moreover, a series of subeffective allele embryos can be generated by gradually reducing gene expression to produce progressively affected phenotypes. Preliminary indications suggest that this model has the potential to provide predictive power at least as good as existing models, and possibly even better.

9.7.2 Application of the Weight of Evidence Method in the Evaluation of Developmental Toxicity of Biologics

Historically, the method for assessing the potential risk of human embryonic developmental toxicity has been based on standard embryonic developmental toxicity studies conducted in pregnant animals. The toxicity signals identified in these studies are used for human risk assessment and product labeling. With ongoing advancements in understanding the biological and physiological processes related to reproduction and developmental biology across different species, there are now alternative approaches to studying potentially harmful effects targeting specific molecules, pathways, cells, tissues, organ functions, and target regulation through targeted biological research. These advancements directly impact risk assessment and provide an alternative to administering substances to pregnant animals for developmental toxicity risk safety evaluation. In this context, the issue driving the safety evaluation becomes: how much and what type of data are needed to reasonably assess the potential embryotoxicity in patient populations [34].

Currently, in some late-stage cancer indications, an alternative approach is used to understand patient risk, and these methods could also be considered for other patient populations. The ICH S9 guideline (Nonclinical Evaluation of Anticancer Pharmaceuticals) has now acknowledged the role of expected pharmacological effects in developmental toxicity risk assessment. This guideline clearly states that for drugs targeting rapidly dividing cells (such as crypt cells and bone marrow), or those falling into categories known to cause developmental toxicity, fertility, and early embryonic developmental toxicity studies are not required. ICH S9 offers alternative methods that may be considered, including a thorough literature review, placental transfer evaluation, direct or indirect effects of biologic drugs, and the evaluation of other developmental factors. These factors may include human genetic expression, gene alteration data from animals, and data from studies involving the same molecular approach in pregnant animals. In cases where sufficient data are available to assess the risk without conducting studies in pregnant animals, such studies may not be necessary.

For example, ICH S9 states that toxicological studies evaluating EFD (embryo–fetal development) for anticancer drugs should be provided when submitting a market authorization application, and that EFD is not considered critical for clinical trials supporting patients with advanced cancer. In fact, EFD studies can be completely omitted from market application data because anticancer drugs are genotoxic, target rapidly dividing cells, or belong to a class that has already been fully described as causing developmental toxicity.

Additionally, if nonhuman primates (NHP) are the only species relevant to pharmacology and the mechanism of action is expected to pose a reproductive toxicity risk, and/or when knockout (KO) animals or alternative biologic agents used in rodents have proven reproductive risks, a weight-of-evidence (WoE) assessment indicating reproductive risks can be provided instead of conducting reproductive toxicity studies. In fact, NHP studies assessing EFD hazards should not be considered the default method, as WoE clearly outlines the risk, meaning that EFD studies in NHP are not always necessary.

The reproductive risk assessment using WoE can be conducted through a comprehensive review of public databases and literature to evaluate the biology, expression, and pharmacological impact of targets on EFD. This includes reviewing existing repeated-dose toxicity data of relevant or related molecules and evaluating the direct or indirect effects of dosing on non-pregnant animals and patients, as well as potential placental transfer. The reproductive risk assessment for daratumumab, approved by the FDA, was primarily based on scientific literature, with no reproductive and developmental toxicology studies conducted. This approach is particularly applicable to biologics, such as antibodies, proteins, and modified proteins. The specificity and limited off-target activity of biologics, especially monoclonal antibodies, increase confidence in predicting potential embryotoxicity based on established pharmacological target biology data. Although ICH S9 and S6 allow for alternative methods, the content of sufficient WoE assessments has not been clearly described [35].

Three case studies of bispecific T-cell engagers (BiTEs) can be presented to illustrate the WoE method, with these molecules exhibiting cross-reactivity only in nonhuman primates.

9.7.2.1 The BiTE1 Molecule has been Identified to Have Potential Non-Tumor Target Expression During EFD

Consistent with the broader expression pattern during development, gene mutations in the target have been associated with malformations in mice. Therefore, the applicant concluded that published studies clearly indicate that the target is expressed during EFD and is involved in normal bone formation, suggesting that embryo exposure to the BiTE1 molecule could lead to embryonic and fetal toxicity. Consequently, EFD studies in nonhuman primates (NHPs) are unnecessary, or the EFD studies in NHPs would not provide additional data that would significantly alter the human risk assessment based on WoE. However, the FDA does not agree with this conclusion, asserting that although the target of the BiTE1 molecule is highly important during EFD, the data on target expression and the data from KO mice are insufficient to inform the risk of BiTE1 molecules during development.

9.7.2.2 The BiTE2 Molecule Targets Tumor Antigens Specific to Certain Blood Cell Types or Populations, and No Off-Target Binding has been Detected in Normal Human Tissues

All effects observed in repeated-dose toxicity studies represented expected pharmacodynamic (PD) effects and were reversible. In the KO mouse EFD study, it was observed that the target does not appear to be essential for EFD, as the offspring of KO mice appeared normal, survived without abnormal complications, and had normal major organs. Because this specific BiTE2 molecule lacks an Fc portion and high molecular weight proteins (>5 kDa) do not cross the placenta by simple diffusion, it is expected that there will be minimal fetal exposure. Even if a very small amount of BiTE2 molecules is transported through passive diffusion, the exposure of the developing embryo/fetus is not expected to cause any effects beyond the known PD effects, such as the depletion and re-proliferation of target cells in bone marrow stem cells after treatment cessation. It is estimated that only about 3% of the female population of reproductive age among cancer patients with this disease is fertile. Furthermore, this drug is likely to be used in combination with other teratogenic and embryotoxic drugs. Based on this WoE evaluation, both the FDA and EMA granted an exemption, allowing the applicant to forgo EFD studies in nonhuman primates.

9.7.2.3 The BiTE3 Molecule Targets Cancer that, Except in Rare Cases, Occurs Only in Adult Populations

Repeated-dose data indicate that administering BiTE3 molecules to nonhuman primates for more than 3 weeks leads to a high incidence of antidrug antibody (ADA) formation, followed by reduced exposure. The applicant submitted a pediatric investigation plan (PIP), with two reasons for a product-specific exemption: ① the disease does not occur in any specified pediatric population and ② some products treating the cancer in pediatric populations have been granted product-specific exemptions due to "the disease occurring only in adult populations." However, the EMA disagreed with the case and, considering its mechanism of action and potential therapeutic benefits in other indications, requested the applicant to provide more comprehensive information to assess the potential use of the product in pediatric populations, focusing on other pediatric malignancies that overexpress the target.

9.7.3 The Artificial Intelligence Platform for Predicting Developmental Toxicity

In recent years, the application of artificial intelligence (AI) methods to reveal quantitative structure–activity relationships (QSAR) has become increasingly important. Successful applications have been made in predictive toxicology, drug discovery, molecular optimization, and novel drug design. The interpretability of AI methods is the most crucial aspect, especially when dealing with high-dimensional data and nonlinear relationships. In such cases, AI models can become very complex and unfriendly, affecting the transparency of the algorithms and their actual applicability to case studies. Therefore, the ideal model should strike a balance between information content and uncertainty estimation, as well as between generalization and transparency [36].

Historically, from the perspective of AI performance evaluation, the measurement of information content and uncertainty estimation has played an important role and has been the cornerstone of all AI models over the years. Today, there is increasing attention on generalization ability, which refers to the ability of an individual or system to quickly learn and adapt to new, previously unencountered situations based on existing knowledge and experience. For AI, this refers to the reliability and transparency of machine learning algorithms' predictions on novel samples, or, in other words, the extent to which the decision-making process of the model is understandable by humans. One of the most prominent challenges in machine learning is dealing with generalization ability: accurate classifiers often adapt perfectly to training data, but their performance on unseen data is often unsatisfactory. Therefore, for life sciences, it is crucial to emphasize the interpretability of both precise and general models.

Therefore, "Explainable Artificial Intelligence" (XAI) has been proposed to provide a unified perspective and strategy for information content, uncertainty estimation, generalization, and transparency. Especially in the past decade, benefiting from the vast amount of data stored in publicly available databases, more and more research has focused on these issues. Currently, there are studies attempting to generate in vitro models for developmental toxicity research, but such studies are rare, and the available high-quality data is extremely limited. Although developmental toxicity is one of the most important toxicological endpoints, and the use and development of alternative methods, such as in vitro assays and computer simulations, is strongly encouraged, there are still significant challenges due to the non-generalizability of models, inability to provide specific indicators, and high costs. As a result, very few models are available. The most popular ones are the CAESAR and Consensus models. CAESAR can be accessed for free through the VEGA platform, while Consensus estimates toxicity by averaging predictions from multiple QSAR methods. In 2022, a literature review summarized a comprehensive dataset of 1244 chemicals extracted from public databases and literature sources. This work provided a strategy for predicting early developmental toxicity based on bioassay clustering, revealing potential links between biological mechanisms and structural features. XAI applications in the biomedical industry can be initially summarized as follows: ① For developers, AI regulations summarize information and data; ② for regulators, models comply with ethical and regulatory requirements, ensuring high reliability and transparency; ③ for users, models are visualized and semantically enhanced with medical knowledge graphs; and ④ for application users, the reasonableness and understandable diagnostic results of model outputs.

Togo et al. proposed a more robust and reproducible XAI method for predicting developmental toxicity. In this study, a training set consisting of 234 chemicals was used for model learning, and validation and generalization were performed using two test sets containing 585 chemicals. This model has been publicly available in TIRESIA for use by independent researchers for further improvement.

Ethical Approval

This chapter is a review of previously published accounts; as such, no animal or human studies were performed.

References

1. Cui Yanjun TY, Li Z et al (2021) Selection of positive drugs for non-human primate embryo-fetal toxicity studies. Chin J New Drugs 30(14):12661273
2. Chellman GJ, Bussiere JL, Makori N et al (2009) Developmental and reproductive toxicology studies in nonhuman primates. Birth Defects Res 86(6):446462
3. Van Esch E, Cline JM, Buse E et al (2008) Summary comparison of female reproductive system in human and the cynomolgus monkey (*Macaca fascicularis*). Toxicol Pathol 36(7suppl):171S172S
4. Zhang XL, Pang W, Hu XT et al (2014) Experimental primates and non human primate (NHPs) models of human diseases in China: current status and progress. Zool Res 35(6):447464
5. Weinbauer G, Fuchs A, Luetjens C M et al (2012) Nonhuman primates as preclinical models for developmental and reproductive toxicity evaluation. In: Developmental and reproductive toxicology: a practical approach, 3rd edn, p 464478

6. Rayburn ER, Gao L, Ding J et al (2018) FDA approved drugs that are spermatotoxic in animals and the utility of animal testing for human risk prediction. J Assist Reprod Genetics 35(2):191212
7. Cappon GD, Potter D, Hurtt ME et al (2013) Sensitivity of male reproductive endpoints in nonhuman primate toxicity studies: a statistical power analysis. Reprod Toxicol 41:6772
8. Vidal JD, Colman K, Bhaskaran M et al (2021) Scientific and regulatory policy committee best practices: documentation of sexual maturity by microscopic evaluation in nonclinical safety studies. Toxicol Pathol 49(5):977989
9. Yoshida T, Hanari K, Fujimoto K et al (2010) Female reproduction characteristics in a large scale breeding colony of cynomolgus monkeys (*Macaca fascicularis*). Exp Anim 59(2):251254
10. Jeanine L, Bussiere G, Moffat L, Zhou et al (2013) Assessment of menstrual cycle length in cynomolgus monkeys as a female fertility endpoint of a biopharmaceutical in a 6 month toxicity study. Regul Toxicol Pharmacol 66:269–278
11. Gerhard FW, Joerg L, Antje F (2012) The enhanced pre- and postnatal development study for monoclonal antibodies. Methods Mol Biol 947:185–200
12. Weinbauer GF, Fuchs A, Niehaus M et al (2011) The enhanced pre and postnatal study for nonhuman primates: update and perspectives. Birth Defects Res C 93(4):324333
13. Bowman CJ, Breslin WJ, Connor AV et al (2013) Placental transfer of Fc containing biopharmaceuticals across species, an industry survey analysis: placental transfer of Fc biopharmaceuticals. Birth Defects Research B 98(6):459485
14. Moffat GJ, Retter MW, Kwon G et al (2014) Placental transfer of a fully human IgG2 monoclonal antibody in the cynomolgus monkey, rat, and rabbit: a comparative assessment from during organogenesis to late gestation. Birth Defects B 101(2):178188
15. Prell RA, Dybdal N, Arima A et al (2018) Placental and fetal effects of onartuzumab, a Met/HGF signaling antagonist, when administered to pregnant cynomolgus monkeys. Toxicol Sci 165(1):186197
16. Philip J, Shiela S, Elvira V et al (2010) The cynomolgus monkey as a model for developmental toxicity studies: variability of pregnancy losses, statistical power estimates, and group size considerations. Birth Defects Res B 89:175–187
17. Luetjens CM, Fuchs A, Baker A et al (2020) Group size experiences with enhanced pre and postnatal development studies in the long tailed macaque (*Macaca fascicularis*). Primate Biol 7(1):14
18. Ishihara Hattori K, Barrow P (2016) Review of embryo fetal developmental toxicity studies performed for recent FDA approved pharmaceuticals. Reprod Toxicol 64:98104
19. Barrow P (2018) Review of embryo fetal developmental toxicity studies performed for pharmaceuticals approved by FDA in 2016 and 2017. Reprod Toxicol 80:117125
20. Barrow P, Clemann N (2021) Review of embryo fetal developmental toxicity studies performed for pharmaceuticals approved by FDA in 2018 and 2019. Reprod Toxicol 99:144151
21. Barrow P (2022) Review of embryo fetal developmental toxicity studies performed for pharmaceuticals approved by FDA in 2020 and 2021. Reprod Toxicol 112:100108
22. Ackley D, Birkebak J, Blumel J et al (2023) FDA and industry collaboration: identifying opportunities to further reduce reliance on nonhuman primates for nonclinical safety evaluations. Regul Toxicol Pharmacol 138:105327
23. Denny KH, Faqi AS (2015) Nonclinical safety assessment of developmental and reproductive toxicology: considerations for conducting fertility, embryo–fetal development, and prenatal and postnatal developmental toxicology studies. In: Faqi A. Developmental and reproductive toxicology. Humana Press, New York, NY
24. Rachel A, Jean F, Gardin JA, Tooze et al (2022) Organ weights in relation to age and sex in cynomolgus monkeys (*Macaca fascicularis*). Toxicol Pathol 50:574–590
25. Mirsky ML, Portugal S, Pisharath H et al (2016) Utility of orchidometric parameters for assessing sexual maturation in male cynomolgus macaques (*Macaca fascicularis*). Compar Med 66(6):480488

26. Iwasaki K, Uno Y, Utoh M et al (2019) Importance of cynomolgus monkeys in development of monoclonal antibody drugs. Drug Metab Pharmacokinet 34(1):5563
27. Brennan FR, Cavagnaro J, Mckeever K et al (2018) Safety testing of monoclonal antibodies in non human primates: case studies highlighting their impact on human risk assessment. mAbs 10(1):117
28. Thomas K, Guenter B, Andreas B et al (2021) Challenges of non-clinical safety testing for biologics: a report of the 9th BioSafe European Annual General Membership Meeting. MAbs 13:1938796
29. Bowman CJ, Evans M, Cummings T et al (2015) Developmental toxicity assessment of tanezumab, an anti nerve growth factor monoclonal antibody, in cynomolgus monkeys (*Macaca fascicularis*). Reprod Toxicol 53:105118
30. Wang C, Liu S, Liu F et al (2022) Application of nonhuman primate models in the studies of pediatric anesthesia neurotoxicity. Anest Analg 134(6):12031214
31. Cavagnaro J, Berman C, Kornbrust D et al (2014) Considerations for assessment of reproductive and developmental toxicity of oligonucleotide based therapeutics. Nucleic Acid Therap 24(5):313325
32. Alessandro S D, Menegola E, Parapini S et al (2020) Safety of artemisinin derivatives in the first trimester of pregnancy: a controversial story. Molecules 25(15):3505
33. Niethammer M, Burgdorf T, Wistorf E et al (2022) In vitro models of human development and their potential application in developmental toxicity testing. Development 149(20):dev200933
34. Rocca M, Morford LL, Blanset DL et al (2018) Applying a weight of evidence approach to the evaluation of developmental toxicity of biopharmaceuticals. Regul Toxicol Pharmacol 98:6979
35. Frank RB, Joy C, McKeever K et al (2017) Safety testing of monoclonal antibodies in non-human primates: case studies highlighting their impact on human risk assessment. MAbs 10:1–17
36. Togo MV, Mastrolorito F, Ciriaco F et al (2023) TIRESIA: an explainable artificial intelligence platform for predicting developmental toxicity. J Chem Inf Model 63(1):5666

Appendix 1 Map of Reproductive and Developmental Toxicology of Cynomolgus Monkeys

I. Preparation of double-stained bone specimens of cynomolgus monkey fetuses

1. Solution preparation: See Table A.1.1.

Table1 Solution preparation methods

Solutions needed	Preparation methods
Fixative solution	95% Ethanol
Alcian blue solution	80 mL of 95% Ethanol was added to 15 mg of Alcian blue, then 20 mL of glacial acetic acid was added
Alizarin red solution	0.1 g of Alizarin red solution was added to 10 g of KOH, then ultra-pure water was added till 1000 mL
1% KOH solution	10 g of KOH was dissolved in 1000 mL of ultra-pure water
Transparent liquid I	400 mL of 70% Ethanol was added into 400 mL of glycerol, then 200 mL of benzyl alcohol was added
Transparent liquid II	1000 mL of 70% Ethanol was added to 400 mL of glycerol
Preservation solution	Glycerol

2. Operating steps: Pregnant monkeys were examined by cesarean section on GD_{100}. The fetuses were taken out, skinned, eviscerated, and the adipose tissues of the neck and back were removed. Then, they were fixed with 95% ethanol for at least 3 days for staining. After 3 days, 95% ethanol was replaced with Alcian blue staining solution for staining. After 5–7 days, 95% ethanol was used again. After 1–3 days, 95% ethanol was removed and the cynomolgus monkey fetuses were immersed in Alizarin red for 2–4 days. The staining solution was removed and treated with 1% potassium hydroxide solution for 1–7 days. The fetuses were transferred into transparent solutions I and II for 30 days each. If the transparency was not good enough, the time in the transparent solution could be

L. Zhou and Z. Sun (eds.), *Reproductive and Developmental Toxicology on Macaca Fascicularis*, https://doi.org/10.1007/978-981-92-3834-7

appropriately extended. Then, the fetuses were replaced with 100% glycerol for preservation.

II. Preparation of visceral specimens of cynomolgus monkey fetuses

(1)Examine the viscera of fresh specimens.
(2)Take out the viscera of cynomolgus monkey fetuses, fix them in 10% formalin solution for at least 48 h, and then conduct a visceral examination.

III. Map of common malformations in experimental cynomolgus monkeys

1. See Figs. A.1.1–A.1.43 for appearance abnormalities.
2. Visceral abnormalities are shown in Figs. A.1.44–A.1.51.
3. Skeletal abnormalities
1. 95% Ethanol: see Figs. A.52–A.60.
2. Alcian blue staining: see Figs. A.1.61–A.1.70.
3. Alizarin red staining: see Figs. A.1.71–A.1.77.
4. Transparent solution I and transparent solution II: see Figs. A.1.78–A.1.96.
4. Abnormal bone density: see Figs. A.1.97–A.1.110.

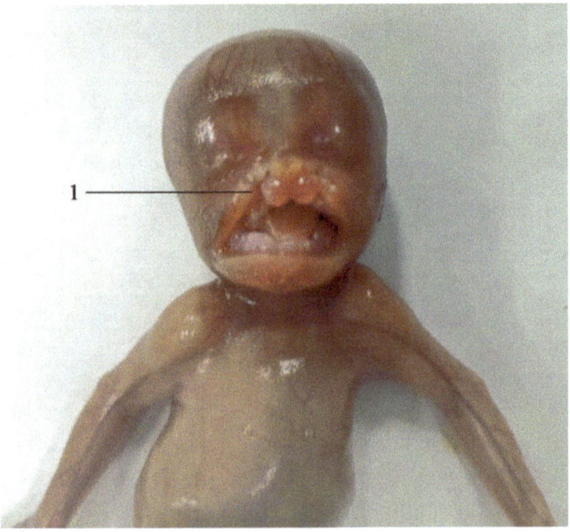

Figure 1 Abnormalities of the lip (front view). Fetal monkey, cyclophosphamide (CP), 20 mg/kg, subcutaneous injection (sc) on GD_{24-28}, cesarean section examination on GD_{100}. 1. Abnormalities of the lip

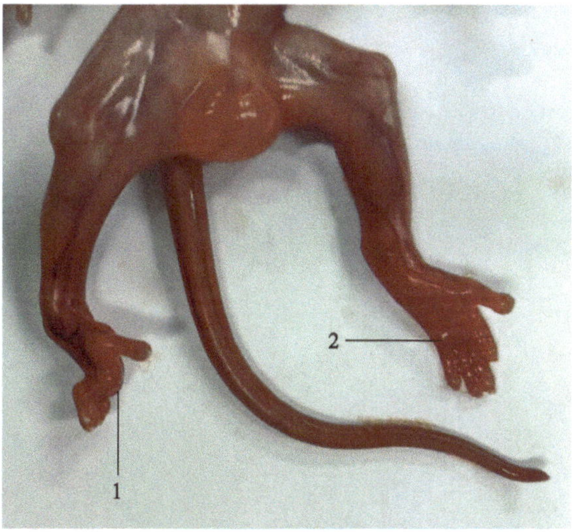

Figure 2 Eversion of the right hind toe and normal toes (front view). Fetal monkey, cyclophosphamide (CP), 20 mg/kg, subcutaneous injection (sc) on GD_{24-28}, cesarean section examination on GD_{100}. 1. Eversion of the right hind toe. 2. Normal toes

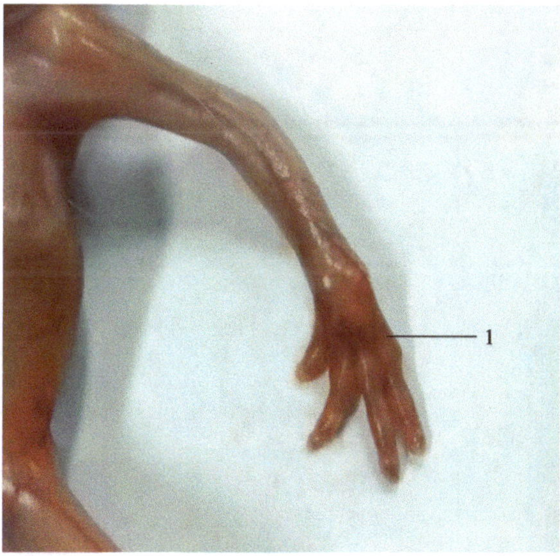

Figure 3 Oligodactyly (front view). Fetal monkey, cyclophosphamide (CP), 20 mg/kg, subcutaneous injection (sc) on GD_{24-28}, cesarean section examination on GD_{100}. 1. Oligodactyly

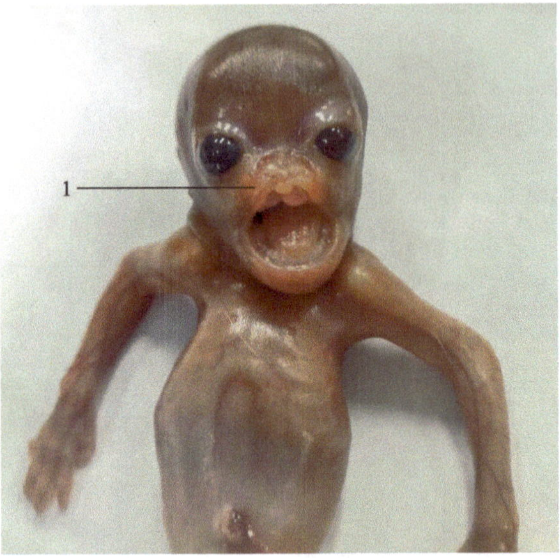

Figure 4 Abnormalities of the lip (front view). Fetal monkey, cyclophosphamide (CP), 20 mg/kg, subcutaneous injection (sc) on GD_{24-28}, cesarean section examination on GD_{100}. 1. Abnormalities of the lip

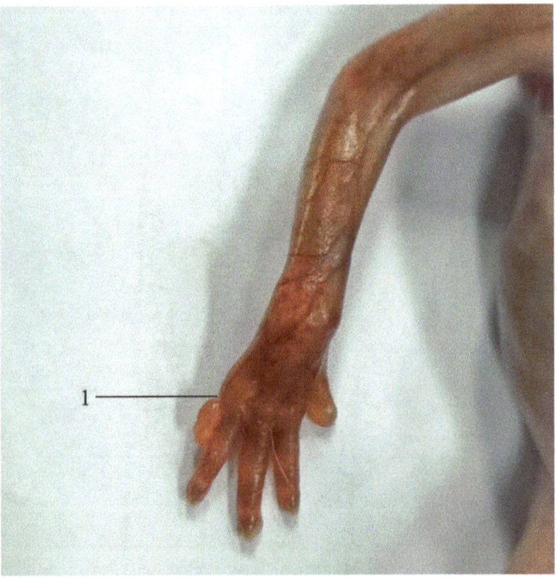

Figure 5 Abnormalities of the little finger (front view). Fetal monkey, cyclophosphamide (CP), 20 mg/kg, subcutaneous injection (sc) on GD_{24-28}, cesarean section examination on GD_{100}. 1. Abnormalities of the little finger

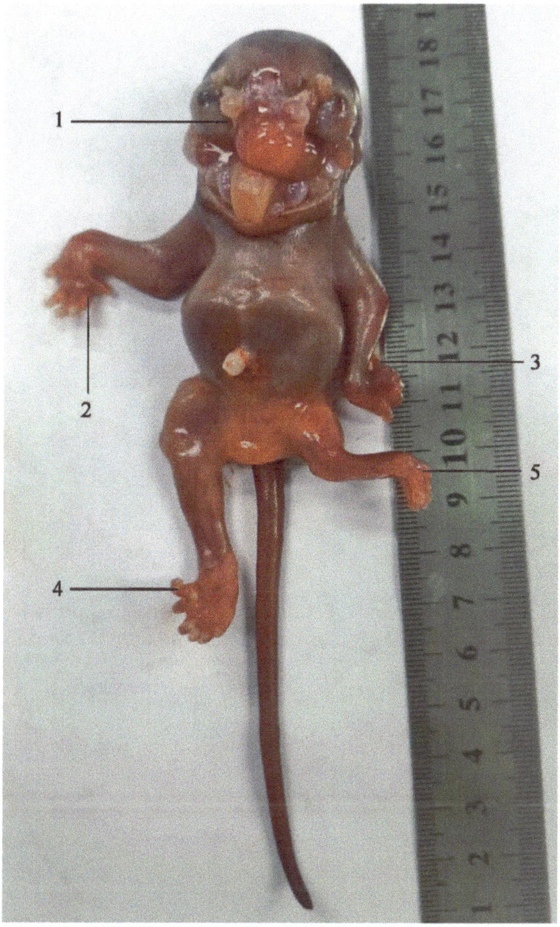

Figure 6 **Facial abnormalities and valgus of fingers and toes (front view). Fetal monkey, cyclophosphamide (CP), 20 mg/kg, subcutaneous injection (sc) on GD_{24-28}, cesarean section examination on GD_{100}. 1. Facial abnormalities. 2–5. Varus or valgus of fingers and toes**

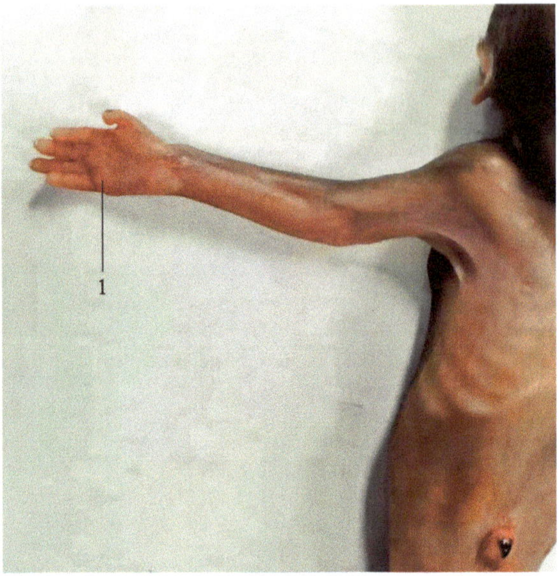

Figure 7 Normal fingers (front view). Fetal monkey, sodium chloride injection, 1 mL/kg, gavage administration (ig) on GD_{24-30}, cesarean section examination on GD_{100}. 1. Normal fingers

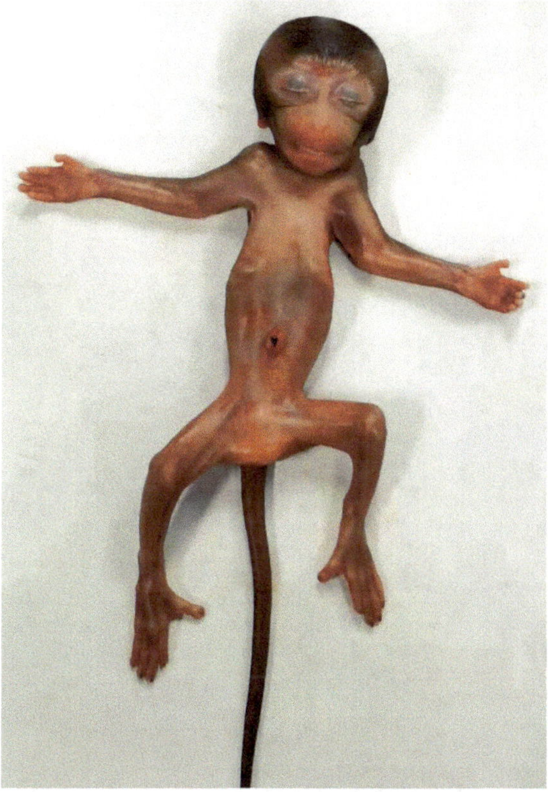

Figure 8 Normal fetus (front view). Fetal monkey, sodium chloride injection, 1 mL/kg, gavage administration (ig) on GD_{24-30}, cesarean section examination on GD100

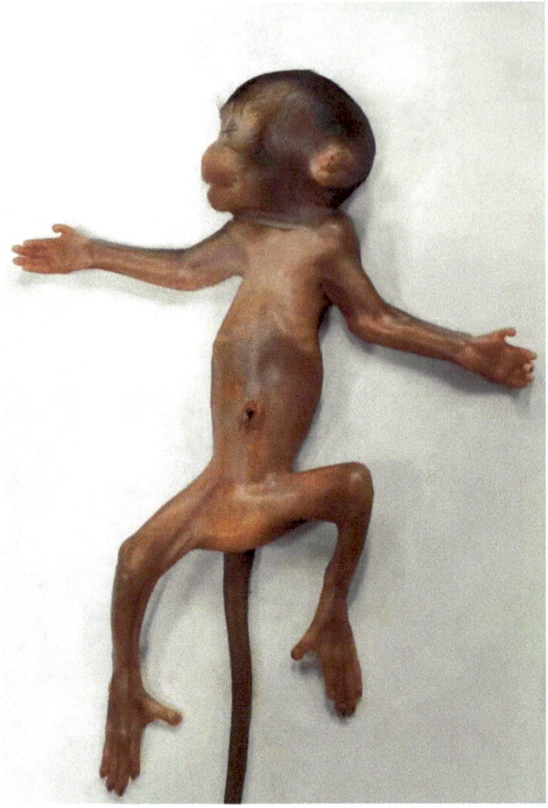

Figure 9 **Lateral view of a normal fetus. Fetal monkey, sodium chloride injection, 1 mL/kg, gavage administration (ig) on GD_{24-30}, cesarean section examination on GD_{100}**

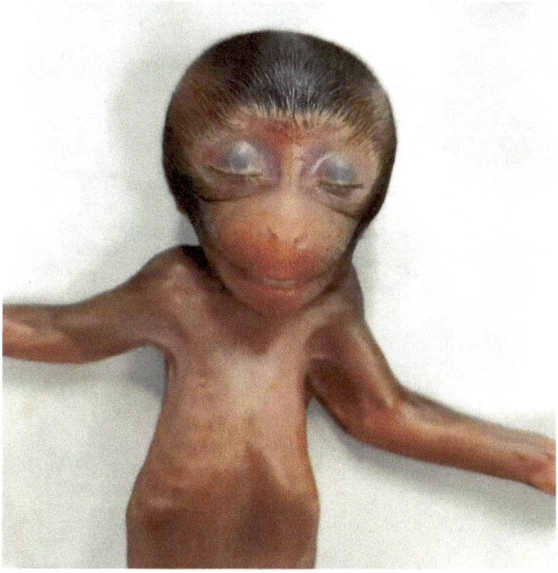

Figure 10 **Front view of a normal fetus. Fetal monkey, sodium chloride injection, 1 mL/kg, gavage administration (ig) on GD_{24-30}, cesarean section examination on GD_{100}**

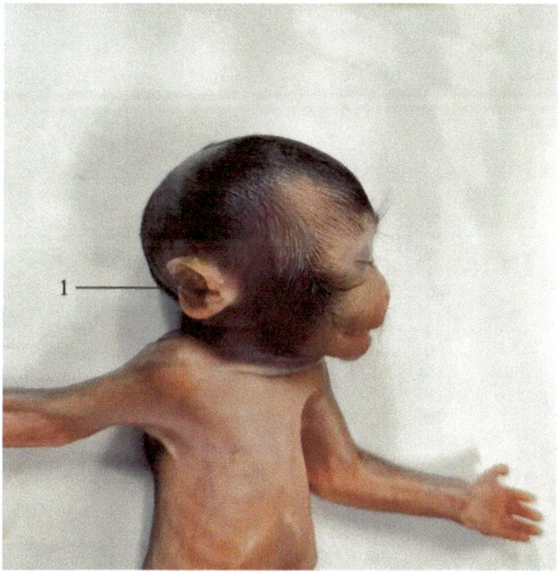

Figure 11 **Ears of a normal fetus. Fetal monkey, sodium chloride injection, 1 mL/kg, gavage administration (ig) on GD_{24-30}, cesarean section examination on GD100. 1. Ears**

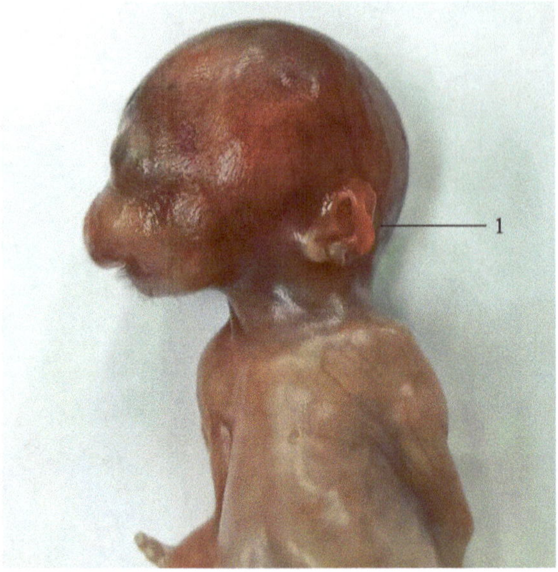

Figure 12 **Adhesion between the auricle and the brain (lateral view). Fetal monkey, thalidomide, 15 mg/kg, gavage administration (ig) on GD_{24-30}, cesarean section examination on GD_{100}. 1. Adhesion between the auricle and the brain**

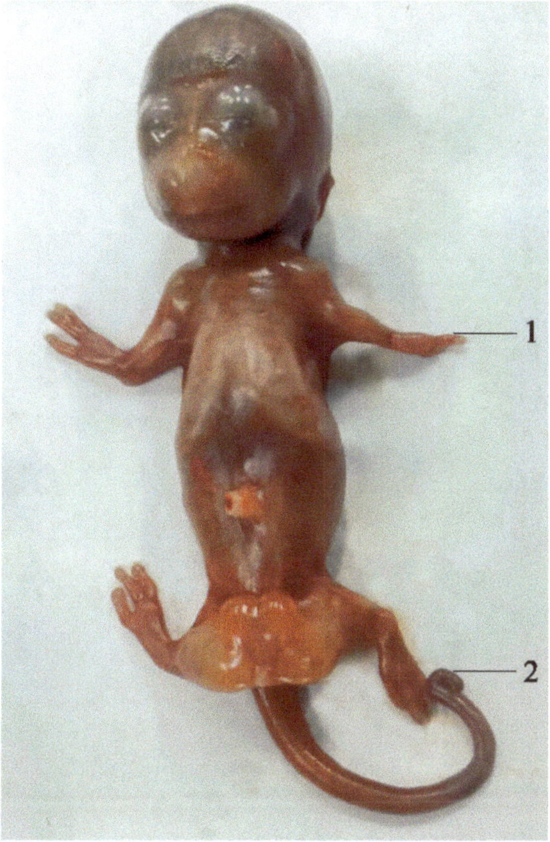

Figure 13 Phocomelia and curly tail (front view). Fetal monkey, thalidomide, 15 mg/kg, gavage administration (ig) on GD_{24-30}, cesarean section examination on GD_{100}. 1. Phocomelia. 2. Curly tail

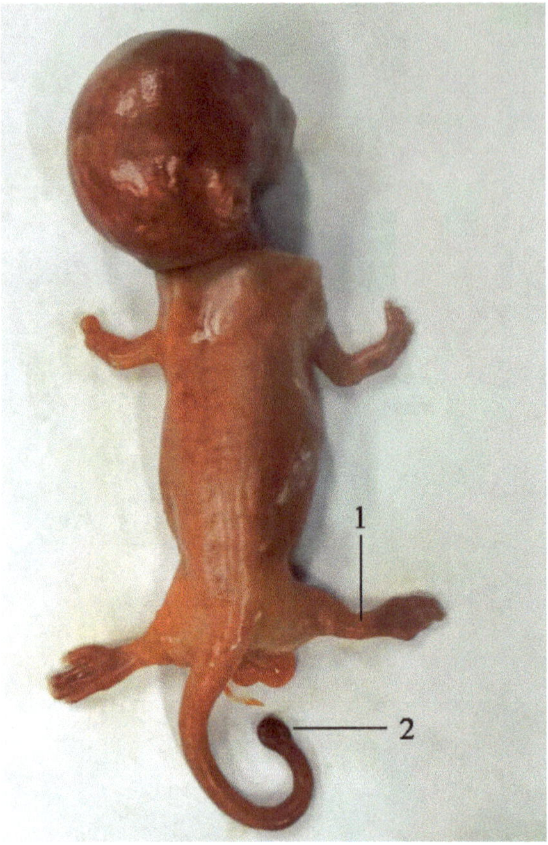

Figure 14 Phocomelia and curly tail (back view). Fetal monkey, thalidomide, 15 mg/kg, gavage administration (ig) on GD_{24-30}, cesarean section examination on GD_{100}. 1. Phocomelia. 2. Curly tail

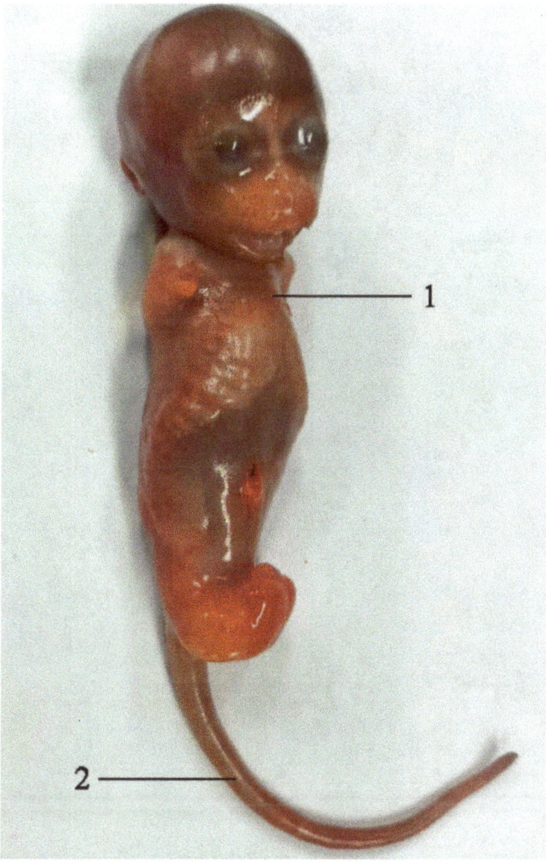

Figure 15 Phocomelia and normal tail (front view). Fetal monkey, thalidomide, 15 mg/kg, gavage administration (ig) on GD_{24-30}, cesarean section examination on GD100. 1. Phocomelia. 2. Normal tail

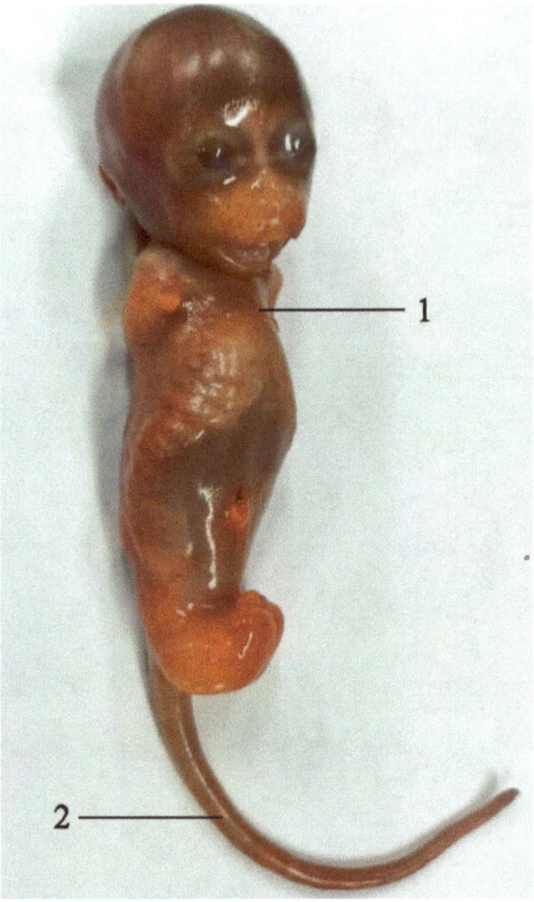

Figure 16 **Phocomelia and normal tail (lateral view). Fetal monkey, thalidomide, 15 mg/kg, gavage administration (ig) on GD_{24-30}, cesarean section examination on GD_{100}. 1. Phocomelia. 2. Normal tail**

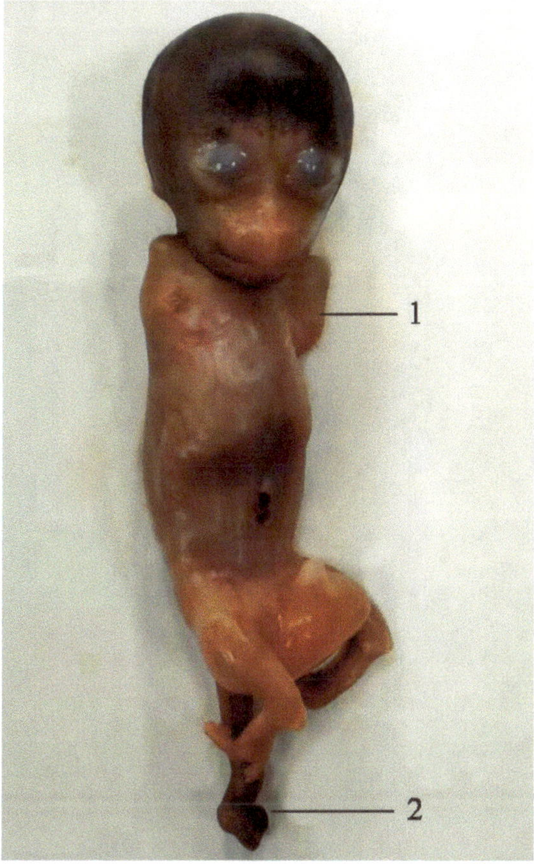

Figure 17 **Phocomelia and curly tail (front view). Fetal monkey, thalidomide, 15 mg/kg, gavage administration (ig) on GD_{24-30}, cesarean section examination on GD_{100}. 1. Phocomelia. 2. Curly tail**

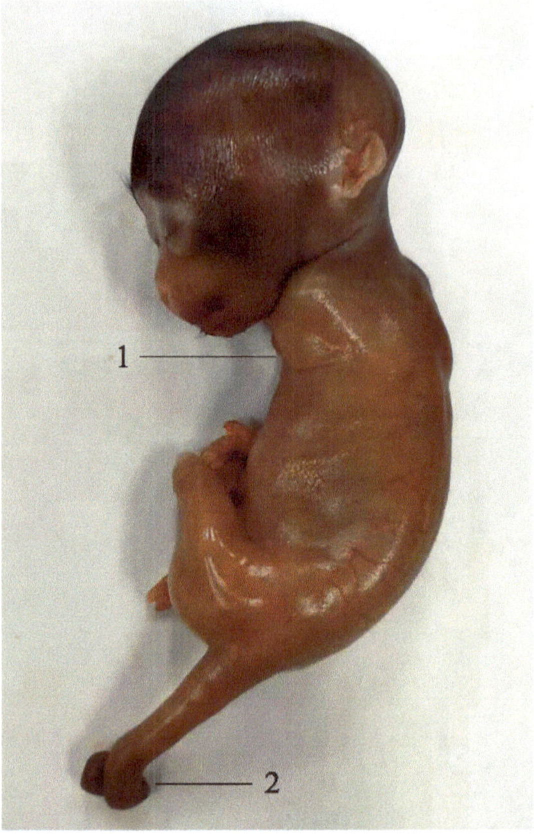

Figure 18 **Phocomelia and curly tail (lateral view). Fetal monkey, thalidomide, 15 mg/kg, gavage administration (ig) on GD_{24-30}, cesarean section examination on GD_{100}. 1. Phocomelia. 2. Curly tail**

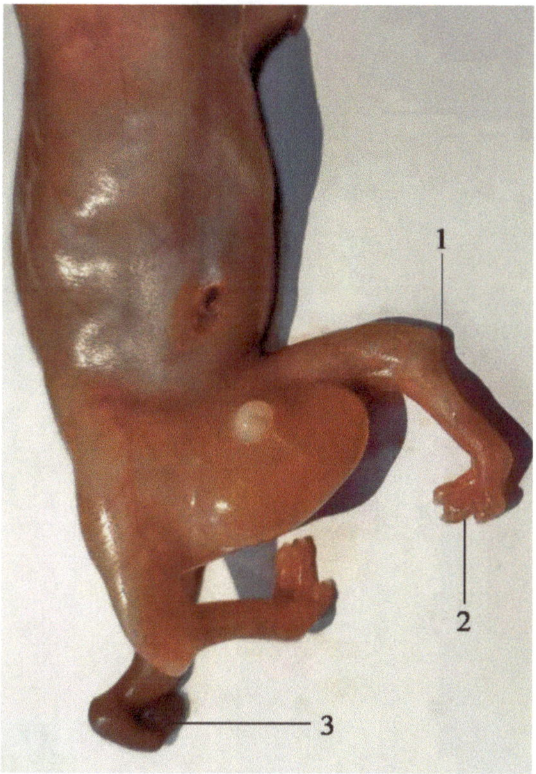

Figure 19 **Phocomelia, curly tail, and varus of the foot (front view). Fetal monkey, thalidomide, 15 mg/kg, gavage administration (ig) on GD_{24-30}, cesarean section examination on GD_{100}. 1. Phocomelia. 2. Varus of foot. 3. Curly tail**

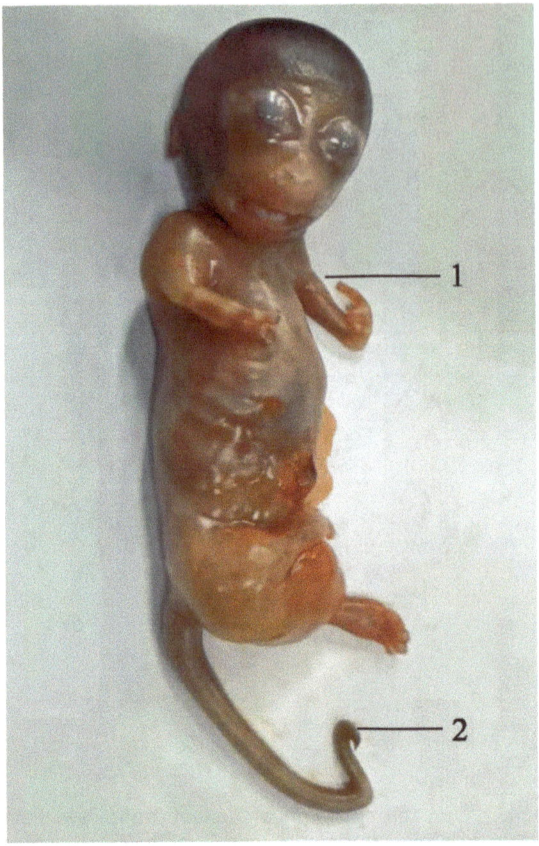

Figure 20 **Phocomelia and curly tail (front view). Fetal monkey, thalidomide, 15 mg/kg, gavage administration (ig) on GD_{24-30}, cesarean section examination on GD_{100}. 1. Phocomelia. 2. Curly tail**

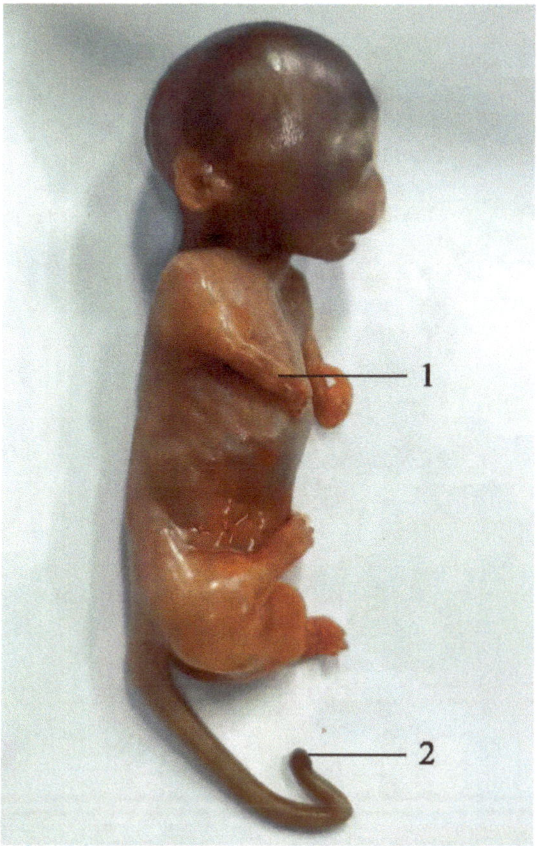

Figure 21 Phocomelia and curly tail (lateral view). Fetal monkey, thalidomide, 15 mg/kg, gavage administration (ig) on GD_{24-30}, cesarean section examination on GD_{100}. 1. Phocomelia. 2. Curly tail

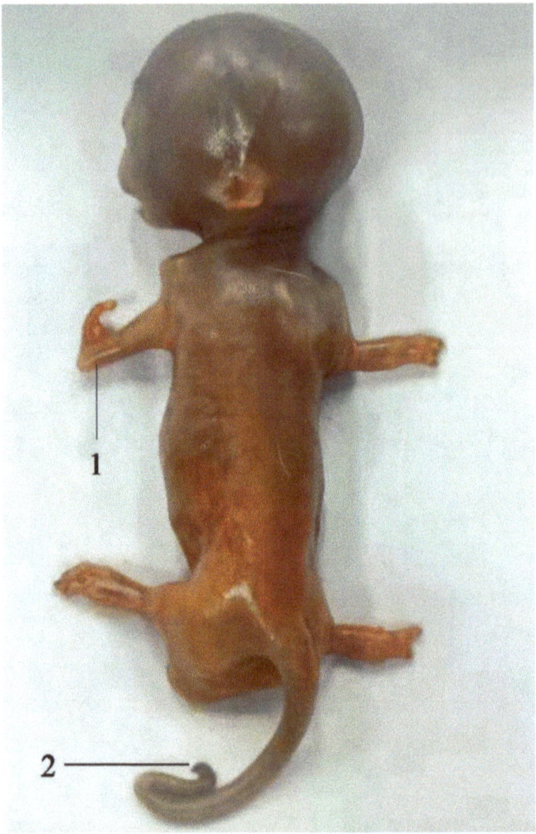

Figure 22 Phocomelia and curly tail (back view). Fetal monkey, thalidomide, 15 mg/kg, gavage administration (ig) on GD_{24-30}, cesarean section examination on GD_{100}. 1. Phocomelia. 2. Curly tail

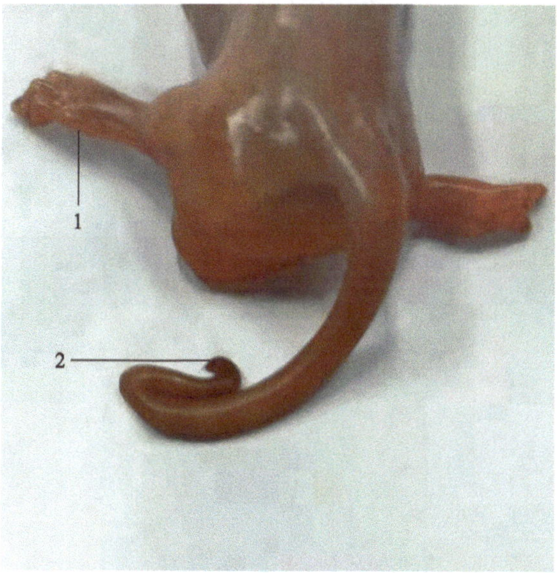

Figure 23 Phocomelia and curly tail (back view). Fetal monkey, thalidomide, 15 mg/kg, gavage administration (ig) on GD_{24-30}, cesarean section examination on GD_{100}. 1. Phocomelia. 2. Curly tail

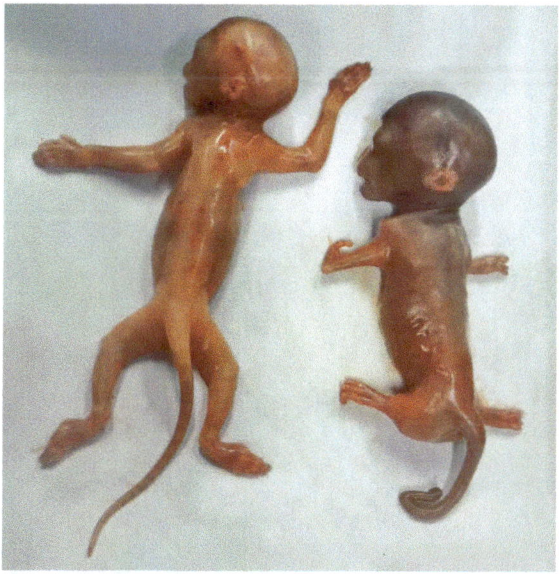

Figure 24 Normal fetus on the left side, phocomelia on the right side (back view). Fetal monkey on the left side, sodium chloride injection, 1 mL/kg, gavage administration (ig) on GD_{24-30}, cesarean section examination on GD_{100}. Fetal monkey on the right side, thalidomide, 15 mg/kg, gavage administration (ig) on GD_{24-30}, cesarean section examination on GD_{100}

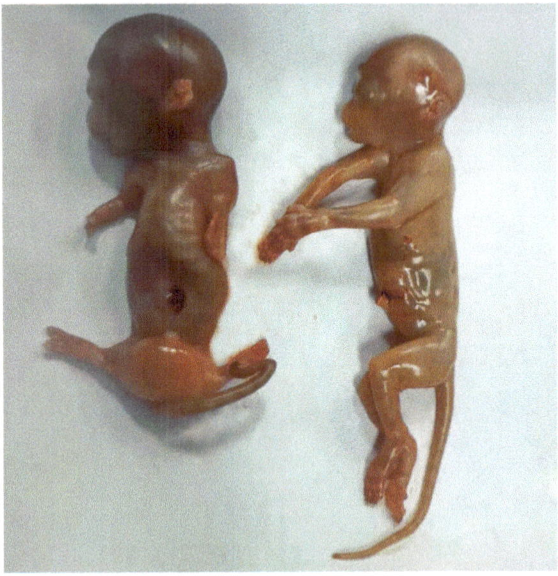

Figure 25 Normal fetus on the right side, phocomelia on the left side (lateral view). Fetal monkey on the right side, sodium chloride injection, 1 mL/kg, gavage administration (ig) on GD_{24-30}, cesarean section examination on GD_{100}. Fetal monkey on the left side, thalidomide, 15 mg/kg, gavage administration (ig) on GD_{24-30}, cesarean section examination on GD_{100}

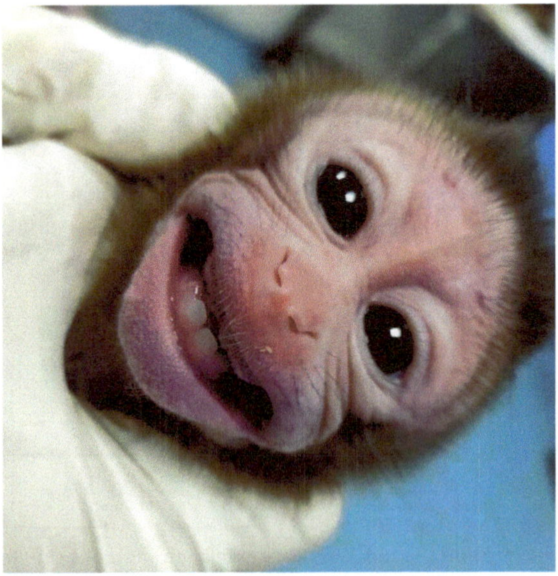

Figure 26 Tooth eruption of a normal fetus (front view). Fetal monkey, sodium chloride injection, 1 mL/kg, gavage administration (ig) on GD_{24-30}, PND_5

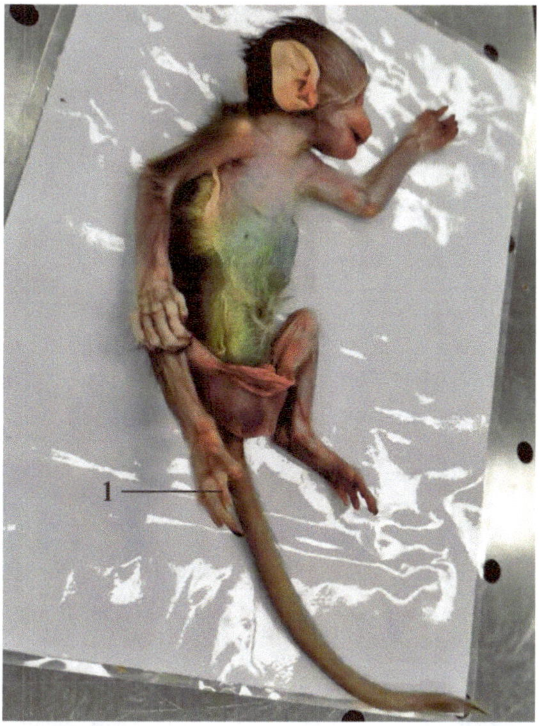

Figure 27 Short toes (lateral view). Fetal monkey, cyclophosphamide (CP), 20 mg/kg, subcutaneous injection (sc) on GD_{24-28}, died on PND_5. 1. Short toes (front view)

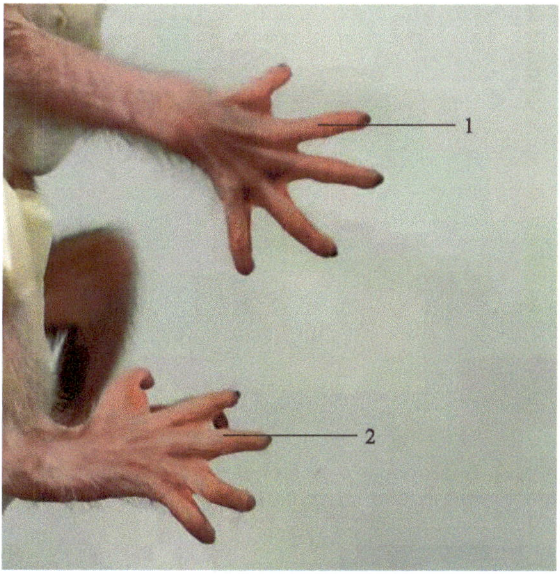

Figure 28 Fingers and toes of a normal fetus. Fetal monkey, sodium chloride injection, 1 mL/kg, gavage administration (ig) on GD_{24-30}, PND_0. 1. Fingers. 2. Toes

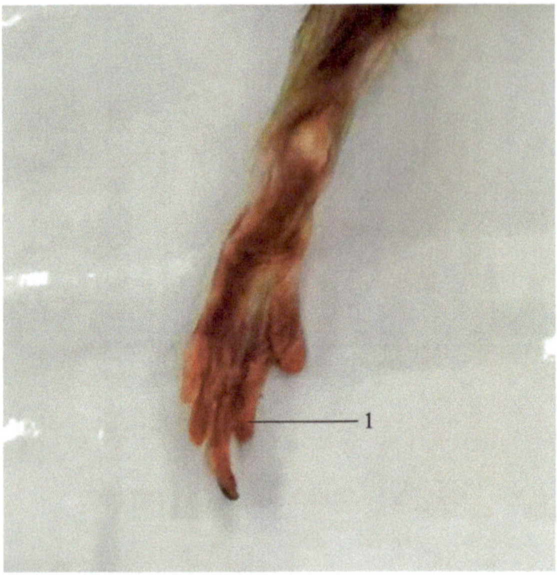

Figure 29 Short toes. Fetal monkey, cyclophosphamide (CP), 20 mg/kg, subcutaneous injection (sc) on GD_{24-28}, died on PND_5. 1. Short toes (back view)

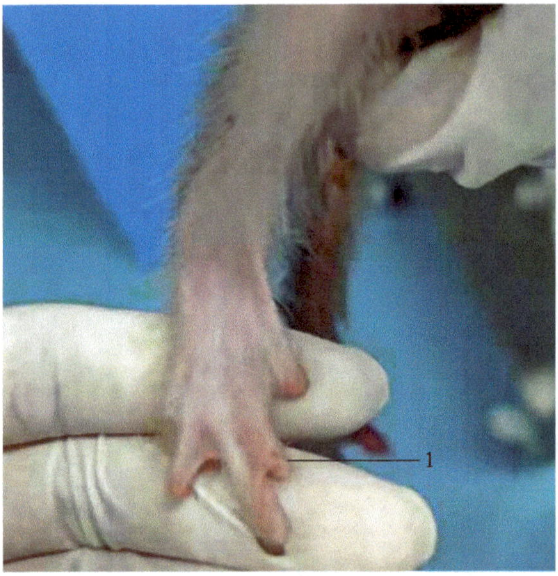

Figure 30 Short toes. Fetal monkey, cyclophosphamide (CP), 20 mg/kg, subcutaneous injection (sc) on GD_{24-28}, PND_0. 1. Short toes (back view)

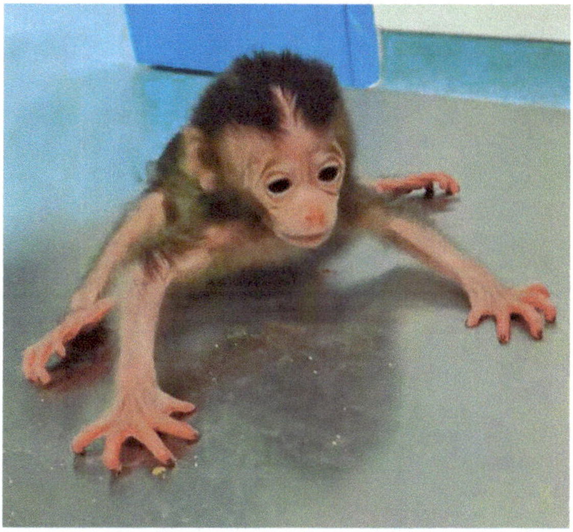

Figure 31 Normal fetus (front view). Fetal monkey, sodium chloride injection, 1 mL/kg, gavage administration (ig) on GD_{24-30}, PND_0

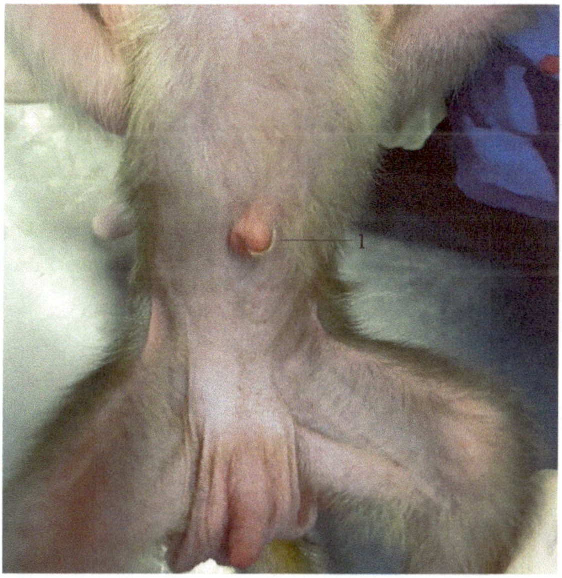

Figure 32 Umbilical cord of a normal fetus. Fetal monkey, sodium chloride injection, 1 mL/kg, gavage administration (ig) on GD_{24-30}, 1. Umbilical cord on PND_5

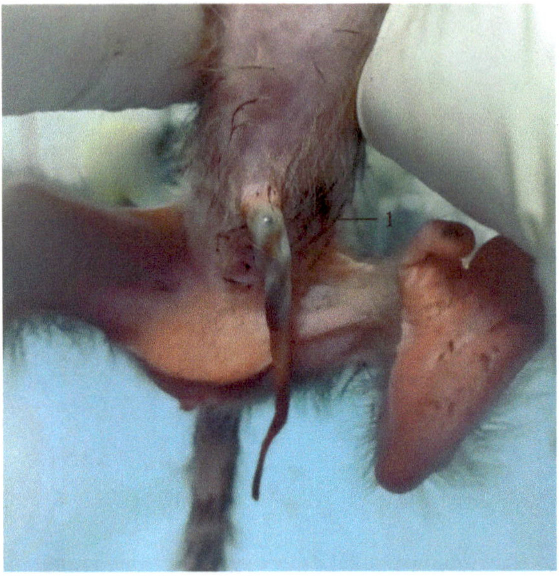

Figure 33 Umbilical cord of a normal fetus. Fetal monkey, sodium chloride injection, 1 mL/kg, gavage administration (ig) on GD_{24-30}, 1. Umbilical cord on PND_0

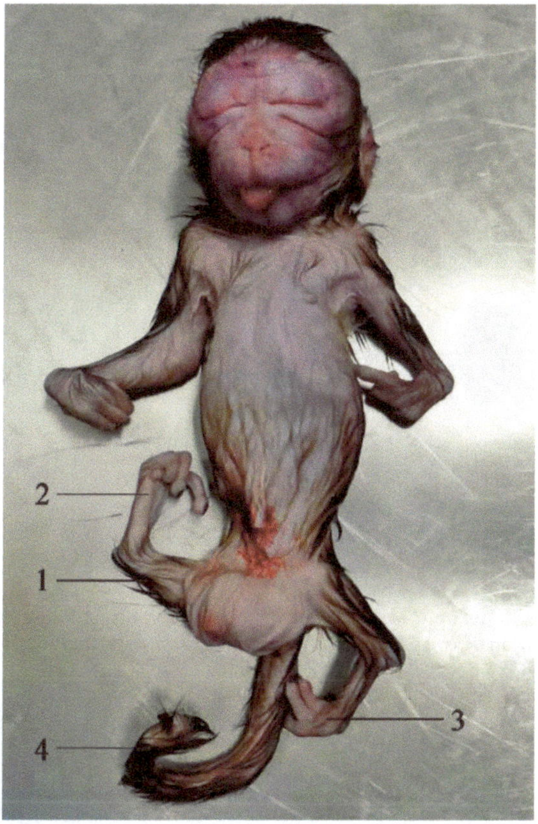

Figure 34 **Fetus with phocomelia, oligodactyly, varus of the foot, and short tail (front view). Fetal monkey, thalidomide, 15 mg/kg, gavage administration (ig) on $GD_{24\text{-}30}$, PND_0. 1. Fetus with phocomelia. 2. Oligodactyly. 3. Varus of foot. 4. Short tail**

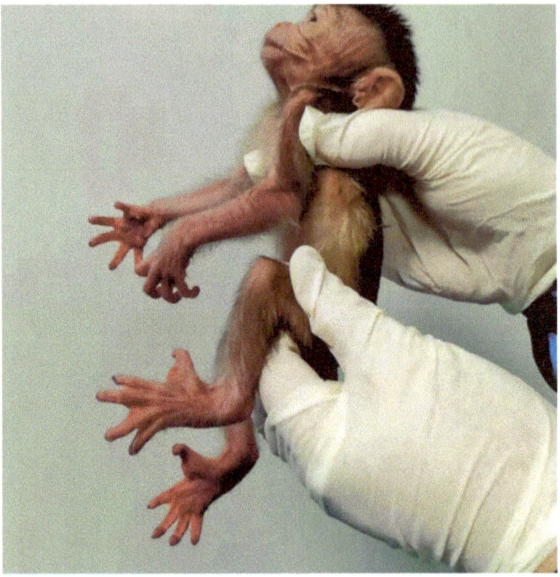

Figure 35 Normal fetus (lateral view). Fetal monkey, sodium chloride injection, 1 mL/kg, gavage administration (ig) on GD_{24-30}, normal fetus (lateral view) on PND_0

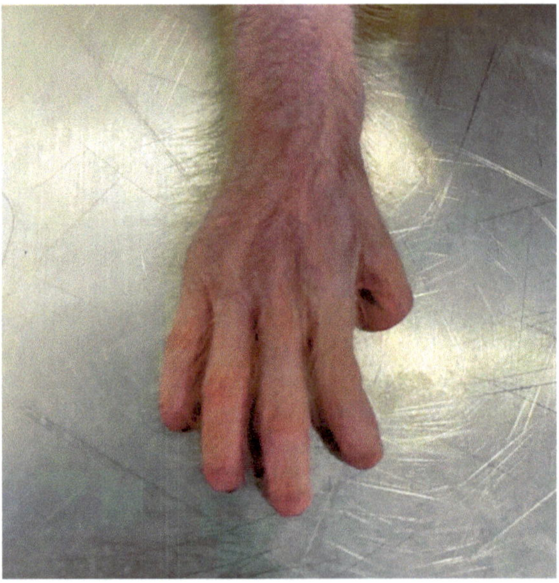

Figure 36 Fingers of a normal fetus. Fetal monkey, sodium chloride injection, 1 mL/kg, gavage administration (ig) on GD_{24-30}, fingers of normal fetus on PND_0

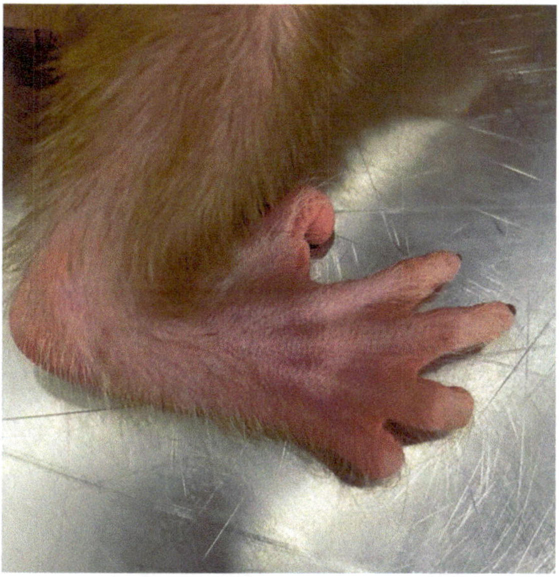

Figure 37 Toes of a normal fetus. Fetal monkey, sodium chloride injection, 1 mL/kg, gavage administration (ig) on GD_{24-30}, toes of normal fetus on PND_0

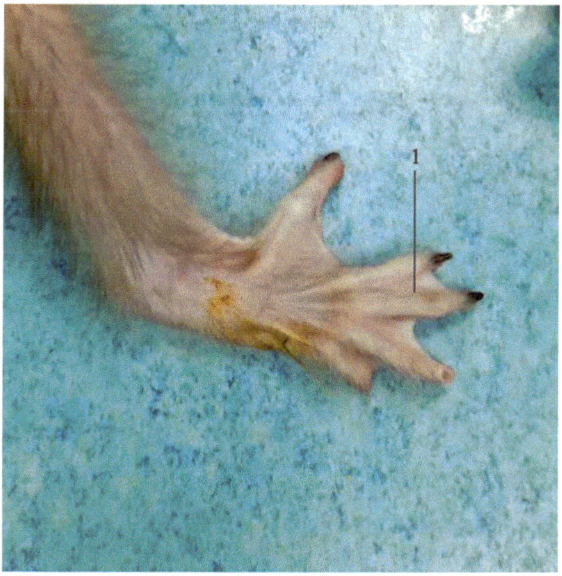

Figure 38 Adhesion of index finger, middle finger, ring finger and little finger. Fetal monkey, cyclophosphamide (CP), 20 mg/kg, subcutaneous injection (sc) on GD_{24-28}, PND_0. 1. Adhesion of fingers

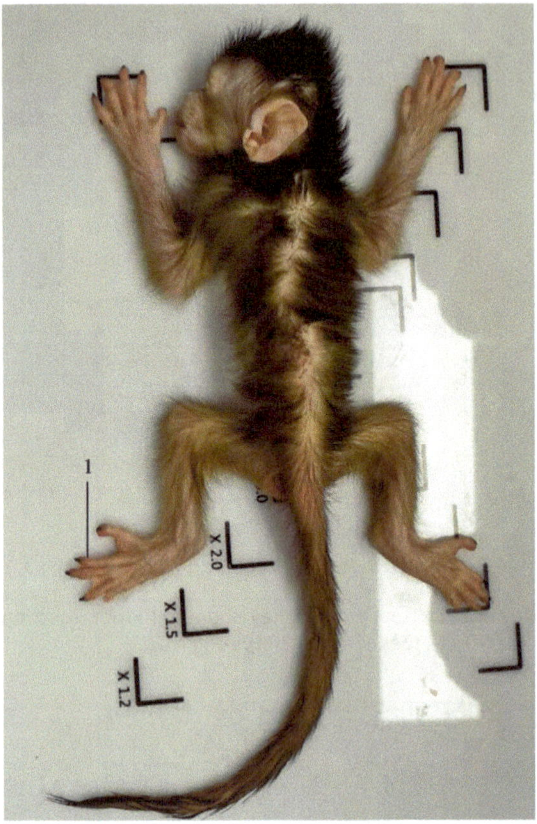

Figure 39 Adhesion of toes (back view). Fetal monkey, cyclophosphamide (CP), 20 mg/kg, subcutaneous injection (sc) on GD_{24-28}, PND_0. 1. Adhesion of toes

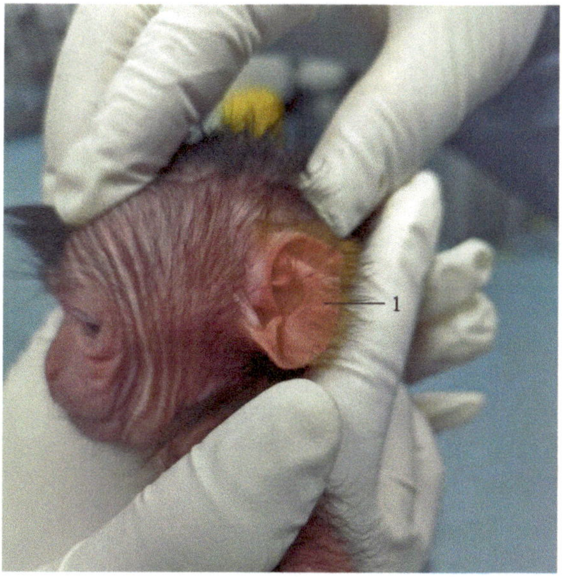

Figure 40 Ears of a normal fetus (lateral view). Fetal monkey, sodium chloride injection, 1 mL/kg, gavage administration on GD_{24-30} (ig). 1. Ears of a normal fetus on PND_0

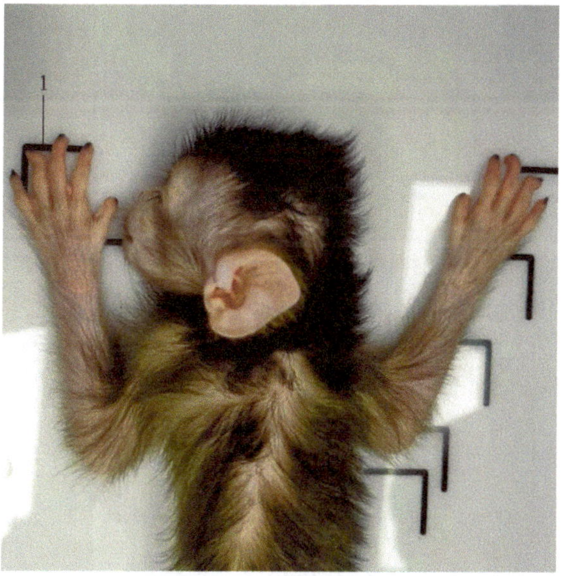

Figure 41 Curvature of the ring finger (back view). Fetal monkey, cyclophosphamide (CP), 20 mg/kg, subcutaneous injection (sc) on GD_{24-28}, PND_0. 1. Curvature of the ring finger

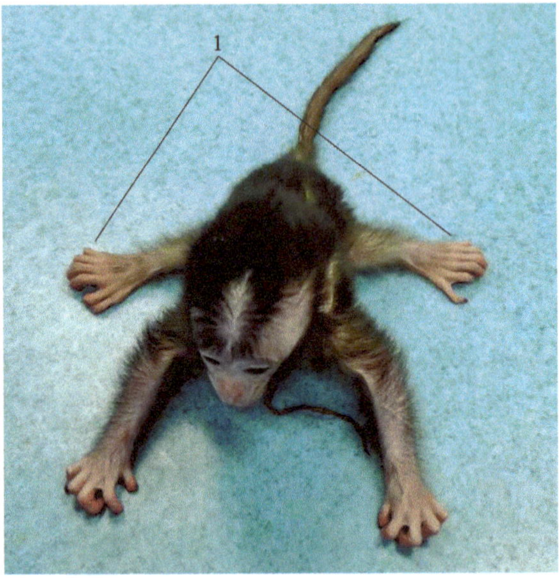

Figure 42 Polydactyly (top view). Fetal monkey, thalidomide, 15 mg/kg, gavage administration (ig) on GD_{24-30}, PND0. 1. Polydactyly

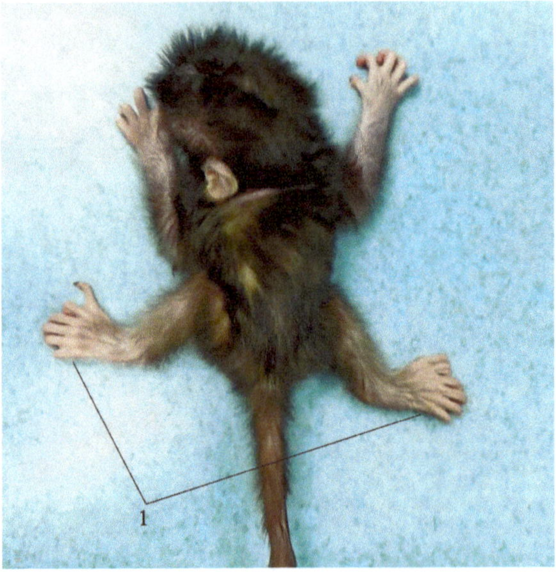

Figure 43 Polydactyly (back view). Fetal monkey, thalidomide, 15 mg/kg, gavage administration (ig) on GD_{24-30}, PND0. 1. Polydactyly

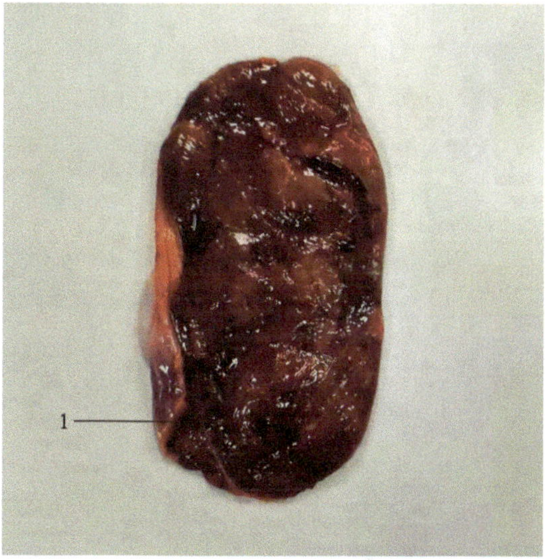

Figure 44 Maternal surface of the placenta of a normal fetus. Fetal monkey, sodium chloride injection, 1 mL/kg, gavage administration (ig) on GD_{24-30}, cesarean section examination on GD_{100}. 1. Maternal surface of the placenta of a normal fetus

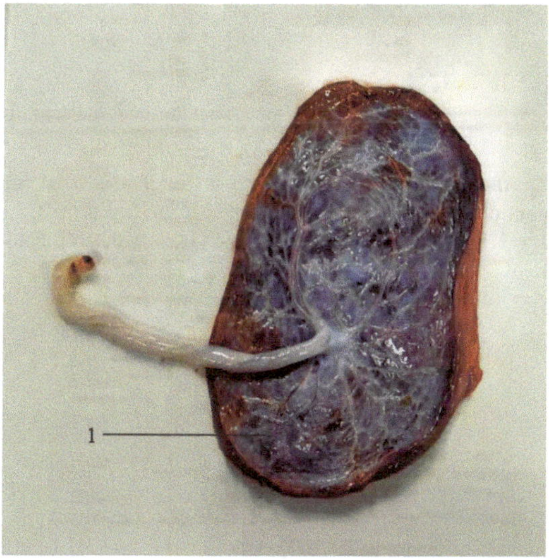

Figure 45 Fetal surface of the placenta of a normal fetus. Fetal monkey, sodium chloride injection, 1 mL/kg, gavage administration (ig) on GD_{24-30}, cesarean section examination on GD_{100}. 1. Fetal surface of the placenta of a normal fetus

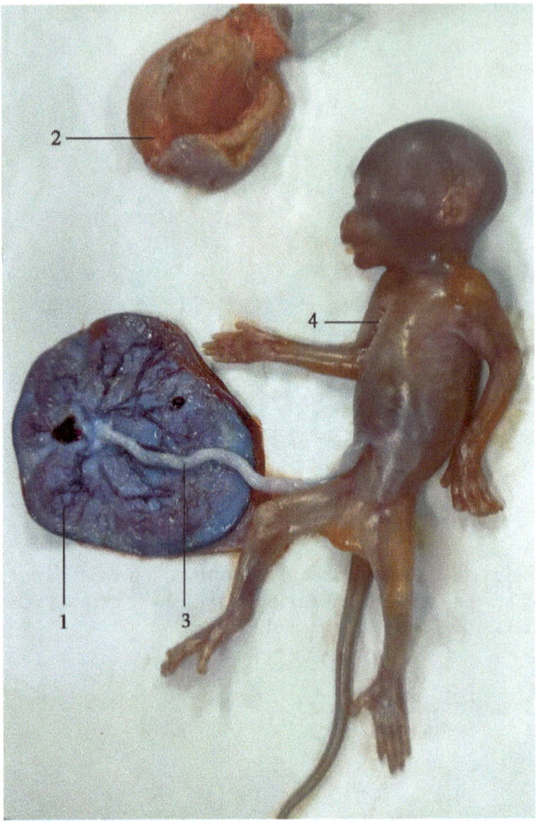

Figure 46 Placenta, uterus, umbilical cord, and fetus of a normal fetus. Fetal monkey, sodium chloride injection, 1 mL/kg, gavage administration (ig) on GD_{24-30}, cesarean section examination on GD_{100}. 1. Placenta of a normal fetus. 2. Uterus. 3. Umbilical cord. 4. Fetus

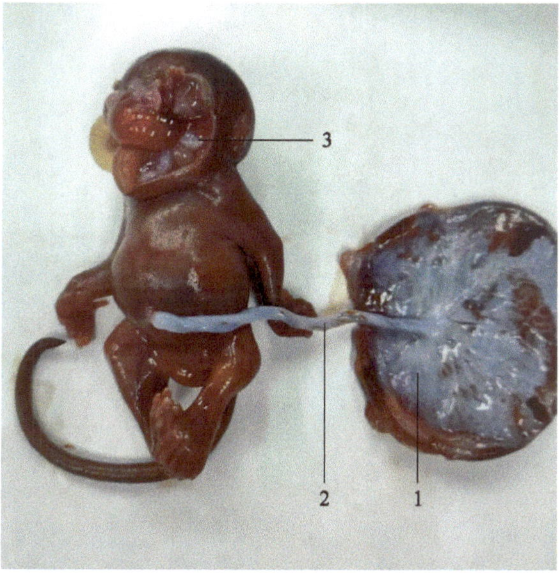

Figure 47 **Placenta, umbilical cord, and fetus of a cyclophosphamide fetus. Fetal monkey, cyclophosphamide (CP), 20 mg/kg, subcutaneous injection (sc) on GD_{24-28}, cesarean section examination on GD_{100}. 1. Placenta of the fetus. 2. Umbilical cord. 3. Fetus with facial abnormalities**

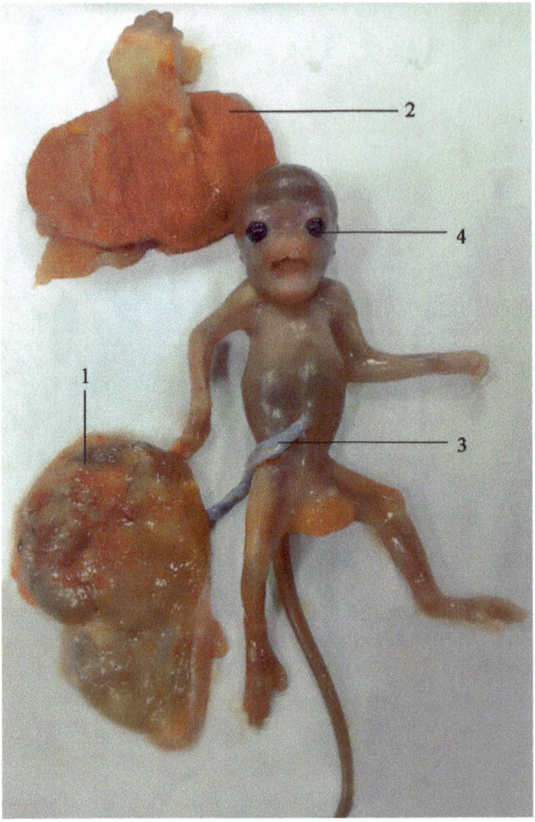

Figure 48 **Placenta, uterus, umbilical cord, and fetus of a cyclophosphamide fetus. Fetal monkey, cyclophosphamide (CP), 20 mg/kg, subcutaneous injection (sc) on GD_{24-28}, cesarean section examination on GD_{100}. 1. Placenta of the fetus. 2. Uterus. 3. Umbilical cord. 4. Fetus with exophthalmos**

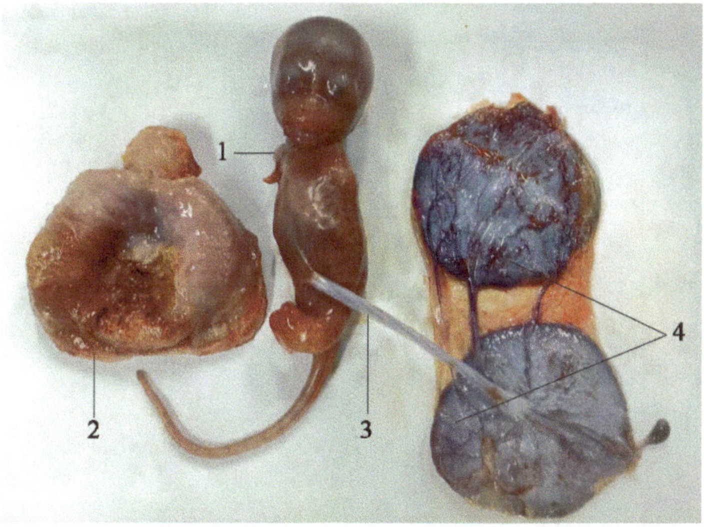

Figure 49 Thalidomide phocomelic fetus, uterus, umbilical cord, and double placentas. Fetal monkey, thalidomide, 15 mg/kg, gavage administration (ig) on GD_{24-30}, cesarean section examination on GD_{100}. 1. Phocomelic fetus. 2. Uterus. 3. Umbilical cord. 4. Double placentas

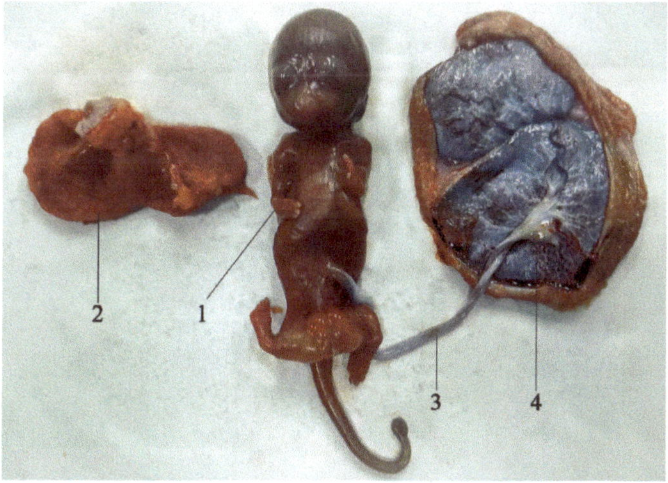

Figure 50 Thalidomide phocomelic fetus, uterus, umbilical cord, and double placentas. Fetal monkey, thalidomide, 15 mg/kg, gavage administration (ig) on GD_{24-30}, cesarean section examination on GD_{100}. 1. Phocomelic fetus; 2. Uterus; 3. Umbilical cord; 4. Double placentas

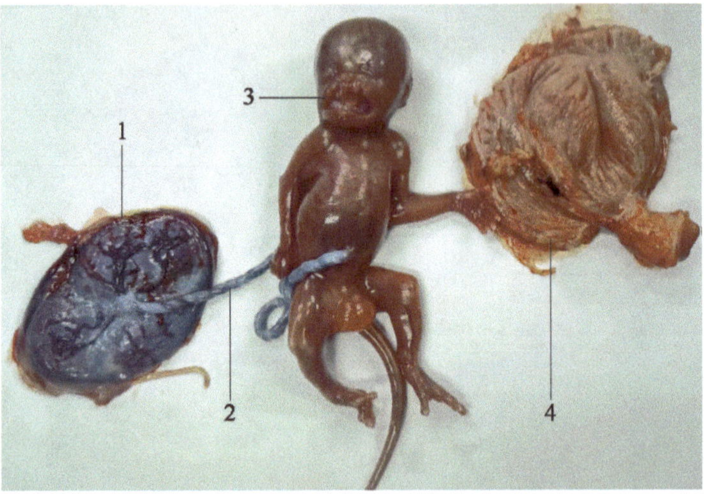

Figure 51 Cyclophosphamide fetus, placenta, umbilical cord, fetus, and uterus. Fetal monkey, cyclophosphamide (CP), 20 mg/kg, subcutaneous injection (sc) on GD_{24-28}, cesarean section examination on GD_{100}. 1. Placenta of the fetus. 2. Umbilical cord. 3. Fetus with facial abnormalities. 4. Uterus

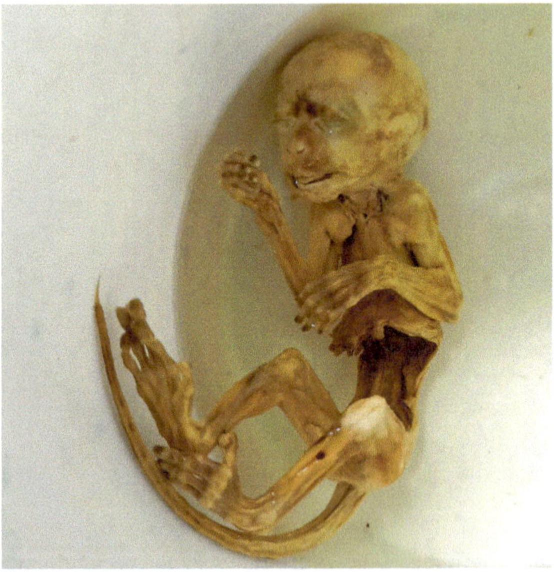

Figure 52 Normal fetus (front view). Fetal monkey, sodium chloride injection, 1 mL/kg, gavage administration (ig) on GD_{24-30}, cesarean section examination on GD_{100}

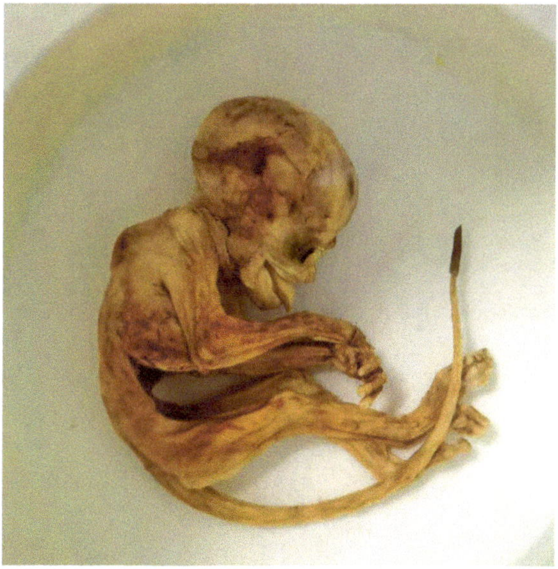

Figure 53 Normal fetus (lateral view). Fetal monkey, sodium chloride injection, 1 mL/kg, gavage administration (ig) on GD_{24-30}, cesarean section examination on GD_{100}

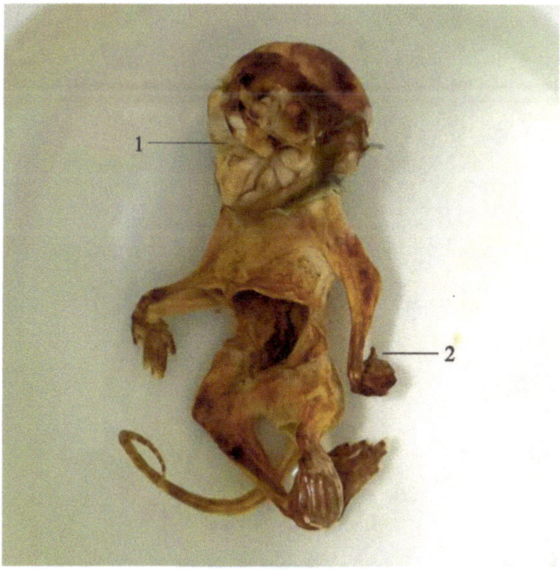

Figure 54 Facial abnormalities, eversion of upper and lower limbs (front view). Fetal monkey, cyclophosphamide (CP), 20 mg/kg, subcutaneous injection (sc) on GD_{24-28}, cesarean section examination on GD_{100}. 1. Facial abnormalities. 2. Eversion of the upper limb

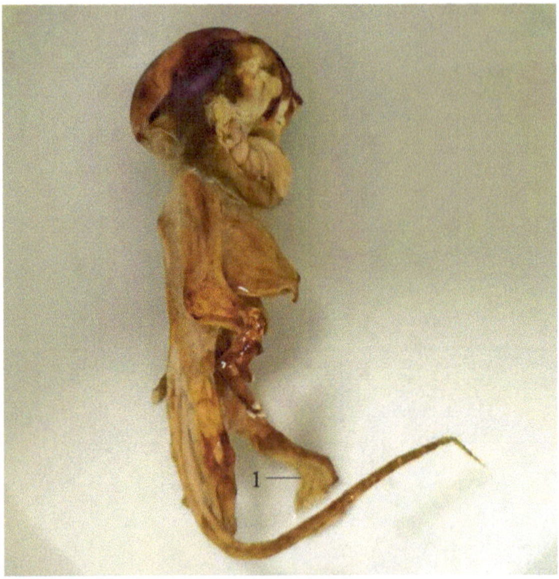

Figure 55 Facial abnormalities, eversion of upper and lower limbs (lateral view). Fetal monkey, cyclophosphamide (CP), 20 mg/kg, subcutaneous injection (sc) on GD_{24-28}, cesarean section examination on GD_{100}. 1. Eversion of the lower limb

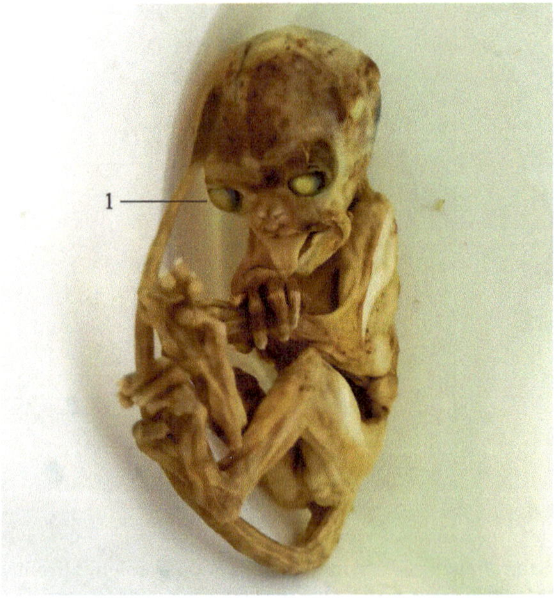

Figure 56 Exophthalmos (top view). Fetal monkey, cyclophosphamide (CP), 20 mg/kg, subcutaneous injection (sc) on GD_{24-28}, cesarean section examination on GD_{100}. 1. Exophthalmos

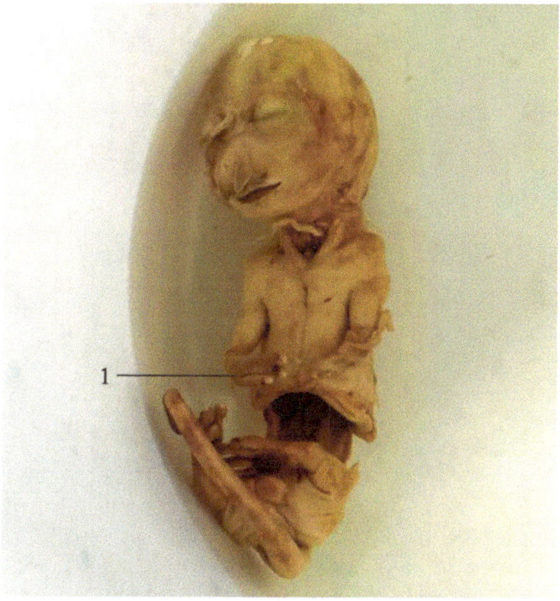

Figure 57 Phocomelia, oligodactyly (front view). Fetal monkey, thalidomide, 15 mg/kg, gavage administration (ig) on GD_{24-30}, cesarean section examination on GD_{100}. 1. Phocomelia, oligodactyly

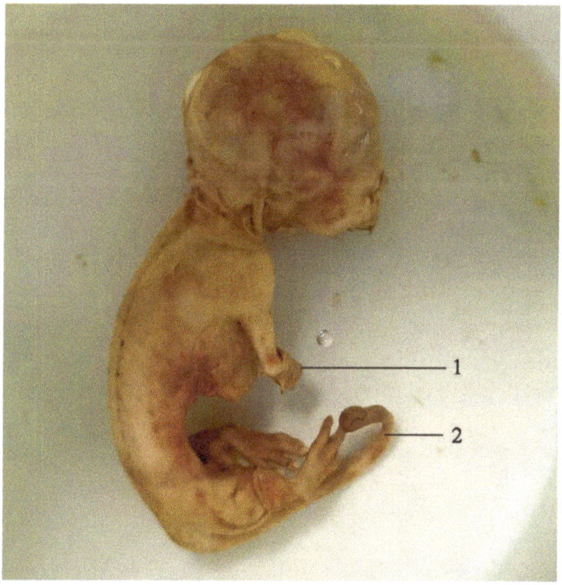

Figure 58 Phocomelia, oligodactyly, curly tail (lateral view). Fetal monkey, thalidomide, 15 mg/kg, gavage administration (ig) on GD_{24-30}, cesarean section examination on GD_{100}. 1. Phocomelia. 2. Curly tail

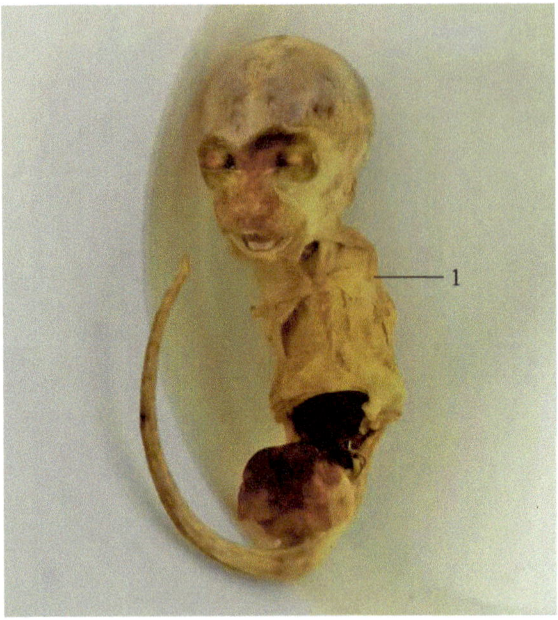

Figure 59 Phocomelia (front view). Fetal monkey, thalidomide, 15 mg/kg, gavage administration (ig) on GD_{24-30}, cesarean section examination on GD_{100}. 1. Phocomelia

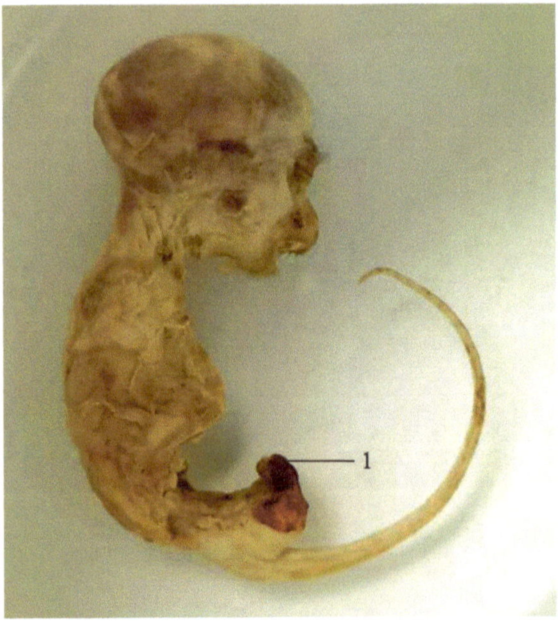

Figure 60 Phocomelia (lateral view). Fetal monkey, thalidomide, 15 mg/kg, gavage administration (ig) on GD_{24-30}, cesarean section examination on GD_{100}. 1. Phocomelia

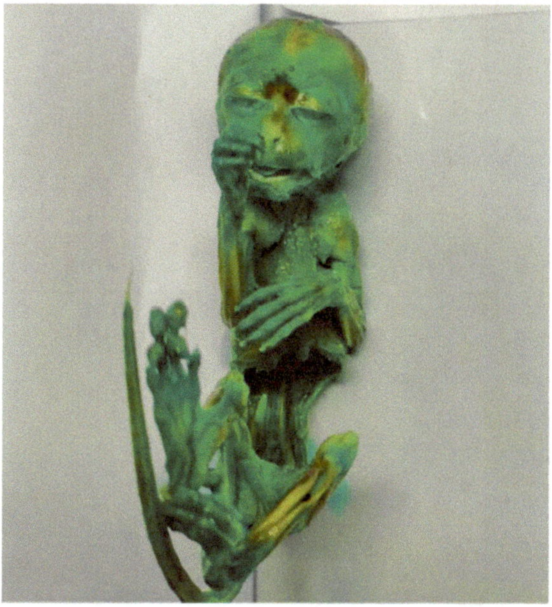

Figure 61 Normal fetus (front view). Fetal monkey, sodium chloride injection, 1 mL/kg, gavage administration (ig) on GD_{24-30}, cesarean section examination on GD_{100}

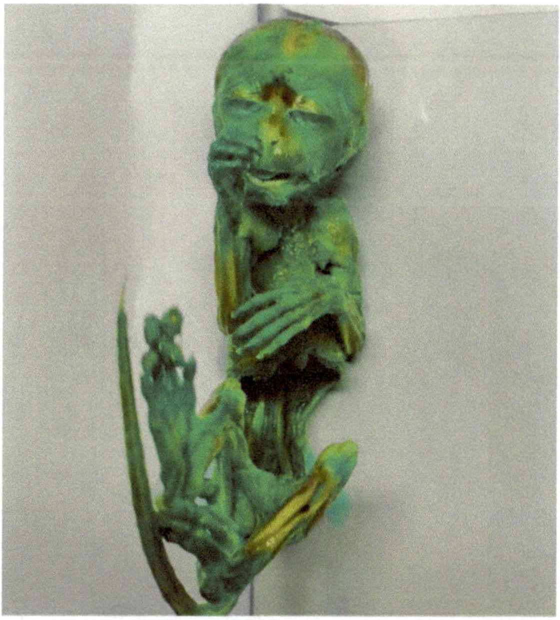

Figure 62 Normal fetus (lateral view). Fetal monkey, sodium chloride injection, 1 mL/kg, gavage administration (ig) from GD_{24-30}, cesarean section examination on GD_{100}

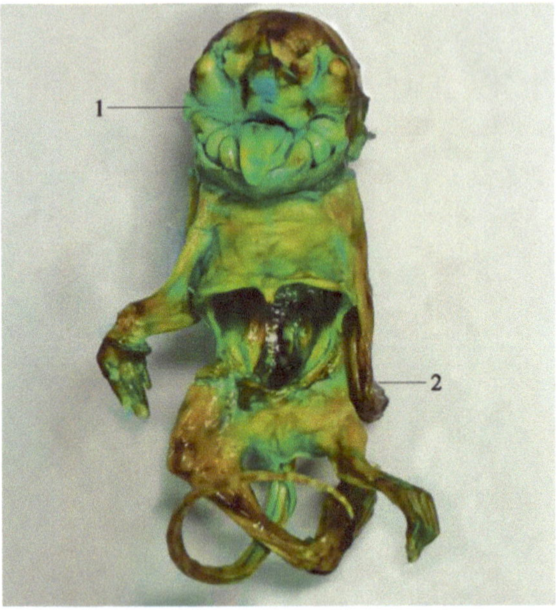

Figure 63 Facial abnormalities, eversion of upper and lower limbs (front view). Fetal monkey, cyclophosphamide (CP), 20 mg/kg, subcutaneous injection (sc) on GD_{24-28}, cesarean section examination on GD_{100}. 1. Facial abnormalities. 2. Eversion of the upper limb

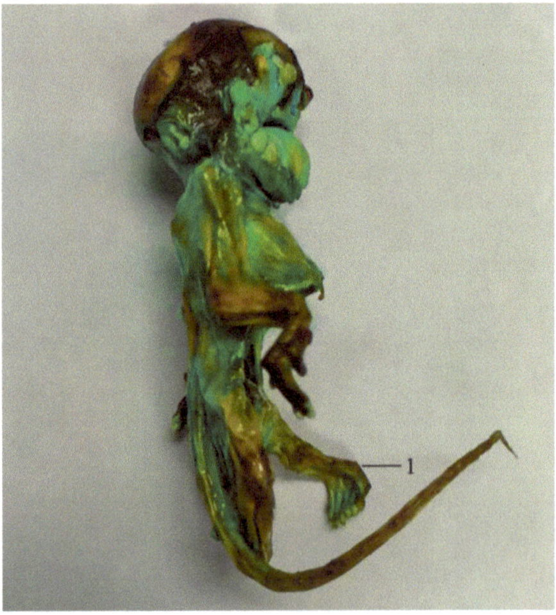

Figure 64 Facial abnormalities, eversion of upper and lower limbs (lateral view). Fetal monkey, cyclophosphamide (CP), 20 mg/kg, subcutaneous injection (sc) on GD_{24-28}, cesarean section examination on GD_{100}. 1. Eversion of the lower limb

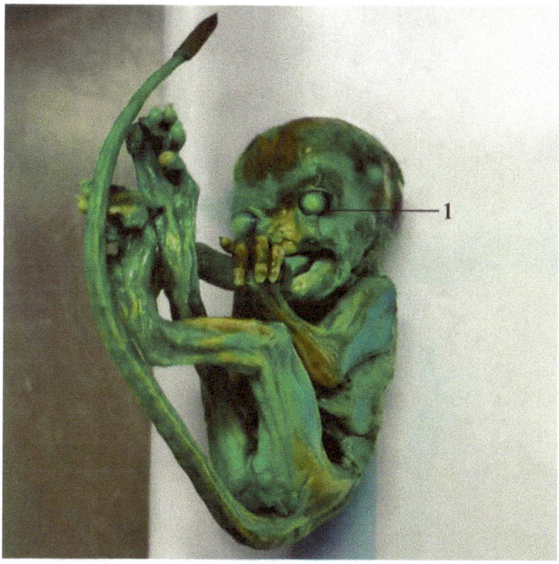

Figure 65 Exophthalmos (front view). Fetal monkey, cyclophosphamide (CP), 20 mg/kg, subcutaneous injection (sc) on GD_{24-28}, cesarean section examination on GD_{100}. 1. Exophthalmos

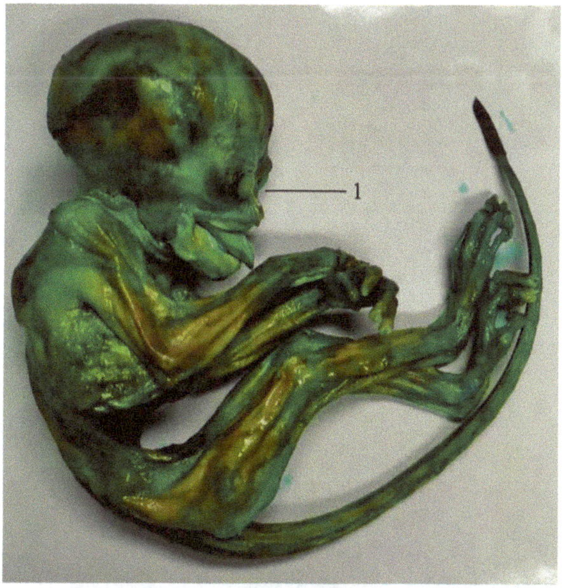

Figure 66 Exophthalmos (lateral view). Fetal monkey, cyclophosphamide (CP), 20 mg/kg, subcutaneous injection (sc) on GD_{24-28}, cesarean section examination on GD_{100}. 1. Exophthalmos

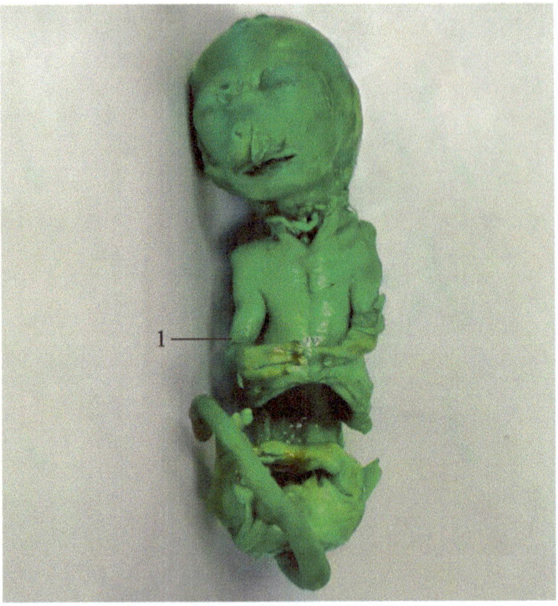

Figure 67 Phocomelia, oligodactyly (front view). Fetal monkey, thalidomide, 15 mg/kg, gavage administration (ig) on GD_{24-28}, cesarean section examination on GD_{100}. 1. Phocomelia, oligodactyly

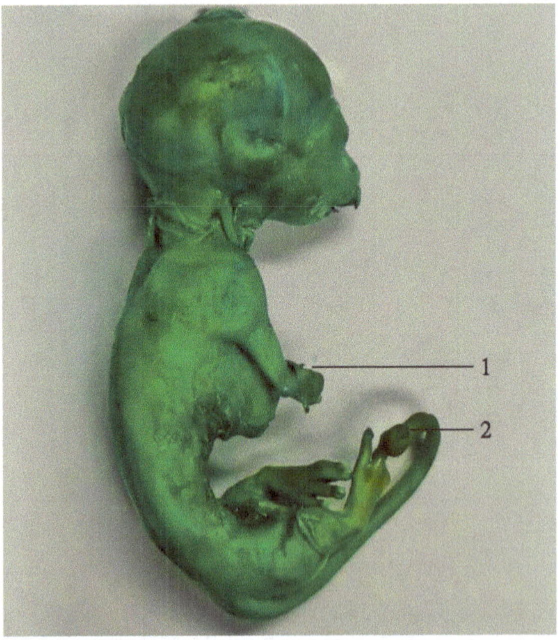

Figure 68 Phocomelia, oligodactyly, curly tail (lateral view). Fetal monkey, thalidomide, 15 mg/kg, gavage administration (ig) on GD_{24-28}, cesarean section examination on GD_{100}. 1. Phocomelia. 2. Curly tail

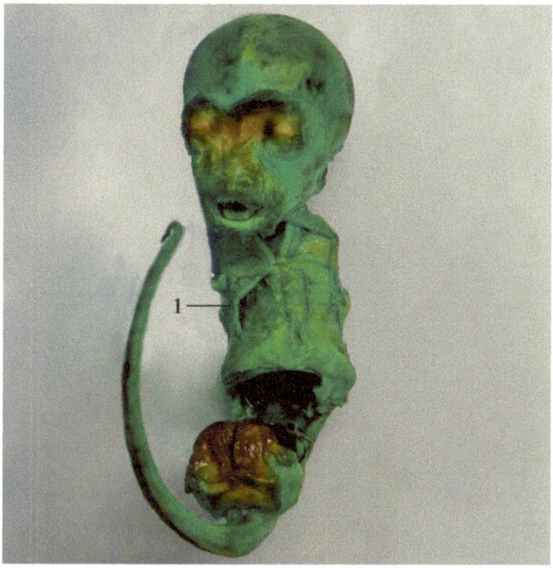

Figure 69 Phocomelia (front view). Fetal monkey, thalidomide, 15 mg/kg, gavage administration (ig) on GD_{24-28}, cesarean section examination on GD_{100}. 1. Phocomelia

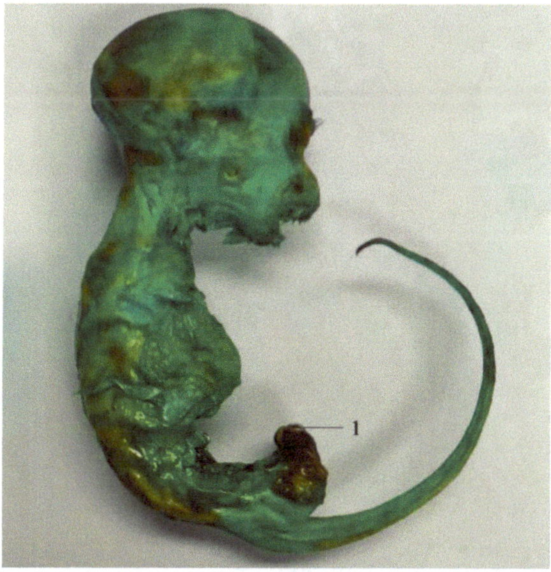

Figure 70 Phocomelia (lateral view). Fetal monkey, thalidomide, 15 mg/kg, gavage administration (ig) on GD_{24-28}, cesarean section examination on GD_{100}. 1. Phocomelia

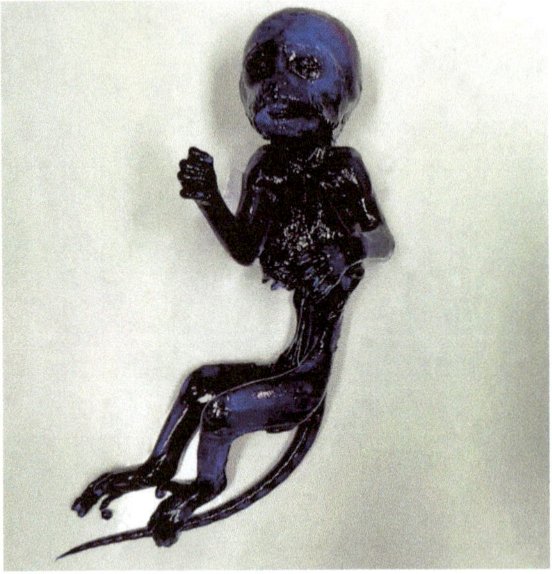

Figure 71 Normal fetus (front view). Fetal monkey, sodium chloride injection, 1 mL/kg, gavage administration (ig) on GD_{24-30}, cesarean section examination on GD_{100}

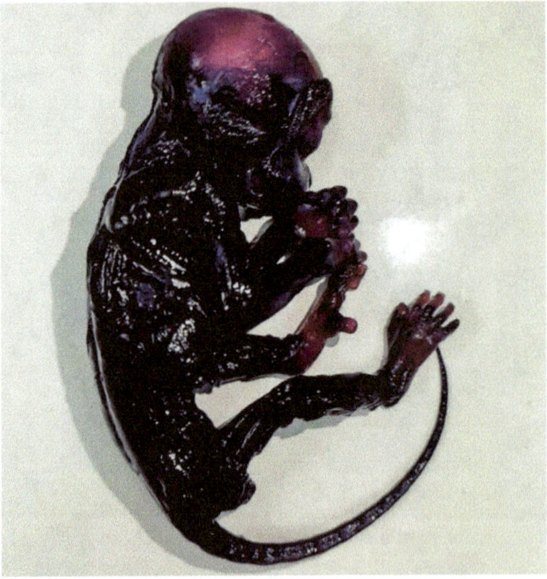

Figure 72 Normal fetus (lateral view). Fetal monkey, sodium chloride injection, 1 mL/kg, gavage administration (ig) on GD_{24-30}, cesarean section examination on GD_{100}

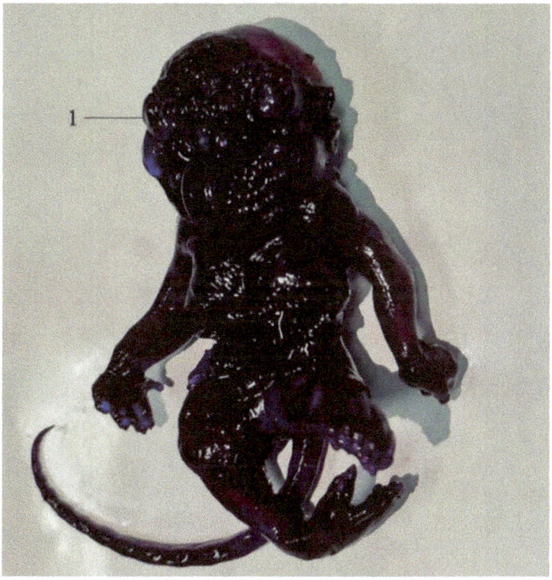

Figure 73 Facial abnormalities, eversion of upper and lower limbs (front view). Fetal monkey, cyclophosphamide (CP), 20 mg/kg, subcutaneous injection (sc) on GD_{24-28}, cesarean section examination on GD_{100}. 1. Facial abnormalities

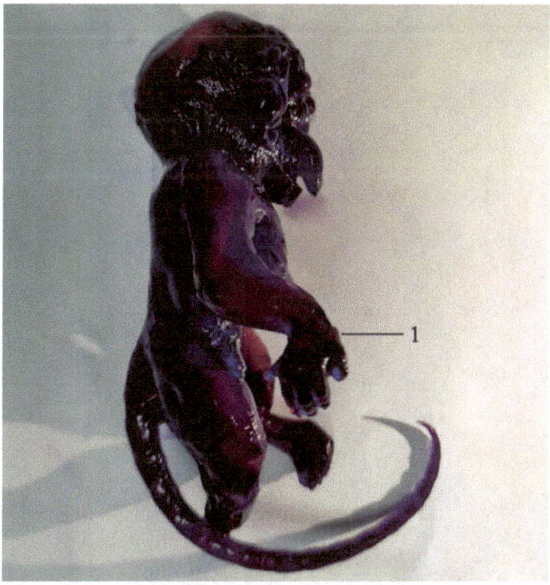

Figure 74 Facial abnormalities, eversion of upper and lower limbs (lateral view). Fetal monkey, cyclophosphamide (CP), 20 mg/kg, subcutaneous injection (sc) on GD_{24-28}, cesarean section examination on GD_{100}. 1. Eversion of the upper limb

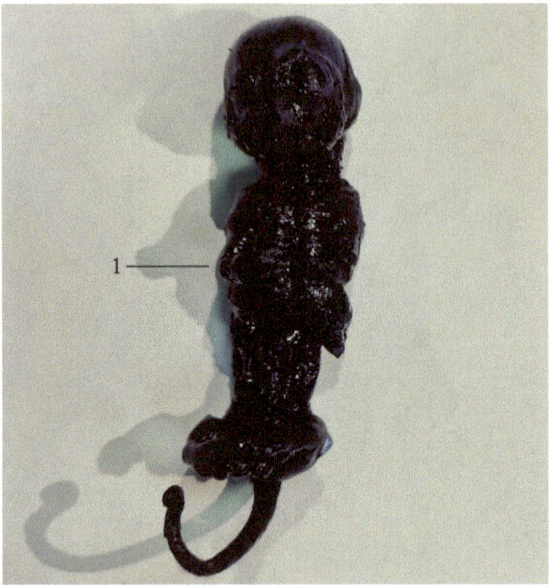

Figure 75 Phocomelia, oligodactyly (front view). Fetal monkey, thalidomide, 15 mg/kg, gavage administration (ig) on GD_{24-30}, cesarean section examination on GD_{100}. 1. Phocomelia, oligodactyly

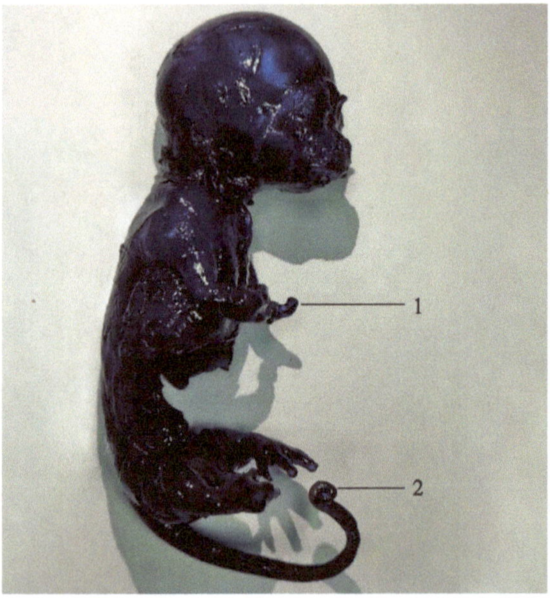

Figure 76 Phocomelia, oligodactyly, curly tail (lateral view). Fetal monkey, thalidomide, 15 mg/kg, gavage administration (ig) on GD_{24-30}, cesarean section examination on GD_{100}. 1. Phocomelia. 2. Curly tail

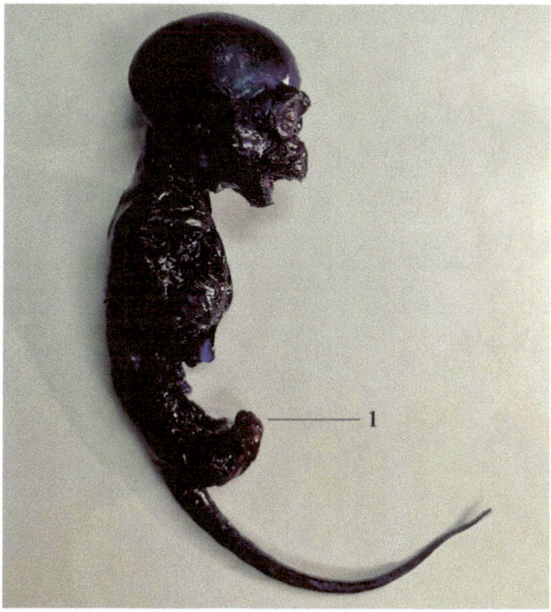

Figure 77 Phocomelia (lateral view). Fetal monkey, thalidomide, 15 mg/kg, gavage administration (ig) on GD_{24-30}, cesarean section examination on GD_{100}. 1. Phocomelia

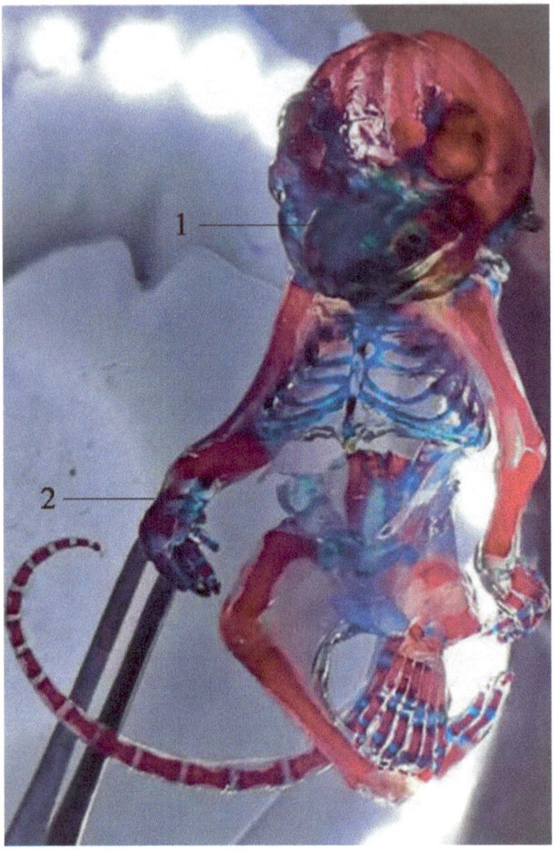

Figure 78 Facial abnormalities, eversion of the upper limb (front view). Fetal monkey, cyclophosphamide (CP), 20 mg/kg, subcutaneous injection (sc) on GD_{24-28}, cesarean section examination on GD_{100}. 1. Facial abnormalities. 2. Eversion of the upper limb

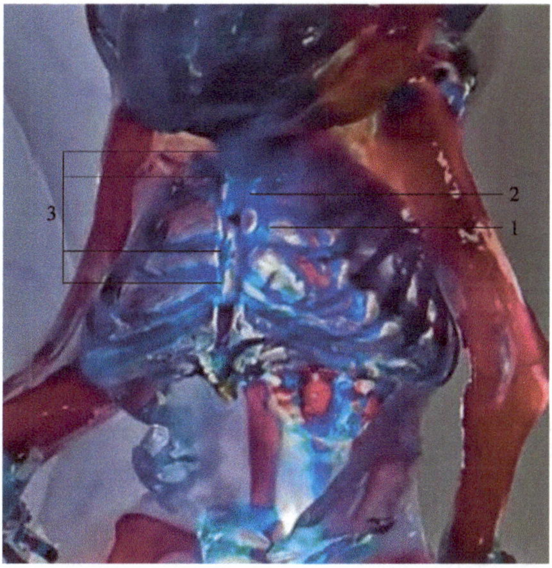

Figure 79 Rib fusion, H-shaped rib, absence of sternum (front view). Fetal monkey, cyclophosphamide (CP), 20 mg/kg, subcutaneous injection (sc) on GD_{24-28}, cesarean section examination on GD_{100}. 1. Disordered, fused, ectopic, and malformed ribs. 2. Rib fusion. 3. Absence of the first, second, fourth, and fifth sternums

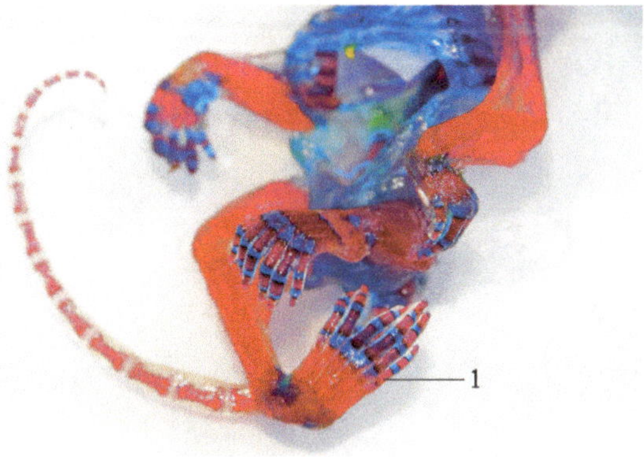

Figure 80 Polydactyly. Fetal monkey, cyclophosphamide (CP), 20 mg/kg, subcutaneous injection (sc) on GD_{24-28}, cesarean section examination on GD_{100}. 1. Polydactyly

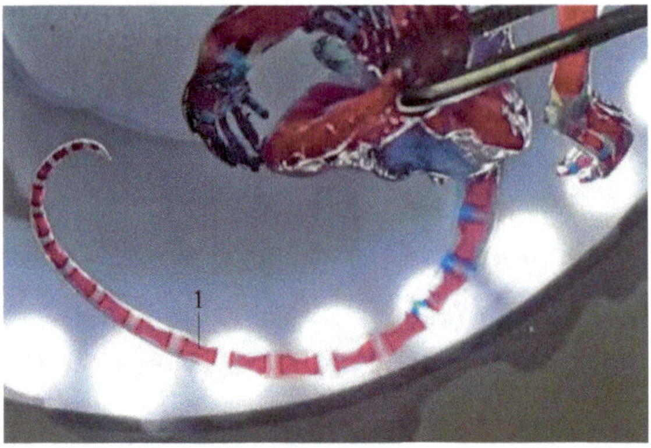

Figure 81 Normal tail. Fetal monkey, cyclophosphamide (CP), 20 mg/kg, subcutaneous injection (sc) on GD_{24-28}, cesarean section examination on GD_{100}. 1. Normal tail

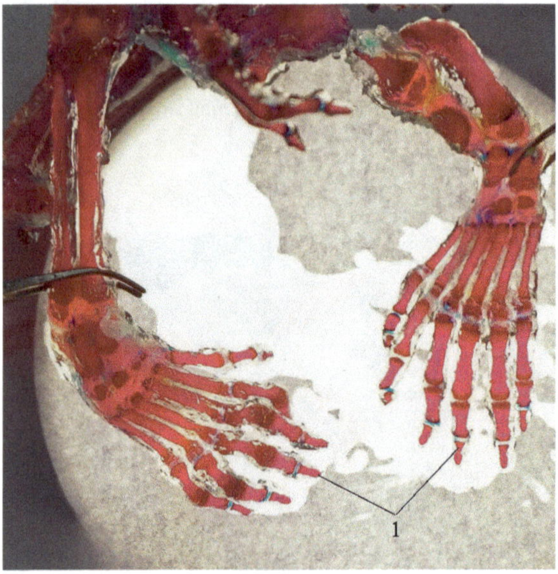

Figure 82 Fetal monkey, thalidomide, 15 mg/kg, gavage administration (ig) on GD_{24-30}, cesarean section examination on GD_{100}. 1. Polydactyly

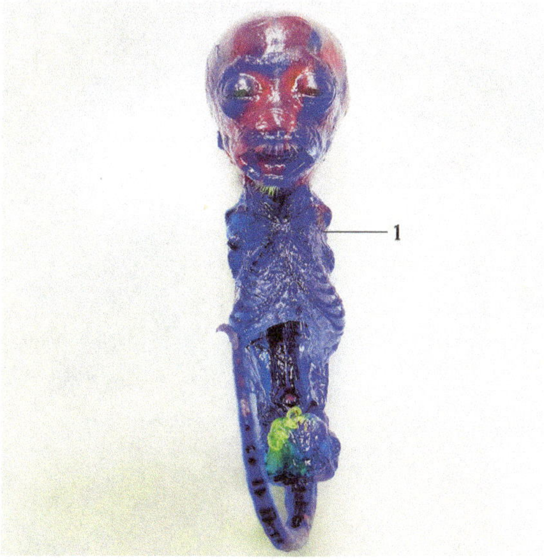

Figure 83 Phocomelia (front view). Fetal monkey, thalidomide, 15 mg/kg, gavage administration (ig) on GD_{24-30}, cesarean section examination on GD_{100}. 1. Phocomelia

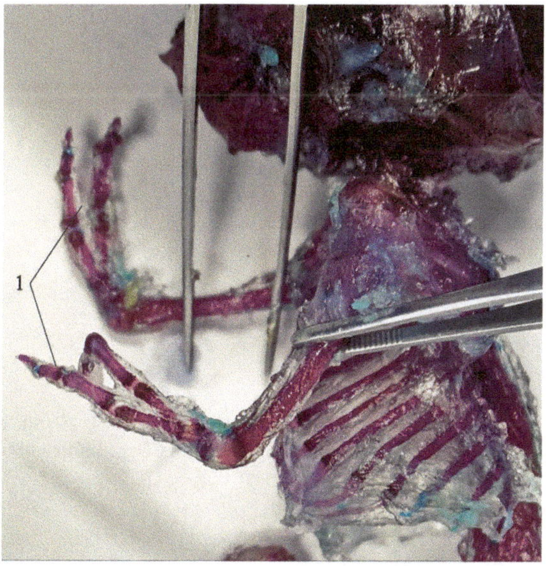

Figure 84 Oligodactyly (lateral view). Fetal monkey, cyclophosphamide (CP), 20 mg/kg, subcutaneous injection (sc) on GD_{24-28}, GD_{100}. 1. Oligodactyly

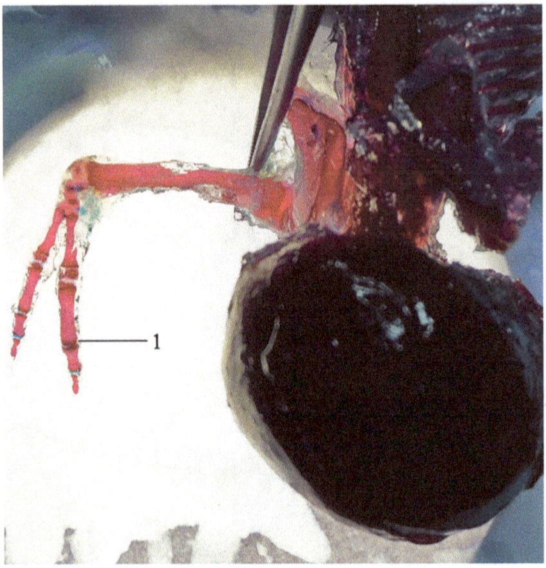

Figure 85 Oligodactyly. Fetal monkey, cyclophosphamide (CP), 20 mg/kg, subcutaneous injection (sc) on GD_{24-28}, GD_{100}. 1. Oligodactyly

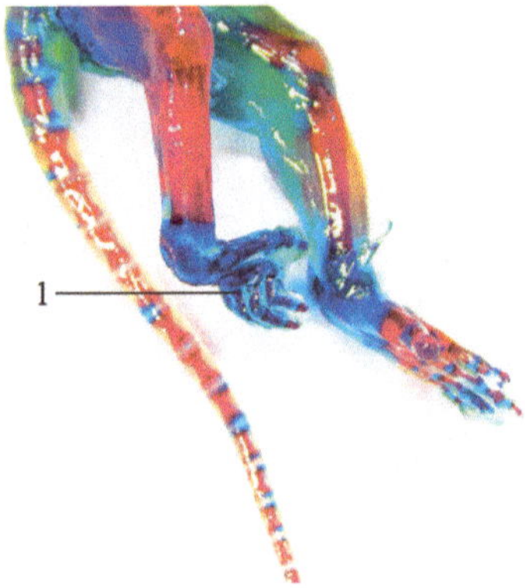

Figure 86 Curved toes. Fetal monkey, cyclophosphamide (CP), 20 mg/kg, subcutaneous injection (sc) on GD_{24-28}, cesarean section examination on GD_{100}. 1. Curved toes

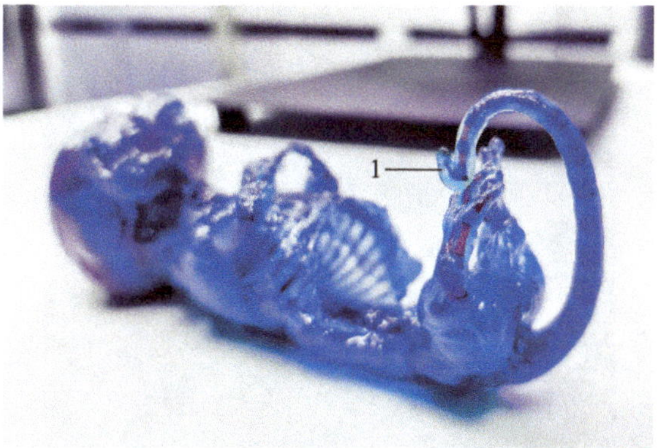

Figure 87 Curly tail (ventral view). Fetal monkey, thalidomide, 15 mg/kg, gavage administration (ig) on GD_{24-30}, cesarean section examination on GD_{100}. 1. Curly tail

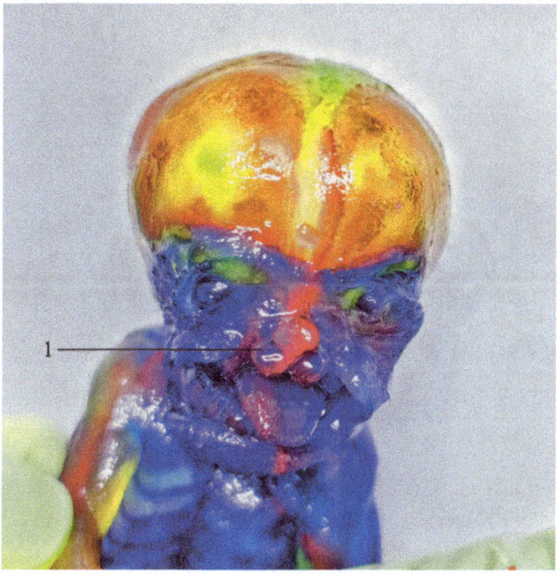

Figure 88 Abnormal lips (front view). Fetal monkey, cyclophosphamide (CP), 20 mg/kg, subcutaneous injection (sc) on GD_{24-28}, cesarean section examination on GD_{100}. 1. Abnormal lips

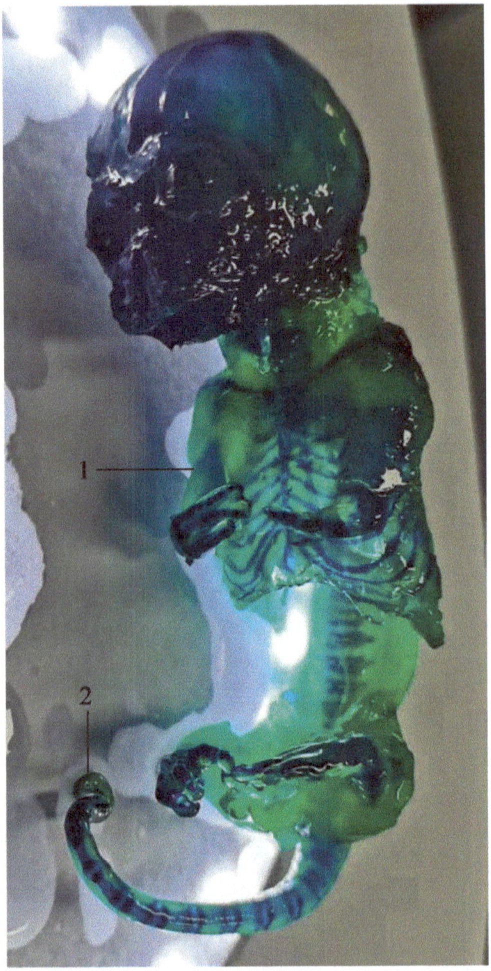

Figure 89 Phocomelia, curly tail (front view). Fetal monkey, thalidomide, 15 mg/kg, gavage administration (ig) on GD_{24-30}, cesarean section examination on GD_{100}. 1. Phocomelia. 2. Curly tail

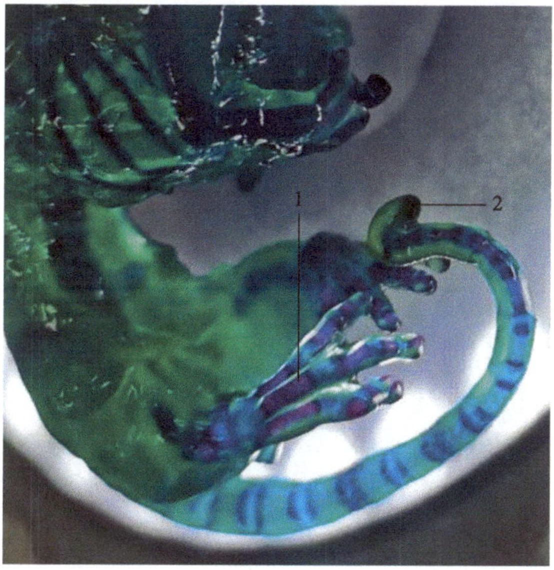

Figure 90 Oligodactyly of toes, curly tail (lateral view). Fetal monkey, thalidomide, 15 mg/kg, gavage administration (ig) on GD_{24-30}, cesarean section examination on GD_{100}. 1. Oligodactyly of toes. 2. Curly tail

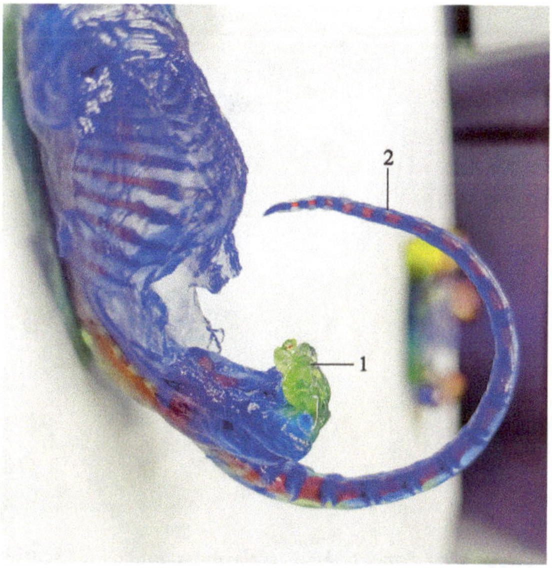

Figure 91 Phocomelia, normal tail (lateral view). Fetal monkey, thalidomide, 15 mg/kg, gavage administration (ig) on GD_{24-30}, cesarean section examination on GD_{100}. 1. Phocomelia. 2. Normal tail

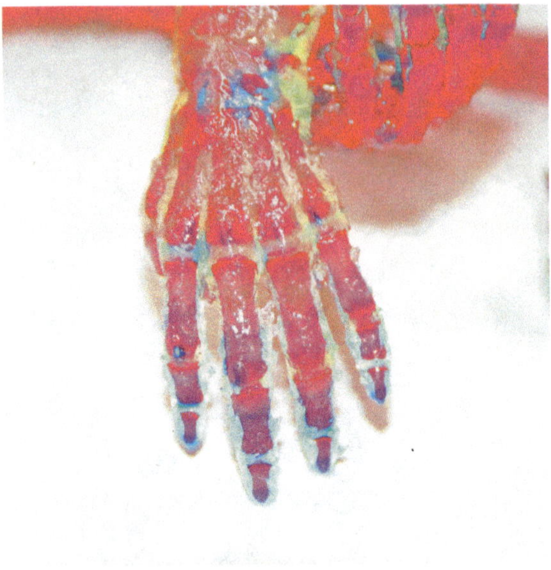

Figure 92 Fingers of a normal fetus. Fetal monkey, sodium chloride injection, 1 mL/kg, gavage administration (ig) on GD_{24-30}, cesarean section examination on GD_{100}

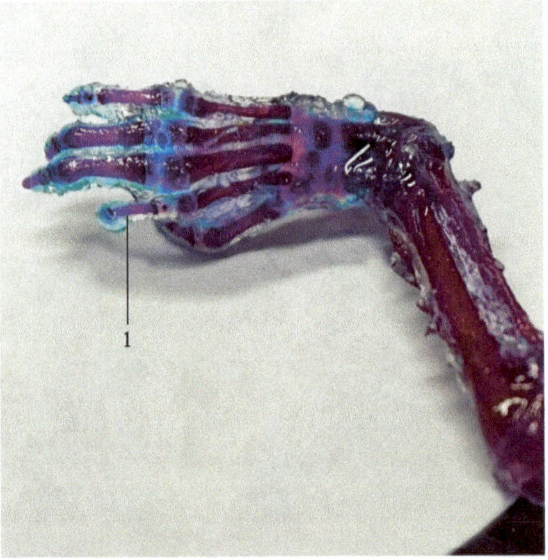

Figure 93 Short index finger. Fetal monkey, cyclophosphamide (CP), 20 mg/kg, subcutaneous injection (sc) on GD_{24-28}, cesarean section examination on GD_{100}. 1. Short index finger

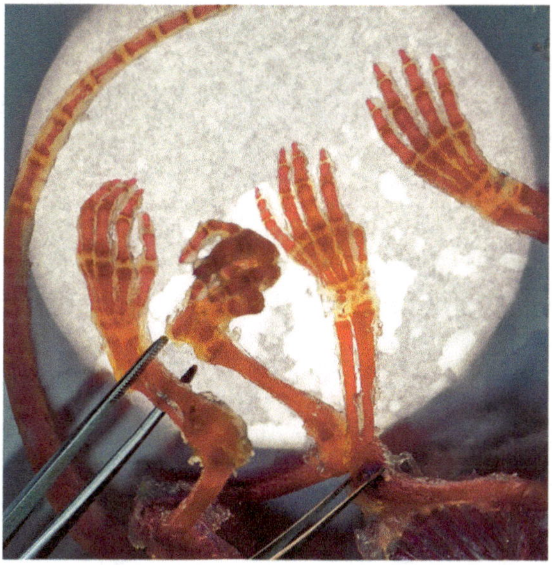

Figure 94 Fingers and toes of a normal fetus. Fetal monkey, sodium chloride injection, 1 mL/kg, gavage administration (ig) on GD_{24-30}, cesarean section examination on GD_{100}

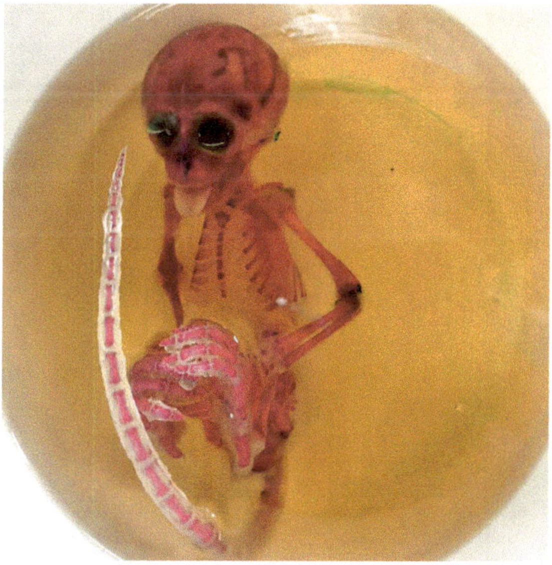

Figure 95 Normal fetus (front view). Fetal monkey, sodium chloride injection, 1 mL/kg, gavage administration (ig) on GD_{24-30}, cesarean section examination on GD_{160}

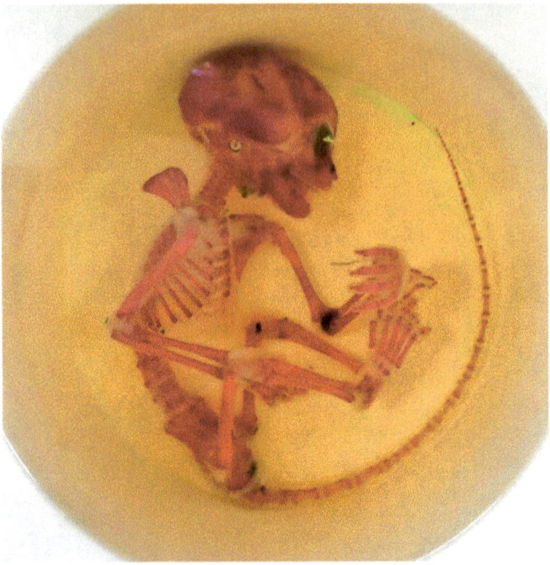

Figure 96 **Normal fetus (lateral view). Fetal monkey, sodium chloride injection, 1 mL/kg, gavage administration (ig) on GD_{24-30}, cesarean section examination on GD_{160}**

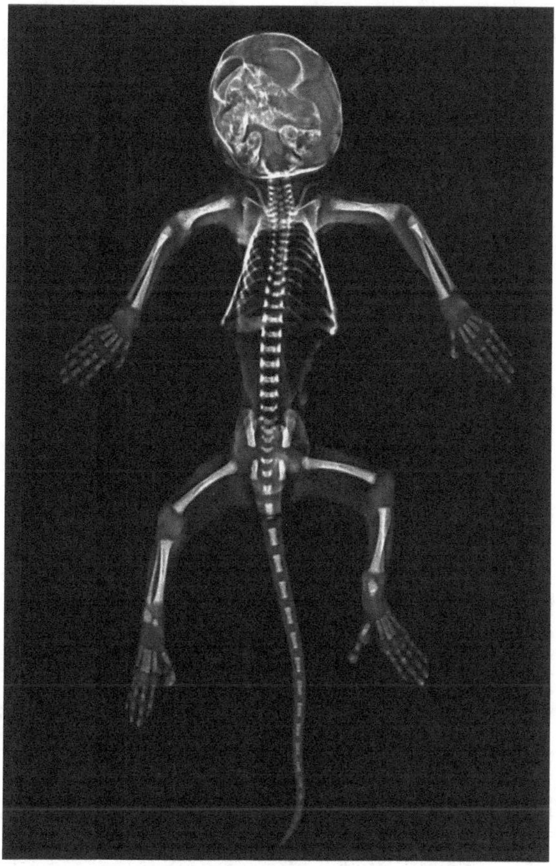

Figure 97 **Normal fetus (back view). Fetal monkey, sodium chloride injection, 1 mL/kg, gavage administration (ig) on GD_{24-30}, cesarean section examination on GD_{100}**

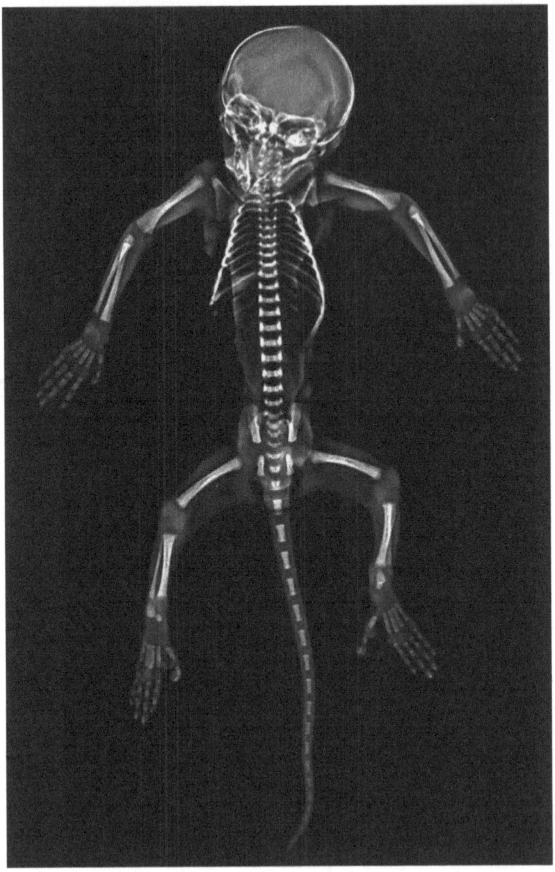

Figure 98 Normal fetus (front view). Fetal monkey, sodium chloride injection, 1 mL/kg, gavage administration (ig) on GD_{24-30}, cesarean section examination on GD_{100}

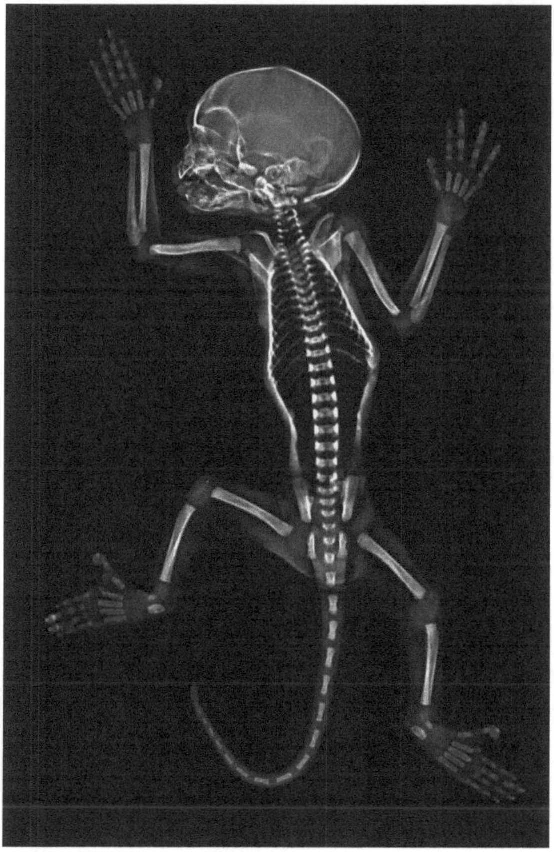

Figure 99 **Normal fetus (back view). Fetal monkey, sodium chloride injection, 1 mL/kg, gavage administration (ig) on GD_{24-30}, cesarean section examination on GD_{100}**

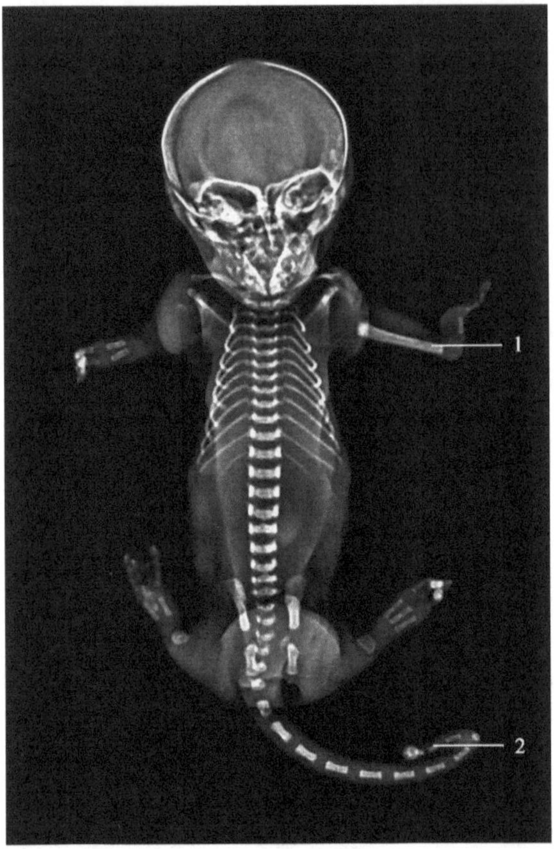

Figure 100 Phocomelia (front view). Fetal monkey, thalidomide, 15 mg/kg, gavage administration (ig) on GD_{24-30}, cesarean section examination on GD_{100}. 1. Phocomelia. 2. Curly tail

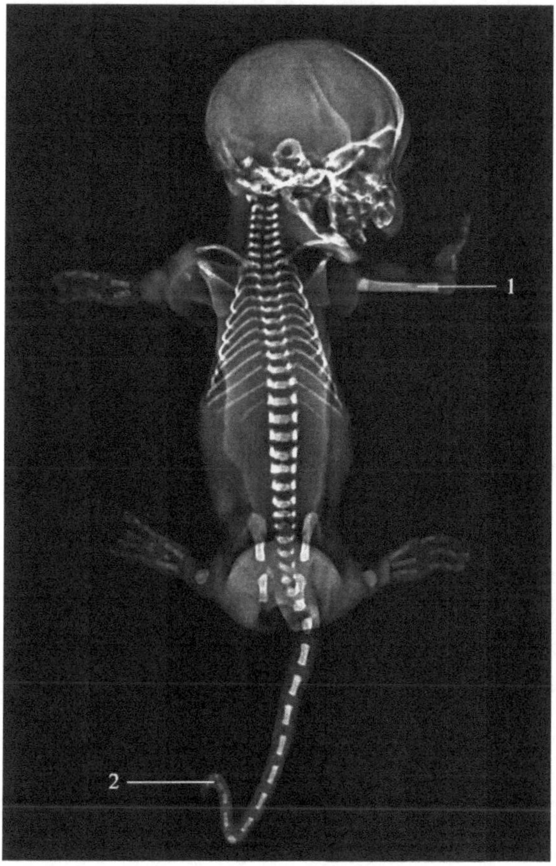

Figure 101 **Phocomelia (back view). Fetal monkey, thalidomide, 15 mg/kg, gavage administration (ig) on GD_{24-30}, cesarean section examination on GD_{100}. 1. Phocomelia. 2. Curly tail**

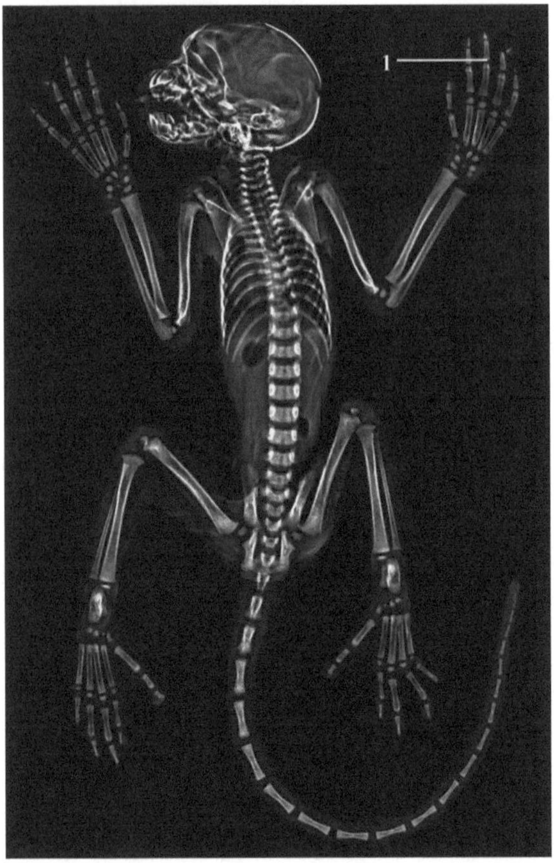

Figure 102 **Curved fingers (back view). Fetal monkey, cyclophosphamide (CP), 20 mg/kg, subcutaneous injection (sc) on $GD_{24\text{-}28}$, cesarean section examination on GD_{100}. 1. Curved fingers.**

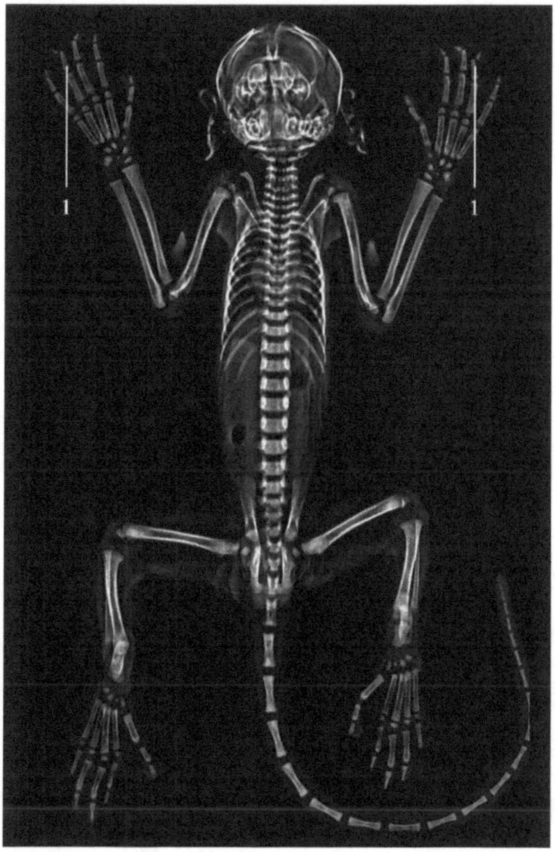

Figure 103 Curved fingers (front view). Fetal monkey, cyclophosphamide (CP), 20 mg/kg, subcutaneous injection (sc) on GD_{24-28}, cesarean section examination on GD_{100}. 1. Curved fingers

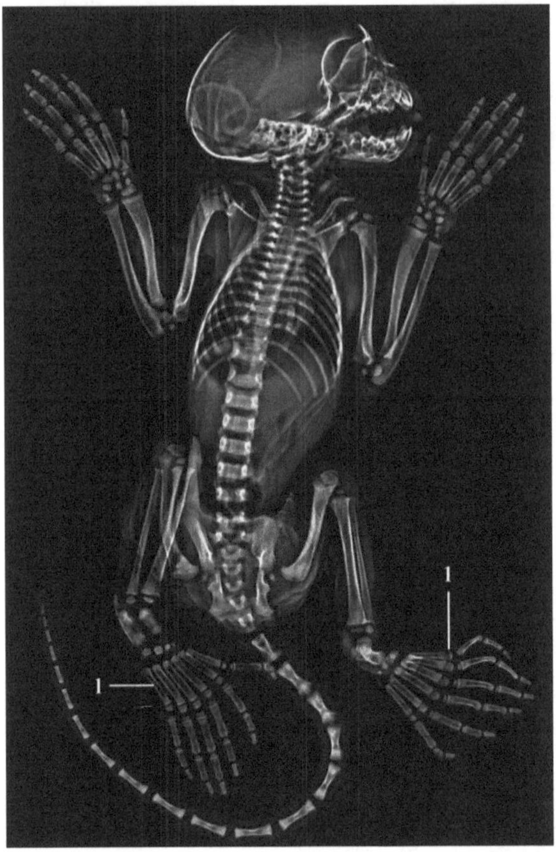

Figure 104 Polydactyly (back view). Fetal monkey, thalidomide, 15 mg/kg, gavage administration (ig) on GD_{24-30}, cesarean section examination on GD_{100}. 1. Polydactyly

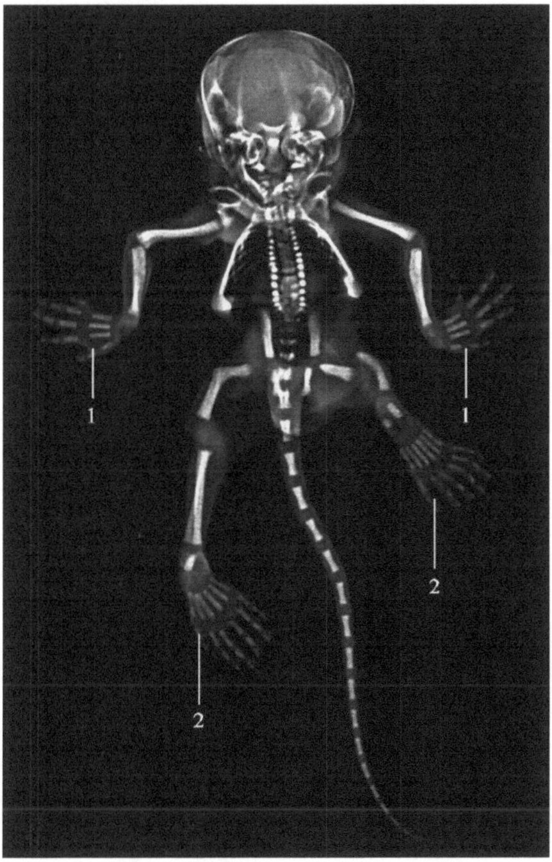

Figure 105 Eversion of forelimb, polydactyly (back view). Fetal monkey, cyclophosphamide (CP), 20 mg/kg, subcutaneous injection (sc) on GD_{24-28}, cesarean section examination on GD_{100}. 1. Eversion of forelimb. 2. Polydactyly

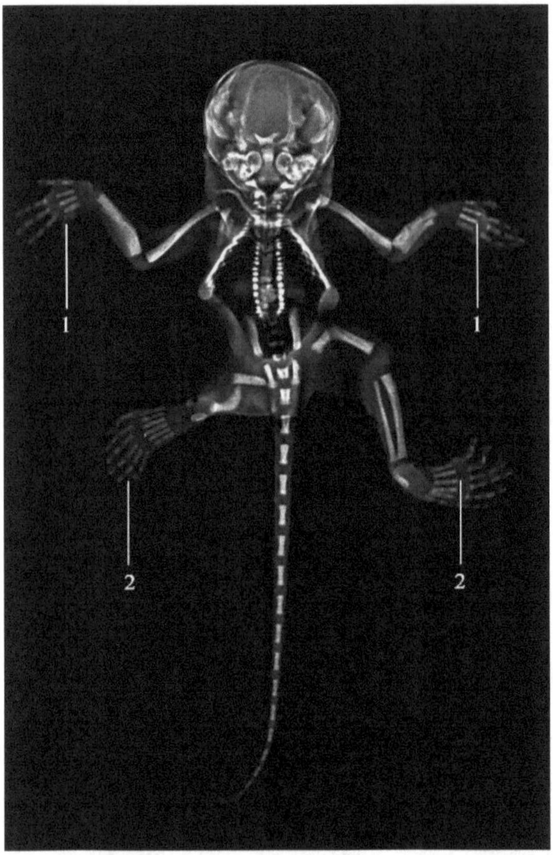

Figure 106 Eversion of forelimb, polydactyly (front view). Fetal monkey, cyclophosphamide (CP), 20 mg/kg, subcutaneous injection (sc) on GD_{24-28}, cesarean section examination on GD_{100}. 1. Eversion of forelimb. 2. Polydactyly

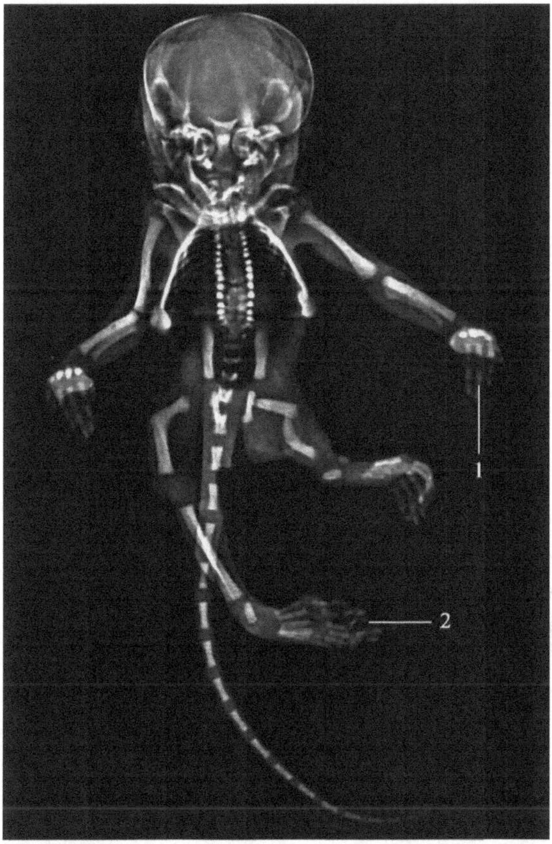

Figure 107 Eversion of forelimb, polydactyly (front view). Fetal monkey, cyclophosphamide (CP), 20 mg/kg, subcutaneous injection (sc) on GD_{24-28}, cesarean section examination on GD_{100}. 1. Eversion of forelimb. 2. Polydactyly

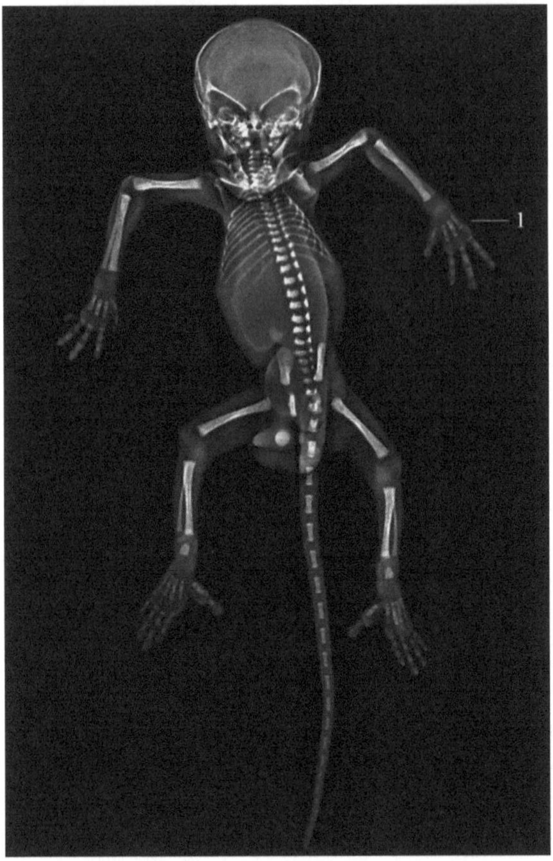

Figure 108 Oligodactyly (back view). Fetal monkey, cyclophosphamide (CP), 20 mg/kg, subcutaneous injection (sc) on GD_{24-28}, cesarean section examination on GD_{100}. 1. Oligodactyly

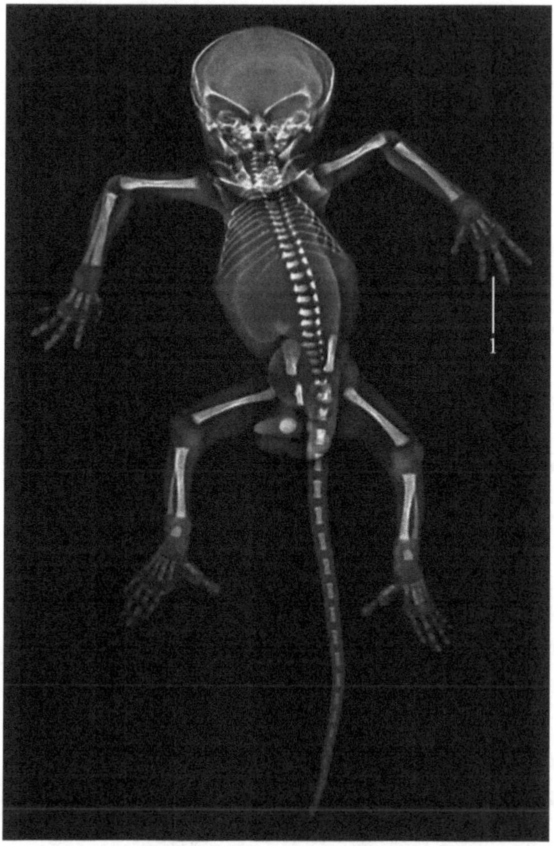

Figure 109 **Oligodactyly (front view). Fetal monkey, cyclophosphamide (CP), 20 mg/kg, subcutaneous injection (sc) on GD_{24-28}, cesarean section examination on GD_{100}. 1. Oligodactyly**

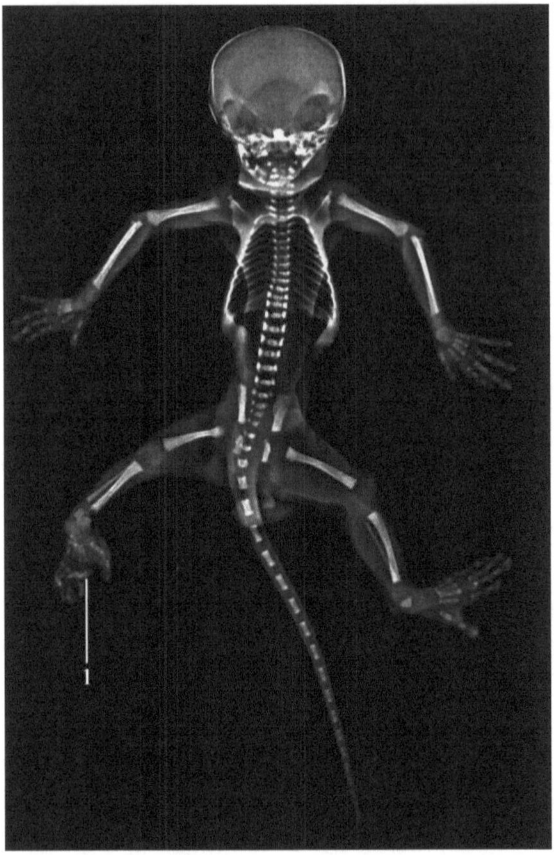

Figure 110 **Varus of the left hindlimb (back view). Fetal monkey, cyclophosphamide (CP), 20 mg/kg, subcutaneous injection (sc) on GD_{24-28}, cesarean section examination on GD_{100}. 1. Varus of the left hindlimb**

Appendix 2 Ultrasound Images of the Uterus and Fetuses of Pregnant Cynomolgus Monkeys

See Figs. A.2.1–A.2.18 for the ultrasound images of the uterus and fetuses of pregnant cynomolgus monkeys at different gestational times.

No Queries

L. Zhou and Z. Sun (eds.), *Reproductive and Developmental Toxicology on Macaca Fascicularis*, https://doi.org/10.1007/978-981-92-3834-7

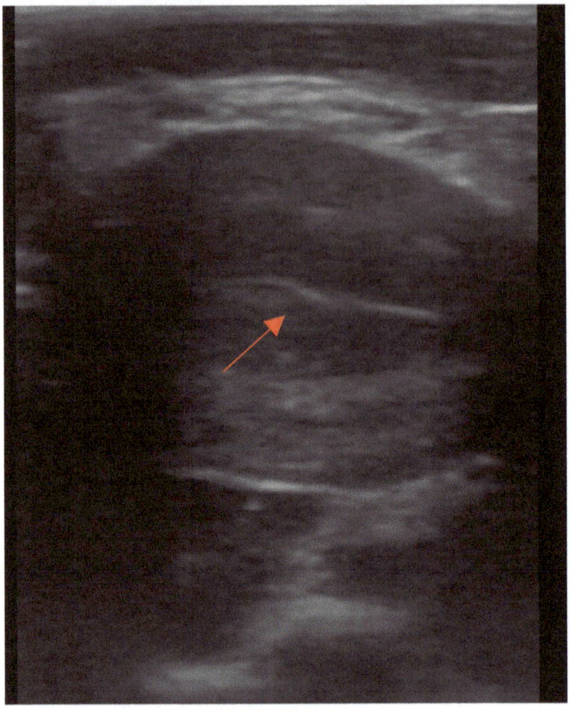

Figure 1 **Gestation GD_{15} uterine wall**

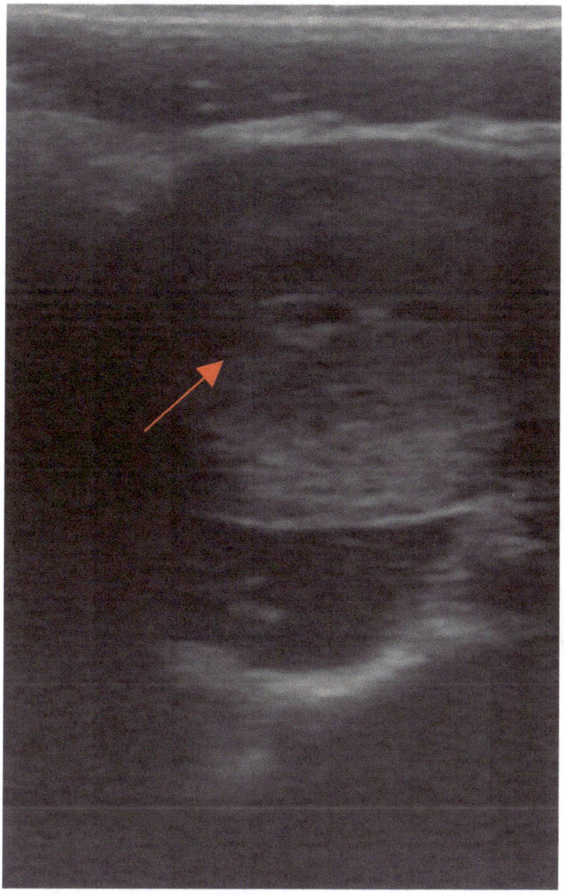

Figure 2 Gestation GD_{17} gestational sac appears

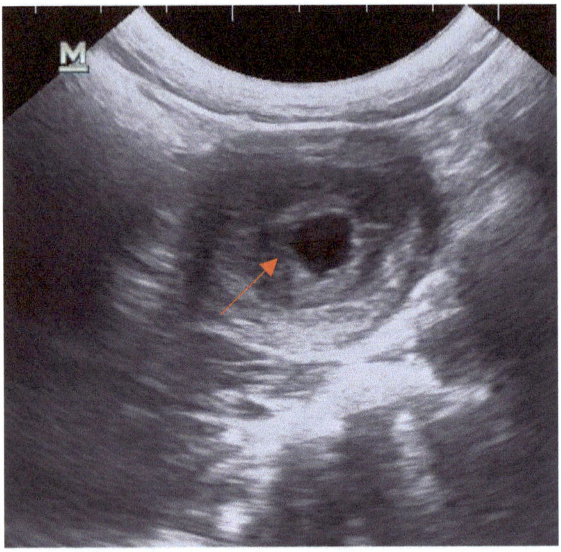

Figure 3 Gestation GD_{18} implantation of the fertilized ova

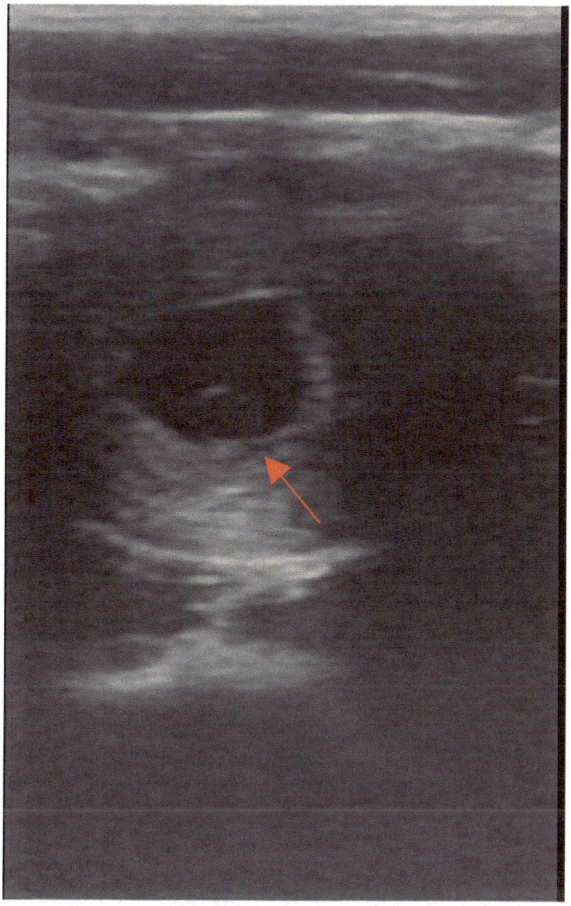

Figure 4 **Gestation GD_{20} formation of the yolk sac**

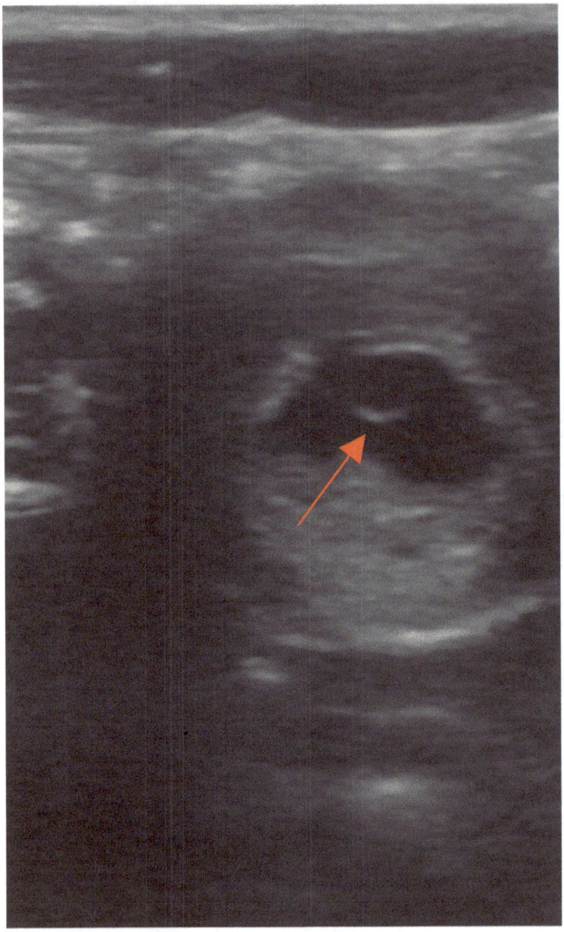

Figure 5 Gestation GD_{22} enlargement of the yolk sac

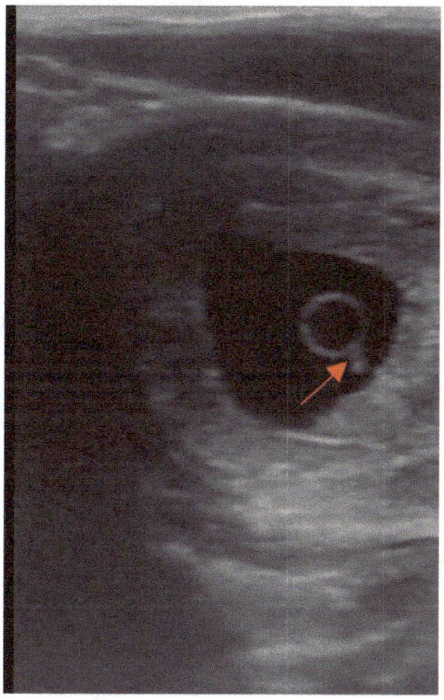

Figure 6 Gestation GD_{25} fetal bud

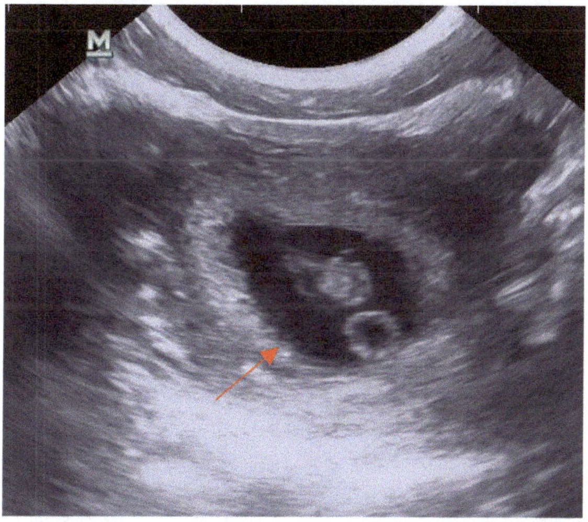

Figure 7 Gestation GD_{30} embryo

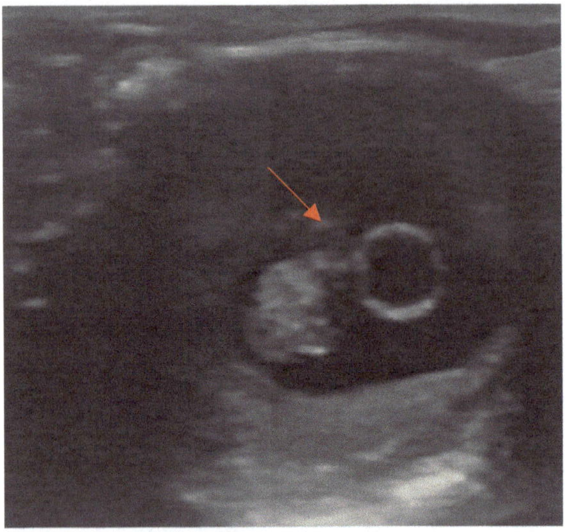

Figure 8 Gestation GD_{35} embryo initially shows the shape of a fetus

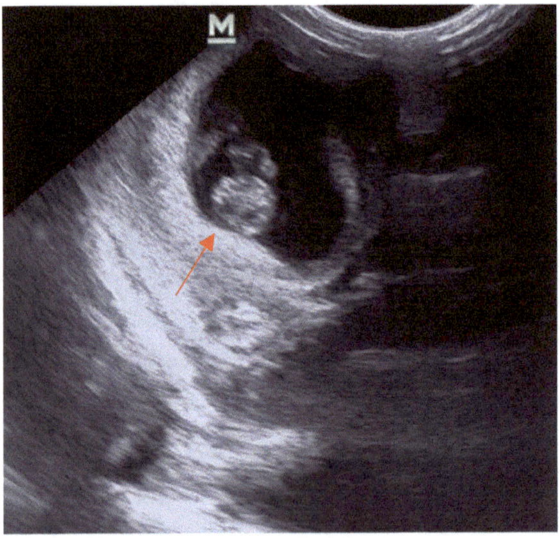

Figure 9 Gestation GD_{40} embryo

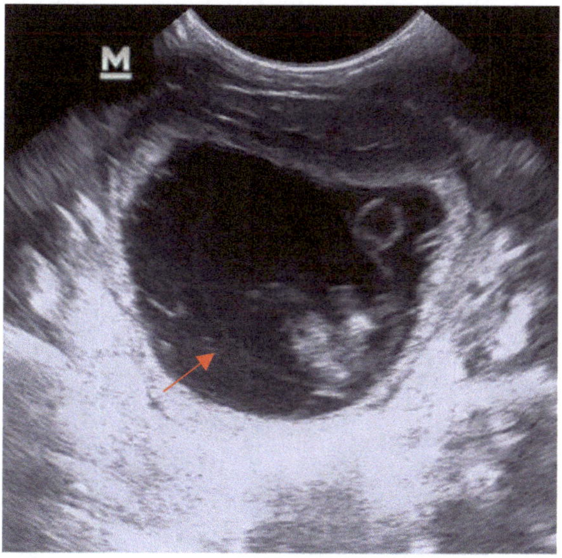

Figure 10 Gestation GD_{50} amniotic sac

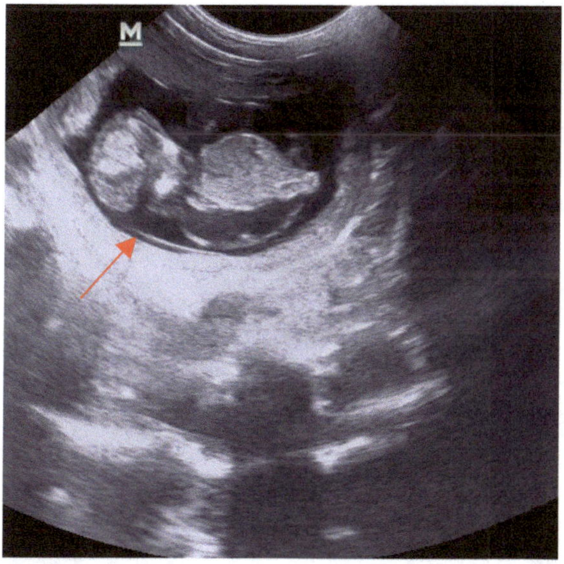

Figure 11 Gestation GD_{60} embryo (with an appearance like a "little seahorse")

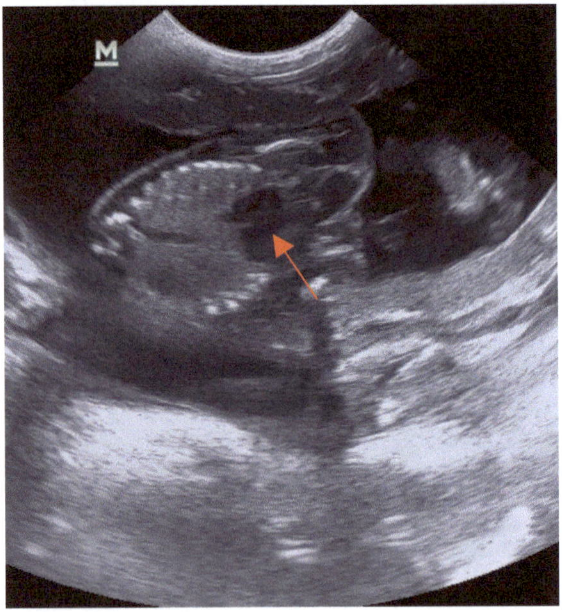

Figure 12 Gestation GD_{70} fetal heart

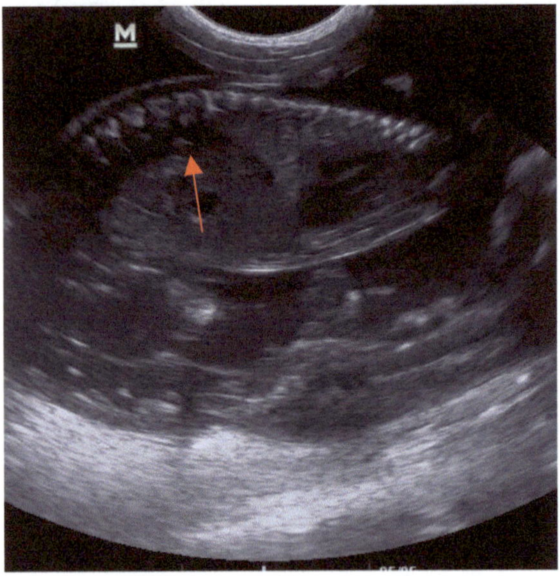

Figure 13 Gestation GD_{80} embryonic bones

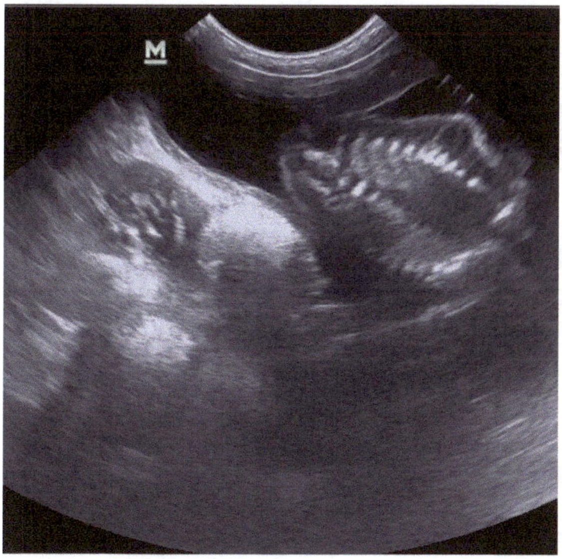

Figure 14 **Gestation GD_{90} embryo appearance**

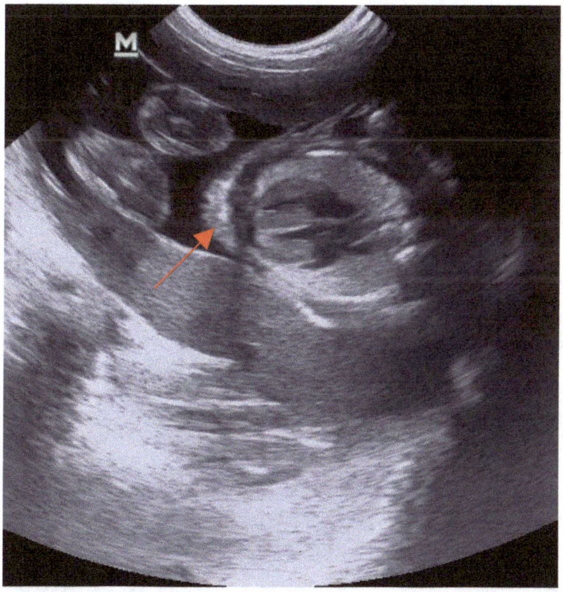

Figure 15 **Gestation GD_{100} embryo thoracic cavity**

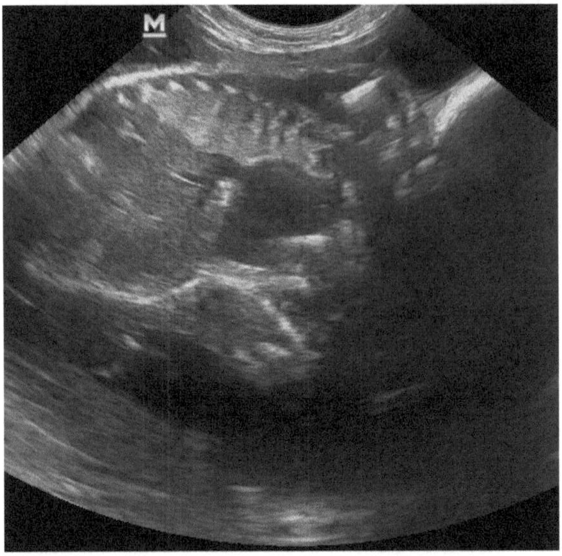

Figure 16 Gestation GD_{110}

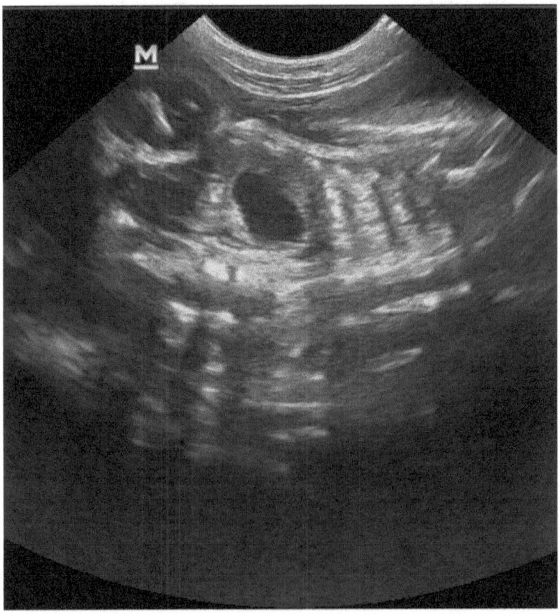

Figure 17 Gestation GD_{120} embryonic heart

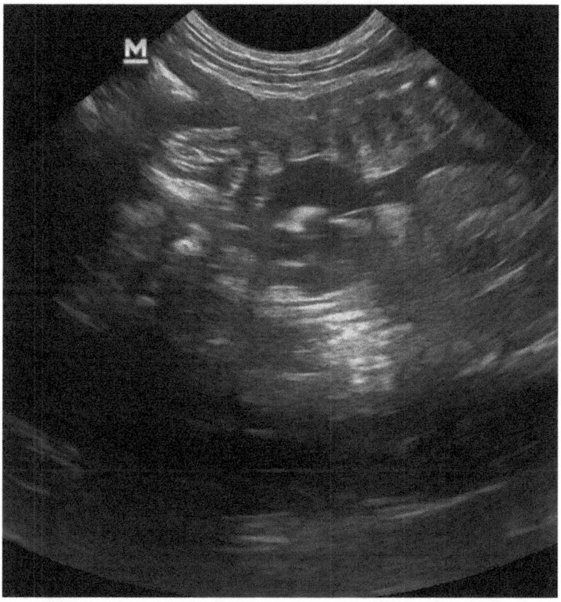

Figure 18 Gestation GD_{130}

FSC
www.fsc.org
MIX
Papier | Fördert gute Waldnutzung
FSC® C083411

Kolibri 360 GmbH
Ferdinand-Jühlke-Straße 7
99095 Erfurt, Deutschland
produktsicherheit@kolibri360.de